ASPERGER SYNDROME

ASPERGER SYNDROME

Edited by

Ami Klin
Fred R. Volkmar
Sara S. Sparrow

Foreword by Maria Asperger Felder, MD

THE GUILFORD PRESS
New York London

© 2000 The Guilford Press
A Division of Guilford Publications, Inc.
72 Spring Street, New York, NY 10012
www.guilford.com

Printed in the United States of America

This book is printed on acid-free paper.

Last digit is print number: 9 8 7 6 5 4 3 2

Library of Congress Cataloging-in-Publication Data

Asperger syndrome / edited by Ami Klin, Fred R. Volkmar,
Sara S. Sparrow; foreword by Maria Asperger Felder.
     p. cm.
    Includes bibliographical references and index.
    ISBN 1-57230-534-7
    1. Asperger's syndrome. I. Klin, Ami. II. Volkmar, Fred R.
III. Sparrow, Sara S.
    [DNLM: 1. Autistic Disorder. WM 203.5 A8388 2000]
RC553.A88 A788 2000
616.89'82—dc21   99-054492

To Siomara, Ian, and Liana;
Lisa, Lucy, and Emily; and Dom

About the Editors

Ami Klin, PhD, is the Harris Associate Professor of Child Psychology and Psychiatry at Yale University's Child Study Center. Dr. Klin is the author of more than 60 articles and chapters in the field of autism and related disorders, and has coordinated a series of federally funded research studies focused on Asperger syndrome. His main research interests involve the neuropsychology and social cognition of disorders of socialization.

Fred R. Volkmar, MD, is Professor of Child Psychiatry, Psychology, and Pediatrics at Yale University's Child Study Center. Dr. Volkmar is the author of more than 150 articles, chapters, and books in the field of autism and related disorders. He is an editor of the second edition of the *Handbook of Autism*, chair of the American Academy of Child and Adolescent Psychiatry's committee on autism, as well as an associate editor of the *Journal of Autism and Developmental Disorders* and the *Journal of Child Psychology and Psychiatry*.

Sara S. Sparrow, PhD, is Professor of Psychology and Chief Psychologist at Yale University's Child Study Center. Dr. Sparrow is the author of more than 100 articles and chapters in the fields of psychological assessment and developmental disabilities, and is the senior author of one of the most widely used psychological instruments, the Vineland Adaptive Behavior Scales. Her main research interests involve the assessment of adaptive behavior, child neuropsychology, and developmental disabilities.

Contributors

D. V. M. Bishop, DPhil, Department of Experimental Psychology, University of Oxford, Oxford, United Kingdom

Alice Carter, PhD, Department of Psychology, University of Massachusetts at Boston, Boston, MA

Matthew G. Foley, MEd, LPC, Lubbock, Texas

Susan E. Folstein, MD, Department of Psychiatry, Tufts University School of Medicine, Boston, Massachusetts; Eunice Kennedy Shriver Center, Waltham, Massachusetts

Elizabeth McMahon Griffith, MA, Department of Psychology, University of Denver, Denver, Colorado

DeAnn Hyatt-Foley, MEd, Lubbock, Texas

Ami Klin, PhD, Yale Child Study Center, Yale University School of Medicine, New Haven, Connecticut

Rebecca Landa, PhD, CCC-SLP, Center for Autism and Related Disorders of the Kennedy Krieger Institute, Department of Psychiatry and Behavioral Sciences, Johns Hopkins Medical Institutions, Baltimore, Maryland

Wendy D. Marans, MA, CCC-SLP, Yale Child Study Center, Yale University School of Medicine, New Haven, Connecticut

Andrés Martin, MD, Yale Child Study Center, Yale University School of Medicine, New Haven, Connecticut

Sally Ozonoff, PhD, Department of Psychology, University of Utah, Salt Lake City, Utah

David K. Patzer, MD, Department of Psychiatry, University of Arizona Health Sciences Center, Tucson, Arizona

Linda Rietschel, BA, Brookfield, Connecticut

Lizabeth M. Romanski, PhD, Section of Neurobiology, Yale University School of Medicine, New Haven, Connecticut

Byron P. Rourke, PhD, FRSC, Department of Psychology, University of Windsor, Windsor, Ontario, Canada; Yale Child Study Center, Yale University School of Medicine, New Haven, Connecticut

Susan L. Santangelo, ScD, Department of Psychiatry, Tufts University School of Medicine, and Department of Epidemiology, Harvard University School of Public Health, Boston, Massachusetts

Robert T. Schultz, PhD, Yale Child Study Center, Yale University School of Medicine, New Haven, Connecticut

Lori S. Shery, BS, Asperger Syndrome Education Network, Inc. (ASPEN®), Edison, New Jersey

Isabel M. Smith, PhD, Department of Pediatrics, Dalhousie University, and IWK Grace Health Centre for Children, Women and Families, Halifax, Nova Scotia, Canada

Sara S. Sparrow, PhD, Yale Child Study Center, Yale University School of Medicine, New Haven, Connecticut

Peter Szatmari, MD, Department of Psychiatry and Behavioural Neurosciences, McMaster University, Hamilton, Ontario, Canada

Digby Tantam, PhD, FRCPsych, Department of Psychotherapy, University of Sheffield, Sheffield, United Kingdom

Katherine D. Tsatsanis, PhD, Yale Child Study Center, Yale University School of Medicine, New Haven, Connecticut

Fred R. Volkmar, MD, Yale Child Study Center, Yale University School of Medicine, New Haven, Connecticut

Jeanne Wallace, MD, University of California at Los Angeles School of Medicine, Los Angeles, California

Lorna Wing, MD, FRCPsych, National Autistic Society's Centre for Social and Communication Disorders, Bromley, Kent, United Kingdom

Sula Wolff, FRCP, FRCPsych, (Formerly) Department of Psychiatry, University of Edinburgh, and Royal Hospital for Sick Children, Edinburgh, Scotland, United Kingdom

Acknowledgments

A number of individuals have aided in the preparation of this volume. We thank the contributors for their effort in making this project a valuable resource to all those involved in the field. We also thank the families who over the years have shared their experiences with us and allowed us to serve their children's needs. They have taught us much, including the wisdom of recognizing what we do not clearly know. We also acknowledge with deep appreciation the important support provided to our program of research by the National Institute of Child Health and Human Development, the National Institute of Mental Health, the Korczak Foundation for Autism Research, the Autism Society of America Foundation, the National Alliance for Autism Research, the Learning Disabilities Association of America, the Asperger Syndrome Coalition of the United States, Inc. (ASC–U.S.), and the Asperger Syndrome Education Network, Inc. (ASPEN®). We extend particular thanks to our colleagues Tammy Babitz, MA, Joel Bregman, MD, Alice Carter, PhD, Dom Cicchetti, PhD, Kathy Koenig, MSN, Jason Lang, BA, James Leckman, MD, Wendy Marans, MA, CCC-SLP, Andrés Martin, MD, Rhea Paul, PhD, David Pauls, PhD, Larry Scahill, PhD, Robert Schultz, PhD, Shannon Smith, BA, Mikle South, BA, Kenneth Towbin, MD, and, most particularly, our department chair, Donald Cohen, MD. It is Dr. Cohen's leadership by example and longstanding commitment to the tradition of clinical work that informs research which has molded and inspired our own work in this area. Finally, we acknowledge the support of our families—Siomara, Ian, and Liana Klin, Lisa Wiesner and Lucy and Emily Volkmar, and Dom Cicchetti. They have been steadfast in their support and tolerant of the occasional spouse or father who was preoccupied with this project.

Foreword

Hans Asperger used to love telling the story of his life; thus all I have to do is retell it. He was born in Vienna in 1906. His grandfather's family had been farmers east of the capital of the Austrian–Hungarian Monarchy for many generations. As a high school student, he became acquainted with the "German Youth Movement." It was in this movement that this achievement-oriented and intellectual young man was to find all those things he valued most throughout his lifetime. There he discovered friendship, mountaineering, nature, art as a source of strength and repose, and literature—the medium in which he moved and lived.

In 1931 he graduated from medical school and started working for the Children's Hospital of the University of Vienna, the institution to which he devoted most of his working years. He remained a pediatrician at heart until the end of his life. However, his first publication (Siegl & Asperger, 1934) already showed that his primary interest was not in symptoms and treatment methods only but, rather, in the child who was suffering, his or her environment, and the interplay between constitutional and environmental factors. This approach to medicine and his work as the director of the Unit for Special Education ("Heilpädagogik") at the Children's Hospital led him to coin the term "autistic psychopathy," which he first used in the article "Das psychisch abnorme Kind" (Asperger, 1938). Despite the fact that considerations of genetic hygiene or racial determinism severely undermined human values at the time, Hans Asperger favored unpredictability and the notion that development resulted from the interplay between genetic and environmental factors ("predisposition is not fate but rather a possible fate").

In 1944, Hans Asperger published his postgraduate thesis, "Die 'Autistischen Psychopathen' im Kindesalter (" 'Autistic Psychopathy' in Childhood"), an excellent and comprehensive description of the children who deeply interested him. By describing the ways they expressed themselves, he tried to gain insight into their being, consciously refusing to impose any underlying system of explanation:

> The path [to understanding] necessarily begins with the individual himself . . . [it] looks for parallels between an outer region and an inner one, between physical constitution and emotional factors, motor activity, facial expression and gestures, between autonomic effects (that reflect emotions), between speech modulation and manner of speaking—and character traits. (Asperger, 1944, p. 44)

Hans Asperger (1944) believed that this disorder was determined by genetic factors:

> In light of the homogeneity and the distinctiveness of this type of mentally disturbed children, the question of genetic determination necessarily must emerge. The question as to whether abnormal conditions are determined by constitution and are thus heritable has long been resolved. . . . Over the past 10 years, we have studied over 200 children who evidence a more or less severe autistic disorder. In the process we also got to know their parents and other relatives of theirs and found abnormal traits in their relatives.

During the war, Hans Asperger served as a medical officer in Croatia (1944–1945). After the war he returned to Vienna. In 1957 he became the director of the Children's Hospital of the University of Innsbruck and in 1963 he was named director of the Children's Hospital of the University of Vienna. Although he kept abreast of the treatment of physical illnesses and the rapid developments in the field of medicine, children themselves and their emotions were his main interest. He tried to adopt an intuitive approach to understanding them rather than an intellectual one:

> A doctor . . . needs more than mere book knowledge; he needs not to have lost the ability to "look," which is a very holistic function of recognition and in which intuitive, instinctive, pre-intellectual skills play an important role. They lead us to the innermost regions of the child to be assessed because whatever a child expresses comes out of the innermost parts of him or herself. (Asperger, 1975, p. 8)

This is what he referred to as "medical art," a skill he considered to be important not only for physicians but also for all those working in the field of education, particularly special education. Thus, although the medical approach seemed to be particularly useful in diagnosing and understanding a child's personality and disorders, pedagogical methods were the first and foremost methods of treating them:

> We believe that an exclusively medical approach to the treatment of mentally disturbed children, even psychiatric therapy, can only be effective to a

limited extent. Only pedagogical methods in the broadest sense of the word can really change people to the better, or put more precisely, can pinpoint the best of the developmental alternatives that are at a child's disposal and make it possible for him or her to develop along these lines. (Asperger, 1950, p. 105)

From 1949 onward, Hans Asperger published several articles comparing the disorder he had been describing with the one that Leo Kanner had called "early infantile autism". He pointed out not only the characteristics that both disorders had in common (impairment in social responsiveness or interest in others, and serious communicative impairment) but also the differences in personality structure and cognitive skills. Yet, despite their common interests, Kanner and Hans Asperger were never to meet.

Hans Asperger was never to lose his lifelong interest in and his curiosity about all living creatures (*naturae curiosus*), which explained why he was elected to the Academy of Nature Researchers in Halle. However, what interested him was not conducting large studies as a method of gaining insight into the meaning of things but, rather, the act of watching as a means to gain insight into the underlying laws that govern life. That is why the words spoken by Lynkeus, the tower watchman in Goethe's *Faust*, meant a great deal to him and guided him:

> Born to see
> Called for to watch
> Pledged to the tower
> I like the world.

Hans Asperger died in Vienna in 1980, after a short illness. He was an active, interested, and committed person until the very end.

MARIA ASPERGER FELDER, MD
Kinder und Jugendpsychiatrie–Psychotherapie
Zurich, Switzerland

REFERENCES

Asperger, H. (1938). Das psychisch abnorme Kinde. *Wiener Klinische Wochenschrift, 51,* 1314–1317.

Asperger, H. (1944). Die "Autistischen Psychopathen" im Kindesalter. *Archiv für Psychiatrie und Nervenkrankheiten, 117,* 76-136.

Asperger, H. (1950). Die medizinischen Grundlagen der Heilpädagogik. *Monatsschrift für Kinderheilkunde, 99*(3), 105–115.

Asperger, H. (1975). Erlebte Heilpädagogik. In H. Asperger (Ed.)., *Heilpädagogik Gegenwart und Zukunft.* Berlin: Springer.

Siegl, J., & Asperger, H. (1934). Zur Behandlung der Enuresis. *Archiv fur Kinderheilkunde, 102,* 88-102.

Contents

V. PERSPECTIVES ON RESEARCH
AND CLINICAL PRACTICE, AND PARENT ESSAYS

Introduction

AMI KLIN

FRED R. VOLKMAR

SARA S. SPARROW

Although first described more than 50 years ago, interest in Asperger syndrome (AS) was slow to develop. Indeed publications about this condition were quite uncommon until the 1980s. Since that time, interest in AS has seemed to increase exponentially—particularly following its "official" recognition in the U.S. diagnostic system—*Diagnostic and Statistical Manual of Mental Disorders,* fourth edition (DSM-IV; American Psychiatric Association, 1994)—and the international one—*International Classification of Diseases,* 10th edition (ICD-10; World Health Organization, 1993). Despite this dramatic increase in interest, however, final answers to essential research questions remain to be resolved. This volume offers a current account of AS against the quickly shifting backdrop of clinical research and clinical practice. The many uncertainties involved in the ongoing research debate of whether or not AS should be seen as a valid condition in its own right has tended to discourage investigators and has been a source of confusion for parents and clinicians alike. While the confusion has continued, the social disabilities of children, adolescents, and adults with this, and similar, conditions have increasingly been recognized as an important clinical problem. Our purpose in producing this volume was twofold. First, we hoped to compile the available research and clinical knowledge as it presently exists. We do not necessarily promise or expect to provide all the answers, but we do hope to highlight both the promising leads and those that can probably now be discarded (either because they are not seen as particularly relevant or because the issue has been resolved). Second, we hoped to assemble the best possible current guidelines for research and clinical practice. Only guidelines that are systematically defined and researched can be proven right or wrong. And it is of little help to those immediately involved with individuals with AS to be told that nothing can be said because there is nothing definitive to be said.

In editing this volume we are aware of the growing interest in the condition and the dramatic upsurge in referrals, public policy discussions, and, to a lesser extent, research publications on AS. Since the tentative inclusion of AS as a formal diagnostic category in DSM-IV (American Psychiatric Association, 1994) and ICD-10 (World Health Organization, 1993), there has been a widening gap between the way researchers speak about the condition and the way the diagnostic label is used in the community. Whereas researchers, many represented in this volume, generally stress the temporary status of current definitions, the lack of validation data, and the limitations of available studies, clinicians have been rather less reserved in their use of the diagnostic category. Often proceeding "full steam ahead" with the desire to secure appropriate services for their patients, clinicians, again many represented in this volume, have diagnosed AS in what now is probably many thousands of children, adolescents, and adults in this and other countries. The families of these individuals are often baffled by the current gap between clinical use of the term (which is frequent) and research (which is relatively rare). That notwithstanding, parents, teachers, and others are forming national and regional support groups that coalesce around the term "AS." As a result, in part, of this increased attention, educational authorities are being asked to provide adequate services to an increasing number of children diagnosed with this condition. Clinicians have had to incorporate AS in their consideration of differential diagnosis, and parents have had to struggle with understanding how this particular label captures some important aspects of their child's difficulties. The *de facto* establishment of AS in the community makes the need for better research and for better guidelines for clinical practice all the more urgent.

In the close to 50 years during which children with autism and related conditions have been evaluated at the Yale Child Study Center, a relatively large number of individuals for whom the diagnosis of AS might apply have been followed up, some for more than 30 years. More recently, however, our research projects focused on AS have enrolled, to our surprise, over 800 families nationwide, leading to close contacts with national and regional parent support agencies such as the Learning Disabilities Association of America (LDAA), the Asperger Syndrome Coalition of the United States, Inc. (ASC–U.S.), the Asperger Syndrome Education Network, Inc. (ASPEN®), as well as many other groups in the United States and abroad. This has resulted in an exponential growth in our commitments and responsibilities toward more able individuals with severe social disabilities and their families. Our awareness of the urgent need for a report on the current status of AS led us to invite a distinguished group of researchers, clinicians, and parents to join us in writing this volume. Even though the present volume is limited in some ways in terms of its scope, our hope is that the contributions of most leading researchers in the field and of the major advocates are reasonably well represented here. We were concerned that this volume address what appear to us to be issues important for both research and intervention.

RESEARCH ON ASPERGER SYNDROME

Ever since Lorna Wing (1981) introduced Hans Asperger's work to a larger English-speaking readership, a great deal of the research on AS has focused on whether the syndrome described by Asperger (1944)—"autistic psychopathy"—differed from that described by Leo Kanner (1943)—"early infantile autism." That this distinction still occupies us today is reflected in the various contributions to this volume, including our own. While it is understandable that the nosologic status of AS vis-à-vis autism be a priority, particularly after the tentative inclusion of AS in DSM-IV and ICD-10, it is important that the field moves ahead and away from the more sterile aspects of this discussion.

First, vague definitions no longer suffice when investigators are describing participants in their studies. Although the rather general semantics of classification systems might work well for children who show a severe or prototypical form of a disorder (e.g., autism associated with moderate levels of mental retardation), the situation is different in the case of more able children or children who show atypical forms of the disorder (e.g., individuals with higher-functioning autism or AS). There is no clear and fast solution to this problem, particularly because many diagnostic criteria refer to negative symptoms (e.g., "lack of" or "relative failure to"), which in the realm of social and communication functioning can span a wide range of expressions, leaving room for subjective decisions that may vary from clinician to clinician. It is in fact remarkable that interrater reliability for the diagnosis of autism is as high as it is (Volkmar et al., 1994); however, it is also well-known that reliability decreases significantly in the case of nonprototypical children (severely retarded or higher-functioning individuals with autism, and children with nonautistic pervasive developmental disorders, including AS), particularly when diagnostic assignment is made by nonexperienced clinicians (Klin, Lang, Cicchetti, & Volkmar, in press). This situation is acute in the case of AS. Hence, attempts to compare research findings across studies when the participants are insufficiently described become an impossible task. There is a need, therefore, for researchers to provide detailed and operationalized characterization of participants, including the procedures used in diagnostic assignments and their reliability. Ideally, however, important aspects of the condition, including social and communication disabilities, should be quantified following standardized procedures for data collection and coding. Important progress has been made in this area with the advent of valid and reliable instruments to collect and code historical and observational data (e.g., Lord et al., 1989, 1994). However, because these instruments have been developed for use with individuals with autism, there is still much work to be done to make them equally useful in the work with related conditions such as AS.

A second trend to be avoided is the path of what can be called "exegetic" research, or the tendency to resort to Kanner's and Asperger's works in search of solutions to current nosological problems. Despite the different settings and priorities of these two pioneers, they both shared a certain distaste for the rather convoluted, unreliable, and theory-based descriptions of mental disorders prevalent during their times, advocating instead descriptive observations that stayed true to the clinical phenomena they were observing. As a result, their papers are as instructive now as they were at the time of their publication. However, the original 11 children described by Kanner, or the 4 children described by Asperger should not be expected to cover the wide range of manifestations of social disabilities. In a way, their early publications described fairly prototypical cases, brilliantly delineating the hallmarks of the syndromes they intended to portray. However, later publications revealed that even a master of scientific observation like Kanner could not immediately extend his diagnostic concept to children who had a presentation more consistent with the children described by Asperger (Kanner, 1954); similarly, Asperger went through great pains to draw lines of distinction between his and Kanner's syndrome (Asperger, 1968) with only partial success (Bosch, 1970, pp. 126–130). Neither men had available current research methodologies to validate their observations. Further belaboring of the original descriptions in the hope that they will yield solutions are unlikely to be fruitful without the help of external validation data. It is up to current investigators, therefore, to assess the utility of different diagnostic constructs on the basis of factors such as predictability of outcome, genetic liabilities, and neuropsychological or neurobiological findings. It is only in the context of such research that the role of potential mediating factors such as intellectual and language functioning, or of specific mechanisms of socialization such as social motivation and social cognitive abilities, can be truly evaluated.

Finally, in the face of absence of strong validation data for AS, some researchers have opted for what is thought to be the conservative approach, namely to regard autism and AS along a continuum, possibly with individuals with autism representing the more cognitively challenged and those with AS the more cognitively able. This approach, however, hardly solves our problem of how to understand AS. Just as investigators who believe the two diagnostic constructs are different need to show the validity and utility of the factors the two conditions are purported to be different on, investigators who believe the two can be placed along a continuum need to show the validity and utility of the dimension(s) along which the two conditions are hypothesized to be related. Neither hypothesis is simpler than the other, and neither circumvents the need for external validation.

Beyond the "same or different" debate, however, a new and valuable research trend transcends categorical classifications by focusing on the behavioral manifestations of psychological or neurobiological mechanisms. Complex syndromes such as autism and AS are likely to result from complex combinations of factors variably affecting the different components of social development. Traits or profiles of genetic vulnerabilities and resiliences, behavioral, neuropsychological, or neurobiological, as well as combinations thereof, may result in different clinical syndromes showing a form of social disability. This possibility ties together the research on AS with the basic effort of the newly emerging social neurosciences. Just as the more prototypical forms of autism have been, over the years, the battleground for a wide range of theories of socialization, the present expansion into relatively milder forms of social disability is bound to profit from this new wave of genetics and neuroscience research. Still, we enter the new millennium knowing less about sociability than about most other psychological functions.

These new developments are likely to bring us closer to etiological factors. But we should not believe that with the advent of etiological discoveries the need for research of clinical syndromes will abate. On the contrary: Similar etiologies may lead to different syndromes; different profiles of development, needs, and assets; and, consequently, different treatment interventions. In this sense, the "same or different" debate will not go away, but we might be much better equipped to intervene earlier and more effectively.

CLINICAL PRACTICE RELATED TO ASPERGER SYNDROME

Our expanded contacts with hundreds of families and with parent support organizations hitherto less involved in the field of autism such as LDAA have taught us that the primary factor accounting for the emergence of AS-related support organizations has been the perception of a void of services for and knowledge about more able children and adolescents with severe social disabilities (i.e., children who generally function within the normal range intellectually—or even in the gifted range—but who have marked and severe deficits). Clearly the prototypical disorder in this regard is autism because it is clear that perhaps 20% of individuals with autism function in normal or above-normal intellectual range cognitively. Decades of effective parent action in autism on the one hand and learning disabilities on the other hand have resulted in a relatively rich infrastructure of services for children with these conditions and their families, including better special education resources, entitlement programs, and, more generally, increased awareness in the mental health and educational communities. Children and adults with AS and related disabilities have problems which appear to fall in between these more generally recognized categories of disability. On the one hand, programs for children with autism are often geared toward individuals who are more cognitively and behaviorally challenged, whereas programs for children with learning disabilities concentrate on academic skills. Neither place suits the unique needs and assets of individuals with AS. Although they require some aspects of the former (e.g., individualized programming and social and communication skills building), their unique profiles mean a different set of social, educational, and behavioral challenges and opportunities. Similarly, whereas the learning disabilities setting offers the opportunities for their unique strengths to blossom, its focus on academic skills misses the point entirely by moving the intervention away from the areas of most need, namely, social and real-life adaptive skills.

But the predicament faced by parents goes beyond that. We have collected countless accounts from parents of children who were denied services because they appeared "too bright" and articulate or were doing well academically. The same children were often characterized as behaviorally or emotionally disturbed because of their inappropriate social behaviors and eccentricities. Ignorance of the fact that such behaviors are part and parcel of a neurobiologically based disorder implied forms of intervention that blamed children for their disability, including ineffective disciplining or placement together with children who indeed can navigate the social environment quite well but cannot restrain themselves from exhibiting conduct problems. Adults with AS have shared with us years of hardship in such settings: Their social naivety made them the perfect victims; the placement made their peers the perfect victimizers.

Clearly, this has not been a universal experience among individuals with AS and their parents, but the frequency with which this pattern occurs is enough to energize a movement advocating more awareness of AS and related conditions, more knowledge from mental health and educational professionals, and a more appropriate infrastructure of resources and services. Not unlike the history of services for children with autism, when parents created schools in their home basements and later activated their congressional representatives to increase resource allocation, this new wave is likely to follow a similar path. It will be important for leading researchers and clinicians to pave the way for this effort. For years, research on the more able individuals with social disabilities has been slow in coming. The notion that only about less than a quarter of individuals with autism were cognitively more able disregarded to some extent a sizable proportion of children seen in clinics who had nonautistic forms of social impairment. In the United States until 1994, the only diagnostic category available for these children was pervasive developmental disorder not otherwise specified (PDD-NOS). A residual category meant to cover only a small percentage of children with PDD disorders, PDD-NOS has become as large as autism in number of referrals but not as well characterized or researched. It is still the case that PDD-NOS functions as a large repository for complex or atypical cases, tremendously heterogeneous and poorly defined. For research, PDD-NOS has been a kind of *terra incognita*. The clinical practice counterpart of this void has been a paucity of knowledge and awareness of best practices for children with less severe disorders. Thankfully, this is now changing, and awareness, at least, is dramatically increasing. Interestingly, this phenomenon has raised the question of whether the prevalence rates of autism are increasing. Close inspection of new prevalence studies (e.g., Honda et al., 1996) indicate that the increase appears to be primarily in the cognitive extremes of the spectrum: the more severely affected, and, to a greater extent, the more able children (Fombonne, 1998). The stage is set, therefore, for dramatic change of the *status quo* in knowledge about and services for these children and their families. Judging by the number of inquiries for information, consultation, and referrals we ourselves are receiving, the mental health community appears to be demanding such a change. Finally, although obvious to parents and experienced clinicians, it is important to note that the "less severe" in less severe social disabilities is a relative term: The untold hardships endured by individuals with AS and related conditions are only "less severe" relative to the challenges brought about by more severe forms of autism.

TO PARENTS

Discussions about the potential for stigmatization notwithstanding, most parents find a great deal of relief in the clinician's validation of something they knew all along: being asked the right questions, seeing the puzzling nature of chronic social and emotional maladaptive behaviors demystified, finding that they are not alone, and being reassured that there are professionals who are interested in their child's problem and have something to offer by way of recommendations. The awareness of what appear to be strong neurobiological mechanisms underlying the disorder may also be the source of some relief. And, at least to some extent, the degree to which educational and support services are conditional on a diagnosis, the provision of a label that implies the need for an adequate education and treatment program is important. It is in the more personal realm, however, that we have seen the clinical process contribute the most. Thankfully, parents of individuals with AS are not being blamed for their children's disability with the same acrimony reserved for parents of children with autism in the 1950s and 1960s. Nevertheless, many parents are left to grapple with their worries and questions by themselves. One mother, for example, mentioned that her son often asked her why did he need her, or, for that effect, why did he need his family. For years, she took such questions as a form of rejection, feeling particularly hurt for the lack of reciprocity of her love and deep commitment to her son. These questions, however, had little to do with the expression of love or lack thereof. They were logical questions, asked by a hyperlogical young man, who, bewildered by a confusing social world, was attempting to apply the rules of mathematical reasoning (which he had amply mastered) to the realm of social relationships (where he was still very much a beginner). Seen in this light, the affective havoc wreaked by such questions could be ameliorated. The same young man tried to define social relationships in terms of mathematical equations, hoping that their solution would give him an insight into why people reacted in the way they did; he also once confided to us that he saw himself as "a poor computer simulation of a human being."

Such experiences are in fact commonplace. Beyond the rationalistic questions, there are the eccentricities, the social naivety, the rigidities associated with moralisms and inflexible routines, and the all-absorbing interests that often not only occupy the individuals with AS themselves but also those around them. The accompanying letter (see page 9) is one of many one parent receives regularly from her son, a young adult with AS.

Of course, the more pressing bits of information that any parent would like to see mentioned in a letter from a son living away (i.e., personal information) is missing in this correspondence. In its place are volumes of impersonal data. Knowing that this is an important aspect of a neurobiologically based condition goes some way in the process of coping with it. The challenge remains, however, for researchers to better understand these fascinating, yet highly disruptive and potentially painful clinical phenomena, and for interventionists to capitalize on them as a way of advancing the person's potential for better adaptation to the learning, work, and social environment.

Parents of individuals with AS often ask the question, "How far can they go?" The answer to this question is still being researched, although prognosis is thought to be far better than used to be the case. In the field of autism, outcome was usually thought to be bleak, with only a small percentage of individuals reaching independence, a steady job, and a fairly routinized social life. However, one of the major reasons the old data on outcome were so negative was that the studies focused on individuals who had been provided with little in terms of intervention services: In fact, few had received early and intensive forms of educational treatment, the two aspects of intervention known to be central in maximizing outcome (Rogers, 1996). As the major predictors of outcome are intellectual level and communicative speech, the outlook is likely to be better for more able individuals with autism and AS (Howlin & Goode, 1998). The intellectual and language assets of individuals with AS are likely to be associated with increased social, vocational, and independent living opportunities. The challenge, however, is to ensure that the forms of intervention currently thought to be effective (e.g., social and communication skills training, focus on real-life skills, academic and vocational programs tailored to maximize the individual's capacities

Dom   Mom

Have you heard about sunglasses that come in all styles? The solarshields are the big ones and come in all colors to suit the users' preference. All must claim to block 100% UV rays. Polycarbonate is plastic and not as good as Borosilicate glass at 1 cm. thick to block ultraviolet radiation. The tinted, hard, thick glass with gold particles (as in space suit blocks UV and X rays.) New picture tubes are that way also to reduce X-rays.

The color filter of sunglasses are grey, clear, neutral, which reduce all colors violet (reduces yellow), blue (reduces orange) green (reduces red, but still see traffic lights safely) yellow/amber (reduces violet) orange (reduces blue) red/pink (reduces green). All colors you see must combine to be white. The tint you see on white is the color of the sunglasses.

The "blue-blocks" filter, sunglasses (amber colored) absorbs blue so effectively that you can hardly destinguish the blue. It makes blue light greenish. Fluorescent tubes yellow, incandescent bulbs orange, sun yellow, red still red.

Blue is more blury and harder to see than yellow by over 400% on the naked eye. There is no blue traffic light.

The police car uses powerful blue flashers with the red flashers.

It's harder to see blue with coteracts. A professional treatment makes blue and violet easier to see. A new artificial lens inserted can make even Ultraviolet visible in a deep violet light.

The blue-white light comes from 3- basic ways. Daylight fluorescent tubes are bluish white with a lot of blue. A blue-white star far away also radiate bluish white light.

In a supernatural way, the Virgin Mary can also issue bluish white light in some ways. Blue is a lovely color which appears almost everywhere.

The sky is blue, on a clear day you can see for.

while providing compensatory tools to deal with areas of weakness) are indeed provided to them. One of the priorities for advocates is to aggressively target the expansion of resources available in the community (school and clinical services), whereas researchers need to urgently begin empirical evaluations of current treatment guidelines and techniques. We have followed up individuals with AS who have been generally successful in their lives, acquiring paying jobs, and, in a few instances, building a family life. However, we have also seen many individuals whose natural talents are wasted due to their untreated social disability and other weaknesses (e.g., inability to manage the practical aspects of independent living, such as managing a bank account; to use public transportation; and to know how to behave in job interviews), having to rely on their families for total or partial support. Both instances—of success and of frustration—forcefully suggest that more knowledge of the factors maximizing better adaptation and more resources of the kind required by individuals with AS and their families are urgently needed.

TO THE PERSON WITH ASPERGER SYNDROME

To use a term that has become popular on the Internet, from the perspective of the individual with AS and related conditions, the world of "neurotypicals" is an extraordinarily confusing and peculiar one. Fraught with irrationalities, truncated messages, and a wealth of implied vocal and gestural signaling, this is a world in which people prefer to talk about themselves, their feelings, and their relationships rather than concrete information that can be mastered in a reliable fashion, explicitly and totally. The unrelenting demand to decode implicit meanings, intuitive judgments, and nonverbal and nonliteral forms of communication poses a great deal of stress and often begs questions such as why people say what they do not mean while meaning things they do not say? A lack of an insider's view into the surrounding social world makes that world quite inaccessible and sometimes hostile. Relationships are harder to come by, job prospects are more limited and often grossly undershoot the person's vocational credentials and abilities; attempts at accessing the social or vocational world are often met with frustrating results, which can, cumulatively, lead to a sense of despondency.

   To bridge the gap between these two worlds there is a need for an approximation between them. The neurotypical world needs to value diversity, allowing for special people with behaviors and views different from the mainstream to contribute to and enjoy the resources of the larger society. Not only is there room for difference, but it should be valued. On the opposite pole, individuals with AS and related conditions need to bring themselves closer to the mainstream, and they should be provided with supportive help to do so. There is no need for obliteration of uniqueness or for an inexorable push toward conformity. The life dangers to individuals who could not conform, were different in any respect, or had a disability, which were prevalent at the time and place of Asperger's early work, are thankfully gone. But the danger remains of moving toward the periphery of society and its resources, of undesirable work and living conditions, and of isolation. To see AS as a profile of strengths and weaknesses means that social skills need to be supported and strengthened, often by means of intensive programs of skill building involving practice and generalization. Most worthwhile educational and job opportunities involve personal interviews; most social relationships involve a measure of mutual sharing and understanding. The acquisition of such skills does not mean a capitulation to a foreign world; rather, it means realizing a right for better opportunities.

ORGANIZATION OF THIS VOLUME

The chapters comprising this volume can be divided into five different sections. *The first section focuses on behavioral aspects of AS.* Volkmar and Klin, in Chapter 1, open this section with an overview of the diagnostic debate, tracing the development of the concept from Asperger's original work to the inclusion of AS in current official diagnostic systems. A comparison of different approaches to the diagnosis of AS is made, including a critique of the DSM-IV and ICD-10 definitions. Finally, the authors review the issues involved in validation of AS as a diagnostic concept as well as the validation data currently available, concluding with a set of guidelines for future research that will expand promising leads while avoiding methodological pitfalls from the past.

Some of the promising leads suggesting differential neuropsychological profiles as a potential external validator of AS vis-à-vis higher-functioning autism (HFA) suggested by Volkmar and Klin are reviewed in detail by Ozonoff and Griffith in the following Chapter 2. Ozonoff and colleagues have for years focused on neuropsychological research, with particular emphasis on "executive functions" (EFs) or the navigational skills involved in organizing one's experiences, in profiting from environmental feedback, and in flexibly adjusting one's thoughts to the tasks at hand. Their contributions have highlighted the profound impact of EF impairment in basic processes of learning and social behavior. In Chapter 2, Ozonoff and Griffith provide a framework for the validation debate and proceed to review motor, visual–spatial EFs, and theory-of-mind research in AS. Their conclusion is a sobering one. Data in this area of research are consistent with some guarded optimism, but past methodological shortcomings make it impossible to draw any definitive summary. Emerging from their excellent discussion is a painstaking set of methodological guidelines that should be adopted by investigators of the neuropsychology of AS and related conditions.

Among the various neuropsychological assets and deficits described in AS, none has received as much attention while being the subject of as little systematic research as motor functioning. Asperger (1944) described "motor clumsiness" as one of the essential features of his syndrome; both ICD-10 and DSM-IV include this as an associated feature of AS. Leading authors in the field have debated less about whether motor deficits are present in individuals with this condition than whether this feature could differentiate individuals with AS from those with higher-functioning autism. Issues of diagnosis and lack of operationalization and quantification of the term "motor clumsiness" have plagued this debate. In Chapter 3, Smith raises this loose discussion on motoric functioning to the level of scientific enquiry. Drawing on the extraordinary review she published with Bryson on imitation and action in autism (Smith & Bryson, 1994), she provides a comprehensive critical review of the literature in this area, quickly moving to fascinating conceptual and empirical questions that radically transform the current discussion on "clumsiness." Once the limitations of current knowledge are forcefully laid bare, she offers a framework to study the components of skilled motor behavior. In this light, the discussion is made relevant not only to diagnosis and subtyping of the pervasive developmental disorders but also to a discussion of etiology and the neurofunctional mapping of strengths and deficits that integrates motor, imitation, and other related cognitive skills and behavioral features of this group of conditions. One important lesson from this chapter is the way in which past unfruitful discussions neglected crucial considerations, for example, that profiles of motoric functioning are predicated on developmental factors (e.g., early strengths might become later deficits and environmental demands at age 3 are different from those at age 16) as well as on complex interactions with other related skills (e.g., the social and cognitive requirements for a given act of motoric performance and how motoric functioning exhibited by a child compares with his or her strengths and deficits in other areas). She concludes the chapter with a useful discussion of implications of this area of research to clinical intervention.

Among the behavioral features of individuals with AS, possibly the most conspicuous aspect of their presentation is the severe deficits in the social use of language despite relatively formal language strengths. Because of the latter, however, there are no attempts in either DSM-IV or ICD-10 to include abnormalities of communication in the definition of the condition. To some extent, this decision reflects the paucity of available data in this crucial area. In Chapter 4, Landa reviews what is known about pragmatic language skills in more able individuals with autism and those with AS. By grounding her discussion in overviews of normative development, she highlights the centrality and severity of pragmatic deficits in these conditions; and by documenting the various aspects of language use that are affected, she establishes a blueprint for studies of pragmatics which are only now beginning to appear in the literature. The importance of this area of research is further emphasized by the various leads pointing to ways in which social language use is related to other aspects of psychological functioning and to profiles of genetic vulnerabilities. It is to a great extent thanks to Landa and her colleagues that pragmatics is now seen as an avenue of genetic exploration into the etiologies of autism and related conditions, including AS. Unfortunately, there has not, to date, been enough extracted from this knowledge to decisively change clinical assessment and intervention practices related to social language use. Hence Landa's attempt to derive the clinical implications of her detailed discussion is both timely and enormously useful.

The second section of this book focuses on genetic and neurobiological research in AS. In the first chapter in this section, Folstein and Santangelo review the available data on family genetic studies in AS and related conditions. In the past few years, research on the genetics of autism have moved forward at a very fast pace, culminating recently with the first full genome screen (International Molecular Genetic Study of Autism Consortium, 1998) which revealed one, and possibly three susceptibility loci in autism. Unfortunately, with possibly the exception of epidemiology, no other area of research is as greatly affected by definition issues as family genetics. Clearly, just as rates of a disorder in the general population are affected by how stringent or broad one is in operationalizing the definition of the disorder, so are the rates of aggregation of the disorder in families of the identified patient. Given the current definition issues in regard to AS, Folstein and Santangelo do a remarkable job at delineating what is known and what is not in this area; less courageous investigators might despair at the very attempt. Their intimate knowledge of this field comes, of course, from the fact that they lead one of the foremost teams in the world currently working on the genetics of autism. The importance of this effort cannot be exaggerated: First, familial transmission of symptoms and traits may become an important source of external validation of AS; second, knowledge of genetic mechanisms may considerably advance our understanding of the pathogenesis of AS (and other related conditions); and, third, there is a tremendous need for knowledge in this area for the purpose of genetic counseling. Folstein and Santangelo's conclusion is clear: although there is little doubt that there are strong genetic contributions to AS, the size and nature of these contributions cannot be firmly established as yet. In this context, they provide a discussion of the term "broader autism phenotype," which has been increasingly used in genetic research of autism. This term brings together a wide range of symptoms or traits that may be present (in varying degrees) in a given person; the assumption is that a combination of these "components" of the autism phenotype may be responsible for different manifestations of social disabilities, at times resulting in autism but at other times resulting in a condition similar in one or many aspects of autism. This research framework has allowed investigators to transcend the current debates on categorical definitions, focusing instead on specific "phenotypes" that may, by themselves, result in psychopathology. One of the exciting points of this approach is that such phenotypes can be derived empirically and may refer to any aspect of the condition (vulnerabilities or strengths) shown to have an impact on social functioning. A similar approach has already yielded remarkable findings in the field of reading disabilities (Grigorenko et al., 1997); unfortunately, we know much more about what might be the "components" of reading skills than about what might be the "components" of social competency.

The enthusiasm generated by current genetic research has probably been matched only by that resulting from developments in neuroimaging research. Not only do current techniques allow us to measure the way the brain looks (i.e., structure), but more and more commonly they also allow us to measure the way the brain works (i.e., function). Both of these avenues of neurobiological research offer myriad opportunities which are only now being explored. In Chapter 6, Schultz, Romanski, and Tsatsanis review the small number of neuroimaging studies available in AS and related conditions and present some preliminary work on the way the normal brain finds social meaning in visual displays. This and other similar paradigms currently being developed in neuroscience laboratories around the world are giving investigators a privileged view indeed: They can see the brain thinking. By applying this new technology to the research of how individuals with severe social disabilities understand and process the social world, the field is likely to make a significant dent into the vast need for more neurobiological knowledge of sociability. And there is little doubt that the more we know about the neurobiology of social processes, the closer we will be to the roots of autism and AS. In this context, the discussion provided in Chapter 6 on what we know about a group of structures in the brain functionally centered around the amygdala is of great interest given the confluence of data implicating these structures in the pathogenesis of autism and related conditions.

Our limited knowledge of the neurobiological processes of socialization has also meant over the years that there is no psychopharmacological treatment for autism or AS insofar as the core symptoms are concerned. Nevertheless, an increased awareness of comorbid conditions such as depression and anxiety, among others, in the more able individuals with pervasive developmental disorders has gone hand in hand with an increased use of psychotropic agents to ameliorate these symptoms. Unfortunately, the paucity of research in this area has also meant that patients often receive medication following a regime that has little basis on empirical data; in fact, at times they receive many different medications simultaneously, eluding even further any attempt to search for a reasonable rationale. In Chapter 7, Martin, Patzer, and Volkmar review the limited research on this area and provide important guidelines for future work. Their own research has revealed troubling facts in clinical practice, making the research of psychopharmacological treatments even more urgent. To summarize, absence of good data has not affected prescription patterns. In a new world of a mental health system that requires fast therapeutic effects, there is a heavy burden on the physician to act first and think later about more reasonable approaches or about other forms of intervention. Leaving such general practice guidelines unresearched is the best way of perpetuating the *status quo*. In Chapter 7, Martin, Patzer, and Volkmar begin to piece together a better rationale for studies in this area, reflecting, to some extent, an increased awareness by research funding agencies that the time has come for a concerted effort to ameliorate treatable symptoms that may have devastating effects in otherwise chronic and medically untreatable groups of conditions.

The third section of this book focuses on diagnostic concepts associated with AS. Over the years, several concepts originating from neuropsychology, psycholinguistics, and psychiatry (among other disciplines) have been used to describe groups of children and adults who share, to some extent, aspects of the presentation seen in individuals with AS. Although the investigators proposing these concepts have all made important contributions in their areas of expertise, a great deal of confusion has resulted from the use of disparate names to what might be an overlapping sample of individuals with disabilities. Parents and clinicians alike often ask whether or not a given child may have condition *A* and condition *B*, or whether these conditions should be considered mutually exclusive. Underlying this question is the notion that each diagnostic construct is a "disease entity," with its own etiology, pathogenesis, behavioral profile, and outcome. In reality, these constructs all have in common the fact that their proponents address forms of social disability associated with their chosen area of research (e.g., a neuropsychological or language/communication profile of strengths and deficits). Unless a common framework of reference is adopted, it is quite improbable that the boundaries (or lack thereof) between these constructs will be delineated. Their inclusion in this volume was an attempt to begin to establish such a common frame of reference. However, another reason for their inclusion here is the fact that the specialized foci adopted by these investigators have made major theoretical and methodological contributions in their own discipline, which we would like to claim for the study of social disabilities such as AS.

The first chapter in this section describes a profile of neuropsychological assets and deficits termed Nonverbal Learning Disabilities (NLD). Initially described in the mid-1970s and extensively researched by Rourke and colleagues, NLD has been shown to be associated with social disabilities not unlike those seen in individuals with AS. Our own interest in NLD came from the hypothesis that it represented a neurocognitive model of AS: To put it succinctly, given the heavy dependence of social development on processing and understanding of nonverbal forms of communication (e.g., gaze, facial emotions, and voice inflection) from the earliest phases of development, a person with NLD would be likely to present with a social presentation not unlike that seen in persons with AS (i.e., overreliance on the rote, verbal, and explicit and neglect of holistic, nonverbal, and implied). Clearly, this association is much more complex. For example, although individuals with AS may often show the NLD profile, the converse is not true. However, the work of Rourke and colleagues has shown some ways in which NLD might be viewed as a mediator in developmental trajectories or as reflective of specific mechanisms of socialization which are associated with their own behavioral phenotypes. In Chapter 8, Rourke and Tsatsanis review these various issues, including the association between NLD and syndromes other than AS and some neurobiological hypotheses purported to lead to the neuropsychological profile. The developmental impact of NLD on social development is discussed in detail, with a view to providing suggestions for future experimental research and to delineate guidelines for intervention affecting learning and socialization.

That one of the aspects commonly associated with AS may represent a mediator for behavioral manifestations of social disabilities, or a possible component of the broader autistic phenotype, is further elaborated by Bishop, whose work on "semantic pragmatic disorder" (SPD) has greatly refined the classification system proposed by Rapin and Allen (1983), the originators of this term. Initially, the term highlighted the need to contrast children whose main difficulties in language functioning were in unusual word choices and pragmatic deficits rather than in phonology and syntax. As this is generally the pattern observed in children with autism and related conditions, particularly in the more able ones, the question whether SPD overlapped with autism was raised by investigators in this area. Moreover, the possibility that the severity of semantic–pragmatic deficits would be strongly associated with the severity of the social disability (i.e., a dimension defining a continuum) was raised. Bishop's work, however, quickly dispels any simple notion of a unidimensional space along which one can place the various forms of pervasive developmental disorders (PDDs). Specifically, pragmatic impairments may exist in children with autism and related conditions but also in children who do not show a social disability as severe as to justify their inclusion in the PDD category. Clearly, our exploration of the borderlands of autism and AS needs to be more complex and multifaceted: Different component phenotypes should be studied, as well as the viability of multiaxial classification systems of autism and related conditions (e.g., with IQ, formal language skills, and social language use representing different dimensions to be considered). Such an exploration depends heavily on better instruments to quantify these various dimensions, particularly the ones related to aspects of social functioning. It is in this regard that Bishop's contribution has been most decisive: Only recently available, her Children's Communication Checklist is capable of profiling different aspects of pragmatic functioning on the basis of extended observations of children's daily communication patterns. This instrument is likely to help us better understand the topography of the broader autistic phenotype. If pragmatic impairments can be found in children with and without autism, comparisons of other developmental aspects across such groups are likely to teach us a great deal about the nature of pragmatics and socialization, how they intersect, and how they might be dissociated.

The overemphasis of the field as a whole on the validation of AS vis-à-vis higher-functioning autism has neglected the kinds of comparisons suggested by Bishop. For the same reason, other comparisons have been neglected that may be as problematic, if not more, than the distinction between AS and autism. For several decades, Wolff and colleagues have followed a group of children into adult life whom they described as having schizoid personality in childhood. Probably not as severely socially impaired as individuals characterized as having AS in ICD-10 and DSM-IV, these individuals nevertheless present social and other impairments that may include aspects of AS as well as aspects from other diagnostic constructs such as schizotypal personality disorder (e.g., Nagy & Szatmari, 1986) and multiplex developmental disorder (Cohen et al., 1986); these concepts, in turn, may at times overlap with PDD-NOS. Wolff's remarkable longitudinal studies forcefully suggest that efforts to validate AS need to take on board these various conditions. Also, insofar as the broader autistic phenotype is proposed to explain the wide variability of syndrome expression in autism and related conditions, Wolff's discussion leads to an important question: Could the vulnerability for developing a thought disorder be part of such a broader phenotype? Wolff's speculation that schizoid personality in childhood may be a possible link between schizoid personality traits and autism on the one hand and schizophrenia on the other would suggest so. However, current data on the comorbidity rates of autism and schizophrenia and studies of family members of autistic individuals would contradict this hypothesis. Nevertheless, the convergence between PDD symptomatology and thought disturbances (as captured in the term "multiplex developmental disorder") has not as yet been adequately researched; therefore, Wolff's hypothesis cannot be dismissed. Aside from this hypothesis, however, nothing highlights the thorny validity issues in AS as much as Wolff's detailed life histories of the children she has followed for so many years.

The fourth section of this book focuses on practical issues related to assessment, treatment, and other supports to the child, adolescent, and adult with AS. Both parents and clinicians often ask for "an evaluation protocol for Asperger syndrome." The expectation is that if the protocol is properly completed, the diagnosis of AS can then be reliably made. Such a protocol, however does not yet exist; considerable clinical experience is required. More importantly, however, assignment of a diagnosis is only one component of the evaluation defining the priorities of the intervention program, and probably not the most important one. In Chapter 11, on assessment, Klin, Sparrow, Marans,

Carter, and Volkmar emphasize the importance of a detailed characterization of the child's strengths and deficits for creating individualized programs. Important principles underlying a clinical evaluation include a transdisciplinary framework, the need for both standardized procedures and other detailed clinical observations, and inclusion of parents and educational professionals familiar with the child's day-to-day patterns of behavior so that reliable measures of real-life skills can be obtained. Specific guidelines for history taking, neuropsychological, communication, and behavioral assessments are given in detail, including a description of assessment instruments known to be useful in the evaluation of individuals with severe social disabilities.

The quality of a given assessment should be judged in terms of its utility for creating an individualized program for intervention. Without detailed recommendations, educational and other interventionists may be at a loss on how to program for a given child. Without baseline data on the child's functioning, it may be impossible to gauge his or her rate of progress, leaving undocumented the extent to which the applied strategies of intervention are, or are not, being effective. In Chapter 12, Klin and Volkmar make the bridge between assessment and intervention, describing in detail a blueprint for treatment programs for individuals with AS. The discussion includes aspects of educational settings to be considered in placement, general teaching strategies, social and communication skills building, and real-life skills. Unfortunately, the data on effectiveness of different treatment strategies are scant. Therefore, the authors rely primarily on their own clinical experience as well as on emerging and exciting literature on social and communication skills training and adaptive technology, among other forms of intervention thought to be particularly well suited to the needs of this population. AS and related conditions are chronic and lifelong disorders; nevertheless, appropriate intervention can make an important difference in a person's life trajectory. Regrettably, the lack of research data in this area is only matched by the shortage of well-trained personnel and resources. Thankfully, awareness of best practices is increasing, partly because of parent action and partly because of a genuine interest on the part of school administrators on how to better serve the unique needs of their more cognitively able students with social disabilities.

The closing chapter in this section focuses on adolescents and adults with AS. Since Kanner's adoption of the term "early infantile autism," a great deal of the literature on autism and related conditions spoke of children, almost as if children with autism did not grow up to become adults. In clinical practice and educational work, with their respective emphases on diagnostic assessments and school-based interventions, we are all at risk of neglecting the unique needs of our older clients. As individuals with AS graduate from their school life, there is always a danger that they might move further and further to the periphery of society, living isolated lives, or move inward into their families, increasing the dependency on, at times, aging parents who are now left with the full responsibility for their son's or daughter's future, including vocational prospects, living arrangements, and other independent living challenges. Clearly, there is a need for a strong and concerted effort on the part of parents, professionals, and advocates to ameliorate this situation. The first step, however, is to make late adolescence and adulthood a more popular subject of investigation, so that new knowledge can guide us more directly in our effort to fill in this void. Several years ago, Schopler and Mesibov (1983) compiled the state of knowledge on autism in adolescents and adults. Although this work focused primarily on more cognitively challenged individuals, there were ample guidelines that could apply to individuals with AS; still, we need more knowledge about the unique challenges and opportunities facing them. Since the mid-1980s, Tantam (e.g., 1988) has been one of the field's primary sources of such knowledge. In Chapter 13, Tantam provides a close view of adolescence and adulthood in AS, weaving his rich clinical experience with research data while addressing, almost in a first-person style, the challenges faced by his adult clients and their families.

The final section of this book presents some thoughtful perspectives on research and clinical practice in AS. Maybe more than in other fields of inquiry, there is some extra need for reflections on the state of knowledge and on plans for future research in AS. With this in mind, we requested two leading investigators and clinicians to provide us with their perspectives on the past and future of research in AS. In the first chapter of this section, Szatmari presents a thought-provoking essay on classification issues in child psychiatric disorders in general, and specifically in the case of the "same or different" debate involving AS and autism. By asking the question "why do we classify," we are led through a series of important considerations that are rarely raised in nosological discussions. In a way, Szatmari's "meta-nosology" makes us think more carefully about what we mean by stating that two conditions are the same or different (e.g., in terms of etiologies, natural history, and response to treatment). Interestingly, his argument also leads to questions on the clinical usefulness (rather than validity) of classification systems for those who are primarily affected by them, namely, the families of individuals with AS and related disabilities, who should be seen as partners in the diagnostic debate.

In Chapter 15, Wing provides an incisive summary of past research in AS and, more importantly, her views of how the field should move forward in the future. Her unique perspective comes from years of service to the community of individuals with autism and related conditions in the United Kingdom and around the world, in the capacity of master clinician, fierce advocate, and leading researcher. Having introduced Asperger syndrome to a large English-speaking readership, and having accompanied the development of the field in the 18 years since, Wing's thoughts on the state of knowledge and the future ahead are required reading for those involved in research of severe social disabilities.

The section closes with four essays written by parents of individuals with AS. These personal experiences go much further than the lives of these four families, as they represent the trials and tribulations, as well as the joys and the victories, of many other affected families we know. The specific challenges and the resourcefulness contained in these accounts, however, are deeply individual; in fact they are as individual as the personal histories of their affected children, whose unique personalities defy any notion of representing their lives with a simple diagnostic category.

REFERENCES

American Psychiatric Association. (1994). *Diagnostic and statistical manual of mental disorders* (4th ed.). Washington, DC: Author.

Asperger, H. (1944). Die "Autistischen Psychopathen" im Kindesalter. *Archiv für Psychiatrie und Nervenkrankheiten, 117,* 76–136.

Bosch, G. (1970). *Infantile autism.* New York: Springer-Verlag.

Cohen, D. J., Paul, R., & Volkmar, F. R. (1986). Issues in the classification of pervasive developmental disorders: Toward DSM-IV. *Journal of the American Academy of Child and Adolescent Psychiatry, 25,* 213–220.

Fombonne, E. (1998). Epidemiology of Autism and related conditions. In F. R. Volkmar (Ed.), *Autism and pervasive developmental disorders* (pp. 32–64). Cambridge, England: Cambridge University Press.

Grigorenko, E. L., Wood, F. B., Meyer, M. S., Hart, L. A., Speed, W. C., Shuster, A., & Pauls, D. L. (1997). Susceptibility loci for distinct components of developmental dyslexia on chromosomes 6 and 15. *American Journal of Human Genetics, 60,* 27–39.

Honda, H., Shimizu, Y., Misumi, K., Niimi, M., & Ohashi, Y. (1996). Cumulative incidence and prevalence of childhood autism in children in Japan. *British Journal of Psychiatry, 169,* 228–235.

Howlin, P., & Goode, S. (1998). Outcome in adult life for people with autism and Asperger's syndrome. In F. R. Volkmar (Ed.), *Autism and pervasive developmental disorders* (pp. 209–241). Cambridge, England: Cambridge University Press.

International Molecular Genetic Study of Autism Consortium. (1998). A full genome screen for autism with evidence for linkage to a region on chromosome 7q. *Human Molecular Genetics, 7*(3), 571–578.

Kanner, L. (1943). Autistic disturbances of affective contact. *Nervous Child, 2,* 217–253.

Kanner, L. (1954). Discussion of Robinson and Vitale's paper on "Children with circumscribed interests." *American Journal of Orthopsychiatry, 24,* 764–766.

Klin, A., Lang, J., Cicchetti, D. V., & Volkmar, F. R. (in press). Inter-rater reliability of clinical diagnosis and DSM-IV criteria for autistic disorder: Results of the DSM-IV autism field trial. *Journal of Autism and Developmental Disorders.*

Lord, C., Rutter, M., Goode, S., Heemsbergen, J., Jordan, H., Mawhood, L., & Schopler, E. (1989). Autism diagnostic observation schedule: A standardized observation of communicative and social behavior. *Journal of Autism and Developmental Disorders, 19*(2), 185–212.

Lord, C., Rutter, M., & Le Couteur, A. (1994). Autism Diagnostic Interview—Revised: A revised version of a diagnostic interview for caregivers of individuals with possible pervasive developmental disorders. *Journal of Autism and Developmental Disorders, 24*(5), 659–685.

Nagy, J., & Szatmari, P. (1986). A chart review of schizotypal personality disorders in children. *Journal of Autism and Developmental Disorders, 16*(3), 351–367.

Rapin, I., & Allen, D. (1983). Developmental language disorders. In U. Kirk (Ed.), *Neuropsychology of language, reading and spelling.* New York: Academic Press.

Rogers, S. J. (1996). Brief report: Early intervention in autism. *Journal of Autism and Developmental Disorders, 26*(2), 243–246.

Schopler, E., & Mesibov, G. (Eds.). (1983). *Autism in adolescents and adults.* New York: Plenum Press.

Smith, I. S., & Bryson, S. E. (1994). Imitation and action in autism: A critical review. *Psychological Bulletin, 116*(2), 259–273.

Tantam, D. (1988). Annotation: Asperger's syndrome. *Journal of Child Psychology and Psychiatry, 29,* 245–255.

Volkmar, F. R., Klin, A., Siegel, B., Szatmari, P., Lord, C., Campbell, M., Freeman, B. J., Cicchetti, D. V., Rutter, M., Kline, W., Buitelaar, J., Hattab, Y., Fombonne, E., Fuentes, J., Werry, J., Stone, W., Kerbeshian, J., Hoshino, Y., Bregman, J., Loveland, K., Szymanski, L., & Towbin, K. (1994). DSM-IV Autism/Pervasive Developmental Disorder Field Trial. *American Journal of Psychiatry, 151,* 1361–1367.

Wing, L. (1981). Asperger's syndrome: A clinical account. *Psychological Medicine, 11,* 115–129.

World Health Organization. (1993). *International classification of diseases: Tenth revision.* Chapter V. Mental and behavioral disorders (including disorders of psychological development). Diagnostic criteria for research. Geneva: Author.

I

Behavioral Aspects

1

Diagnostic Issues in Asperger Syndrome

FRED R. VOLKMAR
AMI KLIN

Asperger syndrome (AS) is a serious and chronic neurodevelopmental disorder which is presently defined by social deficits of the type seen in autism, restricted interests as in autism, but, in contrast to autism, relative preservation of language and cognitive abilities—at least early in life. By definition (see Table 1.1) criteria for autistic disorder according to the fourth edition of the *Diagnostic and Statistical Manual of Mental Disorders* (DSM-IV; American Psychiatric Association, 1994) or childhood autism according to the tenth revision of the *International Classification of Diseases* (ICD-10; World Health Organization, 1993) are not met. The narrative text in both official diagnostic manuals notes that motor awkwardness and/or clumsiness is commonly associated with the condition and that the nature of the restricted interests often relates to an unusual, intense, and highly circumscribed interest or interests. Although not as explicitly discussed, the implication of current diagnostic criteria is that generally the onset of AS (or at least its recognition) is usually after age 3 and, if before that age, problems in social interaction, communication, and responses to the environment must not be of the type seen in autism or must not be accompanied by the characteristic behavioral features of autism.

Although keeping some important historical continuities with Asperger's (1944) original description, the current definitions do differ from it in important ways. Current diagnostic approaches to this disorder and indeed to the question of whether it reserves diagnostic status at all (apart from autism and other conditions with which it shares some common diagnostic fea-

TABLE 1.1. ICD-10 (World Health Organization, 1993) Research Diagnostic Guidelines for Asperger Syndrome

A. There is no clinically significant general delay in spoken or receptive language or cognitive development. Diagnosis requires that single words should have developed by 2 years of age or earlier and that communicative phrases be used by 3 years of age or earlier. Self-help skills, adaptive behavior, and curiosity about the environment during the first 3 years should be at a level consistent with normal intellectual development. However, motor milestones may be somewhat delayed and motor clumsiness is usual (although not a necessary diagnostic feature). Isolated special skills, often related to abnormal preoccupations, are common, but are not required for the diagnosis.

B. There are qualitative abnormalities in reciprocal social interaction (criteria as for autism).

C. The individual exhibits an unusual intense, circumscribed interest, or restricted, repetitive, and stereotyped patterns of behaviour interests, and activities (criteria as for autism, however it would be less usual for these to include either motor mannerisms or preoccupations with part objects or nonfunctional elements of play materials).

D. The disorder is not attributable to other varieties of pervasive developmental disorder; simple schizophrenia schizotypal disorder; obsessive–compulsive disorder, anakastic personality disorder; reactive and disinhibited attachment disorders of childhood.

Note. From World Health Organization (1993, pp. 154–155). Copyright 1993 by World Health Organization. Reprinted by permission.

tures) is not yet adequately resolved. Although described the year after autism, the body of research on AS is much less advanced than that on autism. It is certain that if the concept is retained, improvements in the definition of this condition will be made. This may well parallel the evolution of autism as a diagnostic concept, for example, from Kanner's original prose to Rutter's (1978) definition to that employed in DSM-III (American Psychiatric Association, 1980) and then in DSM-III-R (American Psychiatric Association, 1987) and finally in DSM-IV. During the 1970s and 1980s considerable progress occurred in the attempt to provide better definitions of autism, and it is on this body of work that current defining criteria rest. The official definition of autism was revised twice in the 14 years separating DSM-III from DSM-IV, and even when it appeared in DSM-III for the first time a considerable body of work on diagnosis and definition of autism had accumulated. This is clearly not yet the case with AS; its definition should still be considered tentative and in need of empirical validation. In this chapter we review the rationale for and limitations of the current diagnostic approaches, the limited data regarding validity of the concept, and current controversies in diagnosis. Although we cannot hope to predict the future evolution of the diagnostic concept with certainty, we hope to highlight the issues which are presently of the greatest interest either because they are controversial or because they are critical to supporting the validity of the concept. We first consider the development of the diagnostic concept, its relationship to other conditions, and the development of current definitions, later proceeding with an overview of studies of diagnostic validity and attempts to further refine the diagnostic concept. Many of these issues are discussed in more detail in subsequent chapters of this volume.

EVOLUTION OF THE DIAGNOSTIC CONCEPT

Current official definitions of AS have evolved in important ways in the years since Asperger's (1944) original description of the syndrome of *autistic psychopathy*. This evolution has not been straightforward for several reasons. As with autism modifications in Asperger's description were proposed, most notably by Wing (1981). Some of these changes moved the concept away from the one originally envisioned by Asperger, who clearly regarded the condition as quite separate from autism (Asperger, 1979). Partly because of its ambiguous diagnostic status, markedly divergent views of the condition have arisen. Sometimes these alternative views are only of minimal interest from the point of view of nomenclature, but in other cases the issues proposed are more critical. For example, the convention of viewing AS as a synonymous term for adults with autism is of little interest in that such a convention simply reifies an existing diagnostic concept around an important but nonessential characteristic (in this case age). Similarly, the convention of equating AS with either pervasive developmental disorder not otherwise specified (PDD-NOS) or higher-functioning autism has little importance from the point of view of nomenclature because it simply substitutes one term for another. The much more critical questions are whether AS differs in some important way or ways from autism, PDD-NOS, and other conditions in terms of its natural history, course and outcome, family history or genetic involvement, neuropsychological profiles, and important associated features and in terms of specific implications for treatment and intervention strategies. These differences must be truly "external" ones, avoiding circularity of reasoning or of research strategy in that differences, if found, must reflect factors independent of original diagnostic assignment. A condition for these various questions to be asked is, of course, the requirement that AS can be separated from autism and other conditions in a reliable and empirical fashion. Practical issues involved in diagnostic practice associated with AS have not yet fully benefitted from recent improvements in diagnostic instrumentation seen in autism (e.g., Lord et al., 1989; Lord, Rutter, & Le Couteur, 1994).

Finally, another set of complicating issues has arisen because various alternative diagnostic concepts have been proposed which share at least some fundamental similarity with AS, such as semantic–pragmatic disorder, right-hemisphere learning disability, nonverbal learning disability, and schizoid disorder. These conditions, all of which refer to difficulties that involve some aspect of more complex social skills, have their own histories from diverse disciplines and may have relevance to the validity or definition of AS. Before considering the uses and limitations of current official diagnostic approaches to AS, we, therefore, consider the various alternatives to definition of the condition which have arisen over the years, as well as the potential overlap between AS and these alternative diagnostic concepts.

Alternative Diagnostic Concepts

Professionals from diverse disciplines have dealt, over the years, with individuals with significant problems in social interaction who did not seem to precisely fit Kanner's (1943) concept of infantile autism. For example, Robinson and Vitale (1954) reported three children with patterns of unusual circumscribed interests who talked incessantly about their topic of interest and had significant social difficulties. Similarities and differences were described between these children and the ones described by Kanner (1954) and the authors noted the possibility that the cases might represent a different diagnostic concept. Investigators from fields such as neurology, neuropsychology, and adult psychiatry did propose such concepts. On the one hand, the number of labels available and the diversity of disciplines from which they arose are a testament to the robustness of the underlying clinical phenomena; on the other hand, these various labels have the potential for introducing confusion in this discussion and for inhibiting the kinds of interdisciplinary research that could provide an integrated and comprehensive understanding of individuals with AS. This is particularly an issue for parents whose child might receive any of several different diagnostic labels depending on the training and discipline of the clinician with whom they consult. Given that the various conditions described reflect primarily differences in origins and, at times, emphasis, and that there has not been systematic research on the extent to which they actually describe overlapping populations, it is unclear at present what is the area of overlap between them. What is clear is that these are not mutually exclusive concepts, and that there is need for integrating the better methods originating from each one of them in the effort to better understand aspects of the social, communicative, and neuropsychological disabilities evidenced in individuals with AS.

Schizoid Personality

Originally described by Sula Wolff, a child psychiatrist, the term "schizoid personality in childhood" has been employed by Wolff and colleagues (Wolff & Barlow, 1979; Wolff & Chick, 1980) in their description of children with social isolation and emotional detachment, unusual communicative style, and rigidity of thought and behavior (see Chapter 10, this volume). Originally the term was used because the children described resembled accounts of patients with this personality disorder available in the adult psychiatric literature. Although this initial emphasis on the condition as a personality disorder resulted in more sketchy accounts of developmental course, some attempts at reconstructing the developmental history of these children have been made (e.g., Wolff, 1991). It is still the case, however, that in contrast with children with autism and AS, less is known about the early history of children characterized as having this condition. Several longitudinal follow-up studies (e.g., Wolff, 1991; Wolff, Townshend, McGuire, & Weeks, 1991; Wolff, 1995) have documented that problems of these children typically persist into adulthood where there is also an increase in risk for schizophrenia. The relation of schizoid personality disorder to AS has been somewhat controversial. Several attempts (e.g., Tantam, 1988a; Nagy & Szatmari,1986) have been made to compare these diagnostic concepts. Although there are some areas of similarity (e.g., abnormalities in empathy and nonverbal communication) there have also been areas of difference, primarily in terms of level and pervasiveness of social disability (more severe in AS), outcome (less positive in AS), and relatedness to the schizophrenia spectrum of disorders (the association is stronger in schizoid personality in childhood).

Nonverbal Learning Disability

The concept of Nonverbal Learning Disabilities (NLD) was originally proposed by Johnson and Myklebust (1971; Myklebust, 1975) and subsequently has been elaborated by Rourke (1989). NLD refers to a *profile* of neuropsychological assets and deficits which appears to have a significant negative impact on a person's social and communication skills (see Chapter 8, this volume). Deficits in neuropsychological skills such as tactile perception, psychomotor coordination, visual–spatial organization, and nonverbal problem solving occur in the presence of preserved rote verbal abilities. The particular profile of strengths and deficits result in a characteristic learning style (e.g., the tendency to overly rely on overlearned behaviors when dealing with novel or complex situations. Poor pragmatics and prosody in speech are seen in the presence of relatively preserved formal language skills (e.g., vocabulary and syntax) and single-word reading abilities. Difficulties in appreciating the subtle, and sometimes obvious, nonverbal aspects of social interaction lead to major deficits in social perception and judgment which often result in social isolation and rejection and increased risk for social withdrawal and serious mood disorders (Rourke, Young, & Leenaars, 1989).

The NLD profile is interesting for several reasons. Although potentially associated with a number of different conditions (see Rourke, 1995) it is of much interest that the NLD profile may serve as a neurocognitive model for AS but not for autism (e.g., in autism visual–spatial skills are usually an area of strength) (Siegel, Minshew, & Goldstein, 1996). This has suggested to us and others (e.g., Klin, Volkmar, Sparrow, Cicchetti, & Rourke, 1995a; see

Chapter 8) that the NLD profile may result in a learning style that significantly contributes to the social disability evidenced in AS but not in autism (Klin & Volkmar, 1996). This would represent a potential external validator of AS relative to autism (but see also Chapter 2, this volume, for arguments against this hypothesis). In our experience, although AS is often associated with NLD, the converse is not true. Other important aspects of Rourke's work on NLD include his emphasis on developmental changes in the expression of this profile, its practical implications for intervention, and the association with increased risk for mood disorders in adolescence (as result of frustration accruing from repeated experiences of failure in establishing social relationships).

Developmental Learning Disability of the Right Hemisphere

From the neurological field, attempts have been made to describe many of the same clinical features observed in NLD and AS using the terms "right-hemisphere learning disability," "developmental learning disability of the right hemisphere," or "social–emotional learning disabilities" (Denckla, 1983; Weintraub & Mesulam, 1983). Individuals with this condition exhibit major problems processing information of a social–emotional nature, which is postulated to be a result of underlying right-hemisphere dysfunction, and as a result have major difficulties in understanding and interpreting affective expression and other interpersonal skills (Voeller, 1986). In addition, a possible familial component has been suggested (Weintraub & Mesulam, 1983), as well as a possible overlap with AS (Voeller, 1991).

Semantic–Pragmatic Disorder

This condition has been described in the work on children with language disorders for whom it has been clear that despite adequate speech some individuals have language which is ultimately impoverished in terms of its actual communicative value (e.g., Blank, Gessner, & Esposito, 1979). Rapin and Allen (1983) used semantic–pragmatic deficit disorder to describe cases in which speech and language skills were adequate in form (syntax and phonology) but impoverished in content and use (semantics and pragmatics). Bishop (1989, 1998) has considerably refined the descriptions and assessment instrumentation used in the characterization of communicative difficulties exhibited by these children (see Chapter 9, this volume). Similarities with the communicative style exhibited by individuals with AS are particularly observed in the area of conversational skills, where individuals with this condition show deficits in the ability to introduce, maintain, or shift topics; verbosity without effectively conveying a coherent message; and difficulties in suppressing ongoing thoughts (e.g., might talk aloud to no one in particular). Recent research in this area (see Chapter 9) has shown that the association between semantic and pragmatic deficits is not a necessary one, and that a term such as "pragmatic language impairment" might be preferable to refer to these children. This research has also shown that pragmatic impairments, in themselves, are not necessarily associated with important aspects of AS, such as marked difficulties in social relationships or evidence of restricted interests.

APPROACHES TO DIAGNOSIS OF ASPERGER SYNDROME

Asperger's Views

At the time of Asperger's (1944) original work there was not, of course, the considerable interest in operational definitions which has concerned psychiatry so much since the 1970s (Spitzer, Endicott, & Robbins, 1978). As with Kanner (1943), Asperger provided a clinical account of what appeared to him to be a new syndrome. His description of this condition was inspired by his work with four boys, ages 6 to 11 who had marked problems in social interaction despite having what appeared to be good language and cognitive skills (see Frith, 1991, for an English translation). These four boys, however, were said to be representative of a much larger sample of children presenting with the profile described. In addition to the problems in social interaction, which Asperger emphasized by the use of the word "autism" in his original name for the condition (*Autistischen Psychopathen im Kindesalter*, or autistic personality disorders in childhood), he also noted other features which were commonly present. These included egocentric preoccupations with unusual and circumscribed interests that were the focus of much of the child's life and which interfered with acquisition of skills in other areas (e.g., the child might be fascinated with train schedules but be unable to plan or anticipate his own daily routine). Affectively, Asperger noted that these children had difficulties in dealing with their feelings, often tending to intellectualize them, and had poor empathy and difficulties in understanding social cues. In addition, Asperger mentioned that they were motorically awkward and clumsy, with odd posture and gait and generally poor awareness of the movement of their body in space; graphomotor skills were poor and the ability to participate in group sports activities was compromised. In terms of language and communication skills, Asperger noted that the children he described were like little professors who talked (often at great length) about the topic of their interest but who had difficulties with nonverbal and pragmatic aspects of communication (e.g., in use of facial expressions and gestures, in modulation of their voice, and in responding appropriately to the nonverbal cues of their conversational partners). Behavioral difficulties included noncompliance and negativism which led to aggression and other conduct problems. These difficulties often stemmed from the marked egocentrism and highly circumscribed interests as well as from the poor social understanding and peer relations these children exhibited at school.

In terming this condition "autistic personality disorder," Asperger used Bleuler's (1916/1951) earlier term "autism," which was created to capture "a loss of contact, a retirement into self and a disregard of the outside world" observed in schizophrenia (Asperger, 1979, p. 46). In his use of the term, Asperger was careful to contrast the condition he described from schizophrenia by noting its earlier onset, usually after age 3 years. Asperger's original paper also emphasized familial factors (i.e., similar traits were seen in relatives, particularly fathers).

Initially, Asperger (1944) was rather optimistic in his speculations regarding course and ultimate outcome (e.g., expecting that many of his patients would be able to use their special interests in obtaining employment). His observation of similar traits in family members may also have led him to be more optimistic about ultimate outcome. As time went on Asperger was somewhat less optimistic about outcome.

Early History of the Diagnostic Concept

Asperger published his paper unaware that Leo Kanner had published a description of 11 children with "autistic disturbances of affective contact" the year before. Although Kanner's "early infantile autism" quickly became the focus of much clinical interest in the English speaking world, interest in Asperger's diagnostic concept was limited to Germany and Austria, and to a lesser extent in the Netherlands and Soviet Union. Despite the lack of awareness of his work, some case reports with what we now might recognize as AS did appear in English (e.g., Robinson & Vitale, 1954); in fact, we now know that accounts of children similar to those described by Asperger had appeared in the literature (primarily in German) before Asperger's paper (see Wing, 1998, for a review). However, Asperger's work received vanishingly little attention in the English-speaking world.

In 1962, Van Krevelen and Kuipers attempted to distinguish AS from Kanner's autism, suggesting that the latter was present from first months of life, that language was absent or delayed, that there was a lack of interest in others, and that prognosis was poor. They contrasted this with the later onset/recognition of AS as well as the often precocious language development ("the child talked before he walked"), the one-sided, eccentric social style, which caused problems in social interaction despite social interest, and the apparently better prognosis (see also Van Krevelen, 1963). These views were elaborated by van Krevelen again in 1971 in an article in the first issue of the *Journal of Autism and Childhood Schizophrenia* where he again attempted to draw clear distinctions between autism and AS. Similar attempts had been made in the German literature, some of which were translated into English at around the same time (e.g., Bosch, 1970).

Despite Van Krevelen's attempt to distinguish between the two conditions, considerable confusion arose about AS as a diagnostic concept. This confusion stemmed from several sources. First, it took several decades before investigators and clinicians were sure of the validity of autism (e.g., apart from childhood schizophrenia), and indeed it was not until 1980 that autism was first officially recognized as a diagnosis. Second, as research on autism was conducted in the 1950s and 1960s, it became clear that Kanner's original concept had to be modified in certain ways; for example, Kanner originally thought autism was probably associated with normal intellectual levels but it became apparent that about three-fourths of individuals with autism functioned in the mentally retarded range. The final source of confusion stemmed, understandably, from the use of the same word, "autism," by Asperger and Kanner. This term reflected the core disability, namely, a lack of or inadequate social relatedness present in the children described in their accounts. In addition, both groups of patients had difficulties in the areas of affective reaction, nature and range of interests, and social use of language. The main differences in the two conditions appeared to be that in AS early speech and formal language skills were acquired on time if not precociously, that motor deficits were more common in AS, and that, in contrast to autism, the apparent onset of the condition was after the first several years of life. In addition, all the original cases described by Asperger had been boys whereas Kanner had noted some girls with autism. Other areas of divergence in the accounts included later speech and language skills, motor mannerisms, circumscribed interests, and ultimate outcome. Some of the differences in the original syndrome descriptions may relate to the nature of differences in the groups being reported, that is, while Kanner was describing more impaired and younger children, Asperger was describing older and apparently less impaired individuals. These differences contributed to the subsequent tendency to equate Kanner's syndrome with the "classically" lower-functioning autistic child and Asperger's description with the nonretarded and verbal child with autism.

Wing's Modifications of Asperger's Concept

Lorna Wing's (1981) publication of a review of Asperger's work and a series of cases dramatically increased interest in Asperger's diagnostic concept. Her report of over 30 cases was particularly important in that she was able to identify a group of individuals whose histories and clinical presentations were similar to those in Asperger's account as well as another group of cases in which the current clinical presentation was consistent but early history was not. In addition to summarizing Asperger's original work, Wing proposed some modifications of the concept based on her case series; these modifications were primarily related to the issue of early development and early clinical presentation. Wing suggested that difficulties might be apparent early in life (i.e., in the first 2 years) and might take the form of lack of interest in others, early language deficits, and imaginative play; also, her cases suggested that Asperger's speculation that cases talked before they walked was not often correct. Finally, she noted that in some cases the condition was apparently associated with mild mental retardation, and it was not limited exclusively to males. She highlighted the possible continuities with autism and proposed the eponymous label "Asperger syndrome," in order to avoid the use of the word "psychopathy" adopted by Asperger, as this word was now synonymous with antisocial behavior rather than denoting a personality disorder which was Asperger's original intention.

Wing's (1981) description markedly increased interest in this condition so that now more than 100 publications devoted to the topic have appeared (see Chapter 14, this volume). It also prefigured much of the subsequent work which has been concerned about the boundaries, or lack thereof, with autism. Wing emphasized that despite her interest in Asperger's description, she fundamentally viewed the disorder as clearly on the autistic spectrum and was more concerned with broadening, rather than narrowing, Asperger's original concept. Not surprisingly, the modifications she proposed tended to blur the distinctions between AS and autism originally suggested by Van Krevelen (1971) and reinforced by Asperger (1979).

Asperger Syndrome: 1981–1994

In her summary, Wing (1981) did not provide explicit guidelines for diagnosis but, as noted, she did argue that various modifications in Asperger's original description were warranted. Based on her work, a number of studies (both of single cases and series of cases) have proposed diagnostic guidelines (see Table 1.2). Given that Wing herself had not really attempted to do this and that, indeed, she did not attempt to make a clear distinction between AS and autism, it is perhaps not surprising that the definitions derived from her work diverged from each other in important ways (see Gillberg & Gillberg, 1989; Szatmari, Bartolucci, & Bremner, 1989a; Tantam, 1988a; World Health Organization, 1993; American Psychiatric Association, 1994; Klin et al., 1995a; Klin, Carter, & Sparrow, 1997). Thus different features were seen as necessary, or only supportive of, or not integral to the diagnosis. The differences in approach to diagnosis of AS, not surprisingly, produced major diagnostic discrepancies. For example, Ghaziuddin, Tsai, and Ghaziuddin (1992a) reported a comparison of several diagnostic systems: Asperger (1944), Wing (1981), Gilberg and Gillberg (1989), Tantam (1988a), Szatmari, Bartolucci, and Bremner (1989a), and what was then the draft of ICD-10. One-third of patients who appeared to meet Wing's criteria for the condition did not meet Szatmari et al.'s criteria, and nearly half failed the ICD-10 and Asperger's criteria—usually because the case had exhibited some early language delay/oddity. This is an interesting issue as Wing

TABLE 1.2. Comparison of Six Sets of Clinical Criteria Defining AS

Clinical feature	Asperger (1944, 1979)	Wing (1981)	Gillberg & Gillberg (1989)	Tantam (1988)	Szatmari et al. (1989)	DSM-IV (American Psychiatric Association, 1994)
Social impairment						
Poor nonverbal communication	**Yes**	**Yes**	**Yes**	**Yes**	**Yes**	**Yes**
Poor empathy	**Yes**	**Yes**	**Yes**	**Yes**	**Yes**	Yes
Failure to develop friendship	**Yes**	**Yes**	Yes (implied)	**Yes**	Yes	**Yes**
Language/communication			Yes			
Poor prosody and pragmatics	**Yes**	**Yes**	**Yes**	**Yes**	**Yes**	**Not stated**
Idiosyncratic language	**Yes**	**Yes**	Not stated	Not stated	**Yes**	Not stated
Impoverished imaginative play	Yes	**Yes**	Not stated	Not stated	Not stated	Not stated
All-absorbing interest	Yes	Yes	Yes	Yes	Not stated	Often
Motor clumsiness	Yes	Yes	Yes	Yes	Not stated	Often
Onset (0–3 years)						
Speech delays/deviance	No	May be present	May be present	Not stated	Not stated	No
Cognitive delays	No	May be present	Not stated	Not stated	Not stated	No
Motor delays	Yes	Sometimes	Not stated	Not stated	Not stated	May be present
Exclusion of autism	Yes (1979)	No	No	No	**Yes**	**Yes**
Mental retardation	**No**	May be present	Not stated	Not stated	Not stated	Not stated

Note. Symptoms that are defined as necessary for the presence of the condition are given in **boldface**. Adapted from Klin and Volkmar (1997, p. 100). Copyright 1997 by John Wiley & Sons. Adapted by permission.

(1981) and others (e.g., Gillberg & Gillberg, 1989) have reported cases whom they believed exhibited AS but who had histories of early language delay/ deviance.

The different diagnostic systems for AS take rather different approaches to diagnosis. Some definitions are conceptually very close to autism while others emphasize areas of difference. Even when definitions are close to autism the underlying rationale may be quite different, for example, some authors believe the disorders are fundamentally the same, whereas others wish to emphasize that certain "core" features (such as the social deficit) are present in both disorders. Each of these relevant clinical features is discussed in turn.

Clinical Features Relevant to Diagnosis

Onset of the Disorder

Asperger (1944) emphasized that early development of his cases was apparently normal; in his later publications (1979) he continued to emphasize this as a point of difference from autism where children, even higher-functioning ones, are almost always seen as having problems by 3 years of age (Volkmar, Klin, & Cohen, 1997). In addition two other factors with regard to onset have been reported: the early facility in language development in AS and apparent relative preservation of social skills early on. Asperger (1944) emphasized that language often developed early and that children often had an early interest in language which seemed to serve as a lifeline for them. This notion has persisted in the literature and often is observed clinically, even though the focus has become the preserved nature of *formal* language skills (i.e., phonology, syntax, and semantics) rather than language use (i.e., pragmatics), something Asperger (1979) himself appeared to recognize later on. The possibility that early social skills may be somewhat preserved, at least within the family, is somewhat less clearly established. It does appear that early social skills, including attachment, are not drastically unusual although the absence of delayed or deviant language and the possibility that family members may have similar traits (Volkmar, Klin, & Pauls, 1998) might tend to delay recognition. Indeed a difficulty with current criteria (where autism takes precedence if both it and AS apply to a given case) is that with the wisdom of hindsight and extensive elicitation by an interviewer, mothers (or fathers) may report some early oddity of social, communication, or behavioral functioning. As discussed subsequently, such a report would automatically rule out AS. The lack of interest in others typically reported in autism is, however, not typically reported. Sometimes parents retrospectively recount that the child's social approaches were somewhat awkward or inappropriate and become even more so over time (e.g., as the child enters settings in which his or her tendency to be a "little professor" stands out in the context of a normal peer group). At that time the child with AS might be noted to have very inappropriate or highly unusual approaches to other children, which reflect the child's desire for interaction but marked problems in negotiating it.

Circumscribed Interests. In his original report Asperger (1944) mentioned that children with AS had unusual interests which interfered with their acquisition of normal skills. The notion of special skills was implicit in Kanner's first report of autism; for example, children with autism were noted sometimes to be very adept at tasks which involved, say, puzzle assembly. Subsequently, a body of work on "savant skills" in autism arose as it became clear that some (perhaps 10% of the population of persons with autism) had unusual abilities to draw, play music, or perform mathematical or calender calculations (Treffert, 1989). Although important studies of savant skills have been reported in the literature (e.g., O'Connor & Hermelin, 1989), there has been surprisingly little attention paid to the nature of circumscribed interests of the typed reported by Asperger, and later by Robinson and Vitale (1954), and to the extent to which these interests are all-absorbing and interfere with learning of other skills and with social adaptation (Klin et al., 1997; South, Klin, & Volkmar, 1997). In general it appears that special interests in autism are more likely to involve object manipulation, visual–spatial tasks, music, or unusual savant skills whereas in AS the focus is on amassing large amounts of factual information relative to the child's topic of interest. It does appear that this topic changes over time but usually dominates the life of the child (and often the family) in terms of both the time and energy spent in pursuit of the topic and the content of social interacting with others. The child's early interests may seem somewhat more developmentally appropriate, but as time goes on the child requires extraordinary degrees of knowledge about his or her topic (e.g., railroad telegraph pole line insulators, personal information about all the members of Congress, and knowledge of the passenger list of the *Titanic,* weather information, and various models of deep fat fryers).

Motor Functioning–Praxis

Asperger (1944) noted that his child cases often had delayed motor skills as well as motor incoordination. The impression of motoric awkwardness and motor clumsiness has persisted over time (Tantam, 1988a; Gillberg, 1990) and is listed both in ICD-10 and DSM-IV as an associated (but not necessary) diagnostic feature. In contrast, for younger children with autism, motor abilities may be an area of relative strength (Volkmar et al., 1987). For older individuals, however, the situation is more complex, and motor deficits may be seen in autism as well, making this symptom less discriminating between autism and AS (Ghaziuddin, Tsai, & Ghaziuddin, 1992c; Ghaziuddin, Butler,

Tsai, & Ghaziuddin, 1994; Hallett et al., 1993; Smith & Bryson, 1994; Vilensky, Damasio, & Maurer, 1981). It is very likely that a person's posture, gait, and even specific motor skills involving imitation, learning from demonstration, or interpersonal coordination (such as in group sports) become increasingly more dependent with age on developmental aspects other than simple motor capacities, such as body image, social and self-perception, to name a few (Roy, Elliott, Dewey, & Square-Storer, 1990; see also Chapter 3, this volume, for a comprehensive review).

Social Functioning

The early patterns of social difficulties in autism share some features with Asperger's but also contrast with it. Typically in AS the social presentation differs from that seen in autism in that even though the children have marked social isolation, they are not usually unaware of or disinterested in others (Volkmar et al., 1994). In fact, some of the behavioral difficulties such children exhibit appear to be the result of constant but inappropriate approach to others. On the other hand, this also suggests a point of comparison with Wing's description (Wing & Gould, 1979) of the "active but odd" subgroup of individuals with autism. Nevertheless, clinical reports suggest some areas of potential difference. For example, in AS the child often uses social interaction to engage the conversational partner in long-winded, verbose conversations about his or her topic of special interest, with, however, little attention to the often distancing reactions of others. Individuals with AS may express an interest in having friends, including girlfriends/boyfriends, but usually become frustrated as a result of their frequent failures. In older children and adolescents, the social difficulties observed in AS appear to include problems with spontaneous social interaction, particularly in situations requiring a measure of quick and intuitive social adjustment, even though the individual may be able to describe in great cognitive detail aspects of social conventions. Higher-functioning individuals with autism are more frequently described as withdrawn and are more likely to be seen as unaware of or disinterested in others (Volkmar, Sparrow, Goudreau, Cicchetti, Paul, & Cohen, 1982).

Communication

Although early speech development in AS is typically not of concern, significant abnormalities in communication—especially in pragmatic or conversational skills—are observed as the child matures, likely reflecting the cumulative impact of the child's social deficits. Klin (1994) has noted three ways in which the communication of individuals with AS may be distinctive. First, although prosodic skills may be generally poor as in autism, the degree of abnormal inflection and quality of voice is typically not as pronounced as in autism (Ghaziuddin & Gerstein, 1996). For example, the more markedly monotonic voice typical of individuals with autism is not commonly observed in individuals with AS, who instead may use a small number of inflection patterns without adjusting those to the communicative content of their speech (e.g., making a statement or telling a joke). Abnormalities of rate and volume of speech, however, are frequently observed in both conditions. Thus, the person may not modulate volume regardless of whether he or she is in a classroom, church, or funeral services; he or she may also speak at an erratic speed, which may at times compromise intelligibility. Second, in AS, speech is often tangential and circumstantial and results in a one-sided, egocentric conversational style as the individual engages in unrelenting monologues about his or her topic of special interest. The difficulties with contingency, reciprocity, and other rules of discourses (Grice, 1975), such as topic demarcation (i.e., appropriately introducing a subject, conveying a distinct message, and marking shifts to a new topic), are further compounded by the individual's tendency to verbalize every thought, failing to organize speech in terms of distinct messages to be conveyed to the conversational partner. This phenomenon may result in an impression of incoherent or dissociated speech which can lead to the consideration of the presence of a thought disorder (Caplan, 1994; Dykens, Volkmar, & Glick, 1991). In most cases, however, individuals are able to clarify their speech output, suggesting that this aspect of their presentation can be better understood as part of their communication disability rather than a deterioration of thought processes. We return to this important topic in the subsequent discussion of comorbidity with other psychiatric conditions. Third, throughout their lives, individuals with AS have been reported to be markedly and consistently verbose. Given any opportunity (or even without one), the child may turn to his or her topic of interest (e.g., "Do you know how many people were killed on the *Titanic*"?), moving and enchaining the conversation flow toward the topic in an often didactic fashion. As noted, monitoring of the listener's cues (e.g., lack of interest, obvious boredom, or attempts to shift topic) is typically very poor; as a result, individuals with AS may persist on relating lists of facts without ever coming to a conclusion or communicative closure.

Associated Problems and Conditions

A final area of clinical interest has centered on the possibility that AS and autism differ in terms of associated features and conditions. In his original report, Asperger (1944) noted that the cases often had problems with negativism and conduct. Several subsequent reports have suggested a possible association with violence or criminal behavior (e.g., Baron-Cohen, 1988; Everall & Le Couteur, 1990; Mawson, Grounds, & Tantam, 1985; Tantam, 1988b; Wing, 1986). However, in their review of the literature on this topic Ghaziuddin, Tsai, and Ghaziuddin (1991) found no support for such an association. In contrast, Scragg and Shah (1994) reported an increased rate of AS among individuals in a secure hospital. As we (Klin et al., 1997) have noted elsewhere, our experience has been that individuals with AS are much more likely to be victims rather than victimizers, although emotional insensitivity, pedantic style, and limited social understanding may lead to a perception of lack of concern or empathy and inappropriate social behaviors. For example, in our experience, a blunt style and insensitivity to social rules and expectations have caused an adolescent student to be charged with allegations of sexual harassment. His persistence and inability to understand other people's reactions compounded the situation. His reactions to the young women's rejections, however, were felt as a rebuff of him as a person and of his bids to make friends, resulting in worrisome depression. Rather than being a "sexual pervert," this young man's behaviors were best understood as a consequence of his extremely narrow understanding of the realm and diversity of possible social relationships.

Much interest has also centered on the possibility that individuals with AS are at increased risk for other conditions (e.g., that rates of psychosis and/or schizophrenia may be significantly elevated) (Clarke, Littlejohns, Corbett, & Joseph, 1989; Tantam, 1988a; Taiminen, 1994). Early interest in AS related to the possibility that AS might serve as a condition that linked autism and schizophrenia (Tantam, 1991). The topic of comorbidity is discussed in detail later in this chapter, but it should be noted that the strength and significance of such associations are often questionable (Ghaziuddin, Leininger, & Tsai, 1995). The potential for increased rates of mood disorder does seem high given the individuals' social insight and repeatedly frustrated desire for social relationships, and such associations have been noted (Ellis, Ellis, Fraser, & Deb, 1994; Fujikawa, Kobayashi, Koga, & Murata, 1987; Ghaziuddin, Tsai, & Ghaziuddin, 1992b; Klin, Sparrow, Volkmar, Cicchetti, & Rourke, 1995b; Rourke et al., 1989).

Interpretation of Research Findings

It is unfortunate that comparability of findings reported by different centers is often rendered virtually impossible because of marked differences in diagnostic characterization. Indeed, in some cases, even within a given center, the diagnostic concept appears to have evolved over time. Such evolution poses considerable problems for the interpretation of studies, particularly those attempting to establish the validity of AS relative to higher-functioning autism. In some studies, particularly case reports, issues of diagnosis of AS are addressed minimally, if at all. In some cases, it is only with careful review that readers will discover that AS was used interchangeably with autism, adult autism, PDD-NOS, or nondevelopmental social difficulties. As noted in the introduction to this volume, it is now essential that the field move toward careful, detailed, and explicit characterization of subjects, where systems of classification can be directly and empirically compared. The initial step toward this goal has been made as a result of the inclusion, though still tentative, of AS in "official" diagnostic systems, to which we now turn.

Asperger Syndrome in DSM-IV and ICD-10

Since AS has often been defined in relation to autism, and the definition of autism has evolved over time—that is, from DSM-III (American Psychiatric Association, 1980) to DSM-III-R (American Psychiatric Association, 1987) to DSM-IV (American Psychiatric Association, 1994) and ICD-10 (World Health Organization, 1993)—research on AS was further complicated as a result of the shifting comparison. However, by the late 1980s, a process of revision was under way both for what would become DSM-IV (American Psychiatric Association, 1994) as well as the World Health Organization's ICD-10 (World Health Organization, 1993), and the issue of inclusion or lack of inclusion of AS in these systems became the subject of intense debate. It should be noted that although both of these official diagnostic systems shared some important similarities they also had some important differences. Most important, the ICD system was intended to exist in two versions—the first was meant to be a set of clinical descriptions to be used as guidelines for clinicians, whereas the second was intended as a set of diagnostic criteria for researchers. In contrast, the DSM-IV system was intended to be used for both clinical and research work. At the time that the revisions of these systems were undertaken, it was clear that autism would be officially recognized in both systems, but it was unclear whether the definitions of autism in the two systems would be compatible, and whether other conditions, such as AS, might be included in the pervasive developmental disorders (PDD) class.

As part of the process of revision, considerable preparatory work was conducted. This included preparation of literature reviews on autism and AS (see Rutter & Schopler, 1992; Szatmari, 1992a; Szatmari, 1992b) as well as various data reanalyses (e.g., Volkmar, Cicchetti, Bregman, & Cohen, 1992; Volkmar, Cicchetti, Cohen, & Bregman, 1992). A number of issues were identified; to resolve them a large, multinational field trial was conducted (Volkmar et al., 1994). As part of this international field trial, 21 sites and 125 raters evaluated nearly 1,000 cases. All sites had clinical programs for individuals with autism and PDD and about half the raters were experienced in work with such individuals. Raters completed a set of ratings that included various diagnostic criteria for autism as well as potential criteria for AS and other "new" conditions that might be included in DSM-IV and ICD-10. The ratings also included information on age, IQ, communicative ability, and placement of cases. In the final sample, 48 cases had received a clinical (i.e., clinician assigned) diagnosis of AS.

While the DSM-IV autism field trial was not primarily focused on the definition (much less the validity) of AS, the issues raised by its possible inclusion were relevant to the DSM-IV and ICD-10 definitions of autism, for example, relative to the role of historical information in the diagnosis and narrowness (or broadness) of the final definition of autism. Examination of the 48 cases of AS collected as part of the field trial provided some support for inclusion of AS as an officially recognized category. This was the case when AS was considered relative to higher-functioning autism and PDD-NOS (Volkmar et al., 1994). The cases rated as having AS, either by clinical diagnosis or on the basis of the criteria proposed in ICD-10, were indeed unlikely to have exhibited delays in the development of spoken language. When these individuals with AS were compared with more able (IQ > 85) individuals with autism (based on either clinical or ICD criteria), the AS cases had significantly fewer symptoms of deviance in language and communication. Another interesting contrast emerged in profiles of functioning on intelligence testing. Individuals with AS were more likely to exhibit Verbal IQ scores greater than Performance IQ; the *opposite* result was obtained for higher-functioning individuals with autism. Also, individuals with AS had fewer symptoms of social deviance than did those with autism. A final series of analyses compared cases with AS to those with clinical diagnoses of either atypical autism or PDD-NOS. Compared to individuals with atypical autism and PDD-NOS, those with AS had greater disability in the areas of social deviance and resistance to change.

The draft (and ultimately the final) text in ICD-10 explicitly noted the possibility that AS might be a variant of autism. The framers of ICD-10 and DSM-IV were also aware of the potential difficulties concerning boundaries with other (non-PDD) diagnostic concepts such as Nonverbal Learning Disability (NLD) (Rourke, 1989) and semantic pragmatic disorder (Bishop, 1989). In ICD-10, the condition was noted to differ from autism in terms of a *"lack of any clinically significant general delay in language or cognitive development"* (p. 154). By definition, single words develop by age 2, phrases are used by age 3, and self-help and adaptive behavior are consistent with normal development in the first 3 years of life, although motor development may be delayed. In the draft ICD-10 definition, individuals with AS had to meet the same criteria for qualitative impairments in social interactions as for autism as well as the criteria for restricted, repetitive, and stereotyped patterns of behavior, interests, and activities also of the type exhibited in autism. It was noted, however, that early motor delays and motor clumsiness were usual (but not required for the diagnosis) and that isolated special skills (often related to abnormal preoccupations) might also be present and indeed were more likely than the stereotyped behaviors or preoccupation with part objects exhibited in autism. By ICD definition, AS cannot be attributed to other varieties of PDD or to schizotypal disorder, reactive attachment disorder, simple schizophrenia, obsessional personality disorder, or obsessive–compulsive disorder.

Critique of ICD-10 and DSM-IV

Given the considerable disagreements which have characterized attempts to define AS, it is probably not a great surprise to discover that the present official diagnostic systems have been the subject of debate. Based on research available (e.g., Ghaziuddin et al., 1992a), it does appear that ICD-10 and DSM-IV are, on balance, probably closer to the concept originally proposed by Asperger. This issue is itself the topic of debate as some researchers have complained that AS becomes, they believe artificially, a rather rare disorder. Others would argue that, if anything, both diagnostic systems have tended to err on the side of overinclusiveness as neither circumscribed interests nor clumsiness, both features noted by Asperger (1944), are essential for the diagnosis. We shall return to the issue of diagnostic stringency in the next section, which discusses validity.

Leaving aside this debate for the moment, however, several other complicating issues should be noted. Although conceptually the same, the two systems do differ in terms of text description and level of detail of criteria. ICD-10 provides a somewhat fuller description of the condition in text and explicitly notes the complexities of diagnosis relative to autism; in contrast, DSM-IV essentially restates the criteria in the text. The latter seems particularly unfortunate as it is just when the reader wishes more help in understanding the underlying diagnostic construct that he or she must refer to the text. The ICD-10 research criteria are, as expected, much more detailed, and this allows for greater specification of the nature of the deficits observed; this issue becomes very important in the application of the hierarchical exclusionary rule (i.e., that the case does not meet criteria for autism). Such hierarchical rules are (more or less explicitly) entailed in all aspects of diagnostic systems. In an ideal world, the two disorders would be defined independently. However, given that definitive data are lacking and that it appears that the major point of similarity is the social deficits, AS and autism share the same defining criteria for this critical diagnostic feature. Either of three approaches could have been adopted: AS could have taken precedence over autism if both disorders applied in a given case; the conditions could be defined in such a way as to be mutually exclusive without a hierarchy (leaving the issue to clinical judgment), or autism could take precedence over AS. The latter rule was the one finally adopted. Although this is understandable given the much more established body of research on diagnostic validity of autism as well as the fact that community resources coalesce primarily around this condition, this decision can be problematic in application particularly when it is clear that an individual meets the social criteria for autism/AS and exhibits some unusual aspects of language—especially social use of language or intonation or speech and one of the restricted, repetitive behaviors. In this rather common situation, the critical issue becomes whether the individual's early development was normal or close to normal.

If it was normal, then AS is diagnosed; otherwise autism takes precedence regardless of current clinical presentation. Unfortunately, the wording of the onset criteria for autism in DSM-IV is terse and seems to suggest that any minimal early abnormality in the pertinent areas would be sufficient to justify a diagnosis of autism. The ICD-10 onset criteria are somewhat more detailed and, accordingly, a bit less overencompassing, although even there a thorough review of the child's history with the parents might produce a single recollection of abnormality sufficient to again "move" the child into a diagnosis of autism. Miller and Ozonoff (1997) have criticized this approach and suggest that it is overly restrictive.

To summarize this problem, ICD-10 and DSM-IV appear to differentiate AS from autism almost solely on the basis of the onset criteria regardless of the patient's social impairment later in life; as onset criteria are over-inclusive, the diagnosis of autism rather than AS might often apply, even though the clinician might feel that important differences exist for a given case that would justify the diagnosis of AS. Various cases have been reported (e.g., Gillberg & Gillberg, 1989; Wing, 1981) who were thought to have had AS but who would not have met current onset criteria. It is of interest that the converse problem does not arise, that is, higher-functioning individuals with autism invariably will have had difficulties in the first 3 years of life (Volkmar & Cohen, 1989).

The failure to specify differentiating diagnostic features (e.g., relative to the social or communicative difficulties or relative to restricted interests) is also problematic. Because identical criteria are used for both conditions, features that might carry greater diagnostic precision, particularly positive symptoms (observable deviant behaviors, or observable strengths), are not provided. For example, many clinicians/researchers highlight the nature of circumscribed interests in AS and the direct interference with the individuals' social adjustment, contrasting with typical symptomatology in the areas of "restricted interests" in autism; Tantam (1988a) suggests that a major difference between the two conditions relates to the greater desire and motivation for social interaction in patients with AS. This notion is consistent with earlier reports, such as Van Krevelen's (1971), who emphasized qualitative differences between AS and autism in that in the former there was more social interest.

Finally, neither system makes provision for factors that might arise clinically and potentially affect the application of criteria. For example, it is not clear how a child with cleft palate and some associated though minor language delay who exhibited AS would present clinically. Although some researchers might have hoped that Asperger's own research reports might clarify this issue, it is clearly the case that, as with autism, progress on these issues will only be achieved as more refined and rigorous studies become available.

VALIDITY OF ASPERGER SYNDROME
AS A DIAGNOSTIC CONCEPT

The aims of classification include facilitating communication among professionals, providing information about given disorders that is relevant to treatment and/or to prevention, and providing information useful for research aimed at understanding the pathogenesis of disorders. Classification systems facilitate both clinical work and research by ordering our observations, noting important patterns of regularity, and facilitating communication, prediction, and, ultimately, explanation. It is important to note that simply by assigning a label little progress is made in regard to understanding underlying processes; this is true throughout psychiatry and much of medicine. It also is the case that obtaining a diagnostic label or labels is just one part of a broader *diagnostic process* in which the totality of the individual's strengths and weaknesses are considered in the development of a remedial program (see Chapter 12, this volume). For disorders that first appear in childhood, an additional aspect of classification is the importance of developmental features (e.g., the ways in which conditions are manifest at different ages, change over time as the individual develops and the interrelationship among the various aspects of development).

Classification systems are discussed extensively elsewhere (e.g., Caron & Rutter, 1991; Cohen, Paul, & Volkmar, 1986; Dahl, Cohen, & Provence, 1986; Rutter et al., 1969; Rutter, 1989; Rutter & Gould, 1985; Spitzer et al., 1978; Volkmar et al., 1997). They can be either categorical or dimensional and may vary depending on the purpose of the classification system and the nature of the difficulties being classified. To be recognized as a disorder, the constellation of symptoms, behaviors, signs, or historical features should be a source of significant distress or impairment (DSM-IV), that is, odd or unusual behaviors do not, in and of themselves, constitute a "disorder" unless they are related to a manifestation of serious dysfunction within the individual. Although it is often assumed that mental disorders must have a biological basis, and many indeed probably do, it is also the case that enduring patterns of maladaptive personality traits can be classified as disorders (Morey, 1988). The role of etiology in classification systems is complex because (1) in most cases we presently do not understand underlying pathophysiology, (2) different etiological processes can produce rather similar conditions, (3) identical biological factors can be associated with a range of clinical conditions, and (4) intervention may be more directly related to the clinical condition than to etiology (see also Chapter 14, this volume).

To be useful, classification systems must be usable and reliable. In recent years this has meant that classificatory systems such as DSM and ICD focus on observable clinical features rather than, for example, more theoretical (and less observable and reliable) concepts. In these systems it is also essential that the disorders have some validity. Different types of validity have been identified: The conditions should be described so that they can be readily differentiated from one another (*discriminant validity*); the definition should be written in such a way as to capture the diagnostic construct (*face validity*); the condition should predict some important aspect of subsequent course or response to treatment (*predictive validity*); and the condition as defined in its various criteria should have meaning relative to what it purports to assess (*construct validity*). To summarize these points in the context of AS and autism, to be able to establish that these two conditions differ from each other, they should diverge in important ways *other than those incorporated in the definition*. This could be in regard to response to treatment, natural history in the absence of treatment, familial patterns, biological correlates, or developmental correlates such as neuropsychological profiles. In developing guidelines for diagnosis, the usefulness of alternative approaches and diagnostic criteria is typically assessed relative to some "gold standard" of a prototypical case or cases evaluated by experienced clinicians. For AS, the diversity of previous diagnostic approaches (see Table 1.2), number of potentially overlapping diagnostic concepts, and fundamental differences in diagnostic practice have posed significant problems both for developing and evaluating alternative diagnostic approaches. In reviewing the literature on validity of this condition, it is important that the reader keep in mind several important questions:

- Are any differences found *truly independent* ones? This is essentially the problem of avoiding circularity (Klin, 1994) so that any differences found among two disorders do not simply reflect the diagnostic criteria used to define them in the first place. To state the obvious, if AS is defined, in part, on the basis that early language skills are reasonably normal, reasonable normality of early language skills should not be taken as evidence for the validity of the condition. However, if some feature related to language functioning (e.g., verbosity or exceptional verbal abilities are documented many years later), it might be relevant to the question of validity.
- What specific features are used in making the diagnosis of AS (or autism)? Some studies may indicate that the authors are using Asperger's (1944) or Wing's (1981) criteria, but in neither case do the authors explicitly lay out and operationalize criteria in a way as to make possible replication elsewhere. Given that the diagnosis of AS (or autism for that matter) often relies on the provision of some aspects of developmental history, it is important to understand exactly the process (e.g., who was the informant, who was the interviewer) and quality (e.g., were comprehensive and reliable instruments used) of history taking, and how the underlying question (e.g., onset of disorder) is operationalized in actual practice (e.g., inclusion or exclusion of specific onset criteria). Unfortunately, in many studies of potential interest, these conditions are not fulfilled. In the absence of a systematic at-

tempt to differentiate autism and AS, it is likely that some studies of higher-functioning autism in the past included individuals with AS and vice versa, thus influencing results and affecting conclusions drawn from the data. Also, in the absence of detailed and explicit characterization of subjects, it is likely that some reports comparing AS directly with autism may in fact have studied overlapping samples (e.g., the "autistic sample" includes subjects with autism, whereas the "AS sample" includes subjects with autism and AS). This overlap would affect results in important ways such as, for example, increasing the likelihood of Type II errors (i.e., finding no difference among samples when certain differences exist).

• What are the strengths and weaknesses of the study? Studies of AS have often involved small series of cases or a small number of subjects in case-control studies. If only a handful of subjects are studied, differences in groups may be real but not statistically significant. Conversely, in studies of small samples, one or two outliers may significantly affect group results. Another important quality-control issue involves the extent to which diagnostic assignment process and data collection on the dependent variable are truly independent. For example, if outcome is the measure of interest, the researcher collecting data on outcome should not be the same one who assigned the cases to specific diagnostic groups, as knowledge of the outcome might bias group assignment. Although these are basic methodological safeguards, the research literature on AS has been, unfortunately, plagued by just such shortcomings.

• Was there any attempt to measure the reliability of the research procedures used in the study? Among the various procedures used in research on AS, it is information on the reliability of diagnostic assignments that has been particularly lacking, seriously compromising what we can learn from various studies. If information on interrater reliability (i.e., the extent to which two diagnosticians agree independently on diagnostic assignments) and on the use of diagnostic instruments (both on overall diagnostic algorithms and on specific items) is available, it is not only possible for the reader to judge the quality of a given study but also for the field to assess the status of guidelines for diagnosis of a given condition. For example, it is quite possible for a disorder to have validity but for the current guidelines for its diagnosis to be unreliable.

With these various caveats in mind we can turn to the data on validity of AS. This discussion is organized around the various kinds of evidence which in most cases are examined relative to the validity of AS from higher-functioning autism. In a few instances the comparison is between AS and some other conditions, but such comparisons are much less common. Consistent with the attempt to focus on validity (rather than definitional issues), this discussion focuses on measures *not* included in the definition (e.g., differences in onset and early developmental features have previously been discussed and as they are central in aspects of definition they will not be included here except in so far as they are relevant to selection of groups in the first place).

Neuropsychological Profiles

Wing (1998) notes that a consistent and unique pattern or profile of psychological dysfunction in AS would provide important support for its validity (e.g., relative to autism). A handful of studies have addressed this issue (see Chapter 2, this volume, for a thorough review of these studies with somewhat different conclusions). Although the fact that the studies available have used divergent approaches to the original assignment of the AS diagnosis, thus making comparability of findings difficult, it is also the case that one may use this problem as a way of noticing when differences in neuropsychological profiles did or did not emerge. As noted previously, the applicability of much of the early literature on neuropsychological profiles in individuals with higher-functioning autism (HFA) is questionable given that samples studies may have included individuals with AS, thus increasing heterogeneity and averaging what might have been potentially discrepant profiles. Nevertheless, as Lincoln, Courchesne, Allen, Hanson, and Ene (1998) note, despite the various methodological issues complicating any conclusion drawn on the set of existing studies, it does appear that some generalizations can be made about the available literature which may be relevant to current controversies. In general, individuals with HFA are much more likely to have significant deficits in the areas of verbal comprehension and language (e.g., Lincoln, Allen, & Kilman, 1995; Siegel et al., 1996), and, in general, nonverbal abilities are areas of relative strength (Klin et al., 1997). However, there are important developmental considerations so that, for example, verbal abilities may improve with age in individuals with HFA (Lincoln et al., 1995) and discrepancies between verbal and nonverbal skills may accordingly lessen.

Among the earliest studies of neuropsychological functioning in AS, Szatmari, Tuff, Finlayson, and Bartolucci (1990) used a comprehensive battery of psychological tests in assessing 26 AS and 17 HFA subjects and 36 socially impaired child psychiatric outpatient controls (the groups differed in age but not in terms of overall mean IQ). The approach to diagnosis of AS was a rather broad one in which social and communicative deficits were present but aspects of onset, motor difficulties, and unusual circumscribed interest were not required. There were few differences between the AS and HFA groups; the ones observed included a significantly higher score of the AS group on the Similarities subtest of the Wechsler Intelligence Scale for Children—Revised (WISC-R) and higher scores for the HFA group on a test of motor speed and coordination, with differences also observed in terms of perseverative responses on one test of executive functioning. The conclusion was that AS and HFA had similar neurocognitive deficits which differed from those seen in control subjects.

Ozonoff, Rogers, and Pennington (1991) administered a neuropsycholo-gical battery to 13 HFA subjects and 10 AS subjects and 20 matched nonautistic controls. The groups were similar in terms of Full Scale IQ, Per-formance IQ, and age but did differ relative to Verbal IQ. Criteria used in the study were based on a modification of the ICD-10 definition of AS (*the onset criterion was excluded*). In addition to tests of intelligence, the assessments in-cluded measures of executive function, verbal learning and memory, visual spatial abilities, and theory of mind. Both the HFA and AS groups were im-paired on executive function tests but only the HFA group demonstrated deficits in theory of mind and verbal memory (performing worse than either AS or control cases); however, the high correlation of performance on these measures with verbal abilities (which were significantly higher in the AS group) was a complicating factor in determining the validity of these find-ings. The authors concluded that the data provided some support for differ-entiating HFA and AS.

As noted previously, the DSM-IV field trial for autism (Volkmar et al., 1994), although not focused primarily on AS, did collect information on the cases for which clinicians assigned this diagnosis as part of the sample sub-mitted to the larger field trial. When the 48 cases submitted were compared to those with a clinical diagnosis of autism and IQs in the normative range, individuals with AS were more likely to exhibit higher Verbal than Perfor-mance IQ, whereas the opposite was true for the cases with autism. Al-though these data were limited in various respects, they led our group to undertake a study of neuropsychological profiles in AS and HFA. In this study we (Klin et al., 1995a) found a number of differences between AS and HFA. It is important to note that a major rationale for the study was to eval-uate the presence of such differences in *strictly diagnosed cases* (i.e., if differ-ences were not found using a stricter definition of AS there would be little point in examining the issue of whether a broader and less restrictive defini-tion yielded differences). Accordingly, the groups were diagnosed using ICD-10 research diagnostic criteria with the important additions that for the 19 AS cases, the individual had to exhibit a history of motor clumsiness early in life and marked circumscribed interests had to be present (i.e., con-sistent with Asperger's original description). The 21 cases of HFA were also diagnosed using ICD-10 research criteria. Cases were selected only when ex-tensive psychological testing data had already been collected and cases could be rated independently by a neuropsychologist (blind to diagnosis) for the presence of features suggestive of the NLD profile (which is often as-sociated with significant discrepancies in Verbal–Performance IQ). The groups were comparable in terms of age and Full Scale IQ. They differed, however, in various areas of neuropsychological functioning. Some areas represented areas of strength in AS and weakness in HFA, whereas for other areas the reverse pattern was obtained. Areas predictive of AS included def-icits in fine and gross motor skills, visual motor integration, visual–spatial perception, nonverbal concept formation, and visual memory. Conversely five other areas were negatively related to the diagnosis of AS: These included problems in articulation, verbal output, auditory perception, vocabulary, and verbal memory. Consistent with the DSM-IV field trial results, the study also revealed differences in the pattern of Verbal–Performance IQ for the two groups, with VIQ > PIQ in the AS group and VIQ < PIQ in the HFA group. In addition, 18 of 21 subjects with AS presented with a neuropsychological profile consistent with NLD (Rourke, 1989) while in the HFA group only 1 of 19 did so. The potential overlap between the AS diagnosis and the NLD profile (but not of HFA with NLD) suggested an important point of distinction between HFA and AS.

Commenting on this study, Wing (1998) suggested that at least some of the differences observed were a function of the criteria used (e.g., a history of clumsiness was included as a diagnostic feature of AS and the study did observe differences in certain *current* motor abilities). In addition, Wing rightly notes that not all the 22 neuropsychological items evaluated differed between the groups and that the better verbal output and articulation in the AS group might, again, reflect the selection criteria (i.e., for a diagnosis of AS the child's early language had to be reasonably normal). Her critique raises an interesting and somewhat complicated issue. It is clear that if one defines AS on the basis of *current* motor difficulties or good language abilities and then documents problems in the motor area or strengths in language, the result is simply circular and hence not of much interest. It becomes a more complex issue, however, when the relevant points for diagnosis are *histories* of motor difficulties in early childhood and problems in this area some 15 to 20 years later. Similarly, although early language might be preserved, there is no guarantee that later, particularly much later, language will be preserved (in fact in most cases of AS in this study there were significant problems in *current* language functioning, especially social language use, despite the fact that other aspects of language and language-mediated skills were areas of relative strength). A similar critique of this study points to the relationship between a history of motor clumsiness and current deficits in nonverbal skills such as visual–spatial perception (see Chapter 2, this volume). Although the major results persisted once we reanalyzed the data having excluded the motor criterion in diagnostic assignment, thus substantiating the initial findings, some of these issues will be further elucidated once longitudinal data documenting developmental trajectories and relationships between skills in various areas become available.

Several subsequent reports have appeared in which smaller samples of cases were studied (e.g., Manjiviona & Prior, 1995; Ghaziuddin et al., 1995) or a larger series of cases was evaluated (Lincoln et al., 1995). Lincoln et al. (1998) performed a meta-analysis of these and the earlier results, adding information on seven additional cases. This meta-analysis reported information on 157 individuals with autism (as variously defined) and 117 with AS (also as variously defined) Figure 1.1 presents the results graphically. Lincoln et al. noted that the AS group had higher Verbal than Performance IQ scores whereas the reverse pattern was observed in the autistic group. They also reported a meta-analysis of the IQ scores of another 333 individuals with HFA whose Performance IQ (86) was again higher than the average Verbal IQ (77); values obtained for these autistic cases were similar to those reported in their initial meta-analysis. They concluded that even taking this rather rough approach to the problem (i.e., combining results of diverse studies), it appeared that in autism verbal skills were relatively impaired whereas in AS these skills were more intact. It is of interest that if the cases from Szatmari et al. (1990) and Fine, Bartolucci, Szatmari, and Ginsberg (1994) are excluded (on the presumption that the definition used was less stringent), the IQ differences become more pronounced; that is, for the autistic group the Verbal IQ/Performance IQ difference is 12 points favoring performance while for the AS group the difference is 11 points in the other direction.

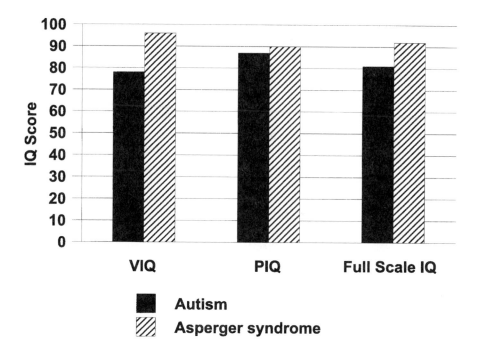

FIGURE 1.1. Meta-analysis of comparisons of IQ scores in reported cases of higher-functioning autism and Asperger syndrome. Data adapted from Lincoln et al. (1998, p. 148).

Another line of work has focused on deficits in other neuropsychological functions, particularly executive functions. Ozonoff (1998) recently reviewed this literature. Although an impressive number of studies have documented deficits in planning abilities, cognitive flexibility, organization, and self-monitoring in autism, only a handful of studies are currently available on individuals with AS. These studies include the Szatmari et al. (1990) report, where the AS group performed less on the Wisconsin Card Sorting Test (WCST) than did controls; however, this difference did not achieve statistical significance. In Ozonoff, Pennington, and Rogers's (1991) study, a composite of performance based on WCST and Tower of Hanoi indicated that significant deficits were shared by these two groups at similar levels of disability.

Finally, a handful of studies have explored an individual's ability to impute mental states such as beliefs, desires, and intentions to others and to self, or to have a theory of other people's (and one's own) subjectivity—a "theory of mind" (ToM) (Baron-Cohen, Tager-Flusberg, & Cohen, 1999; Happé, 1995). In Ozonoff, Rogers, and Pennington's (1991a) study, previously mentioned, group comparisons between the AS and HFA groups revealed significant differences, with the autistic group exhibiting significant impairment in relation to both the AS and an age, and IQ-matched control group; there were no differences between the AS controls. A suggestion was made, therefore, that AS and autism could be distinguished in terms of ToM abilities. Although the finding of no ToM deficits in individuals with AS was replicated in two other studies (Bowler, 1992; Dahlgren & Trillingsgaard, 1996), whether performance on ToM tasks truly differentiates individuals with AS from those with HFA is still open. As previously noted, the AS group in Ozonoff, Pennington, and Rogers's (1991) report also showed higher verbal IQ and verbal memory skills; given the positive correlation between performance on ToM tasks and verbally mediated skills, it is possible that the results reflected differences in the latter rather than in ToM capacities. In addition, Dahlgren and Trillingsgaard (1996) reported no differences in ToM performance between their AS and HFA groups (both performed almost as well as a group of normal controls). Nevertheless, it is possible that the ToM tasks used in these studies were not sensitive enough to capture higher-level and more subtle ToM deficits. For example, Baron-Cohen, Wheelwright, and Jolliffe (1997) reported ToM deficits on two more advanced ToM tasks in their groups of individuals with AS and HFA relative to a clinical and a normative control group, but there was little suggestion that the two groups could be differentiated from one another.

In summary, the available neuropsychological literature does provide some suggestive evidence for meaningful differences in cognitive profiles between individuals with AS and HFA, although a series of problems, especially diagnostic issues, still compromise our ability to derive forceful conclusions from available studies. Data comparing AS to other relevant conditions (e.g., PDD-NOS and schizoid personality disorder) are almost nonexistent. Given the seemingly very different approaches to diagnostic characterization, the differences observed to date between AS and HFA are of great interest and appear to represent an important area for future work. The observed differences, particularly the relative preservation of certain language and verbally mediated skills in AS, may have implications both for understanding the pathophysiology of the condition and for intervention.

It is important, however, to temper this optimism by emphasizing that future studies must strive to provide detailed characterization of subjects and explicit procedures related to diagnostic assignment, including, when possible, quantified information; that circularity in designs is avoided; and that the phenomenological complexity and diversity evidenced in the clinical phenomena are subsumed under vague definitions which blur any potentially important data. In this context, a developmental consideration has often been absent in discussions of, for example, motor deficits or IQ profiles in individuals with AS and autism. Some early strengths may become later weaknesses as the skill studied becomes more dependent on other areas of functioning and increasing environmental demands (e.g., motor skills in individuals with autism), but early deficits may be compensated for as a result of the use of alternative ways of performing a task or as a result of effective intervention (e.g., visual–spatial deficits in individuals with AS). We have seen such an evolution in several cases. For example, one individual (Volkmar et al., 1996) with AS exhibited a major gain in his ability to perform a visual–spatial task (the WISC-R/WISC-III Block Design subtest). When asked to explain the tremendous improvement in his ability to perform that task in adolescence when he had exhibited so much difficulty at it some 5 years earlier, the young man indicated that he had turned the red blocks into 1's, the white blocks into 0's, and the half red and half white blocks into 0.5's; he then created a matrix with these digits and reproduced it on the table using the blocks. His excellent rote memory and facility with numbers allowed him to complete the task using this very unusual route very rapidly, gaining close two standard deviations over his previous score. Such observations highlight the importance of taking developmental change—natural as well as learned coping strategies—into account in our interpretation of neuropsychological profiles. Strengths and deficits should be seen in a dynamic fashion, evolving over time as a result of experience, and ideally, appropriately targeted intervention.

Neurobiological Differences

A handful of studies, often case reports, have focused on possible neurobiological differences between AS and autism. Wing (1981) noted the high rates of perinatal problems in her case series, but Gillberg and Gillberg (1989) reported that obstetrical risk was in fact higher in autism. A few case reports have linked AS with medical conditions of various types (e.g., amino aciduria [Miles & Capelle, 1987], ligamentous laxity [Tantam, Evered, & Hersov, 1990], or specific genetic abnormalities [Anneren, Dahl, Uddenfeldt, &

Janols, 1995; Saliba & Griffiths, 1990; Bartolucci & Szatmari 1987]). In a larger series of cases, Gillberg (1989) reported high rates of various medical abnormalities in samples of both AS and autistic subjects, although subsequent research has questioned these rates (Rutter, Bailey, Bolton, & Le Couteur, 1994). The nature of these reports and common ambiguities in diagnosis make these studies difficult to interpret.

Several studies have, however, speculated on possible central nervous system differences in AS as compared to autism. McKelvey, Lambert, Mottron, and Shevell (1995) suggested that three patients with AS showed abnormalities of right cortical hemisphere functioning using SPECT imaging. Berthier and colleagues (Berthier, Starkstein, & Leiguarda, 1990; Berthier, Bayes, & Tolosa, 1993) have reported various abnormalities on magnetic resonance imaging (MRI) in nine patients with AS studied to date. In one instance a computed tomography (CT) scan performed on a first-degree relative also showed cortical migration anomalies. Other reports have noted left temporal lobe damage (Jones & Kerwin, 1990; CT scan) as well as left occipital hypoperfusion (Ozbayrak, Kapucu, Erdem, & Aras, 1991). Our group (Volkmar et al., 1996) reported a father and son both of whom exhibited AS as well as virtually identical abnormalities on their MRIs. The father's images showed a large, bilateral, V-shaped wedge of missing tissue just superior to the ascending ramus of the Sylvian fissure, at about the level at which the middle frontal gyrus normally intersects with the precentral sulcus. The son's images showed similar dysmorphology in the same area, although it was larger on the right side; his images also showed decreased tissue in the anterior–inferior right temporal lobe, suggesting an atrophic process or a regional neurodevelopmental growth failure. In their recent review, Lincoln et al. (1998) report on a quantitative measurement of specific brain regions on seven cases with AS, indicating more consistent pathology of the cerebellar vermis in autism relative to AS, thinner posterior corpus callosum in autism relative to AS, but larger anterior corpus callosum in AS relative to autism. If confirmed in a larger studies using more rigorous quantitative techniques, these differences would suggest a different pathophysiological basis for these disorders (see also Chapter 6, this volume).

This area of work shows considerable promise for the future given the fast-paced expansion of neuroimaging studies in autism and related conditions. Correlation of any abnormalities with current neuropsychological models (e.g., involving NLD or executive function problems) may be of greatest interest in this regard.

Course and Outcome

In his original paper Asperger (1944) predicted a positive outcome for many of his patients; he thought they would be able to use their special interests and abilities in a gainful way, and he also noted the similarity of personality style to other family members who were possibly doing well in adulthood. By the end of his career Asperger was somewhat more guarded but continued to believe that a more positive outcome was important evidence of a difference between this condition and Kanner's autism. Whereas anecdotal information and case reports have, to some extent, supported his view, few systematic data are available.

Clearly, there is no doubt that if an overall comparison is made between AS and autism (the latter defined to include all cases), outcome would be better in AS (Gillberg, 1991). The more critical question, of course, is whether there are differences in outcome for individual with autism and AS who function at a similar intellectual range.

Tantam (1991) and Newson, Dawson, and Everaard (1984–1985) reported on outcome in young adults with AS and noted that despite relatively good intellectual potential, a majority of those individuals were living at home although several had married and some had jobs. This outcome, however, could be seen as more positive than usually evidenced in autism, although a direct comparison was not made. Gillberg (1998) noted that AS appears to be associated with better outcome than is autism, particularly in regard to the development of self-help skills and academic progress, although he acknowledged the absence of systematic data on outcome of both individuals with AS and HFA. In contrast to these impressions, Szatmari, Bartolucci, and Bremner (1989) noted minimal differences in outcome in a comparison of children with AS and HFA. Reviewing the status of outcome research in regard to these populations, Howlin (Howlin & Goode, 1998) emphasized the limitations of current data and the lack of definitive information on this issue. This is unfortunate given that differences in this crucial area could be seen as strong indicators of the need for making a distinction between AS and autism (e.g., see Kanner, 1971; Lord & Venter, 1992; Lotter, 1978; Venter, Lord, & Schopler, 1992). The need for such studies are, therefore, great. Such research, however, should take into consideration developmental level of the subjects being studied, including primarily IQ and language level, in order to ensure that conclusions reached reflect diagnostic assignment rather than simply variability in central developmental skills.

Comorbidity

Another area of potential difference between autism and AS relates to the issue of comorbidity; that is, are such individuals at greater than expected risk (relative to the general population or to HFA or some other condition) for certain psychiatric problems. Much of the early interest, at least in the English-language literature, on AS related to this issue given early case reports suggesting a link with schizophrenia or violence (see Wolff, 1995; Klin & Volkmar, 1997, for a discussion). Subsequent to these early reports, other papers have suggested associations with psychosis in general as well as schizophrenia in particular (e.g., Clarke et al., 1989; Tantam, 1988a; Taiminen, 1994), Tourette Syndrome (Gillberg & Rastam, 1992; Kerbeshian & Burd, 1986; Littlejohns, Clarke, & Corbett, 1990; Marriage, Miles, Stokes, & Davey, 1993), affective disorders (Berthier, 1995; Fujikawa et al., 1987), and obsessive–compulsive disorder (Thomsen, 1994). Reports of associations with psychotic conditions have included reports of psychotic depression and bipolar disorder (manic–depressive psychosis) (Gillberg, 1985).

Although Tantam (1991), Nagy and Szatmari (1986), and others report associations with schizophrenia in follow-up studies, other research questions these views (Ghaziuddin et al., 1995). It does appear that children who exhibit features suggestive of schizoid personality (not necessarily AS) may be at increased risk for early-onset schizophrenia (Werry, 1992). Asperger (cited in Frith, 1991) noted that only one of his cases had developed schizophrenia, and several considerations suggest some caution in the interpretation of case reports associating AS with other conditions. Individuals with AS often excessively verbalize and have poor social judgment (an adolescent patient of ours was evaluated for psychotic thinking after he responded to a polite offer from a female classmate, "Is there anything I can do to help you," with an explicit sexual request). The tendency of persons with AS to inappropriately verbalize (particularly about their topic of interest) may also lend a somewhat disorganized quality to interaction. The problems of differential diagnosis have been echoed by various other investigators (e.g., Bejerot & Duvner, 1995; Ryan, 1992; Taiminen, 1994).

As Howlin and Goode (1998) reports, a rather more extensive body of work suggests associations of both autism and AS with various disorders of affect (e.g., anxiety or depression) (see also Ellis et al., 1994; Fujikawa et al., 1987; Ghaziuddin et al., 1992b; Grandin, 1990). It is of interest that Rourke et al. (1989) previously suggested that individuals with NLD exhibit high rates of depression and suicidality. On balance, the literature on associated comorbid psychiatric conditions is (1) rather limited and (2) does not clearly provide different patterns of associations with autism or AS.

Various publications, primarily case reports, have associated AS with violent and criminal behavior (e.g., Baron-Cohen, 1988; Everall & Le Couteur, 1990; Mawson et al., 1985; Tantam, 1988b; Wing, 1986). This gave rise to an impression that violent and/or criminal behavior was more frequently associated with AS. This association seemed particularly reasonable given the typical combination, in AS, of high levels of intelligence and verbal ability with problems in empathy and social skills. The data available (which admittedly is limited) generally do not support such associations.

In their review of this issue, Ghaziuddin et al. (1991) found no support for such an association. On the other hand, Scragg and Shah (1994) reported relatively high rates of individuals with AS (about 1.5%) within a secure hospital setting. Our own experience is that rather than being victimizers, individuals with AS are perfect victims. At best, they typically are at the periphery of social interaction, they have emotional insensitivity but are also rather isolated from others. Indeed, in our experience the more typical problem in AS is that the person is overly rigid and moralistic. The story about a man who anxiously monitored the number of items a shopper had in her shopping cart while waiting in the "fast" checkout line to be sure she did not violate the limit of 10-items rule is not at all unrepresentative (Dewey, 1991).

Family History

Both Kanner (1943) and Asperger (1944) noted unusual traits in family members, but Asperger particularly emphasized what appeared to be similar difficulties in fathers of his cases. Rather little systematic research, to date, has been conducted on this aspect of the condition. Similarities could, of course, be due to either genetic or experiential factors or to some combination of both (see Rutter, 1999, for a discussion). It is, however, the possible identification of genetic factors that would be of special interest.

The importance of a potential genetic contribution to autism only began to be appreciated in the late 1970s. The evidence now comes from both twin and family studies (see Rutter, Bailey, Simonoff, & Pickles, 1997, for a review). There is increased concordance in monozygotic (MZ) twins, and rates of autism in siblings are significantly higher than in the general population—probably on the order of 50- to 100-fold. Although precise genetic mechanisms remain to be identified, there is reasonably good evidence to suggest that an epistatic, multilocus form of inheritance will be found in some cases. Although genetic factors are clearly important, it is the case that MZ twin pairs are not always concordant for autism, suggesting a role for nongenetic factors as well. Evidence from various studies also now suggests that it is possible that what we observe as autism is one part of a broader phenotype of social–communicative difficulties (e.g., Bailey et al., 1995; Le Couteur et al., 1996). Studies of families have also suggested possible elevations in rates of other conditions, particularly anxiety and affective disorder in family members (Smalley, McCracken, & Tanguay, 1995).

The available data on the familiarity of AS are essentially limited to a handful of case reports and some preliminary studies (see Chapter 5, this volume). Many case reports have been consistent with Asperger's (1944) original observation of similar traits in family members—particularly fathers (Bowman, 1988; DeLong & Dwyer, 1988; Gillberg, Gillberg, & Steffenburg, 1992; Volkmar et al., 1996). Wing (1981) suggested that inheritance patterns were not limited to fathers and male relatives, and Burgoine and Wing (1983) reported identical triplets with AS. In one of the larger studies to date, we (Volkmar et al., 1997) provided preliminary data based on family self-report (usually maternal report) which had been collected in a preliminary phase of the ongoing Yale studies of AS. These data are limited given their reliance on reports of family history rather than actual assessment by clinicians or data collection with structured diagnostic instruments. The data did, however, provide relatively strong support for a genetic component. In 46% of the 99 families surveyed, the reports indicated that there was a positive family history of AS, or something rather close to it, in first-degree relatives—particularly male relatives. For example, 19% of fathers as opposed to 4% of mothers were reported to be affected, and if the question was broadened to include significant social problems (i.e., without other features more specifically suggestive of AS) the rates increased to 33% and 14%, respectively. On the other hand, only 6% of fathers and 2% of mothers were said to have language problems.

Another line of work relates to the examination of patterns of comorbidity in both probands with AS (and HFA) and their family relatives. The observation of differences in such comparisons would strongly support a distinction between the two conditions. At present, however, no available data address this important issue.

Finally, it should be noted that several reports of autism and AS occurring in different members of the family have appeared (e.g., Wing, 1981). Volkmar et al. (1997) in their preliminary results indicated that 3.5% of siblings of the presumed AS probands also had a diagnosis of autism with rates twice as common in brothers as in sisters. Rates of autism were also increased in first cousins. These findings suggest that regardless of whether or not AS is eventually validated as a condition distinct from autism, there are potentially important genetic links bringing them together, perhaps as part of a spectrum or group of social disabilities.

The implications of the genetic data for the validity of AS can be briefly summarized. Almost all the work available has focused on the comparison of AS relative to autism or HFA. This work is limited in many respects, consisting largely of case reports and preliminary data. However, what is available does appear to suggest that there is an even stronger familial component in AS than in autism, and that there also may be a genetic link between AS and autism. In the absence of better data, the implications of the latter observation for the validity of AS remain unclear. For example, it might eventually be discovered that what we now recognize as AS is to some extent the end result of several genes affecting socialization skills or other related abilities, and that for autism to result the operation of an additional gene or genes (e.g., having an additional impact on communication) is required. At the moment, such models are the topic of speculation. However, as more definitive data become available, it may be possible to derive increasingly more specific predictions about both the nature of underlying genetic mechanisms and similarities and differences between AS and autism. For work in this area to advance, it is clear that a careful diagnostic assessment of both proband and family members is needed and that such an assessment should include various measures not only of psychopathology but also of detailed developmental skills, given the possibility that important aspects of these conditions are mediated by specific deficits or strengths in a developmental area (e.g., language) or more complex profiles associated with social deficits (e.g., NLD).

Treatment

Differential response to treatment would be an important rationale for the validation of AS vis-à-vis related conditions. However, there are no systematic studies examining treatment efficacy or treatment approach to individuals with AS and HFA (Mesibov, 1992). Suggestive information that specificity in treatment approach to these two conditions is warranted comes primarily from unsystematic observations resulting from clinicians' experiences.

In our own observations, it does appear that in some contrast with individuals with autism, individuals with AS experience social isolation but are not withdrawn or devoid of social interest; in fact, they often approach others but in eccentric ways. Their interest in having friends, girlfriends/boyfriends, and social contact may in fact be quite striking. Repeated experiences of failure can and often do lead to clinical depression. This intrinsic motivation for social contact can be a powerful resource in the hands of the interventionist, who may then shape social initiation by means of social and communication skills training with a view to foster social adaptation (see Chapter 12, this volume). Although the same techniques are equally appropriate to individuals with autism, in our experience, the resultant effects for the person's social adaptation tend to be more limited in the case of individuals with autism because of the more withdrawn and disinterested nature of their presentation.

The relatively preserved language skills, which may at times manifest as a preoccupation with definitions, rules, and facts, can be effectively used to foster strategies for learning, acquisition of skills and concepts, cognitive methods for coping, and awareness of behavioral norms which facilitate adaptation. This emphasis on the use of more intact verbal abilities to address areas of deficit is, in our view, of a different magnitude than what one may recommend in the case of individuals with autism, for whom the utilization of visual aids can be especially effective (Hodgdon, 1995). Along these impressions, if there is indeed a unique neuropsychological profile which ultimately is identified as typical of AS, such a profile may lead to other considerations as well, for example, relative to vocational planning where deficits in the motor area may have important implications as may the individual's special interests or skills (Van Bourgondien & Woods, 1992). As an example of misintervention, one adult with AS who had completed a graduate degree in earth sciences could not secure a job in his area of training, primarily because of his extremely poor interview skills. He was advised to seek temporary employment at a carpentry workshop. Because of his marked motor and visual–motor skill deficits, he was unable to perform the simplest carpentry duties. Given his little insight, he continued for several weeks to bring wooden boards, a hammer, and nails to his home in order to practice basic skills. His inadequate performance led to job failure, in a placement he believed to be a "menial," resulting in increased depression. This young man had exceptional skills related to his topic of interest, namely ecology, including associated computer, classificatory, and written skills. Clearly, ignoring his individualized neuropsychological and vocational profiles resulted in great distress to him and his family. Although we have repeatedly argued that from an intervention perspective the wisest course is to program for a specific individual rather than for a diagnosis, it is the case that for research on treatment efficacy to make its essential contribution to the validation of disorders, detailed diagnostic information is crucial.

The new research on comorbid conditions in autism and AS is likely to inform our knowledge of the specificity of treatment approaches in the area of psychopharmacology. Although there are no medications to treat the disorders themselves (see Chapter 7, this volume), the amelioration of associated conditions such as depressions and anxiety can have a decisive impact on a person's well-being (McDougle, Price, & Volkmar, 1994). Greater and more detailed knowledge of associated symptomatology is likely to provide a better rationale for the adoption of specific pharmacological agents. No data are currently available on differential treatment responses to medication in AS and HFA.

To summarize our discussion, the validity of AS as a distinctive diagnostic concept remains to be adequately addressed. Several lines of preliminary evidence, notably the work on neuropsychological profiles and family history, are of great interest in terms of providing validation evidence for this condition. Emerging data on associated features, neuroimaging, treatment response, and outcome would undoubtedly make an important contribution in this regard. Consideration of diagnostic issues remain paramount in all of these efforts. Finally, the vast majority of studies have, probably quite understandably, focused on the question of AS vis-à-vis autism— particularly HFA. Comparisons with other diagnostic concepts have been much less frequent and yet should be seen as equally important to determine the boundaries of AS.

CONCLUSIONS: IMPLICATIONS FOR FUTURE RESEARCH

Several issues are of great importance for future research. In the first place it is clear that to establish both better definitions of AS and the validity of the diagnostic concept it will be important that investigator do the following:

- Avoid circularity.
- Use operational definitions which are explicit and specified in detail.
- Move toward standard diagnostic procedures and standard batteries of information.
- Avoid premature closure of any aspect of research on this and related conditions.
- Begin to consider issues of overlap with conditions other than autism.

Accordingly, it is important that investigators use dependent measures which are independent of diagnosis. Research rigor should include careful attention to aspects of reliability and application of diagnostic guidelines, as well as "blindness" or independence of different lines of data from each other. This consideration is particularly important in research of neuropsychological profiles relative to diagnostic assignment, and of current communication functioning relative to early patterns of language development. The use of explicit, operational definitions is of great importance in order to avoid the mistakes of past research. Given the potential for confusion, the lack of detailed characterization of subjects, preventing the reader from grasping the rationale for diagnostic assignment adopted by the investigators, should be seen as unacceptable. In this context, the recent approach to more precise quantification of diagnostic criteria (e.g., Lord et al., 1989; Lord et al., 1994) in the field of autism, which has made an important contribution to the standardization not only of diagnostic assignment but also of specific observations of pertinent symptomatology, may offer the same opportunities for AS.

The effort to validate AS as a diagnostic concept should not be bound to preconceived, nonempirical ideas as to whether this condition is the same or different from autism. Premature notions of seeing AS and autism as either the same or different, though deceivingly clear-cut to some are in fact quite complex and ultimately begging the availability of good data. To say that the conditions are the same, or on a continuum, implies our knowledge of the continuum on which these conditions place themselves. It is likely that such a continuum space is much more multidimensional than usually argued, bringing together development and psychopathology in the areas of socialization, communication, cognition, and other areas. If viewed in this way, it is clear that this discussion should not involve autism and AS only but other conditions as well which may share to some degree areas of disability. Research on the developmental and familial aspects as well as associated features of AS and autism is likely to illuminate this point, as will a better understanding of specific mechanisms of socialization. Studies should go from diagnosis to specific variables and vice versa (e.g., how common are certain neuropsychological profiles or patterns of onset observed in different conditions and what is the range of resultant phenotype of specific variables of importance).

The repeated suggestion that the nature of the social deficit may take slightly different forms in AS and HFA is also important. Tantam (1988a) noted that in AS, the affected individual often had a wish for social interactions but an inability to engage in them; similarly, Van Krevelen (1971) emphasized the centrality of social avoidance in autism and contrasted this with the eccentric, one-sided interactions of individuals with AS. Such differences may be blurred in the absence of more sensitive measures as a result of all-encompassing, vague definitions.

Advances in the area of epidemiology and natural history are highly dependent on definitional research. Thus, prevalence estimates have varied quite widely from rates of 36/1,000 (Ehlers & Gillberg, 1993) to around 1/10,000 (Wing & Gould, 1979; Wing, 1981) (see Klin et al., 1997, and Fombonne, 1998, for reviews). Estimates of the prevalence of the condition have important implications for service provision as well as research, but the lack of a real consensus on the diagnosis of AS means that present data are, at best, "guestimates" of its prevalence. Asperger himself apparently continued to adopt a relatively stringent view of the diagnosis, and it would appear that in his view the condition was probably not common. The argument, sometimes advanced, that a broad view of AS is needed to "cover" the range of children with problems in social interaction with relatively preserved intellectual skills who do not exhibit the usual features of autism seems to us to be fundamentally wrongheaded. The importance of the disorder would appear to us to be most fruitfully based on research that demonstrates validity rather than on considerations of how frequent the condition "ought" to be. Again, the availability of data should ultimately decide this issue. Practical considerations regarding increased awareness of bright but socially disabled individuals, as well as entitlement for services, creation of support groups, and advocacy effort, are all very important, but the ultimate interest of patients is unlikely to be served through research that is based on loose diagnostic considerations.

Diagnostic issues are also important in the context of research on treatment and on outcome, two crucial variables to be considered in the validation of AS. Although intervention should be individualized, and treatment outcome should be judged in terms of amelioration of detailed symptomatology, any potential benefits accrued by individuals on the basis of their overall presentation would be lost without careful diagnostic considerations, leaving these two essential elements of validation of any medical condition unexplored.

The new upsurge in neurobiological and genetic research in autism is still slow in reaching the group of individuals with AS. Findings in these areas are likely to greatly inform our views of the validity of this and other related conditions and to greatly sharpen our models of developmental psychopathology. For example, the identification of different patterns of cognitive functioning may be related to relatively more specific findings using new procedures, such as functional MRI. Similarly, it is possible that work on the family and molecular genetics of AS may lead us to genes involved in aspects of autism, or vice versa, with increased specification of mechanisms involved in socialization disorders. In this context, researchers of autism and related conditions have much to learn from the recent work on reading disabilities (Grigorenko et al., 1997), which points to the potential of different genes involved in core component processes of the disability, each of which may lead, in combination or perhaps singly, to clinical disorder.

REFERENCES

American Psychiatric Association. (1980). *Diagnostic and statistical manual of mental disorders* (3rd ed.). Washington, DC: Author.

American Psychiatric Association. (1987). *Diagnostic and statistical manual of mental disorders* (3rd ed. rev.). Washington, DC: Author.

American Psychiatric Association. (1994). *Diagnostic and statistical manual of mental disorders* (4th ed.). Washington, DC: Author.

Anneren, G., Dahl, N., Uddenfeldt, U., & Janols, L. O. (1995). Asperger syndrome in a boy with a balanced de novo translocation: t(17;19)(p13. 3;p11) [Letter]. *American Journal of Medical Genetics, 56*(3), 330–331.

Asperger, H. (1944). Die "Autistischen Psychopathen" im Kindesalter. *Archiv für Psychiatrie und Nervenkrankheiten, 117*, 76–136.

Asperger, H. (1979). Problems of infantile autism. *Communication, 13*, 45–52.

Bailey, A., Le Couteur, A., Gottesman, I., Bolton, P., Simonoff, E., Yuzda, E., & Rutter, M. (1995). Autism as a strongly genetic disorder: Evidence from a British twin study. *Psychological Medicine, 25*, 63–77.

Baron-Cohen, S. (1988). An assessment of violence in a young man with Asperger's syndrome. *Journal of Child Psychology and Psychiatry, 29*, 351–360.

Baron-Cohen, S., Tager-Flusberg, H., & Cohen, D. J. (Eds.). (1999). *Understanding other minds: Perspectives from autism* (2nd ed.). Oxford: Oxford University Press.

Baron-Cohen, S., Wheelwright, S., & Jolliffee, T. (1997). Is there a "language of the eyes"? Evidence from normal adults and adults with autism or Asperger syndrome. *Visual Cognition, 4*, 311–331.

Bartolucci, G., & Szatmari, P. (1987). Possible similarities between the fragile X and Asperger's syndrome [letter]. *American Journal of Disorders of Childhood, 141*(6), 601–602.

Bejerot, S., & Duvner, T. (1995). Asperger's syndrome or schizophrenia? *Nordic Journal of Psychiatry, 49*(2), 145.

Berthier, M. (1995). Hypomania following bereavement in Asperger's syndrome: A case study. *Neuropsychiatry, Neuropsychology, and Behavioral Neurology, 8*(3), 222–228.

Berthier, M. L., Bayes, A., & Tolosa, E. S. (1993). Magnetic resonance imaging in patients with concurrent Tourette's disorder and Asperger's syndrome. *Journal of the American Academy of Child and Adolescent Psychiatry, 32*(3), 633–639.

Berthier, M. L., Starkstein, S. E., & Leiguarda, R. (1990). Developmental cortical anomalies in Asperger's syndrome: Neuroradiological findings in two patients. *Journal of Neuropsychiatry and Clinical Neurosciences, 2*(2), 197–201.

Bishop, D. V. M. (1989). Autism, Asperger's syndrome and semantic–pragmatic disorder: Where are the boundaries? *British Journal of Disorders of Communications, 24,* 107–121.

Bishop, D. V. M. (1998). Development of the Children's Communication Checklist (CCC): A method for assessing qualitative aspects of communicative impairment in children. *Journal of Child Psychology and Psychiatry, 39,* 6, 879–891.

Blank, M., Gessner, M., & Esposito, A. (1979). Language without communication: A case study. *Journal of Child Language, 6,* 329–352.

Bleuler, E. (1951). (1951). *Textbook of psychiatry* (A. A. Brill, Trans.). New York: Dover. (Original work *Lehrbuch der Psychiatrie,* published 1916)

Bosch, G. (1970). *Infantile autism.* New York: Springer-Verlag.

Bowler, D. M. (1992). "Theory of mind" in Asperger's syndrome. *Journal of Child Psychology and Psychiatry, 33*(5), 877–893.

Bowman, E. P. (1988). Asperger's syndrome and autism: The case for a connection. *British Journal of Psychiatry, 152,* 377–382.

Burgoine, E., & Wing, L. (1983). Identical triplets with Asperger's syndrome. *British Journal of Psychiatry, 143,* 261–265.

Caplan, R. (1994). Thought disorder in childhood. *Journal of the American Academy of Child and Adolescent Psychiatry, 33*(5), 605–615.

Caron, C., & Rutter, M. (1991). Comorbidity in child psychopathology: Concepts, issues, and research strategies. *Journal of Child Psychology and Psychiatry, 32*(7), 1063–1080.

Clarke, D. J., Littlejohns, C. S., Corbett, J. A., & Joseph, S. (1989). Pervasive developmental disorders and psychoses in adult life. *British Journal of Psychiatry, 155,* 692–699.

Cohen, D. J., Paul, R., & Volkmar, F. R. (1986). Issues in the classification of pervasive developmental disorders: Toward DSM-IV. *Journal of the American Academy of Child and Adolescent Psychiatry, 25,* 213–220.

Dahl, K., Cohen, D. J., & Provence, S. (1986). Clinical and multivariate approaches to nosology of the pervasive developmental disorders. *Journal of the American Academy of Child and Adolescent Psychiatry, 25,* 170–180.

Dahlgren, S. O., & Trillingsgaard, A. (1996). Theory of mind in non-retarded children with autism and Asperger's syndrome. A research note. *Journal of Child Psychology and Psychiatry, 37,* 759–763.

DeLong, G. R., & Dwyer, J. T. (1988). Correlation of family history with specific autistic subgroups: Asperger's syndrome and bipolar affective disease. *Journal of Autism and Developmental Disorders, 18*(4), 593–600.

Denckla, M. B. (1983). The neuropsychology of social–emotional learning disabilities. *Archives of Neurology, 40,* 461–462.

Dewey, M. (1991). Living with Asperger's syndrome. In U. Frith (Ed.), *Autism and Asperger syndrome* (pp. 184–206). Cambridge: Cambridge University Press.

Dykens, E., Volkmar, F. R., & Glick, M. (1991). Thought disorder in high-functioning autistic adults. *Journal of Autism and Developmental Disorders, 21,* 291–321.

Ehlers, S., & Gillberg, C. (1993). The epidemiology of Asperger Syndrome: A total population study. *Journal of Child Psychology and Psychiatry, 34*(8), 1327–1350.

Ellis, H. D., Ellis, D. M., Fraser, W., & Deb, S. (1994). A preliminary study of right hemisphere cognitive deficits and impaired social judgments among young people with Asperger syndrome. *European Child and Adolescent Psychiatry, 3*(4), 255–266.

Everall, I. P., & Le Couteur, A. (1990). Firesetting in an adolescent with Asperger's Syndrome. *British Journal of Psychiatry, 157,* 284–287.

Fine, J., Bartolucci, G., Szatmari, P., & Ginsberg, G. (1994). Cohesive discourse in pervasive developmental disorders. *Journal of Autism and Developmental Disorders, 24*(3), 315–329.

Fombonne, E. (1998). Epidemiology of autism and related conditions. In F. R. Volkmar (Ed.), *Autism and pervasive developmental disorders* (pp. 32–64). Cambridge, UK: Cambridge University Press.

Frith, U. (Ed.). (1991). *Autism and Asperger syndrome*. Cambridge, UK: Cambridge University Press.

Fujikawa, H., Kobayashi, R., Koga, Y., & Murata, T. (1987). A case of Asperger's syndrome in a nineteen-year-old who showed psychotic breakdown with depressive state and attempted suicide after entering university. *Japanese Journal of Child and Adolescent Psychiatry, 28*(4), 217–225.

Ghaziuddin, M., Butler, E., Tsai, L. Y., & Ghaziuddin, N. (1994). Is clumsiness a marker for Asperger Syndrome? *Journal of Intellectual Disabilities Research, 38*(5), 519–527.

Ghaziuddin, M., & Gerstein, L. (1996). Pedantic speaking style differentiates Asperger syndrome from high-functioning autism. *Journal of Autism and Developmental Disorders, 26*(6), 585–595.

Ghaziuddin, M., Leininger, L., & Tsai, L. Y. (1995). Brief report: Thought disorder in Asperger syndrome: Comparison with high-functioning autism. *Journal of Autism and Developmental Disorders, 25*(3), 311–317.

Ghaziuddin, M., Tsai, L. Y., & Ghaziuddin, N. (1991). Brief report: Violence in Asperger syndrome, a critique. *Journal of Autism and Developmental Disorders, 21*(3), 349–354.

Ghaziuddin, M., Tsai, L. Y., & Ghaziuddin, N. (1992a). Brief report: A comparison of the diagnostic criteria for Asperger syndrome. *Journal of Autism and Developmental Disorders, 22*(4), 643–649.

Ghaziuddin, M., Tsai, L. Y., & Ghaziuddin, N. (1992b). Comorbidity of autistic disorder in children and adolescents. *European Child and Adolescent Psychiatry, 1*(4), 209–213.

Ghaziuddin, M., Tsai, L. Y., & Ghaziuddin, N. (1992c). A reappraisal of clumsiness as a diagnostic feature of Asperger syndrome. *Journal of Autism and Developmental Disorders, 22*, 651–656.

Gillberg, C. (1985). Asperger's syndrome and recurrent psychosis: A case study. *Journal of Autism and Developmental Disorders, 15*(4), 389–397.

Gillberg, C. (1989). Asperger syndrome in 23 Swedish children. *Developmental Medicine and Child Neurology, 31*, 520–531.

Gillberg, C. (1990). Autism and the pervasive developmental disorders. *Journal of Child Psychology and Psychiatry, 31*(1), 99–119.

Gillberg, C. (1991). Outcome in autism and autistic-like conditions. *Journal of the American Academy of Child and Adolescent Psychiatry, 30*(3), 375–382.

Gillberg, C. (1998). Asperger syndrome and high-functioning autism. *British Journal of Psychiatry, 172*, 200–209.

Gillberg, C., Gillberg, I. C., & Steffenburg, S. (1992). Siblings and parents of children with autism: A controlled population-based study. *Developmental Medicine and Child Neurology, 34*(5), 389–398.

Gillberg, C., & Rastam, M. (1992). Do some cases of anorexia nervosa reflect underlying autistic-like. *Behavioural Neurology, 5*(1), 27–32.

Gillberg, I. C., & Gillberg, C. (1989). Asperger syndrome—some epidemiological considerations. *Journal of Child Psychology and Psychiatry, 30*, 631–638.

Grandin, T. (1990). Needs of high functioning teenagers and adults with autism: Tips from a recovered autistic. *Focus on Autistic Behavior, 5*(1), 16.

Grice, H. P. (1975). Logic and conversation. In R. Cole & J. Morgan (Eds.), *Syntax and semantics: Speech acts* (pp. 85–102). New York: Academic Press.

Grigorenko, E. L., Wood, F. B., Meyer, M. S., Hart, L. A., Speed, W. C., Shuster, A., & Pauls, D. L. (1997). Susceptibility loci for distinct components of developmental dyslexia on chromosomes 6 and 15. *American Journal of Human Genetics, 60,* 27–39.

Hallett, M., Lebiedowska, M. K., Thomas, S. L., Stanhope, S. J., Denckla, M. B., & Rumsey, J. (1993). Locomotion of autistic adults. *Archives of Neurology, 50,* 1304–1308.

Happé, F. G. (1995). The role of age and verbal ability in the theory of mind task performance of subjects with autism. *Child Development, 66*(3), 843–55.

Hodgdon, L. (1995). Solving social–behavioral problems through the use of visually supported communication. In K. A. Quill (Ed.), *Teaching children with autism: Strategies to enhance communication and socialization* (pp. 265–286). New York: Delmar.

Howlin, P., & Goode, S. (1998). Outcome in adult life for people with autism and Asperger's syndrome. In F. R. Volkmar (Ed.), *Autism and pervasive developmental disorders* (pp. 209–241). Cambridge, UK: Cambridge University Press.

Johnson, D. J., & Myklebust, H. R. (1971). *Learning disabilities.* New York: Grune & Stratton.

Jones, P. B., & Kerwin, R. W. (1990). Left temporal lobe damage in Asperger's syndrome. *British Journal of Psychiatry, 156,* 570–572.

Kanner, L. (1943). Autistic disturbances of affective contact. *Nervous Child, 2,* 217–253.

Kanner, L. (1954) Discussion of Robinson and Vitale's paper on "Children with circumscribed interests." *American Journal of Orthopsychiatry, 24,* 764–766.

Kanner, L. (1971). Follow-up study of eleven children originally reported in 1943. *Journal of Autism and Childhood Schizophrenia, 1,* 119–145.

Kerbeshian, J., & Burd, L. (1986). Asperger's syndrome and Tourette syndrome: The case of the pinball wizard. *British Journal of Psychiatry, 148,* 731–736.

Klin, A. (1994). Asperger syndrome. *Child and Adolescent Psychiatry Clinics of North America, 3,* 131–148.

Klin, A., Carter, A., & Sparrow, S. S. (1997). Psychological assessment of children with autism. In D. J. Cohen & F. R. Volkmar (Eds.), *Handbook of autism and pervasive developmental disorders* (2nd ed., pp. 418–427). New York: Wiley.

Klin, A., Sparrow, S. S., Volkmar, F. R., Cicchetti, D. V., & Rourke, B. P. (1995). Asperger syndrome. In B. P. Rourke (Ed.), *Syndrome of nonverbal learning disabilities: Neurodevelopmental manifestations* (pp. 93–118). New York: Guilford Press.

Klin, A., & Volkmar, F. R. (1995a). Autism and the pervasive developmental disorders. *Child and Adolescent Psychiatric Clinics of North America, 4*(3), 617–630.

Klin, A., & Volkmar, F. R. (1995b, October). *Preliminary data of the Yale-LDA Social Learning Disabilities Project.* Paper presented at the 42nd annual meeting of the American Academy of Child and Adolescent Psychiatry, New Orleans.

Klin, A., & Volkmar, F. R. (1996). The pervasive developmental disorders: Nosology and profiles of development. In S. Luthar, J. Burack, D. Cicchetti, & J. Wiesz (Eds.), *Developmental perspectives on risk and psychopathology* (pp. 208–226). New York: Cambridge University Press.

Klin, A., & Volkmar, F. R. (1997). Asperger syndrome. In D. J. Cohen & F. R. Volkmar (Eds.), *Handbook of autism and pervasive developmental disorders* (pp. 94–122). New York: Wiley.

Klin, A., Volkmar, F. R., Sparrow, S. S., Cicchetti, D. V., & Rourke, B. P. (1995). Validity and neuropsychological characterization of Asperger syndrome. *Journal of Child Psychology and Psychiatry, 36*(7), 1127–1140.

Le Couteur, A., Beiley, A., Goode, S., Pickles, A., Robertson, S., Gottesman, I., & Rutter, M. (1996). A broader phenotype of autism: The clinical spectrum in twins. *Journal of Child Psychology and Psychiatry, 37*(7), 785–801.

Lincoln, A. J., Allen, M., & Kilman, A. (1995). The assessment and interpretation of intellectual abilities in people with autism. In E. Schopler & G. Mesibov (Eds.), *Learning and cognition in autism* (pp. 89–117). New York: Plenum.

Lincoln, A., Courchesne, E., Allen, M., Hanson, E., & Ene, M. (1998). Neurobiology of Asperger Syndrome: Seven case studies and quantitative magnetic resonance imaging findings. In E. Schopler, G. Mesibov, & L. J. Kunce (Eds.), *Asperger syndrome or high-functioning autism?* (pp. 145–166). New York: Plenum.

Lord, C., Rutter, M., Goode, S., Heemsbergen, J., Jordan, H., Mawhood, L., & Schopler, E. (1989). Autism diagnostic observation schedule: A standardized observation of communicative and social behavior. *Journal of Autism and Developmental Disorders, 19*(2), 185–212.

Littlejohns, C. S., Clarke, D. J., & Corbett, J. A. (1990). Tourette-like disorder in Asperger's syndrome. *British Journal of Psychiatry, 156*, 430–433.

Lord, C., Rutter, M., & Le Couteur, A. (1994). Autism Diagnostic Interview—Revised: A revised version of a diagnostic interview for caregivers of individuals with possible pervasive developmental disorders. *Journal of Autism and Developmental Disorders, 24*(5), 659–685.

Lord, C., & Venter, A. (1992). Outcome and follow-up studies of high-functioning autistic individuals. In E. Schopler & G. B. Mesibov (Eds), *High-functioning individuals with autism* (pp. 187–199). New York: Plenum.

Lotter, V. (1978). Follow-up studies. In M. Rutter & E. Schopler (Eds.), *Autism: A reappraisal of concepts and treatment*. New York: Plenum.

Manjiviona, J., & Prior, M. (1995). Comparison of Asperger syndrome and high-functioning autistic children on a Test of Motor Impairment. *Journal of Autism and Developmental Disorders, 25*(1), 23–39.

Marriage, K., Miles, T., Stokes, D., & Davey, M. (1993). Clinical and research implications of the co-occurrence of Asperger's and Tourette syndrome. *Australian and New Zealander Journal of Psychiatry, 27*(4), 666–672.

Mawson, D., Grounds, A., & Tantam, D. (1985). Violence and Asperger's Syndrome: A case study. *British Journal of Psychiatry, 147*, 566–569.

McDougle, C. J., Price, L. H., & Volkmar, F. R. (1994). Recent advances in the pharmacotherapy of autism and related conditions. *Child and Adolescent Psychiatry Clinics of North America, 3*, 71–90.

McKelvey, J. R., Lambert, R., Mottron, L., & Shevell, M. I. (1995). Right-hemisphere dysfunction in Asperger's syndrome. *Journal of Child Neurology, 10*(4), 310–314.

Mesibov, G. B. (1992). Treatment issues with high-functioning adolescents and adults with autism. In E. Schopler & G. B. Mesibov (Eds.), *High-functioning individuals with autism* (pp. 143–156). New York: Plenum.

Miles, S. W., & Capelle, P. (1987). Asperger's syndrome and aminoaciduria: A case example. *British Journal of Psychiatry, 150*, 397–400.

Miller, J. N., & Ozonoff, S. (1997). Did Asperger's cases have Asperger's disorder: A research note. *Journal of Child Psychology and Psychiatry, 38*(2), 247–251.

Morey, L. C. (1988). the categorical representation of personality disorder: A cluster analysis of DSM-III-R personality features. *Journal of Abnormal Psychology, 97*(3), 314–321.

Myklebust, H. R. (1975). Nonverbal learning disabilities: Assessment and intervention. In H. R. Myklebust (Ed), *Progress in learning disabilities,* (Vol. 3, pp. 85–121). New York: Grune & Stratton.

Nagy, J., & Szatmari, P. (1986). A chart review of schizotypal personality disorders in children. *Journal of Autism and Developmental Disorders, 16*(3), 351–367.

Newson, E., Dawson, M., & Everaard, T. (1984–1985). The natural history of able autistic people: Their management and functioning in a social context. *Communication,* 19–21.

O'Connor, N., & Hermelin, B. (1989). The memory structure of autistic idiot-savant mnemonists. *British Journal of Psychology, 80,* 97–111.

Ozbayrak, K. R., Kapucu, O., Erdem, E., & Aras, T. (1991). Left occipital hypoperfusion in a case with Asperger syndrome. *Brain Development, 13*(6), 454–456.

Ozonoff, S. (1998). Assessment and remediation of executive dysfunction in autism and Asperger syndrome. In E. Schopler, G. Mesibov, & L. J. Kunce (Eds.), *Asperger syndrome or high functioning autism?* (pp. 263–289). New York: Plenum.

Ozonoff, S., Pennington, B. F., & Rogers, S. J. (1991). Executive function deficits in high-functioning autistic individuals: Relationship to theory of mind. *Journal of Child Psychology and Psychiatry, 32*(7), 1081–1105.

Ozonoff, S., Rogers, S. J., & Pennington, B. F. (1991). Asperger's Syndrome: Evidence of an empirical distinction from high-functioning autism. *Journal of Child Psychology and Psychiatry, 32*(7), 1107–1122.

Rapin, I., & Allen, D. (1983). Developmental language disorders. In U. Kirk (Ed.), *Neuropsychology of language, reading and spelling.* New York: Academic Press.

Robinson, J. F., & Vitale, L. J. (1954). Children with circumscribed interests. *American Journal of Orthopsychiatry, 24,* 755–764.

Rourke, B. P. (1989). *Nonverbal learning disabilities: The syndrome and the model.* New York: Guilford Press.

Rourke, B. P. (Ed.). (1995). *Syndrome of Nonverbal Learning Disabilities: Neurodevelopmental manifestations.* New York: Guilford Press.

Rourke, B., Young, G. C., & Leenaars, A. A. (1989). A childhood learning disability that predisposes those afflicted to adolescent and adult depression and suicide risk. *Journal of Learning Disabilities, 22,* 169–185.

Roy, E. A., Elliott, D., Dewey, D., & Square-Storer, P. (1990). Impairments to praxis and sequencing in adult and developmental disorders. In C. Bard, M. Fleury, & L. Hay (Eds.), *Development of eye–hand coordination across the life span* (pp. 358–384). Columbia: University of South Carolina Press.

Rutter, M. (1978). Diagnosis and definition of childhood autism. *Journal of Autism and Childhood Schizophrenia, 8*(2), 139–161.

Rutter, M. (1989). Annotation: Child psychiatric disorders in ICD-10. *Journal of Child Psychology and Psychiatry, 30,* 499–513.

Rutter, M. (1999). Two-way interplay between research and clinical work. *Journal of Child Psychology and Psychiatry, 40*(2), 169–188.

Rutter, M., Bailey, A., Bolton, P., & Le Couteur, A. (1994). Autism and known medical conditions: Myth and substance. *Journal of Child Psychology and Psychiatry, 35*(2), 311–322.

Rutter, M., Bailey, A., Simonoff, E., & Pickles, A. (1997). Genetic influences in autism. In D. J. Cohen & F. R. Volkmar (Eds.), *Handbook of autism and pervasive developmental disorders* (2nd ed., pp. 370–387). New York: Wiley.

Rutter, M., & Gould, M. (1985). Classification. In M. Rutter & L. Herson (Eds), *Child and adolescent psychiatry: Modern approaches* (2nd ed., pp. 304–321). Oxford: Blackwell.

Rutter, M., Lebovici, S., Eisenberg, L., Snezhenevsky, A. B., Sadoun, R., Brook, E., & Lin, T. (1969). A triaxial classification of mental disorders in childhood. *Journal of Child Psychology and Psychiatry, 10,* 41–61.

Rutter, M., & Schopler, E. (1992). Classification of pervasive developmental disorders: Some concepts and practical considerations. *Journal of Autism and Developmental Disorders, 22*(4), 459–482.

Ryan, R. M. (1992). Treatment-resistant chronic mental illness: Is it Asperger's syndrome? *Hospital and Community Psychiatry, 43*(8), 807–811.

Saliba, J. R., & Griffiths, M. (1990). Brief report: Autism of the Asperger type associated with an autosomal fragile site. *Journal of Autism and Developmental Disorders, 20*(4), 569–575.

Scragg, P., & Shah, A. (1994). Prevalence of Asperger's syndrome in a secure hospital. *British Journal of Psychiatry, 165*(5), 679–682.

Siegel, D. J., Minshew, N. J., & Goldstein, G. (1996). Wechsler IQ profiles in diagnosis of high-functioning autism. *Journal of Autism and Developmental Disorders, 26*(4), 389–406.

Smalley, S. L., McCracken, J., & Tanguay, P. (1995). Autism, affective disorders, and social phobia. *American Journal of Medical Genetics, 60*(1), 19–26.

Smith, I. S., & Bryson, S. E. (1994). Imitation and action in autism: A critical review. *Psychological Bulletin, 116*(2), 259–273.

South, M., Klin, A., & Volkmar, F. R. (1997, April). *Circumscribed interests in higher functioning autism and Asperger syndrome.* Poster presented at the 1997 biannual meeting of the Society for Research in Child Development, Washington, DC.

Spitzer, R. L., Endicott, J. E., & Robbins, E. (1978). Research diagnostic criteria. *Archives of General Psychiatry, 35,* 773–782.

Szatmari, P. (1992a). A review of the DSM-III-R criteria for autistic disorder. *Journal of Autism and Developmental Disorders, 22*(4), 507–523.

Szatmari, P. (1992b). The validity of autistic spectrum disorders: A literature review. *Journal of Autism and Developmental Disorders, 22*(4), 583–600.

Szatmari, P., Bartolucci, G., & Bremner, R. (1989a). Asperger's syndrome and autism: Comparison of early history and outcome. *Developmental Medicine and Child Neurology, 31*(6), 709–720.

Szatmari, P., Bartolucci, G., Bremner, R., Bond, S., & Rich, S. (1989b). A follow-up study of high-functioning autistic children. *Journal of Autism and Developmental Disorders, 19,* 213–225.

Szatmari, P., Bremner, R., & Nagy, J. N. (1989). Asperger's syndrome: A review of clinical features. *Canadian Journal of Psychiatry, 34*(6), 554–560.

Szatmari, P., Tuff, L., Finlayson, M. A. J., & Bartolucci, G. (1990). Asperger's syndrome and autism: Neurocognitive aspects. *Journal of the American Academy of Child and Adolescent Psychiatry, 29,* 130–136.

Taiminen, T. (1994). Asperger's syndrome or schizophrenia: Is differential diagnosis necessary for adult patients? *Nordic Journal of Psychiatry, 48*(5), 325–328.

Tantam, D. (1988a). Annotation: Asperger's syndrome. *Journal of Child Psychology and Psychiatry, 29*(3), 245–255.

Tantam, D. (1988b). Lifelong eccentricity and social isolation: II. Asperger's syndrome or schizoid personality disorder? *British Journal of Psychiatry, 153,* 783–791.

Tantam, D. (1991). Asperger's syndrome in adulthood. In U. Frith (Ed.), *Autism and Asperger syndrome* (pp. 147–183). Cambridge: Cambridge University Press.

Tantam, D., Evered, C., & Hersov, L. (1990). Asperger's syndrome and ligamentous laxity. *Journal of the American Academy of Child and Adolescent Psychiatry, 29*(6), 892–896.

Thomsen, P. H. (1994). Obsessive–compulsive disorder in children and adolescents: A 6–22-year follow-up study: Clinical descriptions of the course and continuity of obsessive–compulsive symptomatology. *European Child and Adolescent Psychiatry, 3*(2), 82–96.

Treffert, D. (1989). *Extraordinary people*. New York: Bantam.

Van Bourgondien, M. E., & Woods, A. V. (1992). Vocational possibilities for high-functioning adults with autism. In E. Schopler & G. B. Mesibov (Eds.), *High-functioning individuals with autism* (pp. 227–239). New York: Plenum.

Van Krevelen, D. A. (1962). The psychopathology of autistic psychopathy. *Acta Paedopsychiatrica, 29*(1), 22–31.

Van Krevelen, D. A. (1963). On the relationship between early infantile autism and autistic psychopathy. *Acta Paedopsychiatrica, 30*, 303–323.

Van Krevelen, D. A. (1971). Early infantile autism and autistic psychopathy. *Journal of autism and Child Schizophrenia, 1*(1), 82–86.

Venter, A., Lord, C., & Schopler, E. (1992). A follow-up study of high-functioning autistic children. *Journal of Child Psychology and Psychiatry, 33*(3), 489–507.

Vilensky, J. A., Damasio, A. R., & Maurer, R. G. (1981). Gait disturbances in patients with autistic behavior. *Archives of Neurology, 38*, 646–649.

Voeller, K. K. S. (1986). Right-hemisphere deficit syndrome in children. *American Journal of Psychiatry, 143*, 1004–1009.

Voeller, K. K. S. (1991). Social–emotional learning disabilities. *Psychiatric Annals, 21*(12), 735–741.

Volkmar, F. R., Cicchetti, D. V., Bregman, J., & Cohen, D. J. (1992). Three diagnostic systems for autism: DSM-III, DSM-III-R, and ICD-10. *Journal of Autism and Developmental Disorders, 22*(4), 483–492.

Volkmar, F. R., Cicchetti, D. V., Cohen, D. J., & Bregman, J. (1992). Brief report: Developmental aspects of DSM-III-R criteria for autism. *Journal of Autism and Developmental Disorders, 22*(4), 657–62.

Volkmar, F. R., & Cohen, D. J. (1989). Disintegrative disorder or "late onset" autism. *Journal of Child Psychology and Psychiatry, 30*(5), 717–724.

Volkmar, F. R., Klin, A., & Cohen, D. J. (1997). Diagnosis and classification of autism and related conditions: Consensus and Issues. In D. J. Cohen & F. R. Volkmar (Eds.), *Handbook of autism and pervasive developmental disorders* (pp. 5–40). New York: Wiley.

Volkmar, F. R., Klin, A., & Pauls, D. (1998). Nosological and genetic aspects of Asperger Syndrome. *Journal of Autism and Developmental Disorders, 28*(5), 457–463.

Volkmar, F. R., Klin, A., Schultz, R. B., Bronen, R., Marans, W. D., Sparrow, S. S., & Cohen, D. J. (1996). Grand rounds in child psychiatry: Asperger syndrome. *Journal of the American Academy of Child and Adolescent Psychiatry, 35*, 118–123.

Volkmar, F. R., Klin, A., Siegel, B., Szatmari, P., Lord, C., Campbell, M., Freeman, B. J., Cicchetti, D. V., Rutter, M., Kline, W., Buitelaar, J., Hattab, Y., Fombonne, E., Fuentes, J., Werry, J., Stone, W., Kerbeshian, J., Hoshino, Y., Bregman, J., Loveland, K., Szymanski, L., & Towbin, K. (1994). DSM-IV Autism/Pervasive Developmental Disorder Field Trial. *American Journal of Psychiatry, 151*, 1361–1367.

Volkmar, F. R., Sparrow, S. S., Goudreau, D., Cicchetti, D. V., Paul, R., & Cohen, D. J. (1987).

Social deficits in autism: An operational approach using the Vineland Adaptive Behavior Scales. *Journal of the American Academy of Child and Adolescent Psychiatry, 26*, 156–161.

Weintraub, S., & Mesulam, M. M. (1983). Developmental learning disabilities of the right hemisphere: Emotional, interpersonal, and cognitive components. *Archives of Neurology, 40*, 463–468.

Werry, J. S. (1992) Child and adolescent (early onset) schizophrenia: A review in light of DSM-III-R. *Journal of Autism and Developmental Disorders, 22*, 601–624.

Wing, L. (1981). Asperger's syndrome: A clinical account. *Psychological Medicine, 11*, 115–129.

Wing. L. (1986). Clarification on Asperger's syndrome [Letter to the Editor]. *Journal of Autism and Developmental Disorders, 16*(4), 513–515.

Wing, L. (1998). The history of Asperger syndrome. In E. Schopler & G. Mesibov (Eds.), *Asperger syndrome or high-functioning autism?* (pp. 12–28). New York: Plenum.

Wing, L., & Gould, J. (1979). Severe impairments of social interaction and associated abnormalities in children: Epidemiology and classification. *Journal of Autism and Childhood Schizophrenia, 9*, 11–29.

Wolff, S. (1991). "Schizoid" personality in childhood and adult life. III: The childhood picture. *British Journal of Psychiatry, 159*, 629–635.

Wolff, S. (1995). *Loner's: The life path of unusual children.* London: Routledge,

Wolff, S., & Barlow, A. (1979). Schizoid personality in childhood: A comparative study of schizoid, autistic and normal children. *Journal of Child Psychology and Psychiatry, 20*, 19–46.

Wolff, S., & Chick, J. (1980). Schizoid personality in childhood: A controlled follow-up study. *Psychological Medicine, 10*, 85–100.

Wolff, S., Townshend, R., McGuire, R. J., & Weeks, D. J. (1991). "Schizoid" personality in childhood and adult life. II: Adult adjustment and the continuity with schizotypal personality disorder. *British Journal of Psychiatry, 159*, 620–629, 634–635.

World Health Organization. (1993). *International classification of diseases: Tenth revision.* Chapter V. Mental and behavioral disorders (including disorders of psychological development). Diagnostic criteria for research. Geneva: Author.

2

Neuropsychological Function and the External Validity of Asperger Syndrome

SALLY OZONOFF

ELIZABETH McMAHON GRIFFITH

In 1943, Leo Kanner described 11 children with "early infantile autism" who exhibited severe social and communication deficits and restricted, repetitive behaviors. A year later, unaware of Kanner's paper, Hans Asperger (1944/1991) described four socially impaired children with idiosyncratic, narrow interests who suffered from "autistic psychopathy." Asperger's report received relatively little attention in the medical community until the publication of Wing's (1981) influential clinical account of the condition. The similarities to autism, particularly the higher-functioning form, were immediately noted, leading some researchers to suggest that the conditions were essentially the same, differing primarily in severity or degree (Schopler, 1985, 1996; Wing, 1986, 1991). Although Kanner's and Asperger's descriptions were quite similar, they were not identical. Most notably, Asperger emphasized good language and poor motor skills in his cases, whereas Kanner did not. These potential differences have led other researchers to conclude that Asperger syndrome (AS), as it has come to be called, and high-functioning autism (HFA) diverge in clinically meaningful ways (Gillberg & Gillberg, 1989; Green, 1990; Klin, 1994; Szatmari, Bremner, & Nagy, 1989; Tantam, 1988). This chapter explores the validity of the distinction between AS and HFA, focusing on neuropsychological differentiation of the disorders.

SYNDROME VALIDITY ISSUES

It is critical to both research and intervention to determine whether AS and HFA are, as Schopler recently asked, "different labels or different disabilities" (Schopler, 1996, p. 109). If the two are different disabilities it would be inappropriate to group them together for research purposes. Eventual identification of the neural substrate(s) of any psychopathological condition relies on the study of homogeneous samples whose underlying neuropathology is likely to be uniform. In addition, if HFA and AS diverge on meaningful cognitive and behavioral dimensions, then the treatments prescribed for the disorders might differ substantially.

On the other hand, if AS and HFA involve the same fundamental symptomatology, differing only in degree or severity, then retaining the use of different labels for the same disability would be confusing (Schopler, 1996). It has been argued that because the autism label is more familiar, it is also more informative, making the nature of the problem more readily recognizable to parents, teachers, and the public (Happé & Frith, 1991; Schopler, 1996). A diagnosis of autism usually brings with it an acknowledgment that an affected child requires educational support, structured teaching, speech–language therapy, and social skills training, but in some regions of the United States and the world, the less familiar diagnosis of AS may not (Schopler, 1998). If the label is not automatically recognized as an autism spectrum condition by insurance companies, benefits and other coverage may be affected as well (Schopler, 1998). Thus, the debate over whether AS and HFA warrant separate names and classifications is of more than purely academic interest.

One way to determine the relationship between two related conditions is to investigate their external validity. External validation is the process of examining whether disorders differ on external criteria not involved in the original definition of the conditions. The most powerful evidence of external validity is demonstration of disorder by remediation or disorder by task interactions (Fletcher, 1985). Distinct syndromes may require different treatments, demonstrate differential response to the same treatment, or display divergent profiles on cognitive and neuropsychological testing (Fletcher, 1985); all these conditions have been met, for example, in distinguishing learning disability subtypes, such as dyslexia from math disability (Pennington, 1991). In addition, different syndromes may involve different etiologies (e.g., fragile-X syndrome vs. autism), different developmental courses (e.g., autism vs. schizophrenia), or different outcomes (Pennington, 1991).

What is essential to external validation is that the dimensions on which the two conditions are compared fall outside the measurement domain initially used to establish the syndromes. Otherwise, demonstration of syndrome differences will be due primarily to the covariance of tasks within the same measurement domain (Fletcher, 1985). For example, one way that AS and autism are distinguished in the *Diagnostic and Statistical Manual of Mental Disorders,* fourth edition (DSM-IV; American Psychiatric Association, 1994) is on the basis of early language development, with a history of normal language acquisition required for the diagnosis of AS and a history of delayed language more typical (although not required) of individuals with autism. Because early language development is predictive of later language abilities (Paul & Cohen, 1984; Rutter, Greenfield, & Lockyer, 1967; Rutter, Mawhood, & Howlin, 1992), finding that individuals with AS and autism differ in their performance on language tests is not surprising, as the subtypes were originally distinguished, at least in part, on the basis of their linguistic functioning (Kerbeshian, Burd, & Fisher, 1990). Finding that AS and autism differ in terms of their memory capacity or academic skills profile, however, would be more compelling evidence of external validity, as these variables were not involved in originally defining the syndromes. As we will see, few studies that have attempted to distinguish AS from HFA satisfy the criterion that the dependent variables be distinct from the dimensions used in the group definition process.

Another approach that can be helpful in determining the relationship between related conditions is to examine the core and associated characteristics of the disorders. Core or primary deficits of a disorder are those that are universally found among affected individuals, specific to the disorder, present from an early age, and persistent throughout development (Pennington & Ozonoff, 1991). Associated secondary and correlated symptoms, on the other hand, are less central to the diagnosis, as they are found in only a subset of affected individuals, may be present in other conditions, and may disappear during development. If two syndromes do not differ in their core symptoms, even if they do differ in associated characteristics, they may not be true subtypes (Pennington, 1991; Rapin, 1987).

Consensus on the nature of the core symptoms of autism and AS has not yet been reached. Failure to distinguish core from associated symptoms clearly complicates the process of syndrome validation. The strongest case for a core symptom can be made when the probability of the behavior or sign, given the diagnosis, is very high; that is, the sign is universal among those with the disorder. Similarly, when the probability of the diagnosis, given the presence of the sign, is also high (e.g., the sign is specific to the disorder), we again have good evidence that we have identified a core symptom. However, these may be unrealistically stringent criteria to which to hold ourselves. As Meehl (1973a) has so eloquently pointed out, even in organic medicine, there are few pathognomonic signs and few diseases which are invariably associated with a particular symptom. What most clinicians look for is what Meehl (1973b) calls "diagnostic bell ringers," signs that, although perhaps not universal or specific to a disorder, are highly characteristic of it.

Have we identified diagnostic bell ringers for autism? Most would agree that autism characteristically involves some degree of social dysfunction, particularly in social reciprocity. In addition, communication abnormalities are regularly found in autistic individuals. And it has been proposed that cognitive processing abnormalities in the domains of theory of mind and executive function are central to the disorder (Baron-Cohen, 1989; Frith, 1993; Hughes, Russell, & Robbins, 1994; Ozonoff, 1995).

What are the diagnostic bell ringers of AS? It has been suggested that motor deficits may be central to AS, although there is not, as yet, consensus on this. Some diagnostic systems and clinical descriptions consider motor dysfunction to be a core symptom of the disorder (Asperger, 1944/1991; Burgoine & Wing, 1983; Gillberg & Gillberg, 1989; Tantam, 1988; Wing, 1981), whereas others regard it as an associated characteristic that may or may not be present (American Psychiatric Association, 1994; Szatmari, Bremner, & Nagy, 1989; World Health Organization, 1992). It has also been proposed that visual–spatial deficits may be characteristic of AS (Klin, Volkmar, Sparrow, Cicchetti, & Rourke, 1995; Molina, Ruata, & Soler, 1986). Both motor and visual–spatial dysfunction are appealing core symptoms of AS, as they appear to distinguish it from HFA, which is usually described as involving superior abilities in these areas (Kanner, 1943; Shah & Frith, 1993). If a double dissociation is found, in which core deficits of one disorder represent areas of spared functioning in the other condition, and vice versa, this would provide good evidence of external validity. In turn, this might imply that the neural substrates of the two conditions differed and that they required different treatments. However, if no dissociation exists and the disorders appear similar in their core symptoms, differing perhaps only in magnitude or degree, there would be little evidence of external validity for the subtypes.

The approach taken in this chapter is to examine proposed core cognitive symptoms of HFA and AS, as a means of examining the external validity of the syndromes. Four neuropsychological domains were chosen for comparison: motor skills, visual–spatial abilities, executive functions, and theory of mind. Each of these domains has been proposed as being central to either HFA or AS and all are independent of the diagnostic criteria (e.g., DSM-IV) used to define the conditions. Although a number of investigations have documented differences between AS and HFA subjects on language measures (e.g., Klin et al., 1995; Szatmari, Archer, Fisman, Streiner, & Wilson, 1995; Szatmari, Bartolucci, & Bremner, 1989; Szatmari, Tuff, Finlayson, & Bartolucci, 1990), these data are not reviewed in detail here, because positive correlations between early and later language development (Paul & Cohen, 1984; Rutter et al., 1967; Rutter et al., 1992) render any group differences found less informative than studies whose diagnostic and outcome measures are independent. In what follows, we review empirical research that has contrasted AS and HFA in each of these four domains in an attempt to determine the external validity of the subtypes. We end this section with a quote from a highly cited editorial by Schopler (1985): "Since no behavioral distinction between higher-level autism and Asperger Syndrome has yet been demonstrated, diagnostic confusion can be reduced if the Asperger Syndrome label is not used, at least until an empirically based distinction from higher-level autism can be demonstrated for it" (p. 359). This reasonable suggestion was made more than a decade ago. What evidence, if any, has accumulated in the last dozen years of an empirical distinction between autism and AS? We concentrate on cognitive and neuropsychological processes in answering this question in the present chapter.

Before proceeding further, a note of caution is in order. Until only recently, there was little consensus on how to diagnose AS. Prior to the publication of DSM-IV in 1994, a number of different diagnostic systems existed (Gillberg & Gillberg, 1989; Szatmari, Bremner, & Nagy, 1989a; Tantam, 1988; Wing, 1981) and were used with varying consistency by different research teams. It was not uncommon for researchers to modify criteria to suit the needs of particular studies and samples. When six different systems for diagnosing AS were applied to a group of individuals with potential AS, approximately half the subjects met all six sets of criteria; the other half of the sample, however, met only a subset of criteria (Ghaziuddin, Tsai, & Ghaziuddin, 1992a). This tells us that the various diagnostic definitions of AS overlap, but are not identical, and describe somewhat different subsamples of individuals. This makes interpretation of research on AS conducted before the advent of DSM-IV difficult, as the sample identified varies according to the particular diagnostic definition used. Perhaps most problematically, the majority of previous studies have not made clear the criteria for *excluding* a diagnosis of autism in AS subjects and, thus, it is not always certain that the groups defined are mutually exclusive and nonoverlapping.

MOTOR DEVELOPMENT AND FUNCTIONING IN ASPERGER SYNDROME AND HIGH-FUNCTIONING AUTISM

In his original account of the syndrome, Asperger described his index cases as conspicuously clumsy, noting poor balance, ill-coordinated movements, odd posture, and unusual gait in all four boys. Asperger regarded delays in motor development as a primary feature of the syndrome. Kanner, on the other hand, made no mention of motor deficits when he outlined the core symptoms of autism and apparently did not consider them central to the disorder. Since these first accounts, there has been debate about how characteristic clumsiness and motor delays are of AS, with some believing them to be relatively universal (Gillberg & Gillberg, 1989; Klin et al., 1995; Tantam, 1988; Wing, 1981) and others suggesting they are present in only a subset of cases (American Psychiatric Association, 1994; Szatmari, Bremner, & Nagy, 1989; World Health Organization, 1992). In this section, we review the empirical literature that has systematically examined the motor abilities of individuals with autism and AS.

The most explicit test of external validity comes from studies that directly compare AS and HFA subjects on measures of motor skill and coordination. Two investigations by Szatmari and colleagues examined parental reports of early motor development in young children with AS and HFA. Szatmari, Bartolucci, and Bremner (1989) obtained information during a parent interview regarding the child's ability to dress, tie shoelaces, eat with utensils, use a pencil, and complete a puzzle. Both groups demonstrated significantly more delays than did non-autistic psychiatric controls, but no differences were found between the autism and AS groups in their history of achieving motor milestones. In a later study using a standardized measure, the Vineland Adaptive Behavior Scales, to collect early motor history data, the failure to find group differences between AS and HFA was replicated (Szatmari et al., 1995). A third investigation by a different research team also found few motor milestones that distinguished AS from HFA (Eisenmajer et al., 1996); the only significant difference between the groups was later walking in the autistic group, contrary to expectation. These results are mitigated by a high degree of overlap between the autistic and AS samples, however. In Szatmari et al.'s (1995) study, 12 of 21 AS subjects met criteria for autism; using DSM-IV, the diagnosis of autism would normally take precedence, but this criterion was not used in Szatmari's study, conducted prior to the advent of DSM-IV. In Eisenmajer et al.'s (1996) investigation, *all* clinician-diagnosed AS subjects actually met formal criteria for autism according to the *International Classification of Diseases,* 10th revision (ICD-10; World Health Organization, 1992) and the DSM-IV. With such substantial overlap between the two diagnostic constructs, null results are not surprising. As we will see, such modifications in the diagnostic criteria significantly compromise the conclusions that can be drawn, but are unfortunately not rare, affecting interpretation of many of the investigations reported later (including studies from the first author's [SO] own laboratory).

Standardized tests of motor function have also been administered to AS and HFA samples. Within the context of a large neurodevelopmental battery, Gillberg (1989) measured motor clumsiness in children with autism and AS, matched on age and IQ. Using the Griffiths Mental Development Scale, 81% of those in the AS group were found to have motor skills at least 15 points lower than their IQ level, whereas only 22% of the autistic sample met this criterion for clumsiness; this group difference was statistically significant.

Another study found that individuals with AS exhibited significantly more difficulty on the Grooved Pegboard test, a measure of fine motor speed and dexterity, than did autistic individuals matched on IQ (Szatmari et al., 1990), but only when using their nondominant hand (performance of the groups was similar with the dominant hand). Age differences between the groups, with the AS sample being significantly younger, may have contributed to the group differences in fine motor skill, however.

In the most comprehensive investigation of AS–HFA differences to date, Klin et al. (1995) evaluated a broad range of neuropsychological functions, including both fine and gross motor skills (results from other domains assessed are reported later). Subjects with autism and AS were matched on age, sex, and Full Scale IQ. This investigation was one of only a few that explicitly ruled out autism in all AS cases, in accordance with the DSM-IV and ICD-10 "precedence rule." A chart review methodology was employed in which the records of individuals who had previously undergone extensive neuropsychological testing (in both the authors' clinic and elsewhere in the United States) were examined for the presence of neuropsychological strengths and deficits hypothesized to be characteristic of both autism and AS. They found that the percentage of AS subjects whose records contained evidence of motor deficits was significantly greater than in the autistic group. Indeed, fine and gross motor problems were virtually universal in the AS group, with 90% and 100% of the sample demonstrating deficits in the respective areas.

This finding may be related to the manner in which the groups were originally defined. In an effort to make assignment to the AS group on the strictest possible basis, capturing what were thought to be particularly distinctive features of AS in the literature at the time, delayed motor milestones and clumsiness were required for inclusion in the AS group. Finding deficits on standardized measures of motor function might then primarily reflect covariance of tasks within the same measurement domain. There was more to the story, however, and these results cannot be easily dismissed. When the authors reanalyzed their data, dropping the clumsiness criterion for assignment to the AS group, significant differences in motor function remained, with the AS group continuing to demonstrate impairment relative to the HFA group. Thus, the findings of motor deficits in AS in this study were robust and were independent of the diagnostic definition process, providing support for motor clumsiness as a "bell-ringer" of AS.

As noted by Ghaziuddin, Tsai, and Ghaziuddin (1992b), most early studies of AS did not use standardized measures of motor function to identify clumsiness (or, in the Klin et al., 1995, study, did not use one consistent measure to detect motor impairment). Two recent investigations have employed consistent, reliable, valid measures of motor function, however. Ghaziuddin, Butler, Tsai, and Ghaziuddin (1994) compared individuals with AS, diagnosed using ICD-10 draft criteria, to individuals with autism matched on age and Verbal and Performance IQ. They administered the Bruininks–Oseretsky test, a standardized, age-normed measure of gross and fine motor skills and upper limb coordination. Relative to age norms, both groups demonstrated evidence of motor deficits. However, there were no significant differences between the groups, and the AS sample actually performed marginally better than did those with autism on all subtests.

Manjiviona and Prior (1995) replicated this finding in another sample of AS and HFA children, using the Test of Motor Impairment, a standardized measure of motor function explicitly developed to distinguish between clumsy and nonclumsy groups. AS subjects were diagnosed according to ICD-10 draft criteria, modified so that subjects currently exhibiting the classic AS feature of well-developed language were not excluded from the sample if they demonstrated an early history of language delay. This modification may well have permitted overlap between the AS and HFA groups and likely made the groups more similar than they would have been otherwise. No significant group differences were found on subtests of manual dexterity, ball skills, or balance; as in the Ghaziuddin et al. (1994) study, the AS group in fact performed nonsignificantly better than did the HFA group on the motor tests. Mirroring the results of Ghaziuddin et al. (1994), both pervasive developmental disorder (PDD) subtypes demonstrated evidence of clumsiness: 50% of the AS group and 67% of the HFA sample were considered clumsy, relative to age norms. These results do not support the suggestion that motor functioning distinguishes between those with AS and those with HFA. However, the manner in which the groups were defined, permitting overlap between the symptomatology of AS and HFA, likely contributed to the null results. In this case, the failure to find group differences may reflect primarily a failure of diagnostic separation at the level of group assignment rather than true null results.

Direct comparison of individuals with AS and HFA is most informative to the external validity question, but studies comparing either group to a non-PDD comparison sample are also useful. Two studies have done this with AS. Tantam (1991) compared individuals with symptoms of AS (defined by his own criteria; Tantam, 1988) to individuals demonstrating social isolation and eccentricity but who did not meet criteria for AS. One criterion for assignment to the AS group was "an impression of motor clumsiness." Perhaps not surprisingly, results indicated that 91% of the AS sample exhibited motor impairment, as judged by performance on tests of ball skills and balance. A major limitation of this study, however, was that the demarcation between autism and AS was not clear. There was no statement of how the diagnosis of autism was ruled out in the AS sample. In fact, 20% of the AS subjects had been diagnosed with autism in childhood. This degree of overlap is not permitted in DSM-IV, where these diagnoses are mutually exclusive. Thus, we cannot be certain that Tantam was studying AS and not autism.

Miyahara et al. (1997), on the other hand, ruled out autism in all their AS cases and used standard ICD-10 criteria for diagnosis. They administered the Movement Assessment Battery for Children (the most recent revision of the Test of Motor Impairment) to an AS group and learning-disabled controls matched closely on IQ. Contrary to expectation, they found no group differences in ball or balance skills or overall motoric function but significantly better manual dexterity in the AS group relative to the learning-disabled sample.

Although it has long been assumed that the motor skills of children with autism are well preserved, a closer examination of this literature suggests that autism also involves some degree of motor impairment. In fact, some have hypothesized that motor deficits are a primary feature of the disorder (Damasio & Maurer, 1978; Leary & Hill, 1996). Several studies comparing individuals with autism to nonautistic controls have been conducted over the years. Contrary to popular impression, the majority of these studies have documented evidence of motor deficits in children with autism. DeMyer, Barton, and Norton (1972) found that autistic children performed less well than both normal and mentally retarded controls on a variety of gross and fine motor measures, including jumping, hopping, skipping, kicking, throwing, catching, drawing, and assembly tasks. Ornitz, Guthrie, and Farley (1977) and DeMyer (1979) reported that motor milestones, such as rolling over, sitting without support, crawling, and walking, were significantly delayed in autistic children. Jones and Prior (1985) found significantly more neurological "soft signs," such as poor balance, coordination, and gait, in autistic children than controls matched on mental and chronological age. Rumsey and Hamburger (1990) found that nonretarded autistic men performed significantly less well than did normal controls on the Grooved Pegboard test. Hallett et al. (1993) reported mild clumsiness in four of five adults with autism, relative to five healthy, age-matched controls.

Although these studies are consistent in documenting motor deficits in autism, many of them failed to account for group differences in IQ. Because intellectual level and motor ability are significantly correlated, failure to match groups on IQ leaves open the possibility that clumsiness is secondary to lower intellectual functioning in the autistic group. Indeed, one study that did match groups carefully on IQ found no signs of clumsiness or motor deficits on a variety of gross motor tasks (Morin & Reid, 1985). Thus, this literature is difficult to interpret, and a final conclusion about motor skills in autism awaits future research, conducted with careful attention to appropriate control groups and matching.

Summarizing the five investigations directly comparing individuals with AS to those with autism, two demonstrated selective deficits in the AS group (Gillberg, 1989; Klin et al., 1995), two found no group differences (Ghaziuddin et al., 1994; Manjiviona & Prior, 1995), and one reported mixed results (Szatmari et al., 1990). Two of the three studies that examined early motor history suggested that young children with AS and autism demonstrate similar delays in motor development (Szatmari, Bartolucci, & Bremner, 1989; Szatmari et al., 1995) whereas one study found more motor delays in the autistic than the AS group (Eisenmajer et al., 1996). A final determination of the usefulness of motor deficits in differentiating AS from HFA is complicated not only by these mixed results but also by methodological issues.

There is tremendous interstudy variability in diagnostic and group assignment procedures and methods of assessing clumsiness. Both studies documenting and failing to document motor deficits in AS made modifications in diagnostic criteria that may have influenced their results. Those that failed to find any group differences were most likely to have permitted some overlap between the autistic and AS groups whereas some of those that found significant differences modified their samples to include clumsiness as a diagnostic criterion. The only investigation reviewed in this section that used standard diagnostic criteria (ICD-10), without modifications, to define groups, ruled out autism in all AS cases, assessed motor function in a standardized way, and matched groups closely on age and IQ (Miyahara et al., 1997) unfortunately did not make any comparison to autism. However, they found few differences from a learning-disabled control group, with all differences in favor of the AS group. Without further research, it is not possible to make any conclusions about clumsiness as a "diagnostic bell ringer" of AS at the present time.

VISUOSPATIAL FUNCTIONS IN ASPERGER SYNDROME AND HIGH-FUNCTIONING AUTISM

A second potential area of differentiation between autism and AS has been proposed in the domain of right-hemisphere cognitive functions (Klin et al., 1995; Molina et al., 1986). It is generally accepted that the right hemisphere plays a critical role in the processing of spatial information, including object localization and identification, visual and spatial memory, mental rotation, spatial imagery, and visuospatial construction (Stiles-Davis, Kritchevsky, & Bellugi, 1988). In addition, the right side of the brain appears to be involved in the expression and interpretation of emotional material, voice intonation and prosody, and paralinguistic aspects of communication (Kolb & Taylor, 1981; Ross & Mesulam, 1979; Tucker, Watson, & Heilman, 1977; Weintraub, Mesulam, & Kramer, 1981). Acquired lesions of the right hemisphere cause impairments in these areas.

A developmental analog of these difficulties has been described in the literature as a nonverbal or right-hemisphere learning disability (Denckla, 1983; Rourke, 1989; Tranel, Hall, Olson, & Tranel, 1987; Voeller, 1986; Weintraub & Mesulam, 1983). Children with right-hemisphere learning disability (RHLD) exhibit marked impairments in spatial reasoning, mathematics, handwriting, and motor skills, and Performance IQ is typically depressed relative to Verbal IQ (Pennington, 1991; Rourke, 1989). Socially, they are often described as awkward and isolated. Cognitive and behavioral similarities between AS and RHLD were first noted over a decade ago (Denckla, 1983; Molina et al., 1986) but received little research attention until recently. Despite a dearth of empirical study, the idea that AS is associated with visuospatial impairment and higher Verbal than Performance IQ has become generally accepted by many clinicians. In this section, we examine whether this clinical heuristic is justified by the results of recent empirical investigations.

A review of years of cognitive research is consistent in finding preserved visuospatial skills in individuals with autism (see Green, Fein, Joy, & Waterhouse, 1995, for a review). On standard intelligence tests such as the Wechsler scales, most studies report higher Performance IQ (PIQ) than Verbal IQ (VIQ) in autism (see Lincoln, Allen, & Kilman, 1995, for a review). Intersubtest variability is the norm, with scores on the Block Design and Object Assembly subtests typically the highest in a profile (Asarnow, Tanguay, Bott, & Freeman, 1987; Freeman, Lucas, Forness, & Ritvo, 1985; Happé, 1994b; Lincoln, Courchesne, Kilman, Elmasian, & Allen, 1988; Shah & Frith, 1983, 1993). This pattern appears to be independent of IQ level and is present in even high-functioning individuals diagnosed with autism (Fein, Waterhouse, Lucci, & Snyder, 1985; Freeman et al., 1985; Grandin, 1995; Lincoln et al., 1988). In contrast, Wing (1981), in her original description of AS, noted that some of her subjects demonstrated significantly higher VIQ than PIQ. Several case histories have also reported AS individuals who demonstrated significant VIQ > PIQ discrepancies (Baron-Cohen, 1988; Gillberg, 1991; Volkmar et al., 1996). Only a few studies have systematically compared the visuospatial and intellectual functions of AS and HFA, however.

Szatmari et al. (1990) found no AS–HFA group differences in PIQ; in fact, the PIQ of their AS group was nonsignificantly higher than the HFA sample. The predicted VIQ > PIQ discrepancy was not evident in the AS group, nor was the opposite configuration found in the HFA group. On the Beery Developmental Test of Visual–Motor Integration, there were again no significant differences between the groups. As noted previously, the age differences in this sample, with the AS group significantly younger than the HFA sample, may have contributed to these null results. In a later study using a new sample matched on age, however, Szatmari et al. (1995) replicated their earlier results, again failing to find group differences on the Beery test and on the spatial reasoning subtests of the Stanford–Binet Intelligence Scale (e.g., Pattern Analysis, Bead Memory, and Quantitative Reasoning). Similarly, Ozonoff, Rogers, and Pennington (1991) found no AS–HFA differences on three tests of spatial cognition, the Children's Embedded Figures Test, and the Block Design and Object Assembly subtests of the Wechsler Intelligence Scale for Children—Revised. In this study, neither PDD group performed less well than controls. And Manjiviona and Prior (1995) found that the PIQ of their AS sample was actually significantly higher than that of their HFA group. Interpretation of these investigations' results are limited by modifications in the diagnostic process, however. Both Ozonoff, Rogers, and Pennington (1991) and Manjiviona and Prior (1995) eliminated the criterion that AS subjects have no history of language delay, potentially resulting in symptomatic overlap between the AS and HFA samples. In addition, Szatmari et al. (1995) did not rule out autism in their AS cases, with over half the AS sample meeting full criteria for autism according to the Autism Diagnostic Interview—Revised (ADI-R). Clearly, a lack of group differentiation at the diagnostic level could cause a lack of group differentiation at the neuropsychological level.

Ghaziuddin et al. (1994) did rule out autism in their ICD-10-defined AS sample, however, and still did not find the predicted VIQ > PIQ discrepancy. There was a greater than 15-point advantage in both VIQ and PIQ in the AS group, relative to the HFA group. Three of the 11 AS subjects demonstrated VIQ scores significantly greater than their PIQ scores (defined as a split of 12 points or more; Sattler, 1992), but two displayed the opposite pattern, with PIQ significantly higher than VIQ. Similarly, in the HFA group, two (of nine) subjects demonstrated the PIQ > VIQ pattern, whereas two showed the VIQ > PIQ profile. Thus, subjects in each group demonstrated patterns thought to be characteristic of the other group.

In contrast, another recent study has found evidence of visuospatial impairment in AS (Klin et al., 1995). After reviewing the records of forty individuals with AS and HFA, raters blind to diagnosis found evidence of visual–motor integration, visual–spatial perception, nonverbal concept formation, and visual memory deficits in subjects with AS; those with HFA did not demonstrate such impairments but, rather, performed poorly on several tests of language function. In addition, individuals with AS had significantly higher VIQ than PIQ scores (the average size of the discrepancy was 23.8 points), whereas HFA subjects demonstrated Verbal and Performance IQ scores of similar magnitude. It is important that this study be replicated by an investigation that directly tests subjects using consistent measures of visuospatial and intellectual function rather than chart review methods. In addition, future studies should use standard DSM-IV or ICD-10 criteria, without an additional requirement of motor clumsiness for inclusion in the AS group. Because clumsiness and visual–spatial difficulties often co-occur (Henderson, Barnett, & Henderson, 1994; Lord & Hulme, 1987), such modifications in diagnostic criteria potentially weaken this study's evidence of external validity. Given the lack of consistency of findings and great variability in diagnostic procedures across studies, it is again not possible to make firm conclusions about the status of visuospatial impairments in AS at the present time.

THEORY OF MIND IN ASPERGER SYNDROME
AND HIGH-FUNCTIONING AUTISM

A third neuropsychological domain that has been hypothesized to distinguish AS from HFA is theory of mind (ToM). ToM describes a person's ability to think about and act on information about his or her own and others' mental states (beliefs, intentions, desires, etc.). Often a distinction is made between first- and second-order ToM. First-order ToM involves prediction of someone else's mental state, whereas second-order ToM involves recursive processing of one person's mental state about another person's mental state (e.g., "Mary thinks that John thinks that . . . "). One of the most appealing aspects of the ToM hypothesis is its potential to explain the social deficits central to autism spectrum diagnoses. Many studies have found that people with autism exhibit impairments on ToM tasks (Baron-Cohen, 1989; Baron-Cohen, Leslie, & Frith, 1985, 1986; Leslie & Frith, 1988; Perner, Frith, Leslie, & Leekam, 1989; for a review, see Happé, 1994a; Happé & Frith, 1995), and it has been hypothesized to be a core deficit of autism.

In contrast, Asperger (1944/1991), in his original description of the disorder, commented on the good perspective-taking abilities of his subjects. For example, he noted that one of the boys he studied "often surprised us with remarks that betrayed an excellent apprehension of a situation and an accurate judgment of people" (p. 45). In summarizing the features of the disorder, he reported that there was "an ability to engage in a particular kind of introspection and to be a judge of character" (p. 73). This suggests that AS individuals may demonstrate better performance on ToM tasks than do people with autism. In fact, the relatively little research that has been done on ToM skills in AS suggests that this conclusion may be accurate.

As noted previously, the strongest evidence of external validity is gathered when performance of AS and HFA groups is directly compared. A study by Ozonoff, Rogers, and Pennington (1991) is the only one of this type currently in print. A group selected for AS according to modified draft ICD-10 criteria was compared with an HFA group (as noted previously, this modification may have created overlap between the AS and HFA samples). Each sample was also compared to its own non-PDD IQ- and age-matched controls. In line with previous studies, these researchers found evidence of a ToM deficit in the HFA group when compared with appropriate controls (69% performed below the control mean on first-order ToM tasks and 100% on second-order tasks). There was no difference in performance between the AS group and its controls, however. When the direct HFA–AS comparison was made, it was discovered that the AS group performed significantly better than did the HFA group on both first- and second-order measures. These tasks also empirically distinguished the two groups in a discriminant function analysis. The authors proposed that these results provided evidence of a subtype distinction. However, a significant group difference in verbal IQ may have influenced these results. Controlling for this verbal difference attenuated the results, although marginally statistically significant group differences in ToM ability remained.

Bowler (1992) also did not find a ToM deficit in AS. This study compared a group selected for AS according to Wing's (1981) criteria with a control group consisting of socially impaired chronic schizophrenics. The groups were matched on IQ but not on chronological age. These two samples with social impairments were also compared to a "nonhandicapped group" whose background characteristics were not reported. No significant differences were found in the ability to answer key test questions in either first- or second-order ToM stories. In fact, the majority of people with AS were successful on these tasks (93% on first-order and 73% on second-order stories). Although AS subjects typically did not reference higher-order mental states in explaining their answers, neither did subjects in the two control groups.

In a small case series (Berthier, 1995), five AS subjects diagnosed according to ICD-10 criteria were compared with a nonpsychiatric group matched on chronological age and the Vocabulary subtest of the Weschler Adult Intelligence Scale. All but one AS subject performed in the normal range on first- and second-order ToM tasks. This study, although small, again demonstrates spared ToM performance in most subjects with AS.

As with the other neuropsychological domains reviewed earlier, it is difficult to summarize the findings on ToM in autism and AS. Whereas most investigations have found deficient ToM in autism and relatively better skills in AS, only one of these studies directly compared the two groups. In this study (Ozonoff, Rogers, & Pennington, 1991), AS–HFA differences in verbal intelligence may have mediated the group differences in ToM. Recently, in fact, it has been suggested that performance on ToM tasks may be highly dependent on other cognitive abilities, such as verbal skill and executive function. Several investigations of subjects with autism have demonstrated a significant association between verbal mental age and performance on ToM tasks (Eisenmajer & Prior, 1991; Happé, 1995; Ozonoff, Pennington, & Rogers, 1991; Sparrevohn & Howie, 1995; Tager-Flusberg & Sullivan, 1994). The direction of influence in this relationship has yet to be determined, however: Differences in ToM may drive the better verbal abilities of AS subjects or, conversely, ToM skills (or the tasks made to test them) may rely on good linguistic abilities. In support of the latter hypothesis, there has been speculation that subjects who do pass ToM tasks are arriving at their conclusions through more verbally mediated pathways than do nonautistic individuals (Bowler, 1992; Happé, 1995). Because current diagnostic criteria distinguish AS from autism on the basis of language skills, a strong correlation between verbal skills and ToM mitigates the evidence for external validity from this neuropsychological domain.

It has also been proposed that a deficit in executive function underlies the deficits found on ToM tasks (Ozonoff, Pennington, & Rogers, 1991b; Tager-Flusberg & Sullivan, 1994). Russell and colleagues have demonstrated that when the perspective-taking component of ToM tasks is removed but the need to shift set (an executive function) is retained, people with autism continue to be impaired (Hughes & Russell, 1993; Russell, Mauthner,

Sharpe, & Tidswell, 1991). Whether executive function skills can differentiate between autism and AS is explored in the next section. What is relevant here, however, is that if ToM is driven by executive function, it is not a core deficit of either disorder but, rather, a secondary symptom. As discussed previously, if two subtypes demonstrate similar primary symptoms, even if they differ in associated characteristics, there is little evidence for their external validity (Pennington, 1991; Rapin, 1987).

EXECUTIVE FUNCTIONS IN ASPERGER SYNDROME AND HIGH-FUNCTIONING AUTISM

Recent research has suggested that an executive function deficit may underlie symptoms of autism. Executive function (EF) is a broadly defined cognitive construct originally used to describe the deficits found in patients with focal frontal lobe lesions. It refers to the many skills required to prepare for and execute complex behavior, including planning, inhibition, mental flexibility, and mental representation of tasks and goals. Measures commonly thought to tap these abilities include the Wisconsin Card Sorting Test, the Tower of Hanoi, and the Windows task. Executive dysfunction has been consistently found across different ages and ability levels of people with autism when compared with appropriate controls (Ozonoff, Pennington, & Rogers, 1991; Prior & Hoffmann, 1990; Rumsey, 1985; Rumsey & Hamburger, 1988, 1990; Russell et al., 1991; for a review, see Ozonoff, 1995; Pennington & Ozonoff, 1996). Thus, in Meehl's (1973a) terms, the probability of this symptom is high given a diagnosis of autism. Their status as "diagnostic bell ringers" is limited, however, by some lack of specificity to the autism spectrum. EF deficits have been found in a variety of other conditions, including attention-deficit/hyperactivity disorder, obsessive–compulsive disorder, schizophrenia, and various dementias (see Ozonoff, 1997, for a review of this topic). However, the EF impairment of autism does appear to be more severe, of a different type, and of different onset than the EF deficits of other disorders (Pennington & Ozonoff, 1996), providing some specificity for the sign as well.

Given the interest in this domain as a potential core neuropsychological deficit of autism spectrum conditions, there have been surprisingly few studies of the EF skills of AS individuals. One recent study (Berthier, 1995) found that AS subjects performed less well than normal controls on the Wisconsin Card Sorting Test, the Tower of Hanoi, and the Road Map Test; no comparison to autism was made, however. The Ozonoff, Rogers, and Pennington (1991) study discussed in previous sections did directly compare performance on EF tasks in AS and HFA subjects. They found that both groups performed significantly more poorly than their respective controls on the Wisconsin Card Sorting Test and the Tower of Hanoi. Some 100% of the HFA subjects and 90% of the AS group performed below their respective control means on the EF tests. There was no significant difference in the performance of the two groups. These authors concluded that EF was a common deficit shared by all autism spectrum disorders and that performance in this domain did not discriminate between AS and HFA. However, as noted earlier, the modified diagnostic criteria used in this study may have made null results more likely.

Szatmari et al. (1990) examined a group of AS subjects diagnosed according to adapted Wing (1981) criteria, a group of HFA subjects, and a group of outpatient controls with a variety of social difficulties. The AS and HFA groups were matched to each other on IQ, but the HFA group was on average 9 years older than the AS group. In addition, the outpatient controls had significantly higher IQ scores than did both of the other groups. On the Wisconsin Card Sorting Test, the HFA group made significantly more perseverative errors than did the outpatient control group; their performance was, on average, 2 standard deviations worse than that of controls. The AS group also performed more poorly than did the control group on these measures (an average of 1 standard deviation worse), but this group difference was not statistically significant. Most important, when the performance of the HFA and AS groups was directly compared, no significant difference in their performance was found. Whereas a discriminant function analysis indicated that the Wisconsin variables, in addition to two motor variables, best discriminated between the AS and HFA groups, the classification matrix incorrectly classified one-third of each group. In light of the mixed results, the authors decided that EF was not a discriminant factor between the two groups. They concluded that AS was "a very mild form of PDD where the cognitive profiles are virtually identical to autism, suggesting similar deficits in brain organization" (Szatmari et al., 1990, p. 136).

On the whole, there appears to be support for the idea that EF deficits are found across the autistic spectrum. Firm conclusions about EF deficits across the autistic continuum, however, must await future research that carefully uses standardized diagnostic criteria, without modifications, so that the rate of Type II errors (e.g., failing to find group differences that truly exist) is not inflated.

CONCLUSIONS

This chapter examined the neuropsychological evidence that AS is distinct from higher-functioning forms of autism. Although a number of relevant studies have been conducted, the definitive information necessary to make such a determination is not yet available. First, the empirical data are quite mixed, with some studies supporting a distinction between the two disorders and others finding no evidence of a distinction. In addition, few studies reviewed here satisfied the criterion for external validity that the dependent variables be distinct from the group definition process. Of those that did, most investigations remained difficult to interpret due to study-specific modifications in the diagnostic criteria for AS. In many investigations, it was not clear that distinct, mutually exclusive groups were studied; in particular, how autism was ruled out in AS cases was not always obvious. In some studies, there was evidence that the AS group overlapped symptomatically with the autistic sample, increasing the likelihood of Type II errors (failing to find group differences that truly exist) and making the interpretation of results, especially null results, exceedingly challenging. Sadly, more than half a century since the initial descriptions of these conditions, few conclusions about the external validity of AS, as distinct from autism, can yet be made. Until the field surmounts the methodological difficulties just described, it would be as premature to rule out the validity of AS as it would be to treat it as an entity clearly distinguishable from classic autism.

The most consistent evidence of an empirical distinction between AS and autism came from the ToM domain. However, it has been suggested that the well-developed verbal skills of AS may mediate this effect. Several studies have demonstrated a high correlation between verbal mental age and ToM performance (Eisenmajer & Prior, 1991; Ozonoff, Pennington, & Rogers, 1991; Sparrevohn & Howie, 1995; Tager-Flusberg & Sullivan, 1994). Because AS is defined in part by a normal early history of language acquisition and is generally associated with higher VIQ than autism, group differences in ToM may reflect nothing more than the superior verbal abilities of AS. This highlights the difficulty researchers studying external validity face: Even domains that were not used to originally define the groups may be highly correlated with domains that were used in the diagnostic process, rendering them relatively less informative to the external validity question.

It has been suggested that AS may be no more than high-IQ autism. Of the nine investigations reviewed in this chapter that directly compared individuals with AS to those with autism, four found overall IQ or mental age differences (Eisenmajer et al., 1996; Ghaziuddin et al., 1994; Manjiviona & Prior, 1995; Szatmari et al., 1995), whereas five had groups matched on overall IQ (Gillberg, 1989; Klin et al., 1995; Ozonoff, Rogers, & Pennington, 1991; Szatmari, Bartolucci, & Bremner, 1989; Szatmari et al., 1990). Of those finding no IQ differences, two reported a significant VIQ advantage in the AS group (Klin et al., 1995; Ozonoff, Rogers, & Pennington, 1991), two others provided no breakdown of the overall IQ score (Gillberg, 1989; Szatmari, Bartolucci, & Bremner, 1989), and only one found no significant Verbal or Performance IQ differences between the groups. Thus, of the seven investigations with informative data, there was evidence of some type of IQ superiority in the AS group in six. Indeed, it may be difficult to match AS and HFA on IQ, as IQ may capture something fundamental about the difference between the two disorders. The diagnostic criteria for AS mandates normal intellectual functioning. Although IQ, by definition, also falls above the re-tarded range in individuals with high-functioning autism, there is still room for group variation. It may be the case, for example, that the mean Full Scale IQ of people with HFA is significantly lower than that of people with AS. This is an empirical question that is easily addressed (using, of course, strictly defined, nonoverlapping samples with no modifications in diagnos-tic criteria). If this possibility is borne out, the high correlation between IQ and most neuropsychological measures will make it critical that intellectual level always be covaried in future investigations. This will permit research-ers to determine whether AS–HFA neuropsychological differences are pri-mary or are only secondary to preexisting IQ differences.

This chapter focused on group differentiation based on neuropsycholo-gical characteristics. It is certainly possible that evidence of external validity will be provided from other domains, and research in these areas is urgently needed. For example, AS and HFA may differ in terms of the treatment each requires. Or, they may differ in their developmental courses and outcomes, as suggested by a recent study (Szatmari, Bartolucci, & Bremner, 1989). Finally, AS and autism may differ in their underlying neuropathology. The proposed visual–spatial deficits of AS individuals, as well as their difficul-ties producing and interpreting facial expressions, gestures, and prosody (Fine, Bartolucci, Ginsberg, & Szatmari, 1991; Kracke, 1994; Scott, 1985; Tantam, Holmes, & Cordess, 1993), have led to the hypothesis that the right hemisphere is dysfunctional in AS (Denckla, 1983; Goodman, 1989; Klin et al., 1995; McKelvey, Lambert, Mottron, & Shevell, 1995; Molina et al., 1986). Conversely, lateralization work has suggested that the left hemisphere is damaged in autism (Chiron et al., 1995; Dawson, Warrenburg, & Fuller, 1982; Goodman, 1989; Prior, 1979). This suggests a very appealing hypothesis, namely, that AS and HFA result from different patterns of unilateral brain dysfunction.

Unfortunately, however, this right-hemisphere–left-hemisphere dichot-omy does not account for all data (Fein, Humes, Kaplan, Lucci, & Water-house, 1984). First, it has long been evident that classically autistic children exhibit deficits typically considered right hemisphere in origin: For example, they too demonstrate deficits in prosody (Klin et al., 1995) and production and interpretation of facial expression and gesture (Davies, Bishop, Manstead, & Tantam, 1994; Loveland et al., 1994; MacDonald et al., 1989). Second, re-cent studies have documented left-hemisphere damage in AS (El-Badri & Lewis, 1993; Jones & Kerwin, 1990). Therefore, it is too early to conclude that there is evidence of external validity for AS at the neurological level either.

We end this chapter with suggestions for future researchers. The most pressing need in AS research is adoption of a standard set of criteria for making this diagnosis. Many different diagnostic systems were used across the studies presented in this chapter, making interstudy comparisons diffi-cult if not impossible. When samples are ascertained under different diagnostic systems, we cannot be certain of cross-sample agreement on who should be classified as AS. The first step in identifying core cognitive deficits and biological causes of any disorder is to establish clean diagnostic boundaries that can be used reliably to identify homogeneous groups for study. Particularly critical are clear guidelines for how autism is excluded in individuals with AS, whether autism or AS took precedence in the differential diagnostic process, and whether the two groups being studied were truly independent and nonoverlapping conditions.

Future studies should employ research designs in which a variety of different neuropsychological processes are compared in the same samples of AS and HFA individuals. This technique allows researchers to discriminate between diagnostic groups on the basis of differences in profiles of strength and weakness. External validity relies on demonstration of group by task interactions or double dissociations (Fletcher, 1985), with the AS group outperforming the HFA group in some areas but experiencing difficulty relative to them in other domains. Group main effects (e.g., AS outperforming HFA on all tasks) do not constitute good evidence for external validity. Instead, this suggests that AS is similar to autism, differing in severity but not in the essential nature of the disability. If the groups are qualitatively similar, with only quantitative intergroup distinctions, the wisdom of retaining different labels would be questionable. One caution that must be applied with this approach, however, is that the probability of Type I errors (e.g., finding "significant" group differences based on chance alone) increases as the number of comparisons increases. Finally, future research needs to carefully consider the choice of control group and the variables on which to match them. This has proven to be a difficult task when comparing HFA and AS, due to the differences in intelligence, particularly Verbal IQ, found in many studies. More than one control group may be required for adequate comparisons. We hope these methodological improvements will further advance research in this field and provide answers to the many questions that remain.

ACKNOWLEDGMENTS

We would like to thank Judith Miller and Bruce Pennington for their contributions to the work cited in this chapter. Sally Ozonoff was supported in part by a FIRST Award during the writing of this Chapter (No. MH52229) and Elizabeth McMahon Griffith was supported by an NRSA predoctoral fellowship (No. MH11127).

REFERENCES

American Psychiatric Association. (1994). *Diagnostic and statistical manual of mental disorders* (4th ed.). Washington, DC: Author.
Asarnow, R. F., Tanguay, P. E., Bott, L., & Freeman, B. J. (1987). Patterns of intellectual

functioning in non-retarded autistic and schizophrenic children. *Journal of Child Psychology and Psychiatry, 28,* 273–280.

Asperger, H. (1991). "Autistic psychopathy" in childhood. (U. Frith, Trans., Annot.). In U. Frith (Ed.), *Autism and Asperger syndrome* (pp. 37–92). New York: Cambridge University Press. (Original work published 1944)

Baron-Cohen, S. (1988). An assessment of violence in a young man with Asperger's syndrome. *Journal of Child Psychology and Psychiatry, 29,* 351–360.

Baron-Cohen, S. (1989). The autistic child's theory of mind: A case of specific developmental delay. *Journal of Child Psychology and Psychiatry, 30,* 285–297.

Baron-Cohen, S., Leslie, A. M., & Frith, U. (1985). Does the autistic child have a "theory of mind"? *Cognition, 21,* 37–46.

Baron-Cohen, S., Leslie, A. M., & Frith, U. (1986). Mechanical, behavioural and intentional understanding of picture stories in autistic children. *British Journal of Developmental Psychology, 4,* 113–125.

Berthier, M. L. (1995). Hypomania following bereavement in Asperger's syndrome: A case study. *Neuropsychiatry, Neuropsychology, and Behavioral Neurology, 8,* 222–228.

Bowler, D. M. (1992). "Theory of Mind" in Asperger's syndrome. *Journal of Child Psychology and Psychiatry, 33,* 877–893.

Burgoine, E., & Wing, L. (1983). Identical triplets with Asperger's syndrome. *British Journal of Psychiatry, 143,* 261–265.

Chiron, C., Leboyer, M., Leon, F., Jambaque, I., Nuttin, C., & Syrota, A. (1995). SPECT of the brain in childhood autism: Evidence for a lack of normal hemispheric asymmetry. *Developmental Medicine and Child Neurology, 37,* 849–860.

Damasio, A. R., & Maurer, R. G. (1978). A neurological model for childhood autism. *Archives of Neurology, 35,* 777–786.

Davies, S., Bishop, D., Manstead, A. S. R., & Tantam, D. (1994). Face perception in children with autism and Asperger's syndrome. *Journal of Child Psychology and Psychiatry, 35,* 1033–1057.

Dawson, G., Warrenburg, S., & Fuller, P. (1982). Cerebral lateralization in individuals diagnosed as autistic in early childhood. *Brain and Language, 15,* 353–368.

DeMyer, M. K. (1979). *Parents and children in autism.* Washington, DC: Winston.

DeMyer, M. K., Barton, S., & Norton, J. A. (1972). A comparison of adaptive, verbal and motor profiles of psychotic and non-psychotic subnormal children. *Journal of Autism and Childhood Schizophrenia, 2,* 359–377.

Denckla, M. B. (1983). The neuropsychology of social–emotional learning disabilities. *Archives of Neurology, 40,* 461–462.

Eisenmajer, R., & Prior, M. (1991). Cognitive linguistic correlates of theory of mind ability in autistic children. *British Journal of Developmental Psychology, 9,* 351–364.

Eisenmajer, R., Prior, M., Leekam, S., Wing, L., Gould, J., Welham, M., & Ong, B. (1996). Comparison of clinical symptoms in autism and Asperger's disorder. *Journal of the American Academy of Child and Adolescent Psychiatry, 35,* 1523–1531.

El-Badri, S. M., & Lewis, M. A. (1993). Left hemisphere and cerebellar damage in Asperger's syndrome. *Irish Journal of Psychological Medicine, 10,* 22–23.

Fein, D., Humes, M., Kaplan, E., Lucci, D., & Waterhouse, L. (1984). The question of left hemisphere dysfunction in infantile autism. *Psychological Bulletin, 95,* 258–281.

Fein, D., Waterhouse, L., Lucci, D., & Snyder, D. (1985). Cognitive subtypes in developmentally disabled children: A pilot study. *Journal of Autism and Developmental Disorders, 15,* 77–95.

Fine, J., Bartolucci, G., Ginsberg, G., & Szatmari, P. (1991). The use of intonation to communicate in pervasive developmental disorders. *Journal of Child Psychology and Psychiatry, 32,* 771–782.

Fletcher, J. M. (1985). External validation of learning disability typologies. In B. P. Rourke (Ed.), *Neuropsychology of learning disabilities: Essentials of subtype analysis* (pp. 187–211). New York: Guilford Press.

Freeman, B. J., Lucas, J. C., Forness, S. R., & Ritvo, E. R. (1985). Cognitive processing of high-functioning autistic children: Comparing the K-ABC and the WISC-R. *Journal of Psychoeducational Assessment, 4,* 357–362.

Frith, U. (1993). Autism. *Scientific American, 268,* 108–114.

Ghaziuddin, M., Butler, E., Tsai, L. Y., & Ghaziuddin, N. (1994). Is clumsiness a marker for Asperger syndrome? *Journal of Intellectual Disability Research, 38,* 519–527.

Ghaziuddin, M., Tsai, L. Y., & Ghaziuddin, N. (1992a). A comparison of the diagnostic criteria for Asperger syndrome. *Journal of Autism and Developmental Disorders, 22,* 643–649.

Ghaziuddin, M., Tsai, L. Y., & Ghaziuddin, N. (1992b). A reappraisal of clumsiness as a diagnostic feature of Asperger syndrome. *Journal of Autism and Developmental Disorders, 22,* 651–656.

Gillberg, C. (1989). Asperger syndrome in 23 Swedish children. *Developmental Medicine and Child Neurology, 31,* 520–531.

Gillberg, C. (1991). Clinical and neurobiological aspects of Asperger syndrome in six family studies. In U. Frith (Ed.), *Autism and Asperger syndrome* (pp. 122–146). New York: Cambridge University Press.

Gillberg, I. C., & Gillberg, C. (1989). Asperger syndrome: Some epidemiological considerations. *Journal of Child Psychology and Psychiatry, 30,* 631–638.

Goodman, R. (1989). Infantile autism: A syndrome of multiple primary deficits? *Journal of Autism and Developmental Disorders, 19,* 409–424.

Grandin, T. (1995). How people with autism think. In E. Schopler & G. B. Mesibov (Eds.), *Learning and cognition in autism* (pp. 137–156). New York: Plenum.

Green, J. (1990). Annotation: Is Asperger's a syndrome? *Developmental Medicine and Child Neurology, 32,* 743–747.

Green, L., Fein, D., Joy, S., & Waterhouse, L. (1995). Cognitive functioning in autism: An overview. In E. Schopler & G. B. Mesibov (Eds.), *Learning and cognition in autism* (pp. 13–31). New York: Plenum.

Hallett, M., Lebiedowska, M. K., Thomas, S. L., Stanhope, S. J., Denckla, M. B., & Rumsey, J. (1993). Locomotion of autistic adults. *Archives of Neurology, 50,* 1304–1308.

Happé, F. G. E. (1994a). Current psychological theories of autism: The "theory of mind" account and rival theories. *Journal of Child Psychology and Psychiatry, 35,* 215–229.

Happé, F. G. E. (1994b). Wechsler IQ profile and theory of mind in autism. *Journal of Child Psychology and Psychiatry, 35,* 1461–1471.

Happé, F. G. E. (1995). The role of age and verbal ability in the theory of mind task performance of subjects with autism. *Child Development, 66,* 843–855.

Happé, F., & Frith, U. (1991). Debate and argument: How useful is the PDD label? *Journal of Child Psychology and Psychiatry, 32,* 1167–1168.

Happé, F., & Frith, U. (1995). Theory of mind in autism. In E. Schopler & G. B. Mesibov (Eds.), *Learning and cognition in autism* (pp. 177–197). New York: Plenum.

Henderson, S. E., Barnett, A., & Henderson, L. (1994). Visuospatial difficulties and clumsiness: On the interpretation of conjoined deficits. *Journal of Child Psychology and Psychiatry, 35,* 961–969.

Hughes, C., & Russell, J. (1993). Autistic children's difficulty with mental disengagement from an object: Its implications for theories of autism. *Developmental Psychology, 29,* 498–510.

Hughes, C., Russell, J., & Robbins, T. W. (1994). Evidence for executive dysfunction in autism. *Neuropsychologia, 32,* 477–492.

Jones, P. B., & Kerwin, R. W. (1990). Left temporal lobe damage in Asperger's syndrome. *British Journal of Psychiatry, 156,* 570–572.

Jones, V., & Prior, M. (1985). Motor imitation abilities and neurological signs in autistic children. *Journal of Autism and Developmental Disorders, 15,* 37–46.

Kanner, L. (1943). Autistic disturbances of affective contact. *Nervous Child, 2,* 217–250.

Kerbeshian, J., Burd, L., & Fisher, W. (1990). Asperger's syndrome: To be or not to be? *British Journal of Psychiatry, 156,* 721–725.

Klin, A. (1994). Asperger syndrome. *Child and Adolescent Psychiatric Clinics of North America, 3,* 131–148.

Klin, A., Volkmar, F. R., Sparrow, S. S., Cicchetti, D. V., & Rourke, B. P. (1995). Validity and neuropsychological characterization of Asperger syndrome. *Journal of Child Psychology and Psychiatry, 36,* 1127–1140.

Kolb, B., & Taylor, L. (1981). Affective behavior in patients with localized cortical excision: Role of lesion site and side. *Science, 214,* 89–90.

Kracke, I. (1994). Developmental prosopagnosia in Asperger syndrome: Presentation and discussion of an individual case. *Developmental Medicine and Child Neurology, 36,* 873–886.

Leary, M. R., & Hill, D. A. (1996). Moving on: Autism and movement disturbance. *Mental Retardation, 34,* 39–53.

Leslie, A. M., & Frith, U. (1988). Autistic children's understanding of seeing, knowing and believing. *British Journal of Developmental Psychology, 6,* 315–324.

Lincoln, A. J., Allen, M. H., & Kilman, A. (1995). The assessment and interpretation of intellectual abilities in people with autism. In E. Schopler & G. B. Mesibov (Eds.), *Learning and cognition in autism* (pp. 89–117). New York: Plenum.

Lincoln, A. J., Courchesne, E., Kilman, B. A., Elmasian, R., & Allen, M. (1988). A study of intellectual abilities in high-functioning people with autism. *Journal of Autism and Developmental Disorders, 18,* 505–524.

Lord, R., & Hulme, C. (1987). Perceptual judgments of normal and clumsy children. *Developmental Medicine and Child Neurology, 29,* 250–257.

Loveland, K. A., Tunali-Kotoski, B., Pearson, D. A., Brelsford, K. A., Ortegon, J., & Chen, R. (1994). Imitation and expression of facial affect in autism. *Development and Psychopathology, 6,* 433–444.

MacDonald, H., Rutter, M., Howlin, P., Rios, P., Le Couteur, A., Evered, C., & Folstein, S. (1989). Recognition and expression of emotional cues by autistic and normal adults. *Journal of Child Psychology and Psychiatry, 30,* 865–877.

Manjiviona, J., & Prior, M. (1995). Comparison of Asperger syndrome and high-functioning autistic children on a test of motor impairment. *Journal of Autism and Developmental Disorder, 25,* 23–39.

McKelvey, J. R., Lambert, R., Mottron, L., & Shevell, M. I. (1995). Right hemisphere dysfunction in Asperger's syndrome. *Journal of Child Neurology, 10,* 310–314.

Meehl, P. E. (1973a). Some ruminations on the validation of clinical procedures. *Psychodiagnosis: Selected papers* (pp. 90–116). Minneapolis: University of Minnesota Press.

Meehl, P. E. (1973b). Schizotaxia, schizotypy, schizophrenia. *Psychodiagnosis: Selected papers* (pp. 135–155). Minneapolis: University of Minnesota Press.

Miyahara, M., Tsujii, M., Hori, M., Nakanishi, K., Kageyama, H., & Sugiyama, T. (1997). Motor incoordination in children with Asperger syndrome and learning disabilities. *Journal of Autism and Developmental Disorders, 27,* 595–603.

Molina, J. D., Ruata, J. M., & Soler, E. P. (1986). Is there a right-hemisphere dysfunction in Asperger's syndrome? *British Journal of Psychiatry, 148,* 745–746.

Morin, B., & Reid, G. (1985). A quantitative and qualitative assessment of autistic individuals on selected motor tasks. *Adapted Physical Activity Quarterly, 2,* 43–55.

Ornitz, E. M., Guthrie, D., & Farley, A. H. (1977). The early development of autistic children. *Journal of Autism and Childhood Schizophrenia, 7,* 207–229.

Ozonoff, S. (1995). Executive functions in autism. In E. Schopler & G. B. Mesibov (Eds.), *Learning and cognition in autism* (pp. 199–219). New York: Plenum.

Ozonoff, S. (1997). Components of executive function in autism and other disorders. In J. Russell (Ed.), *Autism as an executive disorder* (pp. 179–211). New York: Oxford University Press.

Ozonoff, S., Pennington, B. F., & Rogers, S. J. (1991). Executive function deficits in high-functioning autistic individuals: Relationship to theory of mind. *Journal of Child Psychology and Psychiatry, 32,* 1081–1105.

Ozonoff, S., Rogers, S., & Pennington, B. F. (1991). Asperger's syndrome: Evidence of an empirical distinction from high-functioning autism. *Journal of Child Psychology and Psychiatry, 32,* 1107–1122.

Paul, R., & Cohen, D. J. (1984). Outcomes of severe disorders of language acquisition. *Journal of Autism and Developmental Disorders, 14,* 405–421.

Pennington, B. F. (1991). *Diagnosing learning disorders: A neuropsychological framework.* New York: Guilford Press.

Pennington, B. F., & Ozonoff, S. (1991). A neuroscientific perspective on continuity and discontinuity in developmental psychopathology. In D. Cicchetti & S. L. Toth (Eds.), *Rochester symposium on developmental psychopathology (Vol. 3): Models and integrations* (pp. 117–159). Rochester, NY: University of Rochester Press.

Pennington, B. F., & Ozonoff, S. (1996). Executive functions and developmental psychopathologies. *Journal of Child Psychology and Psychiatry, 37,* 51–87.

Perner, J., Frith, U., Leslie, A. M., & Leekam, S. R. (1989). Exploration of the autistic child's theory of mind: Knowledge, belief, and communication. *Child Development, 60,* 689–700.

Prior, M. R. (1979). Cognitive abilities and disabilities in infantile autism: A review. *Journal of Abnormal Child Psychology, 7,* 357–380.

Prior, M. R., & Hoffman, W. (1990). Neuropsychological testing of autistic children through an exploration with frontal lobe tests. *Journal of Autism and Developmental Disorders, 20,* 581–590.

Rapin, I. (1987). Searching for the cause of autism: A neurologic perspective. In D. J. Cohen & A. M. Donnellan (Eds.), *Handbook of autism and pervasive developmental disorders* (pp. 710–717). New York: Wiley.

Ross, E. D., & Mesulam, M. M. (1979). Dominant language functions of the right hemisphere? Prosody and emotional gesturing. *Archives of Neurology, 36,* 144–148.

Rourke, B. P. (1989). *Nonverbal learning disabilities: The syndrome and the model*. New York: Guilford Press.

Rumsey, J. M. (1985). Conceptual problem-solving in highly verbal, nonretarded autistic men. *Journal of Autism and Developmental Disorders, 15*, 23–36.

Rumsey, J. M., & Hamburger, S. D. (1988). Neuropsychological findings in high-functioning autistic men with infantile autism, residual state. *Journal of Clinical and Experimental Neuropsychology, 10*, 201–221.

Rumsey, J. M., & Hamburger, S. D. (1990). Neuropsychological divergence of high-level autism and severe dyslexia. *Journal of Autism and Developmental Disorders, 20*, 155–168.

Russell, J., Mauthner, N., Sharpe, S., & Tidswell, T. (1991). The "windows task" as a measure of strategic deception in preschoolers and autistic subjects. *British Journal of Developmental Psychology, 9*, 331–349.

Rutter, M., Greenfield, D., & Lockyer, L. (1967). A five- to fifteen-year follow-up study of infantile psychosis: Social and behavioral outcome. *British Journal of Psychiatry, 113*, 1183–1199.

Rutter, M., Mawhood, L., & Howlin, P. (1992). Language delay and social development. In P. Fletcher & D. Hale (Eds.), *Specific speech and language disorders in children* (pp. 63–78). London: Whurr.

Sattler, J. M. (1992). *Assessment of children: Revised and updated third edition.* San Diego: Author.

Schopler, E. (1985). Convergence of learning disability, higher-level autism and Asperger's syndrome. *Journal of Autism and Developmental Disorders, 15*, 359.

Schopler, E. (1996). Are autism and Asperger syndrome different labels or different disabilities? *Journal of Autism and Developmental Disorders, 26*, 109–110.

Schopler, E. (1998). Premature popularization of Asperger syndrome. In E. Schopler, G. B. Mesibov, & L. Kunce (Eds.), *Asperger syndrome or high-functioning autism?* New York: Plenum.

Scott, D. W. (1985). Asperger's syndrome and nonverbal communication: A pilot study. *Psychological Medicine, 15*, 683–687.

Shah, A., & Frith, U. (1983). An islet of ability in autistic children. *Journal of Child Psychology and Psychiatry, 24*, 613–620.

Shah, A., & Frith, U. (1993). Why do autistic individuals show superior performance on the block design task? *Journal of Child Psychology and Psychiatry, 34*, 1351–1364.

Sparrevohn, R., & Howie, P. M. (1995). Theory of mind in children with autistic disorder: Evidence of developmental progression and the role of verbal ability. *Journal of Child Psychology and Psychiatry, 36*, 249–263.

Stiles-Davis, J., Kritchevsky, M., & Bellugi, U. (1988). *Spatial cognition and brain bases and development.* Hillsdale, NJ: Erlbaum.

Szatmari, P., Archer, L., Fisman, S., Streiner, D. L., & Wilson, F. (1995). Asperger's syndrome and autism: Differences in behavior, cognition, and adaptive functioning. *Journal of the American Academy of Child and Adolescent Psychiatry, 34*, 1662–1671.

Szatmari, P., Bartolucci, G., & Bremner, R. (1989). Asperger's syndrome and autism: Comparison of early history and outcome. *Developmental Medicine and Child Neurology, 31*, 709–720.

Szatmari, P., Bremner, R., & Nagy, J. (1989). Asperger's syndrome: A review of clinical features. *Canadian Journal of Psychiatry, 34*, 554–560.

Szatmari, P., Tuff, L., Finlayson, M. A. J., & Bartolucci, G. (1990). Asperger's syndrome and autism: Neurocognitive aspects. *Journal of the American Academy of Child and Adolescent Psychiatry, 29,* 130–136.

Tager-Flusberg, H., & Sullivan, K. (1994). Predicting and explaining behavior: A comparison of autistic, mentally retarded, and normal children. *Journal of Child Psychology and Psychiatry, 35,* 1059–1075.

Tantam, D. (1988). Asperger's syndrome. *Journal of Child Psychology and Psychiatry, 29,* 245–255.

Tantam, D. (1991). Asperger syndrome in adulthood. In U. Frith (Ed.), *Autism and Asperger syndrome* (pp. 147–183). New York: Cambridge University Press.

Tantam, D., Holmes, D., & Cordess, C. (1993). Nonverbal expression in autism of the Asperger type. *Journal of Autism and Developmental Disorders, 23,* 111–133.

Tranel, D., Hall, L. E., Olson, S., & Tranel, N. N. (1987). Evidence for a right-hemisphere developmental learning disability. *Developmental Neuropsychology, 3,* 113–127.

Tucker, D. M., Watson, R. T., & Heilman, K. M. (1977). Discrimination and evocation of affectively intoned speech in patients with right parietal disease. *Neurology, 27,* 947–950.

Voeller, K. K. S. (1986). Right-hemisphere deficit syndrome in children. *American Journal of Psychiatry, 143,* 1004–1009.

Volkmar, F. R., Klin, A., Schultz, R., Bronen, R., Marans, W. D., Sparrow, S., & Cohen, D. (1996). Clinical conference: Asperger's syndrome. *Journal of the American Academy of Child and Adolescent Psychiatry, 35,* 118–123.

Weintraub, S., & Mesulam, M. M. (1983). Developmental learning disabilities of the right hemisphere: Emotional, interpersonal and cognitive components. *Archives of Neurology, 40,* 463–468.

Weintraub, S., Mesulam, M. M., & Kramer, L. (1981). Disturbances in prosody: A right hemisphere contribution to language. *Archives of Neurology, 38,* 742–744.

Wing, L. (1981). Asperger's syndrome: A clinical account. *Psychological Medicine, 11,* 115–129.

Wing, L. (1986). Clarification on Asperger's syndrome. *Journal of Autism and Developmental Disorders, 16,* 513–515.

Wing, L. (1991). The relationship between Asperger's syndrome and Kanner's autism. In U. Frith (Ed.), *Autism and Asperger syndrome* (pp. 93–121). New York: Cambridge University Press.

World Health Organization. (1992). *International classification of diseases and disorders* (draft 10th ed.). Geneva: Author.

3

Motor Functioning in Asperger Syndrome

ISABEL M. SMITH

This chapter has two related purposes. The first is to address the usefulness of motoric features in the differentiation of behavioral phenotypes within the autistic spectrum. In the context of this volume, the relationship between Asperger syndrome (AS) and high-functioning autism (HFA; more prototypical autism accompanied by near-normal IQ) is particularly salient. It has been asserted that motor incoordination (or "clumsiness") might differentiate AS from HFA; the evidence for this claim has been succinctly criticized by Ghaziuddin, Tsai, and Ghaziuddin (1992). The first section of this chapter expands some of their arguments and provides an updated view, emphasizing the methodological and conceptual limitations of this literature.

The second purpose, and the main thrust of this chapter, however, is to argue for a different approach to the investigation of motor functioning in AS and other autistic spectrum disorders. This suggested approach would differ both by considering a wider range of clearly defined motor behaviors and by examining them across the spectrum of autistic disorders. The fundamental recommendation is that investigators adopt a more analytical approach to motor functions in autism.

The position is taken here that motor and perceptual–motor functions are of potential importance in understanding autistic spectrum disorders (Smith & Bryson, 1994). Given the range and complexity of motor phenomena associated with autism and related disorders (Damasio & Maurer, 1978; Jones & Prior, 1985; Smith & Bryson, 1994; DeMyer, 1976), it seems unlikely that a simplistic approach (e.g., "clumsy" vs. "not clumsy") could capture the variability within the autistic spectrum. Instead, an approach is suggested that emphasizes the component processes underlying skilled motor behavior (cf. Henderson, 1987). This alternative view has the potential to contribute not only to issues of diagnosis and subtyping but also to more fundamental questions about the etiology as well as the cognitive and behavioral deficits of autism (Smith, 1996; Smith & Bryson, 1994).

"CLUMSINESS" IN ASPERGER SYNDROME

Ghaziuddin et al. (1992) reviewed 42 papers on AS to determine the empirical status of the claim that clumsiness is particularly characteristic of AS. Their review revealed a number of critical deficiencies in this literature, principal among which was the lack of any attempt to define operationally the concept of clumsiness. Given this, it is not surprising that the assessment of clumsiness was also a major shortcoming of the studies reviewed. Ghaziuddin et al. (1992) also highlighted the importance of considering such factors as age and intellectual level in the evaluation of clumsiness.

Ghaziuddin et al. (1992) identified four studies of AS that incorporated measures of clumsiness (or, conversely, of motor ability) (Gillberg, 1989; Szatmari, Bartolucci, & Bremner, 1989; Szatmari, Tuff, Finlayson, & Bartolucci, 1990; Tantam, 1988b). Two additional studies (Manjiviona & Prior, 1995; Klin, Volkmar, Sparrow, Cicchetti, & Rourke, 1995) recently contributed data that address this issue.

One of Ghaziuddin et al.'s (1992) most fundamental criticisms was that no two studies had used exactly the same diagnostic criteria for AS. Unfortunately, this remains the case. The thorny issues related to inclusionary and exclusionary criteria for AS, especially its distinction from HFA, have been discussed elsewhere in this volume (see Chapter 2). For the purposes of this discussion, however, it is important to highlight the point that motor features undoubtedly will covary with other controversial characteristics of AS (e.g., whether or not a history of early language delay, mental retardation, or indeed classic autism precludes a diagnosis of AS). With every difference in selection criteria, the possibility exists of multiple implications for other domains of functioning.

This discussion of the evidence that motor features might distinguish AS and HFA is presented first in terms of the variations in diagnostic criteria used in the six studies cited previously. Following this comparison, the actual measures of motor skill employed in these studies are contrasted, and the limitations of the findings are reviewed.

Motor Features in Diagnostic Criteria for Asperger Syndrome

When Wing (1981) brought Asperger's work to the English-language literature, problems with motor coordination were identified as a major characteristic of AS. Indeed, the four case histories in Asperger's original paper all described individuals whose movements were awkward (Asperger, 1944/1991). Wing's paper contributed a summary of the characteristics of 34 cases that she had diagnosed based on Asperger's descriptions of the syndrome. Of these, 90% were "poor at games involving motor skills, and sometimes the executive problems affect the ability to write or to draw" (p. 116).

Several important points may be illustrated with reference to Wing's (1981) paper. First, whereas she considered the association with poor motor coordination to be noteworthy, Wing clearly did not consider clumsiness a *necessary* condition for the AS diagnosis (given that 10% of the reported cases were not motorically impaired). Second, although gross motor skills were very frequently affected, fine motor (or more specifically, graphomotor) skill deficits were also sometimes observed (as was also true of Asperger's own cases). Thus, the manifestations of "clumsiness" were heterogeneous. Indeed, Wing (1988; Wing & Attwood, 1987) has held that a variety of motoric dysfunctions exist in individuals with autistic spectrum disorders. For example, Wing (1981) contrasted the poor coordination of "posture, gait and gestures" often observed in AS, with the early presentation of "classic" autism, which was typically associated with relative strength in balance and in gross motor skills such as climbing. However, she also emphasized developmental aspects of autistic symptoms, noting that her clinical experience (supported by the observations of DeMyer, 1979) was that the agility of some children with autism waned with age. That is, by adolescence, the physical presentations of children with HFA and AS might well be indistinguishable. The differential association of clumsiness with AS might then be diagnostically useful only in the early presentation of the disorder. This important point has often been overlooked (but see Ghaziuddin et al., 1992; Smith & Bryson, 1994).

Gillberg (1989), Szatmari et al. (1989), Szatmari et al. (1990), and Tantam (1988b, 1991) all attributed their criteria to the descriptions provided by Asperger (1944/1991) and Wing (1981). However, neither of these two authors clearly stated which clinical features were essential for a diagnosis of AS. Instead, subsequent investigators have abstracted those features they felt were emphasized by Asperger and Wing and developed their own criteria, resulting in considerable variability between studies. Some consensus on the diagnosis of AS has only recently become available, represented by the definitions of the *International Classification of Diseases, Tenth revision* (ICD-10; World Health Organization, 1993) and the *Diagnostic and Statistical Manual of Mental Disorders* (DSM-IV; American Psychiatric Association, 1994). Neither of these definitions counts motor features among the essential criteria for a diagnosis of AS. Instead, poor motor coordination is regarded as an associated feature of AS.

Gillberg (1989) reported clumsiness to be almost universal among the children who met his other criteria for AS (consisting of severe impairment in social interaction, circumscribed preoccupation with a topic, reliance on routines, pedantic language with impaired comprehension, and nonverbal communication problems). In later work, Gillberg included clumsiness as an essential diagnostic feature of AS (e.g., Ehlers & Gillberg, 1993; Gillberg & Gillberg, 1989). It is also noteworthy that, according to Gillberg's (1989) criteria, neither a history of language delay nor the presence of mental retardation would rule out a diagnosis of AS.

Szatmari et al. (1989) defined AS broadly, using the criteria of (1) isolated behavior; (2) impaired social interaction; (3) one of odd speech, impaired nonverbal communication, or bizarre preoccupations; and (4) onset before age 6, with no explicit exclusionary criteria (although all individuals in the study had IQs in the normal range, suggesting that those with mental retardation were excluded). Neither clumsiness nor other motor features were mentioned in the diagnostic criteria, although "gestures are large and clumsy" was noted as a clinical feature under the heading "impaired nonverbal communication" (p. 710). The same criteria were used by Szatmari et al. (1990).

Tantam (1988b) measured clumsiness in his study of 60 adults with histories of eccentricity and social isolation, 46 of whom were described elsewhere as meeting criteria for "an autistic disorder of the Asperger type" (Tantam, 1991, p. 149). These criteria included the following symptoms evidenced in adulthood: impaired nonverbal communication; narrow, obsessive and/or idiosyncratic special interests; difficulty conforming to social conventions; abnormal language pragmatics; and lack of close peer relationships. These, plus an "impression of clumsiness," constitute Tantam's criteria for AS in adults. However, Tantam (1991) stated that 91% of the AS individuals in his study were judged to be clumsy, apparently prior to obtaining direct motor measures. In addition, a childhood history of the same symptom profile, or of autism, and no history of later psychotic disorder were required for individuals to be considered to have AS. It appears that Tantam included the "clumsiness" criterion for AS on the basis of his analysis of the characteristics of the 60 socially impaired adults in his initial sample. It is somewhat unclear from the published record (Tantam, 1988a, 1988b, 1991) how the differential diagnoses of AS and schizoid personality disorder were arrived at for this larger group and, in particular, at what point clumsiness was used as a diagnostic feature.

Klin et al. (1995) and Manjiviona and Prior (1995) both used ICD-10 criteria as their starting points for diagnosis. However, each made different critical modifications to these criteria. Klin et al. (1995, p. 1131) included "delayed motor milestones and presence of motor 'clumsiness' " in their AS criteria. Other modifications were the requirement of an "isolated, unusual all-absorbing skill or activity" (an associated feature in ICD-10, but required by Gillberg, 1989, and by Tantam, 1988b, 1991), and only one symptom, rather than two, indicating "restricted interests and activities."

Manjiviona and Prior (1995) also used ICD-10 diagnostic criteria for AS, but these investigators eliminated the requirement of generally normal language acquisition. Instead, the criterion was applied to *current* language functioning (also see Ozonoff, Rogers, & Pennington, 1991, for an argument in support of this strategy, and Klin et al., 1995, for a contrary viewpoint).

That these differences in selection are critical is highlighted by the striking dissimilarity of the cognitive profiles of the AS groups reported by Klin et al. (1995) and Manjiviona and Prior (1995). In particular, the AS group of Klin et al. displayed a high Verbal–low Performance IQ pattern, while their HFA group's profiles were inconsistent. In contrast, both groups in the Manjiviona and Prior (1995) study displayed a degree of inconsistency comparable to that of the HFA group in Klin et al.'s study. Whereas heterogeneity in the cognitive profiles of HFA individuals has also been reported by Siegel, Minshew, and Goldstein (1996), it may be the inconsistencies between the AS profiles reported by Klin et al. and Manjiviona and Prior that are at issue. Klin and his colleagues reported that the neuropsychological profiles of a significant majority of their AS group matched those found in the syndrome of Nonverbal Learning Disability (NLD; Rourke, 1989). One characteristic of the NLD syndrome is the high Verbal–low Performance IQ pattern, clearly not present in Manjiviona and Prior's AS group (see Manjiviona & Prior, 1995, pp. 32–33, Tables II and III). It is obvious that the criteria used in these two studies have resulted in groups with important differences that are relevant to the issue of motor skills. What is unclear is which differences are critical and what the relationships are between these differences and motor functions.

To reiterate, Klin et al. (1995) have reported that an AS group selected for intact early language and delayed, poorly coordinated motor behavior was distinguished from an HFA group by the high Verbal–low Performance IQ pattern (among other characteristics). In contrast, Manjiviona and Prior (1995) did not eliminate cases with early language delay and did not consider motor behavior in the diagnostic process. Their AS group did not show the consistent IQ profile seen in the Klin et al. sample. Thus, it appears reasonable to conclude that diagnostic differences between studies are a major contributor to conflicting conclusions regarding motor skills in AS versus HFA, although not the only potential source. Another factor is differences in the definition and measurement of the motor characteristics of interest.

Definition and Measurement of Clumsiness

As noted by Ghaziuddin et al. (1992), progress in the task of evaluating whether "clumsiness" is characteristic of AS has been hampered by the lack of any operational definition of the term. It appears that most authors have in mind the colloquial sense of physical awkwardness, with lack of grace or skill in execution of movements (e.g., Gubbay, 1975). However, it is seldom clear whether the term is being used with reference to fine or to gross motor behavior, or to both, or on what sorts of tasks clumsiness should be evaluated (e.g., ratings of "real world" behavior, clinical judgment in a neurological exam, or standardized tasks). Furthermore, it is apparent in the existing literature that there is no consensus regarding what constitutes clumsiness not only in autism but in any population. Dewey (1995) discussed this issue in regard to the use of the term "developmental dyspraxia," which is often used interchangeably with "clumsiness" to describe developmental motor coordination problems (Cermak, 1985). Dewey argued that developmental dyspraxia should be reserved for impairment of complex learned movements (i.e., gestures and pantomime), in keeping with the similar use of the term "apraxia" in the adult neuropsychological literature (Geschwind, 1975; cf. Roy, Elliott, Dewey, & Square-Storer, 1990). Others have argued that clumsiness entails dysfunction in perceptual–motor integration rather than in purely motor skills (e.g., Laszlo, Bairstow, Bartrip, & Rolfe, 1988). In particular, the roles of vision and kinaesthesis in motor control have been investigated in clumsy children (e.g., Piek & Coleman-Carman, 1995; Lord & Hulme, 1988).

Given the lack of consensus on what abilities are impaired when the term "clumsiness" is invoked, variability in methods of measurement is to be expected. Motor ability in AS and HFA has been assessed indirectly, by measures such as parent report (Szatmari et al., 1989), and directly, by methods ranging from clinical judgment (Klin et al., 1995) to formal observations (Tantam, 1988b) to normed tests (Gillberg, 1989; Klin et al., 1995; Manjiviona & Prior, 1995); no study of AS to date has examined systematically the agreement between different types of ratings (e.g., clinical judgments and objective testing) or reported data on the reliability of the measures used.

Keogh, Sugden, Reynard, and Calkins (1979) have shown that within the general population of children, there is poor agreement about who is clumsy. This low reliability is obtained both between observers using the same measures (e.g., two teachers using the same rating scale) and across measures (e.g., teacher ratings and standardized test results). However, once a group of children has been identified as clumsy on the basis of a given set of measures, the evidence indicates that their problems persist (Losse et al., 1991).

Szatmari et al. (1989) used an indirect method to assess clumsiness in AS and HFA (not a direct measure, as reported by Ghaziuddin et al., 1992). Parents rated the degree of difficulty their child had experienced in *acquiring* five skills (dressing, tying shoelaces, using eating utensils, printing with pencils, doing puzzles), as well as their *present* skill level at each of these tasks. A 3-point scale was used: 0, no impairment; 1, mild difficulty; 2, serious difficulty. Children designated as having AS and HFA had equal difficulty learning these adaptive motor tasks, with both groups showing higher difficulty ratings than a control group of children who were outpatients in a psychiatric clinic. Given this, it is somewhat surprising that no differences between groups were observed for present skill levels. This issue of the relationship between skill acquisition and the skill levels eventually attained is not typically addressed but may contribute to the complex picture of motor functioning seen in autistic spectrum disorders (cf. Tantam, 1991).

Szatmari et al. (1990) employed the same diagnostic criteria for AS and HFA as did Szatmari et al. (1989), and apparently tested a subset of the cases from the original series. Szatmari et al. (1990) compared the neuropsychological profiles of a combined group of individuals with AS ($n = 26$, ages 8–18 years) and HFA ($n = 17$, ages 7–32 years) with an outpatient psychiatric control group ($n = 36$, ages 7–18 years). Unlike the previous work by Szatmari's group, this study included a direct measure of motor performance (manual dexterity) using the Grooved Pegboard test (Matthews & Klove, 1964; Knights & Norwood, 1979). The combined group of individuals with autistic disorders (HFA + AS) completed the Grooved Pegboard test more slowly than did controls. These controls, however, had significantly higher Verbal and Performance IQs than did the AS/HFA group. The Szatmari et al. study is therefore inconclusive with respect to the uniqueness of manual motor coordination deficits to autistic spectrum disorders. Their study is somewhat more revealing with respect to comparisons between the HFA and AS groups. These groups were matched for IQ, although unfortunately not for age (the HFA group being significantly older). The HFA and AS groups did not differ in their dominant hand performance on the pegboard, whereas the HFA group was significantly slower with the nondominant hand than was the AS group (which did not differ from controls). Szatmari et al. (1990) also reported that unlike individuals diagnosed with AS, most HFA participants did not show the typical dominant hand advantage. In a discriminant function analysis predicting HFA versus AS diagnoses, both dominant and nondominant hand performance were significant variables (although the overall rate of correct classification was not impressive).

Clumsiness was defined by Gillberg (1989) as a significant discrepancy between the child's IQ and his or her score on the gross motor subscale of the Griffiths scale. Deficient motor skills were therefore defined relative to IQ level (see also Gillberg, 1993) in an attempt to control for any association between poor motor coordination and lower IQ. As previously mentioned, clumsiness thus defined was reported for virtually the entire AS group. No information about the fine motor skills of the sample was presented.

Tantam (1988b, 1991) composed a clumsiness summary score from tasks consisting of (1) copying a meaningless hand gesture, (2) flexing the terminal joint of one finger in imitation, (3) balancing on one leg, and (4) catching a paper ball. Tantam's measures are noteworthy by virtue of directly assessing motor abilities and for the inclusion of both manual and gross motor skills. The inclusion of manual imitation measures is of particular interest, given the strong evidence for gestural deficits in autism (Smith & Bryson,

1994). Tantam (1991) reported that these scores were significantly interrelated, that all indicated poorer performance in AS, and that ball catching produced the greatest difference between AS and non-AS individuals. Recall that the comparison group in this study, however, consisted of nonautistic adults with severe social impairment and eccentric behavior. Thus, Tantam's results address the separation of AS and non-AS patterns within this larger group rather than the distinction between AS and HFA.

Klin et al. (1995) also reported comparative results from neuropsychological examinations of AS and HFA individuals, including assessments of fine and gross motor skills. As mentioned previously, in this study delayed motor milestones and clumsiness were necessary for an AS diagnosis. For their matched HFA group, Klin et al. used the ICD-10 diagnostic criteria for autism and an IQ cutoff of 70. Klin et al. (1995) noted that judgments regarding gross motor skills were based primarily on clinical observations, rather than on the results of normative assessments. The specific fine motor skill measures were not identified, but in a typical neuropsychological battery these would consist of scores on normed tests such as the Grooved Pegboard (as used by Szatmari et al., 1990), the Purdue Pegboard, or the Finger Tapping Test (Lezak, 1983).

Klin et al. (1995) found that a significantly higher proportion of AS than HFA individuals exhibited deficits in both fine and gross motor skills, either relative to norms (fine motor) or by clinical judgment (gross motor). It is unsurprising that all 21 AS cases showed gross motor skill deficits, given that "clumsiness" was a diagnostic criterion. However, 19 of these cases also had impaired manual dexterity, suggesting that poor coordination was indeed a global characteristic of their motor performance. Within the HFA group, for which there was no selection on the basis of motor skill, 12 of 19 individuals also were judged to have gross motor incoordination; only 6 of the 19 exhibited poor dexterity. Thus, although global motor impairment was more often associated with a diagnosis of AS, HFA individuals also showed a high rate of deficit, particularly in gross motor skills. Comparison of this result with those of Szatmari et al. (1990), who found manual dexterity to be poorer for HFA than AS, but only for the nondominant hand, suggests that lateralized differences may be an important discriminator. Comparable data were not included in the Klin et al. (1995) report. Discrepancies between these studies may also stem from diagnostic differences, and from the fact that impairments defined relative to norms and relative to the performance of matched controls are not necessarily congruent. Both types of information are required in order to address the separate issues of subgroup differences and of clinically significant deficits.

Klin et al. (1995) acknowledged the possibility that the use of the "motor delay and clumsiness" criterion for AS may have introduced some bias to their study. However, they reported that the difference between the HFA and AS groups in the frequency of gross motor impairment remained significant even when the six potential AS cases who did not exhibit significant motor problems were included in the analysis. It therefore appears that their finding of deficits in fine and gross motor coordination in AS is not entirely dependent on selection for those problems. What remains to be demonstrated, however, is that other differences in criteria (e.g., regarding early language) are not critical for motor differences to emerge.

Thus, although the available data implicate gross motor delays and/or deficits as being particularly characteristic of AS, and manual dexterity differences may also contribute to the HFA/AS distinction, only Manjiviona and Prior (1995) have systematically assessed a range of gross and fine motor skills using standardized measures in both AS and HFA individuals. Recall that Manjiviona and Prior defined AS using ICD-10 criteria, without the "normal language development" stipulation. The HFA group in this study met either ICD-10 or DSM-III-R (American Psychiatric Association, 1987) criteria; both the HFA and AS groups were selected for IQs at least in the near-normal range. It is noteworthy that although the mean difference between Full Scale IQs was not statistically significant, the mean for the HFA group (84.9) was lower than that of the AS group (104.2) by more than a standard deviation. Other aspects of the cognitive profiles of these groups were discussed earlier in relation to differences between this sample and that of Klin et al. (1995).

Manjiviona and Prior (1995) reported that 50% of the HFA and 67% of the AS groups presented with significant motor impairment, as defined by norms on the Test of Motor Impairment—Henderson Revision (TOMI-H; Stott, Moyes, & Henderson, 1984). However, the two autistic subgroups did not differ, either in total scores, or on any of the three subscales of the TOMI-H (manual dexterity, ball skills, and balance). For all subjects, significant negative correlations were observed between the TOMI-H total scores and both Full Scale and Performance IQs. These relationships were reported to be due mainly to the influence of the AS group. A negative correlation between TOMI-H scores and Verbal IQs was also observed in AS. Analyses of covariance on TOMI-H scores with Full Scale IQ as the covariate did not reveal any significant differences between groups. Thus, it was argued that differences in intellectual functioning were not responsible for the variability in motor scores. Manjiviona and Prior (1995) concluded that no aspect of motor impairment differentiated HFA from AS. Rather, their study provided an illustration of the heterogeneous manifestations of motor difficulties and of their relationships to cognitive profiles in autistic spectrum disorders.

For all the reasons previously mentioned, direct comparisons of findings from the various studies described here are not possible. Nonetheless, it is instructive to outline some of the possible points of departure. One would expect that a similar pattern of relationships would obtain between diagnostic category and the TOMI-H Manual Dexterity score and between diagnosis and the dexterity measures reported by others. Examination of the data presented by Manjiviona and Prior (1995) reveals considerable heterogeneity of performance within both the AS and HFA groups, with no suggestion of group differences, unlike the findings of Klin et al. (1995), in which significant fine motor impairment was more common for AS. The lack of overall differences in manual dexterity between AS and HFA reported by Manjiviona and Prior (1995) is more consistent with the findings of Szatmari et al. (1990), although once again, both diagnostic differences and the lack of information about dominant and nondominant hand performance precludes detailed comparisons.

Similarly, Tantam's (1991) finding that ball skills were particularly problematic for his AS adult group, compared with socially impaired controls, must be contrasted with Manjiviona and Prior's (1995) failure to demonstrate any systematic differences between AS and HFA groups on the comparable subscale of the TOMI-H. These findings highlight the importance of clarifying which comparisons are of interest (for instance, AS vs. nonautistic psychiatric disorders or learning disabilities, as opposed to AS vs. HFA).

The issue of the association of clumsiness with AS remains ambiguous. It seems doubtful whether it will be resolved through the types of studies described previously unless data become available for which there is consistency across all of the following aspects of the studies: diagnostic criteria, motor behaviors (that are clearly operationalized and reliably measured), and control groups. Even if such data were to become available, what would this contribute to our understanding of the spectrum of autism? Although resolution of this long-standing diagnostic debate would be satisfying, larger issues deserve attention. Systematic studies addressing these broader concerns might well provide that resolution.

AN ALTERNATIVE APPROACH TO MOTOR FUNCTIONING IN AUTISTIC SPECTRUM DISORDERS

The foregoing discussion has demonstrated shortcomings in the literature on clumsiness as a feature of AS that are both methodological and conceptual. The focus now shifts to an alternative approach to the study of motoric functioning in autistic spectrum disorders, including AS. An essential feature of this approach is an attempt to specify the processes underlying the motor behavior of interest. That is, it is suggested that future studies must go beyond identifying differences in performance to accounting for differences in performance with reference to underlying mechanisms. It is argued that a better understanding of the quality and degree of motor impairment manifested not only in AS and HFA but across the entire spectrum of autism might shed light on the question of autistic subtypes, as well as on issues at other levels of analysis, such as neurological substrates.

In recent years, the study of nonautistic clumsy or dyspraxic children has been characterized by a search for underlying perceptual and/or motor planning deficits (Henderson, 1987). The virtue of such studies (e.g., Lord & Hulme, 1988; Piek & Coleman-Carman, 1995; van der Meulen, Denier van der Gon, Gielen, Gooskens, & Willemse, 1991) is that they compare directly the performance of groups on tasks that can be clearly specified. The relationship between performance on these tasks and real-world motor behavior can then be addressed empirically. The initial selection of subjects based on clumsiness remains a significant problem for research in this area. There is still a tendency to rely on clinical judgments, with investigators seldom reporting data on the reliability of these. One preferable approach is to use the results of standardized tests (e.g., the TOMI-H) to define clumsiness in terms of motor abilities below those expected for age or intellectual level.

In this section, some of the evidence for impairment on several varieties of broadly defined motor tasks in individuals with autistic spectrum disorders are reviewed. The studies to be described address several areas of motor function: manual dexterity, gait and balance, and praxis. None of the studies to be described in this section directly tests whether the skills in question distinguish AS from other putative autistic subtypes. However, they illustrate the range of motor functions that appear worthy of further investigation in autism and related disorders. Examining the component processes that underlie performance on these measures may enrich our understanding of the interaction of perceptual, motor and cognitive processes in the autistic syndrome.

Manual Dexterity in Autistic Spectrum Disorders

The advantage of using manual dexterity as a measure of motor skill is that it can be operationalized as performance on relatively simple speeded tasks such as pegboards (Lezak, 1983). Pegboard measures have been administered in a number of studies of individuals with autistic spectrum disorders. Those that involved research participants with AS were described in the preceding section (Klin et al., 1995; Szatmari et al., 1990), although Klin et al. did not identify explicitly the fine motor measures referred to in their study.

It is instructive to compare Szatmari et al.'s (1990) findings with those of Rumsey and Hamburger's (1988) neuropsychological study of HFA. The latter study compared 10 adult men with HFA with normal controls on a test battery that included the Grooved Pegboard. Rumsey and Hamburger defined HFA in terms of DSM-III (American Psychiatric Association, 1980) criteria for infantile autism, residual state. That is, these men would have met DSM-III criteria for autism when younger but no longer did so, although they remained socially and behaviorally impaired. Rumsey and Hamburger's IQ cutoff for HFA was 80 (vs. 70 in Szatmari et al.'s study). The HFA group and normal controls were matched for chronological age and for educational levels, and quite closely matched for IQ (with slightly lower mean Verbal and Performance IQs for the HFA group; $p < .06$). A trend ($p < .06$) toward slower performance overall on the Grooved Pegboard for the men with autism was obtained. In addition, the authors described a tendency ($p < .07$) toward slower completion of the pegboard with the nondominant hand for the HFA group.

Despite similarity in overall findings (individuals with HFA tended to show relatively slow performance on the Grooved Pegboard), important discrepancies were found. Each of these studies suggested that dominant–nondominant hand differences on a pegboard task may differentiate HFA, either from normal controls (Rumsey & Hamburger, 1988) or from AS and psychiatric controls (Szatmari et al., 1990). However, it appears that different effects have been demonstrated. Rumsey and Hamburger reported that HFA showed a trend toward slower nondominant performance, and comparable dominant performance, for HFA men relative to normal controls. Szatmari et al. (1990) found that an HFA group did not differ from an AS group with respect to dominant hand speed on the pegboard, although both were slower than psychiatric controls. However, for the nondominant hand, the pattern changed, with the HFA group resembling controls, and the AS group showing slower performance. In considering these differences in findings, it is important to note that Rumsey and Hamburger's sample consisted of adults (ages 19–36 years), whereas Szatmari et al.'s HFA group ranged in age from 7 to 32 years, and their AS group, from 8 to 18 years. As will become apparent, these age differences may account in part for the differences in findings.

Pegboard tasks have also been administered to children with autism by McManus (McManus, Murray, Doyle, & Baron-Cohen, 1992; Cornish & McManus, 1996), McEvoy, Rogers, and Pennington (1993), Rapin (1996), and Smith and Bryson (1998a). McEvoy et al. administered the Wallin pegboards A (round pegs) and B (square pegs) from the Merrill–Palmer Scale of Mental Tests as discriminant tasks in their study of executive functions in preschoolers with autism. There were no differences in speed (on the two pegboards combined) between the children with autism and either nonverbal mental-age-matched or verbal mental-age-matched normally developing children. This finding is consistent with the commonly held view that perceptual–motor skills are unimpaired in autism, although the high degree of individual variability in performance on the tasks was notable (McEvoy et al., 1993).

McManus et al. (1992) also found no significant differences between children with autism and verbal-age-matched normal controls on the Annett pegboard task (Annett, 1970). This measure consists of the time taken to move 10 pegs from one row of holes to another, parallel row. (Children with mental retardation completed the task more slowly than either the autistic or normal groups, but this group had a significantly lower verbal mental age than did the normal controls.) What was of interest in the performance of children with autism in this report was a dissociation between the preferred hand for the task and speed of the hands in completing the task. That is, unlike the case for the majority of children in both control groups (90–92%), the preferred hand often was not the most skillful hand for the children with autism. Only 50% of the autistic group showed the typical concordance of preference and skill. Cornish and McManus (1996) extended this work by testing a younger group of children with autism and additional controls, and reanalyzing the total data set. The study incorporating the new data indicated that children with autism were significantly slower to complete the pegboard, with left and right hands, than were typically developing controls. Nonautistic children with mental retardation were again the slowest group, but the significant difference in level of functioning, with this group scoring much lower than the autistic group on the Merrill–Palmer Scales, still makes this comparison difficult to interpret. The major difference between the new findings and those reported by McManus et al. is that the skill-preference dissociation observed in the original study was not obtained when data from a younger group of children with autism were included.

These findings, especially in combination with the lateralized effects described previously for adults with HFA, highlights the importance of examining motor abilities systematically. The evidence suggests that manual skills that develop asymmetrically in other populations may show an atypical (less lateralized) pattern in autism (see also Bryson, 1990; Soper et al., 1986), but that these effects are ephemeral and appear to depend critically on both the developmental and chronological ages of the samples. Data on the development of lateralized manual skills in autism are needed. Careful attention will need to be paid to choice of controls for such studies, given evidence of reduced skill asymmetry in other developmentally handicapped populations (e.g., Elliott, Weeks, & Jones, 1986).

The largest body of data addressing motor skills in young children with autism is from the Autism and Language Disorders Collaborative Project—Preschool Study Group (Rapin, 1996). This rich data base cannot be done justice here, but a few of the descriptive findings regarding motor measures are summarized. Readers are referred to the monograph edited by Rapin (1996) for additional details of this ambitious work. There were 51 high-functioning children with autistic disorder (HAD; nonverbal IQ of at least 80), and 125 low-functioning children with autistic disorder (nonverbal IQs below 80; LAD). Each of these groups was matched on nonverbal IQ to a group of children. In the case of the HAD group, the matched group consisted of children with developmental language disorders (DLD). For the LAD group, the control group included globally impaired children with nonverbal IQs below 80 but not autism (non-autistic, low nonverbal IQ; NALIQ). Briefly, the measures of motor functioning included the Annett pegboard task, Seguin Formboard, and a test of praxis (the Manual Expression subtest, Illinois Test of Psycholinguistic Abilities; Kirk, McCarthy, &

Kirk, 1968). The results were inconsistent with those of McManus in that children with autism were slow to complete the Annett pegboard relative to norms, but their speed did not differ from that of controls when age and nonverbal IQ were covaried. Both high-functioning groups (HAD and DLD) were significantly faster than the lower-functioning groups (LAD and NALIQ). Compared with norms, children in the HAD group showed particular difficulty completing the task with their right hands. Performance on the Sequin Formboard did not differentiate either the two high-functioning groups or the two low-functioning groups, although the former were much faster than the latter. When age and nonverbal IQ were covaried, the HAD group remained faster than the LAD group.

In addition to issues of obvious importance such as differences in age and level of functioning and the question of skill asymmetry, it is of interest to examine task-related variables that may complicate even the apparently simple domain of manual dexterity. When motor skill differences have *not* been observed for children with autism, the tasks were the Annett pegboard, in which relatively large round wooden pegs are removed from and fitted into identical holes, and the Wallin pegboards, which also use relatively large round or square wooden pegs. Both of these tasks involve relatively simple visual–motor coordination. In contrast, efficient completion of the Grooved Pegboard entails taking into account the orientation of each slot as one approaches with a small key-like metal peg and matching the orientation of the peg to the slot during the movement. In Smith's study, children and adolescents with autism completed the Grooved Pegboard more slowly than did either of two control groups (language-delayed and typically developing children, both matched for receptive language mental age) with both the dominant and nondominant hands (Smith & Bryson, 1998a). One variable that may be important in accounting for differences between studies is that the visual–motor coordination required for this task is considerably greater for the Grooved Pegboard than for these other pegboard tasks. Another factor is the age of the participants in the various studies, with the data from older children and adults tending to show larger differences than the data obtained with child samples. Perhaps the tests used at older ages amplify the more subtle differences that appear in some but not all studies with children. Developmental data from studies that systematically manipulate task variables are needed to resolve these inconsistencies in findings.

Finger-tapping speed is another commonly used measure of fine motor skill (Lezak, 1983). Although this measure has been included in neuropsychological batteries used in studies of individuals with autism (e.g., by Dawson, 1983), the data have not been reported separately. However, the finger-tapping task provides a useful example of an approach to component analysis that has been applied to the study of motor incoordination in nonautistic children.

Component Analysis of a Motor Skill

Two components of performance on motor tasks such as finger tapping are timing and force control (Keele, Ivry, & Pokorny, 1987). Lundy-Ekman, Ivry, Keele, and Woollacott (1991) have reported that two subgroups of clumsy children showed a double dissociation between the signs of clumsiness they exhibited and their performance on independent measures of timing and force control. The two subgroups were distinguished on the basis of their clinically judged movement abnormalities and the neurological structures implicated by these motor signs (basal ganglia for one set of symptoms, cerebellum for the other). On the experimental (tapping) tasks, those children who had exhibited predominantly signs of involvement of the basal ganglia showed deficits in force control but not in timing. In contrast, those with signs of cerebellar dysfunction had deficits in timing behavior (manifested in both perceptual and motor tasks) but not in force control.

Findings such as those of Lundy-Ekman et al. (1991) support the suggestion that clumsiness is not all of a kind, and that classification of individuals as clumsy/not clumsy may obscure other differences. That is, different underlying processes might be impaired in subgroups of children with poor motor coordination. This possibility has particularly interesting implications for the study of motor functioning in autism. First, the heterogeneity of motor impairment within the autistic spectrum and the variety of other characteristics potentially associated with these motor problems (e.g., the quality of early language development, presence of visual–spatial deficits) suggest that various neurological substrates might be involved.

Second, with specific reference to the findings of Lundy-Ekman et al. (1991), autism has been postulated to involve both the basal ganglia (Damasio & Maurer, 1978; Vilensky, Damasio, & Maurer, 1981) and the cerebellum (Courchesne et al., 1994; Kohen-Raz, Volkmar, & Cohen, 1992; Sears, Finn, & Steinmetz, 1994). Some of the variability in motor performance (and perhaps thereby in other characteristics) in autistic disorders may be due to the differential involvement of neural systems associated with these two structures. Tasks that can be used to dissect the relative contributions of these systems to motor performance across the autistic spectrum have the potential to contribute to our understanding of the neuropsychology of this complex syndrome. A few studies of nonmanual motor functions provide data that support the usefulness of this enterprise.

Gait and Balance in Autistic Spectrum Disorders

Following observations by Damasio and Maurer (1978) of autistic motility disturbances, Vilensky et al. (1981), analyzed the gait patterns of a group of children with autism. Using filmed records, they identified gait abnormalities in these children that were not observed in a control group of normally developing children or in a small control group of "hyperactive–aggressive" children. The reported abnormalities were said to resemble those typically associated with Parkinsonism (additional comparative comments were reported by Teitelbaum, Maurer, Fryman, et al., 1996). This preliminary study deserves replication and extension. In particular, it would be important to include children with diagnoses conforming to current research standards and representing the range of functioning in autism. The controls in the Vilensky et al. (1981) study were not matched for level of mental retardation, and specific information regarding intellectual profiles was not provided. Furthermore, the presence or absence of other potentially confounding conditions (e.g., seizures) was not noted for either the autistic or control groups.

These criticisms do not apply to the study by Hallett et al. (1993), who assessed the gait of five high-functioning adults with autism, compared with age-matched normal controls. Using computer-assisted video kinematic techniques, they found that gait was somewhat atypical in these individuals. However, the authors concluded that the overall clinical findings were more consistent with cerebellar rather than basal ganglion dysfunction.

The importance of resolving these discrepancies is underscored by the fact that Jones and Prior (1985) did not observe gait abnormalities in their investigation of neurological "soft signs" in a group of children with autism. The fine-grained movement analyses enabled by current kinematic techniques permits the identification of problems that are not apparent in a clinical examination, as used in the Jones and Prior (1985) study. However, other motor symptoms were noted in association with autism in this study. For example, an elevated frequency of impaired balance was observed, compared with both chronological- and mental-age-matched normally developing children.

Consistent with this, Kohen-Raz et al. (1992) demonstrated that the postural control of children with autism differed from that of matched mentally handicapped and normally developing children, and from that of adults with vestibular pathology. The objective measures were obtained using a computerized "posturographic" technique. Specific findings for the children with autism included paradoxically good stability when assuming postures that are normally stressful (e.g., eyes closed while standing on an unstable surface) and unusual heel–toe weight distribution. The pattern of atypical postural characteristics was reported to be more consistent with mesocortical or cerebellar, rather than vestibular, pathology.

Vilensky et al. (1981), Kohen-Raz et al. (1992), and Hallett et al. (1993) have thus provided independent empirical evidence of basic disturbances in the motor systems of individuals with autism, especially involving postural and lower limb control. These results, derived from objective measurement techniques, provide a starting point for a more systematic examination of motor functions in autistic spectrum disorders. However, as of this writing, none of these findings has been replicated. It would be particularly valuable if performance on measures such as those used in these studies could be related to independent measures of the intactness of the neural structures that control these functions (e.g., from functional magnetic resonance imaging or positron emission tomography) in clearly diagnosed groups of individuals with the range of autistic disorders, including AS.

Dyspraxia in Autistic Spectrum Disorders

One of the largest areas of literature bearing on motor functioning in autism concerns the imitative learning of others' movement patterns. Learned gesture and object use, or praxis, was first suggested to be deficient in autism by DeMyer et al. (1972). Smith and Bryson (1994) reviewed evidence for specific imitative deficits in autism and concluded that although the evidence for poor imitation and pantomime ability in autistic spectrum disorders was compelling (see also Meltzoff & Gopnik, 1993; Rogers & Pennington, 1991), there was little information about the nature of the disability. Rogers (1999) has provided another excellent review.

A number of the outstanding issues raised by Smith and Bryson (1994) have recently been addressed. Rogers, Bennetto, McEvoy, and Pennington (1996) and Smith (1996; Smith & Bryson, 1998a, 1998b) have examined the performance of individuals with autistic spectrum disorders on a wide variety of gesture imitation and object pantomime tasks.

Both Rogers et al. (1996) and Smith and Bryson (1998a) reported that gesture imitation was deficient for their autistic groups relative to clinical controls matched for intellectual level. Data from the Autism and Language Disorders Collaborative Project (Rapin, 1996) confirm this finding in that both the low- and high-functioning groups with autism were more impaired than were the groups matched for nonverbal IQ on the manual praxis subtest of the Illinois Test of Psycholinguistic Abilities. Other recent data from preschool children with autism are consistent with these results (Stone, Ousley, & Littleford, 1997).

To redress unresolved issues from the descriptive literature, both Rogers et al. (1996) and Smith (1996; Smith & Bryson, 1998a, 1998b) introduced control tasks for visual memory, object use, and motor skills. Neither study found any overall differences in recognition memory for the imitation tasks, nor any difficulty with using actual objects (as opposed to pantomiming their uses, which was a significant deficiency of the autistic groups in both studies). Rogers et al. ascertained that each subject could perform the movements needed to perform each gesture; Smith also did so, and in addition administered a standard measure of manual motor skill. As previously mentioned, children with autism in that study were slower to complete the Grooved Pegboard than were either language-delayed or typically developing language-matched controls. Furthermore, manual dexterity accounted for a significant percentage of the variance in nonsymbolic gesture imitation ratings. However, significant group differences in imitation remained such that the performance of the autistic group was poorer than could be accounted for by differences in motor functioning alone.

In both the Rogers et al. (1996) and Smith (1996; Smith & Bryson, 1998a, 1998b) studies, group differences were obtained for imitation of arbitrary manual movements, and for pantomimed use of objects. However, the results of the two studies differed with respect to imitation of meaningful gestures. Rogers et al. found no significant deficits for their autistic group, whereas Smith reported that, for her somewhat younger and lower-functioning group, both symbolic and nonsymbolic gestures were performed poorly relative to controls. This discrepancy is probably attributable to the age and intellectual levels of the children and adolescents, to the levels of difficulty and familiarity of the gestures, and to the methods of scoring.

Following the recommendations of Smith and Bryson (1994), a goal of the Smith (1996) study was to provide descriptive information on gesture imitation by individuals with autism. In addition to clinical controls, the study included typically developing children matched to the autistic group for language level. Furthermore, Smith and Bryson identified a need for more hypothesis-driven research. Therefore, the patterns of errors in imitation by children with autism were examined, as well as the effects of specific stimulus manipulations on imitative performance.

For example, impaired ability to combine visual and kinesthetic information specifying the body positions of self and other has been hypothesized to be critical in the genesis of the imitative deficit in autism (Meltzoff & Gopnik, 1993; Rogers & Pennington, 1991; see also Barresi & Moore, 1996). The data reported by Smith (1996; Smith & Bryson, 1998a, 1998b) are consistent with this suggestion. In this investigation children and adolescents with autism showed a significantly increased tendency to produce a distinctive imitative error. This error involved the 180-degree rotation of the model's gesture such that the child appeared to be matching his or her view of the model's hand to that of his or her own hand. This error was interpreted to indicate a failure to transform the model's gesture using body-centered coordinates; instead the gesture was reproduced directly as seen. The significance of this relatively low-level "error in action" for understanding characteristically autistic patterns in language (e.g., pronoun reversal errors) and social understanding (e.g., failure to appreciate other's perspectives) appears worthy of additional exploration (see also Whiten & Brown, 1999). Understanding the basis for this error may also illuminate another phenomenon, that of the apparent paradox of children who show echopraxic behavior (i.e., the copying of movements in an automatic manner) when "intentional" imitation is lacking. The parallel phenomenon in speech (echolalia, in the absence of verbal imitation on request) has been commented upon by others (e.g., Abrahamson & Mitchell, 1990) and may be of significance for understanding the neuropsychology of autism (Rogers & Pennington, 1991).

A comparison of putative autistic subtypes (e.g., AS and HFA) on measures of praxis would be of particular interest given that Smith (1996; Smith & Bryson 1998b) has interpreted autistic impairment in imitation and pantomime as evidence of atypical representational capabilities that may be fundamental to information processing in autism (see also Smith & Bryson, 1994). The essence of the argument is that in autism, dysfunctional mechanisms of visual–spatial attention (Bryson, Landry, & Wainwright, 1997) may result in the encoding of objects, events, and actions in a relatively rigid manner. This overly specific encoding may occur at the expense of higher-order, integrated representations. One implication of Smith's data for example, is that perhaps representations based primarily on visual information (vs. integrated visual–kinesthetic information) result in characteristic errors in action, including the previously mentioned difficulty with shifting perspective when imitating others' gestures. In contrast to this account, which emphasizes deficits in basic attentional processes and their consequences, Rogers et al. (1996) have suggested that the praxic deficit in autism is a reflection of a general deficit in executive functioning, a domain they and their colleagues have previously reported distinguishes HFA from AS (Ozonoff et al., 1991). These representational and executive functioning accounts might indeed be fundamentally related in that compromised flexibility of thought and action is a common underlying issue. The question then becomes at what level the deficit is specified, with the very real possibility that multiple levels of processing might well be affected, both within individuals and across the spectrum of autistic disorders.

Executive Dysfunction in Autistic Spectrum Disorders

Motor skills in autistic spectrum disorders must be evaluated in the context of evidence of executive dysfunctions (for reviews, see Pennington & Ozonoff, 1996; Bryson et al., 1997). However, as noted by Lezak (1983), "distinctions between disturbances of motor behaviour resulting from a supramodal executive dysfunction and specific disorders of motor functions are clearer in the telling than in fact" (p. 527). Executive functions emphasize formulation of goals and planning of actions but also the ability to initiate actions, to persist toward appropriate goals, and to inhibit inappropriate responses. Work by Hughes and Russell (1993; Hughes, Russell, & Robins, 1994) is consistent with the notion that executive deficits in autism are evident in planning simple actions and not only in relatively complex problem-solving tasks (e.g., the Wisconsin Card Sorting Test or the Tower of Hanoi; for review, see Pennington & Ozonoff, 1996).

In a recent report, Hughes (1996) described impaired motor planning in a group of children with autism. The task entailed making a series of movements to place a rod into a holder, with the requirement that one or the other end of the rod (specified by its color) had to be upright at the conclusion of the action. By manipulating the position in which the rod was presented, each child was made to choose either an efficient or an inefficient approach to the task. The investigator was thus able to assess the child's ability to anticipate the movements required to complete the task. Compared with groups of mentally handicapped and normally developing children, autistic children were significantly less successful at this task. Hughes (1996) suggests several testable hypotheses as to the basis of this deficit. The need for this process-oriented approach is highlighted by the fact that an earlier motor planning study (using a rotary pursuit task) found no differences in performance between an autistic group and normal controls, whereas a specific deficit was found for a third group, children with Down syndrome (Frith & Frith, 1974).

Studies that systematically examine the requirements of these various tasks may result in more specific conceptualization of what is meant by executive functions (Eslinger, 1996) and how they differentiate among various developmental disorders (Pennington & Ozonoff, 1996). The recent volume edited by Russell (1998) is a significant contribution to this effort in the case of autism.

IMPLICATIONS FOR RESEARCH ON MOTOR FUNCTIONS IN AUTISM

A number of research avenues have been suggested throughout this discussion. Among the points worth reiterating is the importance of considering motor functioning in a developmental context. The developmental course of motor abilities and their dynamic relationships with other skills have never been followed in a population of children with autistic disorders. For example, longitudinal data are needed to validate or repudiate clinical observations that motor skills may deteriorate as some children with autism grow up. Conversely, it may be the case that there is a relative acceleration of development in other skill areas for some children, producing an *apparent* dropoff in motor abilities. Standardized measures are necessary to document such effects.

In agreement with the conclusions of Ghaziuddin et al. (1992), both consistency of diagnosis and operationalization of motor skills are essential to research in this area. There is a place for studies of subgroup differences in motoric functions, but the relevant data have yet to be collected. It has been argued that to make significant progress in understanding the relationships among autistic characteristics (motoric or other), tasks must be designed that test specific hypotheses regarding these relationships and the processes and neurological substrates that might underlie them (Smith & Bryson, 1994).

IMPLICATIONS FOR CLINICAL PRACTICE

Much of this chapter has been devoted to discussion of the role of motor features in the diagnosis of disorders on the autistic spectrum, with an emphasis on research issues. However, at least some brief comments are warranted on the clinical value of considering the motor functioning of the individual child, not only for diagnostic purposes but also for treatment implications.

To begin with the clinical history, collecting information about developmental milestones is a standard component of the assessment process. Obviously, the use of retrospective data on the acquisition of developmental milestones is unavoidable. Even in the services with the most rigorous ascertainment, children are not often seen before 2 years of age even with the "classic" presentation of autism (Gillberg et al., 1990; Lord, 1995), and typically much later when a milder autistic spectrum disorder, especially of the AS type, is suspected. Reliance on parental recollection for data concerning early development clearly increases with the time that elapses until an assessment takes place. To use such data for either clinical or research purposes, it is essential that methods are employed that support accurate recall. These include specific descriptions of milestones (e.g., "took first step" vs. "walked"); asking parents to consult "baby books," photographs, or, increasingly, videos; and tying recall to key events such as birthdays or other memorable occasions. Specific questions, rather than global judgments, are also important because parents (especially of firstborn children) may have quite unrealistic expectations of, for example, the dressing skills of the average 2-year-old. The "dawdling" over dressing so prevalent in toddlers and preschoolers may or may not be accompanied by skill deficits. However, the two factors may not be considered separately by parents unless they are cued to do so. Furthermore, in the case of the child with classic autism, the relative normality of gross motor milestones may be very salient. When concerns about the child's development arise later (perhaps not until kindergarten or school age for AS), the parents' focus on milestones is presumably quite different.

In addition to the emphasis on diagnostic criteria and on laboratory measures of motor skills in most of this review, it is important to keep in mind that ultimately it is the real-life implications of these deficits that concern the clinician. The commonly accepted wisdom is that motor skills are unimpaired or even precocious in autism (as opposed to AS; see, e.g., Sigman & Capps, 1997). Many of the written resources for families and teachers of children with autism reinforce this view, resulting in frustration when a child's motor skills are weaker, and some recommended strategies may not be appropriate. In contrast, the imitative deficit in autism is widely recognized, with imitation skills being among the first targeted by most behaviorally based teaching programs (e.g., Maurice, 1996).

It is important to keep in mind that adaptive motor performance is poor overall in autism, even when the children are young (Rapin, 1996), and that a *relative* strength may still be a deficit when compared to normative performance (Klin, Volkmar, & Sparrow, 1992). As previously mentioned, it is the clinical impression of some experts that the deficit becomes more pronounced as individuals with autism get older (e.g., DeMyer, 1979; Wing, 1996). In practical terms, this is a reminder to clinicians to consider the value of occupational or physical therapies for any child with an autistic spectrum disorder when adaptive motor skills are impaired. Although motor skills may not typically be considered priorities for intervention, there may be practical advantages to incorporating remedial activities in these areas into a child's program. For example, observable success in areas such as self-help skills (e.g., dressing) may be achieved more readily than in social or communicative skills, providing reinforcement for parents' and teachers' efforts while promoting the child's independence.

Many occupational therapists employ sensory integration techniques (Ayres, 1979) in working with children with autism. Although the direct efficacy of sensory integration is unsupported by empirical evidence, these methods appear to provide strategies for increasing the comfort of the child with autism with certain sensory experiences as well as enjoyable sensory and motor activities within which to engage the child socially (Siegel, 1996).

The opportunities for socializing presented by the structured interactions of physical games provide another reason to emphasis motor skills for those children for whom this area is not a strength. The possibility that an adapted physical education curriculum may be necessary is often overlooked in the design of individual education plans, especially when assumptions are made about motor skills in autism. Some authors (e.g., Wing, 1996) have suggested that individual sports (e.g., swimming and riding) may have more long-term value as recreational activities for people with autism, as the motor planning requirements are not complicated by the need to coordinate one's own movements with those of others (Tantam, 1991). In addition to the need to tailor activities to each individual's social and recreational needs, there are health implications to consider. Recent data indicate high rates of obesity for children with autism, suggesting that promotion of physical activity should be an important lifelong goal for these individuals (Ho, Eaves, & Peabody, 1997).

There are practical considerations, too, regarding fine motor and graphomotor difficulties for many HFA and AS individuals. Simply allowing more time for activities such as dressing, or promoting the use of keyboards rather than handwriting, may be necessary to reduce frustration for all concerned. As with other skills, breaking down and routinizing the steps in an activity so that the same sequence is followed each time will assist the person with autism. For those with the "clumsy, high Verbal IQ" profile, verbal mediation (talking through the steps) may be particularly helpful. For younger or less verbal children, creating songs or rhymes that outline the steps may promote success. The hand-over-hand technique, or otherwise putting the child through the movements involved in a task (Ricks & Wing, 1975), may be necessary for teaching. For some motor tasks, there is no substitute for repetition with corrective feedback. Anecdotally, success may be obtained for some AS and HFA individuals by practicing motor skills (including gait and posture) with videotape review.

The research discussed in this chapter also has implications for the teaching of motor skills. For example, the praxic errors described here suggest that it might be helpful to demonstrate some skills from beside rather than facing the individual with autism. Similarly, for some individuals, demonstrating a skill in a mirror may help them to translate what is seen into what they must do. Most who work in the field of autism are aware of the unfortunate consequences of facilitated communication, a technique that supposedly compensates for praxic deficits in autism (Biklen, 1990; see Jacobson, Mulick, & Schwartz, 1995, for a history of the phenomenon). The ease with which facilitated communication was accepted by so many perhaps highlights the need for scientific study of dyspraxia in autism and for empirically justified strategies to compensate for any deficits that are identified in individuals.

CONCLUSION

Autism in all its manifestations is a complex disorder; the variety of expressions of the syndrome both between individuals and across the lifespan is freely acknowledged here. One goal of this contribution has been to highlight this heterogeneity with reference to an often neglected domain while pointing out a number of areas in which systematic investigation may reveal some underlying order. It is hoped that increased recognition of the potential relationships between motor dysfunctions and other aspects of the autistic syndrome will both stimulate new experimental approaches and inform clinical practice.

ACKNOWLEDGMENTS

I thank Susan Bryson, PhD, for ongoing stimulating discussions of these and many other issues in autism. Editor Ami Klin, PhD, made many valuable suggestions; these and the comments of William Hayes, PhD, are greatly appreciated.

REFERENCES

Abrahamsen, E. P., & Mitchell, J. R. (1990). Communication and sensorimotor functioning in children with autism. *Journal of Autism and Developmental Disorders, 20,* 75–86.

American Psychiatric Association. (1980). *Diagnostic and statistical manual of mental disorders* (3rd ed.). Washington, DC: Author.

American Psychiatric Association. (1987). *Diagnostic and statistical manual of mental disorders* (3rd ed., rev.). Washington, DC: Author.

American Psychiatric Association. (1994). *Diagnostic and statistical manual of mental disorders* (4th ed.). Washington, DC: Author.

Annett, M. (1970). The growth of manual preference and speed. *British Journal of Psychology, 61*, 545–558.

Asperger, H. (1991). "Autistic psychopathy" in childhood (U. Frith, Trans.). In U. Frith (Ed.), *Autism and Asperger syndrome* (pp. 37–92). Cambridge, UK: Cambridge University Press. (Original work published 1944)

Ayres, J. (1979). *Sensory integration and the child.* Los Angeles: Western Psychological Services.

Barresi, J., & Moore, C. (1996). Intentional relations and social understanding. *Brain and Behavioral Sciences, 19*, 107–122.

Biklen, D. (1990). Communication unbound: Autism and praxis. *Harvard Educational Review, 60*, 291–314.

Bryson, S. E. (1990). Autism and anomalous handedness. In S. Coren (Ed.), *Left-handedness: Behavioral implications and anomalies* (pp. 441–456). Amsterdam: Elsevier North-Holland.

Bryson, S. E., Landry, R., & Wainwright, J. A. (1997). A componential view of executive dysfunction in autism: Review of recent evidence. In J. A. Burack & J. T. Enns (Eds.), *Attention, development, and psychopathology* (pp. 232–259). New York: Guilford Press.

Cermak, S. (1985). Developmental dyspraxia. In E. A. Roy (Ed.), *Neuropsychological studies of apraxia and related disorders* (Vol. 23, pp. 225–248). Amsterdam: Elsevier North-Holland.

Cornish, K. M., & McManus, I. C. (1996). Hand preference and hand skill in children with autism. *Journal of Autism and Developmental Disorders, 26*, 597–609.

Courchesne, E., Townsend, J. P., Akshoomoff, N. A., Yeung-Courchesne, R., Lincoln, A., James, H. E., Haas, R. H., Schreibman, L., & Lau, L. (1994). A new finding: Impairment in shifting attention in autistic and cerebellar patients. In S. H. Broman & J. Grafman (Eds.), *Atypical cognitive deficits in developmental disorders: Implications for brain function* (pp. 101–137). Hillsdale, NJ: Erlbaum.

Damasio, A. R., & Maurer, R. G. (1978). A neurological model for childhood autism. *Archives of Neurology, 35*, 777–786.

Dawson, G. (1983). Lateralized brain dysfunction in autism: Evidence from the Halstead–Reitan Neuropsychological Battery. *Journal of Autism and Developmental Disorders, 13*, 269–286.

DeMyer, M. K. (1976). Motor, perceptual–motor, and intellectual disabilities of autistic children. In L. Wing (Ed.), *Early childhood autism* (pp. 169–193). Oxford: Pergamon Press.

DeMyer, M. K. (1979). *Parents and children in autism.* Washington, DC: Winston.

DeMyer, M. K., Alpern, G. D., Barton, S., DeMyer, W. E., Churchill, D. W., Hingtgen, J. N., Bryson, C. Q., Pontius, W., & Kimberlin, C. (1972). Imitation in autistic, early schizophrenic, and non-psychotic children. *Journal of Autism and Childhood Schizophrenia, 2*, 264–287.

Dewey, D. (1995). What is developmental dyspraxia? *Brain and Cognition, 29*, 254–274.

Ehlers, S., & Gillberg, C. (1993). The epidemiology of Asperger syndrome: A total population study. *Journal of Child Psychology and Psychiatry, 34*, 1327–1350.

Elliott, D., Weeks, D. J., & Jones, R. (1986). Lateral asymmetries in finger-tapping by adolescents and young adults with Down syndrome. *American Journal of Mental Deficiency, 90,* 472–475.

Eslinger, P. J. (1996). Conceptualizing, describing, and measuring components of executive function: A summary. In G. R. Lyon & N. A. Krasnegor (Eds.), *Attention, memory, and executive function* (pp. 307–395). Baltimore: Brookes.

Frith, U., & Frith, C. D. (1974). Specific motor disabilities in Down's syndrome children. *Journal of Child Psychology and Psychiatry, 15,* 293–301.

Geschwind, N. (1975). The apraxias: Neural mechanisms of disorders of learned movements. *American Scientist, 63,* 188–195.

Ghaziuddin, M., Tsai, L. Y., & Ghaziuddin, N. (1992). A reappraisal of clumsiness as a diagnostic feature of Asperger syndrome. *Journal of Autism and Developmental Disorders, 22,* 651–656.

Gillberg, C. (1989). Asperger syndrome in 23 Swedish children: A clinical study. *Developmental Medicine and Child Neurology, 31,* 520–531.

Gillberg, C. (1993). Asperger syndrome and clumsiness [letter]. *Journal of Autism and Developmental Disorders, 23,* 686.

Gillberg, C., & Gillberg, I. C. (1989). Asperger syndrome—Some epidemiological aspects: A research note. *Journal of Child Psychology and Psychiatry, 30,* 631–638.

Gillberg, C., Ehlers, S., Schaumann, H., Jakobsson, G., Dahlgren, S. O., Lindblom, R., Bagenhom, A., Tjuus, T., & Blidner, E. (1990). Autism under age three years: A clinical study of 28 cases referred for autistic symptoms in infancy. *Journal of Child Psychology and Psychiatry, 31,* 921–934.

Gubbay, S. S. (1975). *The clumsy child.* New York: Saunders.

Hallett, M., Lebiedowska, M. K., Thomas, S. L., Stanhope, S. J., Denckla, M. B., & Rumsey, J. (1993). Locomotion of autistic adults. *Archives of Neurology, 50,* 1304–1308.

Henderson, S. E. (1987). The assessment of "clumsy" children: Old and new approaches. *Journal of Child Psychology and Psychiatry, 28,* 511–527.

Ho, H. H., Eaves, L. C., & Peabody, D. (1997). Nutrient intake and obesity in children with autism. *Focus on Autism and Other Developmental Disabilities, 12,* 187–192.

Hughes, C. (1996). Planning problems in autism at the level of motor control. *Journal of Autism and Developmental Disorders, 26,* 90–107.

Hughes, C., & Russell, J. (1993). Autistic children's difficulty with mental disengagement from an object: Its implications for theories of autism. *Developmental Psychology, 29,* 498–510.

Hughes, C., Russell, J., & Robbins, T. W. (1994). Specific planning deficit in autism: Evidence for a central executive dysfunction. *Neuropsychologia, 32,* 477–492.

Jacobson, J. W., Mulick, J. A., & Schwartz, A. A. (1995). A history of facilitated communication. *American Psychologist, 50,* 750–765.

Jones, V., & Prior, M. P. (1985). Motor imitation abilities and neurological signs in autistic children. *Journal of Autism and Developmental Disorders, 15,* 37–46.

Keele, S., Ivry, R., & Pokorny, R. A. (1987). Force control and its relation to timing. *Journal of Motor Behaviour, 19,* 96–144.

Keogh, J. F., Sugden, D. A., Reynard, C. L., & Calkins, J. A. (1979). Identification of clumsy children: Comparisons and comments. *Journal of Human Movement Studies, 5,* 32–41.

Kirk, S. A., McCarthy, J. J., & Kirk, W. D. (1968). *The Illinois Test of Psycholinguistic Abilities.* Urbana: University of Illinois Press.

Klin, A., Volkmar, F. R., & Sparrow, S. S. (1992). Autistic social dysfunction: Some limitations of the Theory of Mind hypothesis. *Journal of Child Psychology and Psychiatry, 33,* 861–876.

Klin A., Volkmar, F. R., Sparrow, S. S., Cicchetti, D. V., & Rourke, B. P. (1995). Validity and neuropsychological characterization of Asperger syndrome: Convergence with Nonverbal Learning Disabilities syndrome. *Journal of Child Psychology and Psychiatry, 36,* 1127–1140.

Knights, R. M., & Norwood, J. A. (1979). *Revised smoothed normative data on the Neuropsychological Test Battery for Children.* Ottawa, Ontario, Canada: Department of Psychiatry, Carleton University.

Kohen-Raz, R., Volkmar, F. R., & Cohen, D. J. (1992). Postural control in children with autism. *Journal of Autism and Developmental Disorders, 22,* 419–432.

Laszlo, J. I., & Bairstow, P. J., Bartrip, J., & Rolfe, U. T. (1988). Clumsiness or perceptuomotor dysfunction? In A. M. Colley & J. R. Beech (Eds.), *Cognition and action in skilled behavior* (Vol. 55, pp. 293–309). Amsterdam: Elsevier North-Holland.

Lezak, M. D. (1983). *Neuropsychological assessment* (2nd ed.). New York: Oxford University Press.

Lord, C. (1995). Follow-up of two-year-olds referred for possible autism. *Journal of Child Psychology and Psychiatry, 36,* 1365–1382.

Lord, R., & Hulme, C. (1988). Patterns of rotary pursuit performance in clumsy and normal children. *Journal of Child Psychology and Psychiatry, 29,* 691–701.

Losse, A., Henderson, S. E., Elliman, D., Hall, D., Knight, E., & Jongmans, M. (1991). Clumsiness in children: Do they grow out of it? A 10-year followup study. *Developmental Medicine and Child Neurology, 33,* 55–68.

Lundy-Ekman, L., Ivry, R., Keele, S., & Woollacott, M. (1991). Timing and force control deficits in clumsy children. *Journal of Cognitive Neuroscience, 3,* 367–376.

Manjiviona, J., & Prior, M. (1995). Comparison of Asperger syndrome and high-functioning autistic children on a test of motor impairment. *Journal of Autism and Developmental Disorders, 25,* 23–39.

Matthews, C. G., & Klove, H. (1964). *Instruction manual for the Adult Neuropsychology Test Battery.* Madison: University of Wisconsin Medical School.

Maurice, C. (Ed.). (1996). *Behavioral intervention for young children with autism: A manual for parents and professionals.* Austin TX: PRO-ED.

McEvoy, R. E., Rogers, S. J., & Pennington, B. F. (1993). Executive function and social communication deficits in young autistic children. *Journal of Child Psychology and Psychiatry, 34,* 563–578.

McManus, I. C., Murray, B., Doyle, K., & Baron-Cohen, S. (1992). Handedness in childhood autism shows a dissociation of skill and preference. *Cortex, 28,* 373–381.

Meltzoff, A. N., & Gopnik, A. (1993). The role of imitation in understanding persons and developing a theory of mind. In S. Baron-Cohen, H. Tager-Flusberg, & D. J. Cohen (Eds.), *Understanding other minds: Perspectives from autism* (pp. 335–366). Oxford: Oxford University Press.

Ozonoff, S., Rogers, S. J., & Pennington, B. F. (1991). Asperger's syndrome: Evidence of an empirical distinction from high-functioning autism. *Journal of Child Psychology and Psychiatry, 32,* 1107–1122.

Pennington, B. F., & Ozonoff, S. (1996). Executive functions and developmental psychopathology. *Journal of Child Psychology and Psychiatry, 37,* 51–87.

Piek, J. P., & Coleman-Carman, R. (1995). Kinaesthetic sensitivity and motor performance of children with developmental co-ordination disorder. *Developmental Medicine and Child Neurology, 37,* 976–984.

Rapin, I. (Ed.). (1996). *Preschool children with inadequate communication* (Clinics in Developmental Medicine No. 139). London: MacKeith Press.

Ricks, D. M., & Wing, L. (1975). Language, communication, and the use of symbols in normal and autistic children. *Journal of Autism and Childhood Schizophrenia, 5,* 191–221.

Rogers, S. J. (1999). An examination of the imitation deficit in autism. In J. Nadel & G. Butterworth (Eds.), *Imitation in infancy* (pp. 254–283). Cambridge UK: Cambridge University Press.

Rogers, S. J., Bennetto, L., McEvoy, R. E., & Pennington, B. F. (1996). Imitation and pantomime in high-functioning adolescents with autism spectrum disorders. *Child Development, 67,* 2060–2073.

Rogers, S. J., & Pennington, B. F. (1991). A theoretical approach to the deficits in infantile autism. *Development and Psychopathology, 3,* 137–162.

Rourke, B. P. (1989). *Nonverbal learning disabilities: The syndrome and the model.* New York: Guilford Press.

Roy, E. A., Elliott, D., Dewey, D., & Square-Storer, P. (1990). Impairments to praxis and sequencing in adult and developmental disorders. In C. Bard, M. Fleury, & L. Hay (Eds.), *Development of eye–hand coordination across the life span* (pp. 358–384). Columbia: University of South Carolina Press.

Rumsey, J. M., & Hamburger, S. D. (1988). Neuropsychological findings in high functioning men with infantile autism, residual state. *Journal of Clinical and Experimental Neuropsychology, 10,* 201–221.

Russell, J. (Ed.). (1998). *Autism as an executive disorder.* Oxford: Oxford University Press.

Sears, L. L., Finn, P. R., & Steinmetz, J. E. (1994). Abnormal classical eye-blink conditioning in autism. *Journal of Autism and Developmental Disorders, 24,* 737–751.

Siegel, B. (1996). *The world of the autistic child: Understanding and treating autistic spectrum disorders.* New York: Oxford University Press.

Siegel, D. J., Minshew, N. J., & Goldstein, G. (1996). Wechsler IQ profiles in diagnosis of high-functioning autism. *Journal of Autism and Developmental Disorders, 26,* 389–406.

Sigman, M., & Capps, L. (1997). *Children with autism: A developmental perspective.* Cambridge, MA: Harvard University Press.

Smith, I. M. (1996). *Imitation and gesture representation in autism.* Unpublished doctoral dissertation, Dalhousie University, Halifax, Nova Scotia, Canada.

Smith, I. M., & Bryson, S. E. (1994). Imitation and action in autism: A critical review. *Psychological Bulletin, 116,* 259–273.

Smith, I. M., & Bryson, S. E. (1998a). Imitation in autism I: Nonsymbolic postures and sequences. *Cognitive Neuropsychology, 15,* 747–770.

Smith, I. M., & Bryson, S. E. (1998b). *Imitation in autism II: Symbolic gestures and pantomimed object use.* Manuscript submitted for publication.

Soper, H. V., Satz, P., Orsini, D. L., Henry, R. R., Zvi, J. C., & Schulman, M. (1986). Handedness patterns in autism suggest subtypes. *Journal of Autism and Developmental Disorders, 16,* 155–167.

Stone, W. L., Ousley, O. Y., & Littleford, C. D. (1997). Motor imitation in young children with autism: What's the object? *Journal of Abnormal Child Psychology, 25,* 475–485.

Stott, D. H., Moyes, F. A., & Henderson, S. E. (1984). *Manual: Test of Motor Impairment (Henderson Revision).* Guelph, Ontario: Brook International.

Szatmari, P., Bartolucci, G., & Bremner, R. (1989). Asperger's syndrome: Comparison of early history and outcome. *Developmental Medicine and Child Neurology, 31,* 709–720.

Szatmari, P., Tuff, L., Finlayson, A. J., & Bartolucci, G. (1990). Asperger's syndrome and autism: Neurocognitive aspects. *Journal of the American Academy of Child and Adolescent Psychiatry, 29,* 130–136.

Tantam, D. (1988a). Lifelong eccentricity and social isolation. I. Psychiatric, social, and forensic aspects. *British Journal of Psychiatry, 153,* 777–782.

Tantam, D. (1988b). Lifelong eccentricity and social isolation. II. Asperger's syndrome or schizoid personality disorder? *British Journal of Psychiatry, 153,* 783–791.

Tantam, D. (1991). Asperger syndrome in adulthood. In U. Frith (Ed.), *Autism and Asperger syndrome* (pp. 147–183). Cambridge, UK: Cambridge University Press.

Teitelbaum, P., Maurer, R. G., Fryman, J., Teitelbaum, O. B., Vilensky, J., & Creedon, M. P. (1996). Dimensions of disintegration in the stereotyped locomotion characteristic of parkinsonism and autism. In R. L. Sprague & K. M. Newell (Eds.), *Stereotyped movements: Brain and behavior relationships.* Washington, DC: American Psychological Association.

van der Meulen, J. H. P., Denier van der Gon, J. J., Gielen, C. C. A. M., Gooskens, R. H. J. M., & Willemse, J. (1991). Visuomotor performance of normal and clumsy children. I: Fast goal-directed arm movements with and without visual feedback. *Developmental Medicine and Child Neurology, 33,* 40–54.

Vilensky, J. A., Damasio, A. R., & Maurer, R. G. (1981). Gait disturbances in patients with autistic behavior: A preliminary study. *Archives of Neurology, 38,* 646–649.

Whiten, A., & Brown, J. D. (1999). Imitation and the reading of other minds: Perspectives from the study of autism, normal children and non-human primates. In S. Braten (Ed.), *Intersubjective communication and emotion in ontogeny: A sourcebook* (pp. 266–280). Cambridge, UK: Cambridge University Press.

Wing, L. (1981). Asperger's syndrome: A clinical account. *Psychological Medicine, 11,* 115–129.

Wing, L. (1988). Autism: Possible clues to the underlying pathology—Clinical facts. In L. Wing (Ed.), *Aspects of autism: Biological research* (pp. 1–10). London: Gaskell/National Autistic Society.

Wing, L. (1996). *The autistic spectrum: A guide for parents and professionals.* London: Constable.

Wing, L., & Attwood, A. (1987). Syndromes of autism and atypical development. In D. J. Cohen & A. M. Donnellan (Eds.), *Handbook of autism and pervasive developmental disorders* (pp. 3–19). New York: Wiley.

World Health Organization. (1992). *International classification of diseases: Tenth revision.* Chapter V. Mental and behavioral disorders (including disorders of psychological development). Diagnostic criteria for research. Geneva: Author.

4

Social Language Use in Asperger Syndrome and High-Functioning Autism

REBECCA LANDA

Impairment in the *social use of language,* or pragmatics, is a hallmark of autism and Asperger syndrome (AS; Asperger, 1944; Kanner, 1943; Dewey & Everard, 1974; Tager-Flusberg, 1981; Volkmar et al., 1987; Baron-Cohen, 1988). Pragmatic impairment may be the most stigmatizing and handicapping aspect of these disorders. From school age onward, individuals with AS report that their social language vulnerabilities give rise to anxiety, avoidance of some social situations, and self-image challenges and are a source of great concern to them. Adults diagnosed with AS report having difficulty at jobs and establishing friendships due to their social communication impairment, despite being professionally productive and otherwise quite capable.

Despite its prominence in AS, pragmatic language impairment is not included in the diagnostic criteria for AS according to the fourth edition of the *Diagnostic and Statistical Manual of Mental Disorders* (DSM-IV; American Psychiatric Association, 1994). There are only two DSM-IV criteria for AS that pertain directly to communication: (1) gross language milestones are achieved within the normal chronological time frame during the first 3 years of life and (2) abnormal nonverbal communication. These criteria are problematic for several reasons. First, the criterion of normal language development during the first 3 years of life is based only on clinical impression of gross markers of language development. Without formal testing during the first 3 years of life, there is no sure way of knowing whether language development was indeed normal during that period. The diagnostic challenge resulting from the existing criteria for AS is illustrated in the following example. A 3-year-old child comes to the clinic for assessment due to parental concerns about his or her social and behavioral patterns. The psychologist identifies the child as having at least normal intellectual functioning but restricted affect and stereotyped patterns of play. The psychiatrist identifies social and behavioral patterns consistent with AS. Because the child produced his first words at 14 months of age and is talking in sentences, the parents and pediatrician have not been concerned about a language disorder.

Next, the child is seen for a speech–language assessment. The interview reveals that the child did not babble until 9 months of age, and even then, babbling did not have the normal rich intonational contours expected. First words were limited in number, consisted mostly of nouns, and were used only to request objects and actions needed by the child. The child did not use his words to express social communicative intentions expected during the first two years of life. During the speech–language assessment, the child scores more than 1.5 standard deviations below the mean on one or more subtests of the standardized tests, displays pragmatic language abnormalities, as well as other language processing difficulties involving word retrieval, restricted patterns of word combinations, restricted range of semantic notions expressed, and failure to understand language patterns within novel social contexts. This places the diagnostic team in a quandary. From a quantitative perspective, the child meets the DSM-IV communication onset criteria for AS. Yet the child's language processing is not normal. Should this child be diagnosed with AS?

This scenario is a common one in our clinical program. A similar problem arises for older individuals as well, where language formulation, abstract language processing, gist formation, and pragmatic language problems may be identified during speech–language assessment. Yet without formal testing, this detail about language and communication function would not have been clearly identified. What features of communication may be impaired and to what degree in association with a diagnosis of AS? More research is needed into the communication features of individuals with AS to resolve these diagnostic dilemmas.

Pragmatic language function is critical to assess as part of the diagnostic process for any developmental disorder, but it is especially relevant when a patient is suspected of having a pervasive developmental disorder. Yet assessment of pragmatic skills is complicated due to the multifaceted, context-bound nature of pragmatics and difficulty of measuring pragmatic functions in an ecologically valid way using standardized pragmatic measures. In this chapter, an attempt is made to demystify the concept of pragmatics and review the rather scant literature on pragmatic-related behavior associated with high-functioning autism (HFA) and AS. In this chapter, reference is made to HFA and AS. During discussions of research reports, the nomenclature used by the researchers is maintained. During more general discussions, "HFA" and "AS" will be used interchangeably since the two phenotypes have not been clearly delineated in the area of pragmatic function.

WHAT IS MEANT BY "PRAGMATICS" OF LANGUAGE?

The pragmatic rule system represents one domain of language functioning. Pragmatic rules guide the use of linguistic constructs (e.g., grammar, semantics) across different contexts for the purpose of communicating one's intended message. It is only when people within a culture follow these rules, or systematically violate them, that we understand when someone is teasing, has a hidden agenda, being polite, humorous, sarcastic, and so on (Grice, 1975). Speakers employ their entire language system (including syntax and semantics) to support their pragmatic competence.

Pragmatics represents an attempt by the linguistic community to embrace an ecologically valid approach to the study of communication. Before pragmatics was recognized as a component of language functioning, students of child language development focused on isolated parts of the language system without regard to how the communication system functioned as a whole. For example, Chomsky (1968) focused on the rules of syntax, which govern how words are arranged into phrase and sentence structures. These rules tell us how to go from a declarative form, such as "John is helping Bob," to an interrogative form, such as "Is John helping Bob?" Early in development, some young children produce phrases for which they do not appear to have developed underlying combinatorial rules (e.g., rules for combining the words with other words to form unique phrases, with the words being flexibly used in any position within the sentence). This gestalt pattern of language learning makes the child appear quite linguistically advanced, but assessment may reveal that the child's language comprehension and phrase structure development are not as sophisticated as might appear. Rather, the child has developed a repertoire of "giant words" (memorized chunk of words) which are used in appropriate contexts. This is analogous to the stereotyped language use and gestalt language learning patterns exhibited by autistic individuals who, unlike unimpaired children, may not develop a truly flexible syntactic rule system. Individuals with AS and HFA are often reported to have intact syntactic abilities, but the flexibility and true productivity of syntactic skills are typically not assessed. Flexible syntactic skills are essential for tailoring the form of message expression to fit the demands of the social context (see the section "Communicative Intentions"). Even if normal syntactic ability is demonstrated on productivity and comprehension measures, the integrity of the entire linguistic system cannot be judged based on intact skills in one isolated linguistic domain. Semantic and pragmatic skills must be examined despite the presence of well-formed sentences. This is because the ability to form intact syntactic structures does not ensure the ability to express meaningful semantic relationships in socially appropriate ways.

Semantic development involves learning how words and word combinations express meaning. Depending on the child's level of functioning, semantic assessment will include some or all of the following: receptive and expressive lexical (vocabulary) development, comprehension and production of a variety of semantic relationships (e.g., existence, locative action; comparative, and temporal), category development, appreciation of synonyms and antonyms, comprehension of the gist of discourse and stories, comprehension and expression of figurative language, and inferencing and prediction skills. Such skills contribute to academic and social success, enabling the child to "get the point" of what has been said or read. This is particularly important to remember when assessing the language system of individuals with AS. Syntactic skills may be relatively intact (at least superficially), but semantic and pragmatic skills are not as well developed (Menyuk & Quill, 1985; Baltaxe, 1977). Careful assessment of the entire language system is of great diagnostic and theoretical importance as we strive to understand the relationship between autism and AS.

Pragmatic development involves learning the rules for tailoring language forms and expression of meaning to fit the social demands of the linguistic and nonlinguistic context. Pragmatic development follows a rather predictable course throughout childhood and adolescence, with specific rules differing from culture to culture. Although most pragmatic rules are tacit, some are explicitly taught. For example, adults often comment on the "honesty" of young children who frankly speak their opinions or thoughts (e.g., openly commenting on someone's weight or appearance). Although this is often viewed as the innocent "honesty" of childhood, it is a reflection of not having learned what statements are taboo in public and how to phrase criticisms in a nonoffensive, indirect way. Violations of theses taboos are clearly identified by caretakers, with more appropriate models often being provided. The acquisition of pragmatic rules relies heavily on other aspects of development such as the other language subsystems (discussed previously), cognitive systems (including social cognition and the executive control functions such as set shifting, inhibiting prepotent responses), social–emotional knowledge, and visually based aspects of information processing. The growing normative pragmatic literature enables clinicians to compare pragmatic development to other aspects of language, social, emotional, and cognitive growth.

One organizational framework for understanding pragmatic language involves three somewhat overlapping domains: the acts of expressing communicative intentions, presupposition, and discourse organization. The next segment of this chapter defines each of these three domains, discusses normal development of pragmatic language within the domains, and reviews patterns of impairment in HFA and AS for each of these three domains. The review of impairment in HFA and AS reflects general trends rather than an enumeration of well-known facts. This is because there are relatively few empirical studies of pragmatic functioning in individuals with AS or HFA and each study focuses on a discrete set of pragmatic skills rather than the whole pragmatic system. Furthermore, researchers approach the study of pragmatics in autism in different ways and focus on different age groups. This makes comparison of discrepancies across studies difficult. Keeping in mind the heterogeneity of autism spectrum disorders and the unclear relationship between HFA and AS, the general trends in pragmatic functioning reported in this population are presented in the next section.

COMMUNICATIVE INTENTIONS

Definition

Utterances produced by a speaker typically have an intended communicative function (Austin, 1962), and thereby perform a speech act (Searle, 1975) or action. Although this is most obvious when we say such things as "I promise to call," where the act of promising has occurred simply by producing the statement, it is also true of nearly every utterance we produce. According to Dore (1977), even the intentional communicative vocalizations and gestures of preverbal children (which begin at around 9 months of age) can be assigned a type of function (e.g., greeting, showing, commenting, rejecting, and protesting). Speakers may communicate different intentions through the production of a single form and, conversely, may use a variety of forms to express a single intention. For example, the form "Can you walk the dog tonight?" may have intended functions of politely commanding, requesting information, or making a sarcastic comment. The intended communicative function of the sentence will be made clear by the context, including shared information between the speakers (e.g., both parties knowing that the listener has tentative plans for the evening that might affect the dog walking routine), cues signaled through intonation (vocal pitch and loudness variations), facial and gestural expressions, and environmental cues.

The use of various forms to express one intention is illustrated by the options to use indirect, polite expressions, such as "Do you have the time?," when in a somewhat formal situation, or a more direct expression, such as "What time is it?," in less formal situations. For social success, it is important to develop the ability to recognize situations in which intentions should be expressed indirectly (e.g., requesting politely rather than commanding an action be completed). It is also important to have the linguistic flexibility to select appropriate forms for expressing the intention. Failure to do so could have dire social consequences, including social isolation, decreased cooperation from others, and school and workplace challenges.

Normal Development

Before words are acquired, children express a variety of declarative (attention getting, socially-oriented) and imperative (efforts to obtain an object or action) communicative intentions through gestures (including pointing), vocalizations, and facial expressions. They actively check the gaze patterns of their communicative partner to determine whether their intent has been accurately recognized (Bates, O'Connell, & Shore, 1987). During the preschool years, children develop increasing options for expressing their intentions and learn how to frame their messages indirectly. Nevertheless, preschoolers tend to be quite forthright in expressing themselves, sometimes to the embarrassment of their parents. A variety of new intentions appears during the preschool years (e.g., teasing), but common forms of communicative intentions (e.g., negotiation, introductions, and clarification requests) are acquired in informal and formal polite forms later, by 9 years of age (Wiig, 1982). Throughout childhood, there is an increase in the means (grammatical, semantic, integration of paralinguistic signals) of expressing intentions and tailoring them to the context at hand.

In Autism and Asperger Syndrome

Most children with autism, even those with a high IQ, exhibit impairment in the development of communicative intentions. Autistic children show idiosyncratic form of expressing intentions, a restricted variety of intentions expressed, and limitations in their ability to flexibly control the degree of directness with which some intentions are expressed. During infancy, some autistic babies have abnormal and idiosyncratic cries (Ricks & Wing, 1975). The idiosyncratic forms of expression make it difficult for caregivers to confidently identify the need or desire being communicated. Idiosyncratic manner of expression continues as intentional communicative ability emerges. Atypical nonverbal strategies for establishing referents involve leading others by the hand to objects of interest rather than using pointing gestures and gaze patterns (Landry & Loveland, 1988). Even when pointing and eye contact are used during request productions, they are not coordinated and do not involve the normal looking from the object of desire to the communicative partner (Mundy, Sigman, Ungerer, & Sherman, 1986).

Abnormality is also observed in many autistic children's use of verbal forms to "point" things out (e.g., use of deictic markers such as personal pronouns and demonstratives such as "here, there") (Fay & Schuler, 1980). That is, autistic children have particular difficulty using forms of language that have no fixed referent but, rather, shift in meaning depending on contextual variables. This difficulty creates a challenge for the communicative partner to determine the child's intended referent and intended meaning.

Another abnormality in autism is the idiosyncratic expression of fear, requests, and other intentions using immediate or delayed echolalia. An illustration of this was one child's use of the phrase "Got a splinter" whenever she was upset or hurt (Prizant & Wetherby, 1987). The child had originally heard the phrase during a painful experience, but then began to use it in contexts she associated with the original experience. Idiosyncratic expression of communicative intentions may manifest in the use of repetitive questions or statements, the function of which may be to sustain interactions in the absence of more creative ways of doing so (Caparulo & Cohen, 1977; Turner, 1995). This contrasts with the purpose for which repetition is used by unimpaired children (e.g., to emphasize a point, express surprise, and acknowledge). The idiosyncratic communications of intended meaning are difficult for listeners to understand, especially if they do not share essential aspects of past experiences with the child. Caregivers' efforts to infer the intention being expressed may be unsuccessful, limiting their ability to soothe and fulfill the child, possibly leading to a cascade of socially unacceptable behavior from the child (e.g., tantrums or aggression) due to the frustration of not making him- or herself understood. A complex, difficult dynamic may result, which may be partly alleviated through the development of an alternative communication system. Such a system may be developed by a speech–language pathologist, in conjunction with the family and educational professionals, to provide a conventional code (pictures, icons, etc.) of shared meaning between the child and his or her communicative partner.

HFA children also differ from the norm in the types of communicative intentions expressed. In the autistic population, expression of social intentions (e.g., greeting and commenting) are greatly outnumbered by instrumental intentions (having own needs met) (Wetherby & Prutting, 1984). The means of communicating social and instrumental intentions may be different, with gaze and pointing occasionally used for instrumental purposes but not for expressing social intentions (Mundy et al., 1986). Thus, the autistic child may experience a fundamentally different challenge in social–affectively based communications compared to communicative efforts intended to obtain an object or action of interest. When social intentions are expressed, inappropriateness or awkwardness is apt to be noted. For example, opinions may be expressed forthrightly rather than in more subtle, socially acceptable indirect ways, leading to impressions of impoliteness, rudeness, or insensitivity. This poses a particular problem for teenage and adult individuals who express their fondness or desire to be near someone of the opposite sex in an offensively direct way. Understanding the intended meaning of others may also pose a problem for the HFA individual, who may interpret indirect expressions literally (Ozonoff & Miller, 1996; Rumsey & Hanahan, 1990). This limits the ability to respond in the socially expected way and sets the stage for communication breakdown.

PRESUPPOSITION

Definition

Presupposition refers to the knowledge, expectations, and beliefs that a speaker postulates to be shared with the conversational partner. When making a "presupposition," a speaker assesses what information he or she shares with the communicative partner and uses this information to plan the content and form of the message to be communicated. Other aspects of the situation are also taken into consideration, including physical qualities (e.g., age) and social status of the partner, setting (e.g., formal office setting vs. a picnic) and contextual variables (e.g., presence or absence of referent), history of shared experiences, and previous content of the discourse. Accurate judgments about amount and type of shared knowledge may enable the speaker to communicate clearly with only one word (Bates, 1976). An example of a presuppositional error is when a speaker uses informal words and speech patterns (e.g., "Wanna soda?") rather than more formal means (e.g., "Would you like something to drink?") when speaking to an authority figure. Another example would be omitting important background information or details that the partner needs to fully understand the message (e.g., giving too few details in directions to get to the airport when the listener has never driven in that part of town before and does not know that the highway splits yet both veins are labeled with the same highway number).

Presuppositional ability requires intact attentional mechanisms, an awareness of social rules, the ability to consider the perspectives of others (Flavell, Botkin, Fry, Wright, & Jarvis, 1968), the ability to consider alternative ways for phrasing ideas, and having the language skills to do so. Presuppositional skills include knowing when and how to be polite, formal, or colloquial; when to elaborate on an idea or to give a condensed version; how much background information to provide; how complex the words and sentence structures should be; and what topics are taboo in what situations. These judgments affect how receptive, motivated, and successful a partner will be in continuing the conversational interaction. Communicative behavior resulting from these judgments also leave an impression on the listener about the overall social appropriateness of the speaker and may have substantial consequences in situations such as job interviews.

Normal Development

Although the precursor skills to presuppositional development have not been empirically defined, many skills that seem important for developing presuppositional abilities are acquired in the first 2 years of life. For example, joint referencing skills (looking in the direction that a partner is looking) are present in an early form at 6 months of age. Joint attention skills are needed to track the changes in referents during conversations, so that inferences about the speaker's intended meaning may be made successfully. Another example is the awareness that young children have of saliency in their environment. They pay attention to what is important. This awareness of saliency is reflected in children's first words, which typically represent a salient person, place, thing, or action such as "ball, kitty, cookie" rather than inanimate objects having little relevance in their lives such as "wall." This seemingly innate detection of salience sets the stage for identifying referents of others' utterances, detecting salient social cues that guide interpretation of ambiguous linguistic input, and, later, recognizing the main topic of someone's utterance or of text.

By 4 years of age, children recognize differences in listeners' ability to process language input. Four-year-olds speak differently to younger children, age peers, and adults, adjusting the complexity of their grammar to their audience (Shatz & Gelman, 1973). They also adjust their language in consideration of a listener's role or occupation (Bates, 1976; Ervin-Tripp, 1977). They recognize the communicative significance of nonlinguistic cues and of requests for them to clarify ambiguous messages. Strategies for clarifying misunderstood messages increase across the preschool years. While 12- to 24-month-old children clarify messages by repeating them more loudly and with more precise articulation, 3-year-olds are able to substitute, delete, or add words in revising their messages (Gallagher, 1977). Rules that certain manners of expression and types of topics are taboo in certain contexts are acquired. Thus, the "openness" of the preschooler who bluntly comments on a stranger's personal features diminishes with age.

In Autism and Asperger Syndrome

A common characteristic of HFA and AS individuals is failure to adjust their language productions in consideration of the ever-changing contextual cues. A classic example is their tendency to use a pedantic, formal speaking style when a more relaxed or colloquial speech register is more appropriate (Kanner, 1943). In part, impaired presuppositional skills may result from impaired comprehension of nonverbal and verbal cues. For example, limited comprehension of affective (Sigman, Yirmiya, & Capps, 1995) and linguistically based intonational (Fine, Bartolucci, Ginsberg, & Szatmari, 1991; Baltaxe & Simmons, 1985) cues may compromise the HFA individual's ability to understand marked syntactic boundaries, judge others' degree of social engagement, judge speakers' attitudes, and recognize that an utterance is not meant to be taken literally (e.g., jokes and sarcasm). Such difficulty, in addition to poor comprehension of implied meaning (as expressed in indirect speech acts), contributes to poor recognition that a request for clarification has been presented by a listener. Indeed, Loveland and Tunali (1991) reported that autistic individuals failed to respond to general inquiries for them to produce additional information, requiring specific prompts to clarify their ambiguous utterances. Even once the clarification request has been comprehended, HFA adolescents reportedly make fewer revisions in their messages compared to controls (Baltaxe, 1977). Baltaxe further reported that when revisions were made, they reflected the developmentally immature strategy of repetition rather than changing the content of the message.

Impaired recognition of nonverbal and indirect verbal cues is also evident in HFA individuals' tendency to repeatedly initiate topics of their special interest without regard for the listener's interest in the topic (Wing & Attwood, 1987). Socially inappropriate topics (e.g., asking a stranger his or her age) may be initiated (Langdell, 1980) and messages may be expressed in an overly direct manner (bluntly). In addition, HFA individuals display poor awareness of contextual rules for discourse behavior. This is illustrated by the experience of a young HFA woman who loudly answered her minister's questions during his sermon on Sundays. She did not appreciate the rule that individual members of an audience do not take the role of responder. From her view, she was simply doing the expected by responding to the questions. Like other HFA individuals, this young woman reported puzzlement at the irritated reactions she sometimes received in response to her social communicative behaviors. Once a discourse rule is explicitly stated, however, such individuals often follow successfully.

Making inferences about the intended meaning of others may also be disrupted by the autistic individual's difficulty understanding nonliteral uses of language (e.g., jokes and metaphor) and of how meaning shifts with changes in context. The literature indicates that HFA individuals' nonliteral language comprehension abilities are impaired, but not globally so. HFA individuals do recognize general differences in different types of speech acts. For example, they understand the formal requirement that jokes end in a humorous way but that stories may not (Ozonoff & Miller, 1996). Furthermore, they are typically able to appreciate simple or slapstick humor (Van Bourgondien & Mesibov, 1987). Comprehension of more complex humor, however, is a challenge, even for HFA individuals. Ozonoff and Miller (1996) hypothesized that the problems many autistic individuals have in understanding more complex jokes lies in a cognitive rigidity that interferes with abandoning initial impressions and reinterpreting the initial information so that a humorous, semantically correct ending may be selected. An alternative explanation is that HFA individuals fail to understand abstract language due to an overall deficit in complex information processing (Minshew, Goldstein, & Siegel, 1995).

Individuals with autism not only have problems appreciating socially relevant signals but often fail to provide signals that would permit their listeners to make appropriate presuppositions about them. The ability to signal intended meaning is partly compromised due to impaired use of intonational cues to express special or novel meanings (Fine et al., 1991; Rumsey, Andreasen, & Rapoport, 1986). Listeners may not know how to "read" what has been said and are then unsure about how to react. Such challenges in the communicative interchange may cause the listener to perceive the autistic individual as odd or rude and to avoid frequent contact with him or her.

DISCOURSE

Definition

Discourse refers to an ongoing series of utterances that create a "text" of sorts. It may have a hierarchy of topics and subtopics (Bates & MacWhinney, 1987) or a series of topics, with digressions from the main topic. There are a variety of types of discourse genres, only two of which are discussed here: social discourse (conversation) and narrative discourse (story telling). Both types of discourse have predictable organizational structures and developmental sequences. Although there have been few empirical studies of either type of discourse in individuals with HFA or AS, there is evidence that aspects of both are atypical in these populations.

Social Discourse

Social discourse is guided by rules for topic management (topic initiation, maintenance, and termination) and conversational repair following a communication breakdown. Information is presented in a predictable way, with speakers giving signals that they are about to speak, relinquish a turn, change a topic, and so on. When basic tacit rules, such as contributing informative and relevant information in the discourse (Grice, 1975), are broken, the coherence of the discourse is likely to decrease.

The organization of information in discourse typically involves providing background information early on. This principle is also followed at the sentence level, where old information precedes new information, providing a context for interpreting new information. Speakers also use words (cohesive devices) to link current information to that presented earlier in the discourse (Halliday & Hassan, 1976). Effective use of cohesion enables conversational partners to avoid confusion about referents. For example, in the two utterances "Tom broke the chair. He felt terrible about it," the cohesive devices "he" and "it" make sense because they refer to words previously presented in the discourse. Using pronouns enables the speaker to avoid redundancy, but if the rules for using cohesive devices are not followed properly, the referent for a pronoun may be difficult to determine and coherence will be compromised.

Cohesion and other strategies are used to maintain topics. Topic maintenance is a complex skill, requiring the ability to flexibly employ grammatical skills, understand and produce meaningful semantic relationships, recognize shared information with conversational partners, notice and interpret the significance of changing contextual cues, and so on.

Normal Development

The rudiments of discourse are seen early in infancy. Infants initiate social communicative interactions as well as respond to and maintain the interactions initiated by others. They engage in reciprocal gaze and affective exchanges (Stern, 1974), setting the stage for later conversational turn taking. The rules for reciprocal verbal turn taking appear to be appreciated very early in development, with rare instances of turn overlap or "interruption" (Ninio & Bruner, 1978). As early as 3 months of age, infants take a vocal turn after being spoken to by their caregivers (Bloom, Russell, & Wassenberg, 1987). Effective verbal turn taking continues once language forms are acquired, as can be observed when 1- and 2-year-olds remain quiet during the conversational turn of their mothers (Schaffer, Collis, & Parsons, 1977). With increasing age, children attend to and recognize signals being sent by multiple conversational partners at once. They become capable of negotiating a three-way conversational exchange by 4 years of age.

Early forms of topic maintenance are observed when infants and their caregivers attend to the same thing at the same time (joint attention). Between 6 and 8 months of age, infants begin to follow their caregiver's line of visual regard (Scaife & Bruner, 1975), setting the stage for later topic maintenance. With the acquisition of words, children become increasingly adept at establishing topics pertaining to themselves and to objects/events outside themselves. At first, adults shoulder the responsibility for developing and maintaining these topics. They do this by building a sort of scaffold (Bruner, 1978) around what the child says. By referring to events, engaging in routines, and using words and sentence structures familiar to the child, adults foster children's development of mental scripts for events with associated socially and semantically appropriate language (Foster, 1981, 1986; Ervin-Tripp, 1979). This both supports the likelihood that the child will maintain the topic and sets a foundation for later topic maintenance skills. As the ability to integrate verbal (linguistic content) and nonverbal (including intonational cues, shared experiences, setting, body language) cues develops, children become increasingly capable of identifying others' topics. During the primary grades, children become quite facile at identifying the gist, or topic, of an entire discourse text, such as a conversation or story, and making inferences and predictions based on that gist. Recognizing topics and gists is paramount to producing topically contingent responses and contributing to the discourse in a coherent and socially acceptable way.

Strategies for maintaining topics increase with development, from repeating part of the partner's utterance to adding new information. A repertoire of topic maintenance strategies is developed, enabling the speaker to select a strategy that is well suited to the context. One set of strategies involves the use of cohesive devices (cohesion). Use of cohesive devices to tie segments of the discourse together and make smooth transitions to new topics increases in sophistication with age. By kindergarten, children make semantic ties between current utterances and previous discourse using phrases (e.g., "*Speaking* of games, I learned a new game today") and cohesive devices (substituting pronouns for nouns, ellipsis, etc.; see above). Competent use of cohesive devices is important for discourse to be coherent, but it is not sufficient. Coherent discourse also depends on factors such as well-organized presentation of information and appropriate signaling of how messages are to be interpreted.

In Autism and Asperger Syndrome

In autism, the early bases of discourse, joint attention, and reciprocal social play are impaired (Mundy & Sigman, 1989; Ungerer & Sigman, 1981). Deficits in joint attention are characterized by absent or decreased use and comprehension of pointing and showing gestures (Mundy et al., 1986), and of eye gaze patterns for engaging in *social* communicative acts (Loveland & Landry, 1986; Mundy et al., 1986). Eye gaze is not used to determine whether the communicative partner is looking at the referent of the child's communication. Early deficits in reciprocal social communicative exchanges appear to linger throughout the lifespan, perhaps in more subtle form for the more able individuals with AS. For example, the communicative value of eye movements and gaze patterns continue to be poorly recognized. This will have an impact on abilities such as establishing co-reference with a partner (leading to topic maintenance difficulties), using eye contact to modulate turn length, and detecting signals (e.g., rolling the eyes) indicating nonliteral language use.

HFA individuals also exhibit difficulty using signals to modulate discourse. Some typical situations in which they inconsistently or inappropriately use signals in discourse include indicating that they are about to speak, clearly identifying the intended recipient of their message, indicating that they are about to relinquish a turn; and indicating an intended transition in the course of the topic (Langdell, 1980). One major consequence of poor signaling is confusion on the part of the listener; the stage has been set for a faulty exchange of information. In some cases, an intended listener may not attend to the speaker at all, which the speaker may interpret as being ignored.

Another difficulty involves maintaining topics of interest to the communicative partner. Individuals with AS and HFA have a reputation for being associative, which may lead them to shift a topic abruptly when the current topic reminds them of something else. Poor maintenance of others' topics stands in stark contrast to their ability to sustain topics of their own special interest for extended periods of time. However, the information shared within these topics tends to be a series of detailed facts rather than a story that leads to a gist or main point. Therefore, conversational partners tend to have difficulty building a reciprocal exchange of information with AS and HFA individuals. The information imparted by the AS and HFA individual may be new and interesting to a listener upon the first encounter, but repeated encounters often reveal that the information is stereotyped in nature, with the same facts being recounted each time the topic is discussed.

Within a discourse event, individuals with HFA and AS have difficulty using linguistic strategies, such as cohesion, for tying new information to previous discourse (Loveland, McEvoy, Kelley, & Tunali, 1990; Baltaxe & D'Angiola, 1992; Fine, Bartolucci, Szatmari, & Ginsberg, 1994). The precise nature of the types of cohesion errors exhibited by these groups are difficult to determine due to differences across studies in comparison groups, in subjects' language functioning and ages, and in type of elicitation task. One study has suggested that HFA and AS subjects differ in their pattern of cohesion use. Fine et al. (1994) compared referential cohesion use in HFA, AS, and nonautistic socially impaired children and teens. The groups differed in the relative frequency with which they used different types of cohesive devices. HFA subjects referred more often to the physical environment and less often to previous discourse, making it difficult to build a reciprocal conversation. The AS group differed from the other groups in the production of more unclear references (using words that have more than one possible referent in the previous discourse or that have no previous referent). Although the specific types of cohesion errors were different in the HFA and AS groups, both groups made significantly more errors than did other socially impaired children. This, together with the findings of other studies of cohesion usage by autistic individuals, indicates that rules for tying units of discourse together often are not appropriately employed by individuals in the autism spectrum. This is likely to result in discourse that is compromised in coherence.

Discourse Function and Thought Disorder in Autism and Asperger Syndrome

The difficulty that autistic individuals have in the use of cohesive devices, in understanding abstract language (e.g., multiple-meaning words and figurative language), and in generating new information may result in reduced coherence and reciprocity of the conversational exchange. This may lead some mental health professionals to conclude that the patient exhibits a thought disorder. The presence of thought disorder in HFA and AS has been suggested in studies using language sampling methods and/or analysis procedures that are standard clinical and research methods used with schizophrenic populations.

Dykens, Volkmar, and Glick (1991) used the Rorschach to elicit stories from HFA adults, then analyzed the stories for positive and negative features of thought disorder using the Thought, Language, and Communication Scale (Andreasen, 1979). HFA subjects reportedly exhibited poverty of speech, poor reality testing, and perceptual distortions as well as several examples of cognitive slippage (incongruous combinations, fabulized combinations, deviant responses, inappropriate logic). However, the HFA subjects exhibited less illogicality than did schizophrenic subjects.

Also using Andreasen's rating scale, Rumsey et al. (1986) compared communication behavior of a group of HFA (residual state) adults with that of adult schizophrenics. The autistic group exhibited a tendency to talk to themselves, perseveration on particular questions or topics, poverty of speech, poverty of content of speech, flat intonation, word or phrase repetition, and use of stereotyped scripts. The schizophrenic group showed more poverty of speech, derailment, illogicality, and loss of goal.

Ghaziuddin, Leininger, and Tsai (1995) explored thought disorder in HFA and AS adolescents using the Rorschach Inkblot Test to elicit and score samples of language output. These researchers used criteria for AS according to the *International Classification of Diseases, Tenth revision* (ICD-10; World Health Organization, 1993), which requires "autistic social dysfunction in the presence of normal intelligence and a history of normal language development" (p. 313). Despite considerable heterogeneity with the AS group, AS subjects produced responses that reflected "more active internal lives involving complex fantasies and cognitive processes compared to persons with HFA" (Ghaziuddin et al., 1995, p. 316). AS subjects were also more introverted than were HFA subjects. The authors concluded that the groups differed in their mechanisms of understanding and processing of new information. This would appear to indicate that a cognitive–linguistic process may contribute to impressions of thought disorder.

Although HFA/AS subjects appear to differ from schizophrenics in aspects of their discourse behavior, they sometimes may be classified as thought disordered (Rumsey et al., 1986; Dykens et al., 1991). However, the communicative oddities reported in studies of thought disorder in HFA/AS seem to be related to the social language deficit that has its beginnings early in life and reflects an impaired developmental process. It seems likely that HFA/AS individuals' deficits in semantic, social language, and cognition (e.g., executive functions) contribute to impressions of thought disorder. Following is a brief summary of semantic, linguistic, and executive function deficits reported in HFA individuals that might be related to the language characteristics associated with thought disorder.

• Impairment in word finding (Boucher, 1988) is likely to result in the production of words that are semantically inappropriate for the immediate context. Difficulty bringing a word to mind may result in the selection of a less preferred choice, resulting in an odd combination of words (e.g., incongruous combinations or fabulized combinations).

• Impaired ability to generate plans specifically formulated to the current, novel context may be inferred from studies of HFA children's play and language productions (Turner, 1995). Although autistic children fail to exhibit advanced forms of make-believe such as object substitutions in spontaneous play (Baron-Cohen, 1987), they are capable of make-believe in structured, prompted situations (Lewis & Boucher, 1995a, 1995b). The difficulty that some HFA individuals have in formulating language in a novel elicitation task has been reported by numerous investigators (Ghaziuddin et al., 1995; Landa, Martin, Minshew, & Goldstein, 1995; Baltaxe & Simmons, 1977; Menyuk & Quill, 1985). Thus, when asked to develop a story from an inkblot stimulus or when being interviewed about psychiatric/emotional experiences (a topic known to be difficult for this population) autistic individuals may have great difficulty generating substantial content. This deficit limits the amount of language output or content that is produced under certain sampling conditions, resulting in codings of poverty of speech or poverty of content of speech. Some HFA individuals produce very little language spontaneously regardless of the sampling procedure used and may represent a more impaired or different subgroup.

• Difficulty shifting cognitive sets will limit the subject's ability to consider alternative, and more contextually appropriate, interpretations of language (Ozonoff & Miller, 1996). This difficulty could also result in stereotypical, rigid language use.

• Reliance on stereotyped, rigid language forms, especially in novel situations, may result in what seem to be contextually unrelated responses or responses that are inadequately adapted to the social context (e.g., deviant responses, inappropriate logic, and stereotyped scripts) (Rumsey et al., 1986; Prizant & Wetherby, 1987; Simmons & Baltaxe, 1975).

• Poor awareness of the type and amount of background information listeners need may lead subjects to produce poorly linked sequences of information. The subject may infer that the listener already knows the conceptual link between segments of information and not bother to articulate it. This results in what may seem to be illogical sequences of information.

• Impaired ability to use cohesive devices handicaps the individual's ability to clearly mark the relationship of current to previous discourse. This could compromise the coherence of the speaker's discourse.

• Impaired understanding of abstract concepts and language (including words having more than one meaning such as "heel" or "run") limits the individual's ability to respond contingently in a conversation.

• Impaired gist comprehension may affect the subject's comprehension of the "main point" of the conversation and interpretation of how the conversational partner's current utterance relates to previous discourse. This could lead to tangential or off-topic responses.

Deficits in language, social–emotional, and cognitive (e.g., executive function, metarepresentational) abilities have a major impact on an AS or HFA individual's discourse behavior. Therefore, classification of thought disorder should be reserved until language, social, and neuropsychological evaluations are completed. Applying the label of thought disorder connotes a set of diagnostic associations, such as schizophrenia, that may be inappropriate for individuals with HFA and AS. Although some children with atypical social features later develop schizophrenia, the relationship between schizophrenia spectrum disorders and HFA and AS is not at all clear. Thought disorder implies a lack of coherence of behavior that may not be applicable to the HFA and AS population. Thus, the classification of thought disorder should be used with caution in the autistic population. Because autism is no longer viewed as a childhood psychosis, differential diagnosis is especially important and will depend on careful and thorough assessment. Such assessment is essential if diagnosticians are to distinguish psychotic from nonpsychotic processes, which have different outcomes, prognoses, and preferred treatments. More collaborative research between communication disorders specialists, neuropsychologists, and psychiatrists is needed to clarify the issue of thought disorder in HFA and AS.

Narrative Discourse in Autism and Asperger Syndrome

Another form of discourse that is relevant here is storytelling, or narrative discourse. Like social discourse, the narrative is a social form of exchanging information. It is an important form of communication on which people rely heavily in their everyday lives. Narratives are used when telling about an event that has been experienced or when making up a story. Like more basic units of language, narratives have a grammar or rule-based form. In mainstream U.S. culture, the grammar of the narrative is characterized by an episode (plot) structure that has several critical parts (Stein & Glenn, 1979), including a problem encountered by the characters, their attempt to resolve the problem, and the outcome of that attempt. Around 6 years of age, children tacitly organize their stories into narrative episode structure.

Narrative discourse analysis permits assessment of how someone organizes information, adheres to basic linguistic rules (phonological, grammatical, semantic), formulates novel text, recognizes the social rules embodied in the narrative, uses cohesion to tie the discourse together, and considers the listener's informational needs. Narrative analysis is a sensitive indicator of subtle discourse deficits. For example, "recovered" traumatic brain-injured patients may score well on standardized tests but have evident problems in producing coherent discourse (Liles, Coelho, Duffy, & Zalagens, 1989). Such difficulty is identifiable and measurable through narrative analysis.

There have been few studies of narrative production in HFA, and none known to this author in AS. Using a story completion procedure, Landa et al. (1995) compared narrative production in HFA teens and adults to that of controls individually matched on age, IQ, and gender. Although no significant between-group difference was detected in story length (number of independent clauses), HFA subjects exhibited much greater variability in story length. Complete episode structures were generated by half the HFA subjects and 75% of the controls. HFA subjects produced significantly more incomplete episodes. Thus, unlike their controls, HFA subjects' stories often included both complete *and incomplete* episodes. Furthermore, HFA subjects produced more irrelevant information and presuppositional errors than did controls. Presuppositional errors involved wording phrases in ways that indicated an assumption that the listener already had certain information rather than stating the information forthrightly. Not surprisingly, HFA subjects' stories were rated as being less coherent than those of controls.

This study reveals several strengths in the social/language abilities of HFA individuals. Like Loveland et al.'s (1990) mentally handicapped autistic youngsters who generated recognizable episode structures in a story retelling task, many of Landa et al.'s (1995) subjects produced conventionally structured stories. This indicates that some HFA individuals form mental representations for events, which may serve as a launching point in intervention. Indeed, Gray and Garand (1993) have reported that using stories to teach social skills to school-age autistic individuals has been successful.

Despite the production of complete episode structures, Landa et al.'s (1995) HFA subjects organized information less well into plot structures and less often expressed information needed to link salient aspects of the story compared to controls. Thus, the relevance of information was not always clear. These problems contributed to an impairment in overall coherence of HFA subjects' narratives and may indicate impaired awareness of how meaningful aspects of events are integrated in creating a gist. The HFA subjects' failure to clearly provide sufficient background information indicates a failure to consider listeners' informational needs, possibly related to theory-of-mind (defined later) deficits. The impaired efficiency and organization of information into plot structures may indicate an impaired executive process of formulating a well-organized plan for generating a goal-based story. This study indicates that HFA individuals have areas of discourse strength, and that areas of weakness in discourse formulation appear to stem from more than a single basic deficit.

ASSESSMENT OF PRAGMATIC SKILLS

Most individuals with AS achieve scores within the normal range on most standardized language tests, which typically focus on grammatical and semantic constructs within linguistic units up to a single sentence in length or, rarely, on comprehension of a short text (story). Yet the language context in which individuals with AS typically experience their greatest challenge is discourse, especially when interacting with unfamiliar people who are not adept at compensating for their social language vulnerabilities. Because the pragmatic language impairment associated with AS is one of the most stigmatizing aspects of the disorder, appropriate pragmatic assessment and intervention are essential. Because valid assessment of pragmatic skills requires observation of an individual in a dynamic social context, most aspects of pragmatic function are difficult, if not impossible, to test using highly structured formats. Two normed tests that tap skills important for pragmatic competence should be included in a language assessment: Test of Language Competence (TLC; Wiig & Secord, 1989) and Test of Problem Solving (Zachman, Huisingh, Barrett, Orman, & LoGiudia, 1994). These tests examine aspects of language and context comprehension that are critical for pragmatic competence. The TLC taps abstract language skills such as multiple-meaning words/sentences, formulating sentences with content appropriate to the pictured context, making inferences, and interpreting figures of speech. This test differentiated HFA adolescents and adults from individually matched controls (Minshew et al., 1995).

The Test of Problem Solving employs photographs of familiar contexts and associated questions to explore comprehension of key vocabulary and social problem-solving skills. The child must integrate pictured cues to appropriately infer the nature of the context and then go on to generate solutions to problems associated with that context. The standardized score generated by this test allows for comparison of a child's performance to that of a normative sample. In addition to this developmental information, the language specialist obtains additional valuable information from the child's responses to test stimuli, including the child's ability to formulate language in response to a novel question (outside the context of scripted conversational routines); ability to express thoughts in a specific way; perspective-taking skills; perseverative tendencies; ability to focus responses on the question at hand rather than an associated or unrelated topic; ability to monitor the adequacy of responses and appropriately modify responses when prompted to provide additional information; ability to speculate on events and outcomes that are within and outside personal life experience; ability to discuss a range of events involving a variety of social settings and different types of people; and impulsivity.

Although poor performance on the tests discussed previously is likely to suggest abnormal pragmatic ability, the assessment of pragmatic skills is not complete without directly observing multiple aspects of pragmatic performance in socially valid contexts. Attempts have been made to develop normed, standardized tests of expressive pragmatic language skills. One measure, the Test of Pragmatic Skills (Shulman, 1985) provides a normed (3 years to 8 years, 11 months), play-based format for eliciting conversational intentions (e.g., requesting information, informing, and calling). This test must be supplemented with another rating scale to code other aspects of pragmatic behavior (e.g., topic initiation strategies, topic maintenance, and presuppositional errors). Another tool, the Test of Pragmatic Language (Phelps-Terasaki & Phelps-Gunn, 1992) (normed for ages 5 years to 13 years, 11 months), involves presenting a picture to establish a social context about which the examiner poses questions. The questions presented are designed to elicit information about the subject's pragmatic skills regarding physical setting, audience, topic, purpose (speech acts), visual–gesture cues, and abstraction. This tool is useful for sampling some aspects of pragmatic function but cannot substitute for a naturalistic observation of the subject in an interaction with a peer or adult. The length of the tool makes it prohibitive in many clinical settings. Due to the length of the verbal stimuli, the role of receptive language skills must be evaluated if a child receives a score that places him or her in the impaired range. Alternatively, this test is likely to have ceiling effects, so an age-appropriate score does not rule out the presence of a pragmatic disorder, especially for AS subjects, who tend to perform best within highly structured situations.

For young children, the Communication and Symbolic Behavior Scales (CSBS; Wetherby & Prizant, 1993) may prove useful in the assessment of pragmatic skills. This test involves presenting elicitation stimuli for a variety of communicative intentions within semistructured play sequences. Norms are available. Other methods use similar elicitation strategies to sample social communicative behavior but focus less on pragmatics compared to the CSBS and the Early Social and Communication Scales (Siebert, Hogan, & Mundy, 1982). These methods require specific training and are mostly used within research contexts.

In combination with the structured testing described earlier, pragmatic rating systems may be used. Observational rating systems may be used within any context to code observations regarding multiple facets of pragmatic behavior. One example of such a system is the Pragmatic Rating Scale (Landa et al., 1990) (for ages 9 years and over). The drawback of observational rating systems is the lack of norms. Clinicians using these forms must rely on their clinical expertise to recognize appropriate and inappropriate pragmatic behavior and to judge whether the threshold of pragmatic disorder has been crossed. The Pragmatic Rating Scale provides a social discourse sampling guide in an attempt to standardize the sampling context and to provide subjects with the opportunity to demonstrate a variety of pragmatic skills or vulnerabilities across the three main pragmatic domains discussed earlier in this chapter. Having a consistent interview format across subjects strengthens the clinician's ability to interpret subject responses because all subjects will receive the sample "presses" or opportunities to demonstrate pragmatic skills across the domains of communicative intentions, discourse management, and presupposition.

WHAT UNDERLIES SOCIAL LANGUAGE IMPAIRMENT?

Numerous theories of autism contribute to an understanding of the pragmatic impairment associated with this disorder. It is unlikely that any one theory could account for all aspects of the pragmatic deficit in autism and Asperger syndrome. Deficits in attention to novel stimuli, affective information processing, and cognitive functions (e.g., establishing higher-order categories, theory of mind, and executive function) would have a substantial impact on pragmatic functioning. Numerous studies report that autistic subjects have abnormal responses to novel stimuli (Courchesne, Lincoln, Kilman, & Galambos, 1985; Palkowitz & Wiesenfeld, 1980). Such an abnormality may be related to poor identification/recognition of contextual cues that signal topics and subtopics, the need to shift to a different level of formality, recognition of cues that a misunderstanding has occurred, and so on. Such a deficit, along with difficulty participating in "intersubjective social experience" (Hobson, 1989, p. 23), would affect the child's ability to express and understand affective cues and to develop an image of others' perspectives. The impaired ability of HFA individuals to express and understand affective intonational cues (Macdonald et al., 1989; Smalley & Asarnow, 1990) will limit their ability to signal emotional reactions to certain topics and thereby elicit a set of expected responses from a listener.

Taking a more cognitive view, some have proposed that autistic individuals fail to develop a theory of mind. This leads to a failure to "attribute mental states (such as beliefs, desires, intentions, etc.) to themselves and other people, as a way of making sense of and predicting behavior" (Tager-Flusberg, Baron-Cohen, & Cohen, 1993, p. 3). The resulting impairment in perspective-taking skills would have a deleterious effect on pragmatics, such as poor awareness of the need to signal preparedness to speak or to relinquish the conversational floor, the need to provide background information, how to revise messages to clarify communication breakdowns, and how to effectively negotiate or persuade. The applicability of the theory-of-mind hypothesis to HFA and AS individuals has been questioned due to the unimpaired performance of some such individuals on complex theory-of-mind tasks (Ozonoff, Rogers, & Pennington, 1991). More research is needed to determine whether such unimpaired performance is related to ceiling effects.

Regardless of whether theory-of-mind deficits exist in HFA individuals, other deficits might explain many of the social deficits previously attributed to deficits in theory of mind. For example, deficits in executive functions (e.g., planning, shifting sets, working memory, and inhibition of prepotent responses) could give rise to deficits in many aspects of pragmatic functioning. As mentioned earlier, impaired planning ability could result in decreased quantity of information as well as the formulation of new information, especially in novel speaking situations. Difficulty shifting sets could result in difficulty considering alternative meanings, leading to misinterpretation of indirect speech acts and nonliteral language (Ozonoff & Miller, 1996). It could also result in difficulty shifting from one style or perspective to a more contextually appropriate one (e.g., from a formal manner of speaking to a more colloquial form). Impaired working memory in HFA individuals (Minshew & Goldstein, 1993; Bennetto, Pennington, & Rogers, 1994) may result in poor ability to formulate a gist of previous discourse, to integrate new information with previously shared information, and to formulate responses that are appropriately semantically tied to previous discourse. Impairment in the executive control function of inhibition ability could underlie the HFA individual's repetitive question asking, failure to terminate topics of their special interest, and overtalkativeness.

Many of the theories of autism have implications for intervention. Each must be considered as an assessment is planned so that appropriate intervention programs are developed. The social communication deficit in autism is a multifaceted phenomenon that will require a multifaceted intervention program incorporating methodologies developed out of a variety of theoretical perspectives.

IMPLICATIONS FOR INTERVENTION

The need for socially-based communication and language intervention with HFA and AS individuals is substantial, despite clear articulation and production of grammatically intact sentences. Strengthening pragmatic skills will improve the ability to negotiate the verbal social world, which is likely to translate into better long-term adjustment and prognosis (Matson & Swiezy, 1994). Early intervention is ideal. However, individuals with HFA and AS may not be appropriately diagnosed until late childhood, or even adulthood. Even in these cases, intervention may be beneficial. A case in point is an adult whose AS had been misdiagnosed as schizophrenia (despite the lifelong absence of delusions and hallucinations). Through social communication intervention, she began to develop an understanding of her difficulties. She learned strategies for dealing with her word retrieval problems and difficulty formulating contextually appropriate language. This led to decreased anxiety and increased self-confidence. She became willing to engage in social organizations of interest to her and remarked that a new world had opened to her. Numerous clinical researchers have reported the effectiveness of socially based interventions with HFA and AS individuals (Mesibov, 1984; Williams, 1989; Ozonoff & Miller, 1995).

Programming for pragmatic skills intervention is based on assessment of cognitive, social, language, and communication skills. Based on the assessment, goals and appropriate methods will be identified. Methods employed in social communication intervention represent a blend of techniques originating from a variety of theoretical perspectives. For example, strategies known to be effective with specifically language impaired individuals (e.g., scaffolding and scripting) are but one part of an intervention program for autistic individuals, whose cognitive, social, and behavioral styles differentiate them from the SLI population.

Aimed at improving areas of weakness, intervention builds on strengths, incorporating materials and activities that are enjoyable and interesting to the individual. Factors that enhance comprehension are identified (level of linguistic input, need for visual supports, familiar routines, favorite activities, etc.) and guide the intervention process. At the same time, basic skills and behaviors needed to support the development of social and communication skills must be addressed within the treatment program. For example, problems with overstimulation, overselectivity, poor set shifting, and rigid styles are addressed through increasing the predictability of the sessions (e.g., establishing communication routines and schedules), gradually increasing the child's repertoire of enjoyable activities, establishing effective contingencies, and so on.

Regardless of the specific methods employed or the specific therapeutic targets, the intervention program must provide systematic opportunities to develop social and communicative skills. For young children, systematic responses to behavior and creating systematic communicative opportunities are necessary to help them recognize their power as communicative beings. They are taught to use conventional means of communicating within communicative routines, incorporating enjoyable activities that can be stopped and reinitiated (e.g., tickling and swinging). Turn taking (beginning with movements that are within the child's repertoire employing favorite activities), social communicative expressions, and means for establishing co-reference (e.g., pointing and understanding pointing) are introduced. Basic social scripts within daily routines and play are developed, with appropriate communicative behaviors taught within those scripts. The child learns to expect a sequence of activity and develops a repertoire of contextually appropriate responses. The cognitive load of attending to novel stimuli is reduced, creating a greater likelihood that attention will be focused on social and communication intervention targets. The routine is systematically varied and can be tailored to address the child's individual social or behavioral challenges. Eventually, mental state terms ("think," "believe," "expect"), perspective taking, shifting speech registers (formal, informal), understanding and using multiple-meaning words and figurative language, and so on are introduced. A full discussion of intervention strategies is beyond the scope of this chapter, but excellent suggestions may be found in a book by Quill (1995).

Naturalistic techniques are insufficient to make the child aware of the rules that other children acquire tacitly. Clearly defined goals and rules for social communication are a necessity. These should be presented to the child in a permanently available form, tailored to the child's developmental level. They should be reviewed within relevant situations that occur naturally and that are contrived. For older children, guided discussions of videotapes of their classmates, sitcoms, and their own interactions may be a critical part of the therapeutic process. The social communication intervention program should extend to the child's social environment, including peers, family members, school personnel, and other important individuals in the child's social world. Environmental supports (Dalrymple, 1995) should be developed. The goal is to create an atmosphere that promotes growth in the child but, at the same time, reduces the social and cognitive demands to avoid overwhelming the child. When problems with behavior, mood, anxiety, obsessiveness, and so on occur, psychiatric evaluation should be sought to determine whether counseling or medical intervention is warranted.

EVIDENCE FOR GENETIC LIABILITY OF SOCIAL COMMUNICATION IMPAIRMENT IN AUTISM

From the earliest reports, researchers and clinicians have reported atypical social features in some parents of individuals with autism. Kanner and Eisenberg (1957) noted that numerous parents of autistic children were "serious-minded, perfectionistic individuals . . . lacking a genuine interest in developing relationships with others" (p. 59). Although this observation may have been interpreted as evidence that parents' personality features caused their children to develop autism, empirical studies indicate a genetic, neurobiological interpretation. Epidemiological, twin, family history, and family studies indicate that hereditary factors play a substantial etiological role in autism (reviewed by Rutter et al., 1990). The prevalence of autism in the siblings of autistic individuals is about 200 times greater than in the general population (Ritvo et al., 1989; reviewed by Folstein & Rutter, 1988). The concordance rate of autism is higher in monozygotic (MZ) than in dizygotic (DZ) twins (Folstein & Rutter, 1977; Bailey et al., 1995; Steffenburg et al., 1989). Reports that social and learning deficits occur in some MZ and DZ nonautistic twins of autistics (Folstein & Rutter, 1977; Bailey, Le Couteur, Gottesman, & Bolton, 1995) suggest a genetic liability to milder but conceptually related impairments in family members of autistic individuals (Folstein & Rutter, 1977). Social and language impairments in siblings and parents may represent a subthreshold manifestation of genetic liability because autistic probands invariably show severe impairment in these domains.

Evidence for social and language difficulties in family members of autistic individuals is increasing. Wolff et al. (1988) interviewed parents of autistic children and parents of nonautistic mentally handicapped children, blind to proband diagnosis. Nearly half of the parents of autistic children, but no controls, were rated as schizoid. Ratings of schizoid were heavily based on decreased empathy and emotional responsiveness, rapport, social openness, and smiling as well as problems with over- and undercommunicativeness, verbal disinhibition, and a single-minded pursuit of special interests (Wolff, Narayan, & Moyes, 1988). In a family study of autism, a subgroup of parents exhibited abnormal conversational behavior (e.g., odd or absent greeting, overly talkative, and terse and ambiguous responses), problems telling well-formed, coherent stories (Landa et al., 1990; Landa, Folstein, & Isaacs, 1991), and problems appreciating social cues (Piven et al., 1994). More research is needed to determine the cause of the social communication difficulties in some parents (e.g., association with stressful situations).

There is also evidence that social and language difficulties occur in siblings. Bailey et al. (1995) report that the learning difficulties reported by parents in nonautistic MZ and DZ twins of autistic probands were overshadowed by social deficits during teen years. Striking social deficits were also reported in adult siblings of Kanner's original autistic patients despite normal intelligence (Piven, Landa, Wzorek, & Folstein, 1990). Our ongoing direct study of siblings (infancy through 17 years of age) of autistic individuals suggests that some siblings exhibit social and specific language processing deficits. Some cases of previously undiagnosed high-functioning autism have been identified in siblings. These impairments occur in the siblings of HFA as well as mentally retarded autistic individuals. More research is needed to understand developmental patterns in siblings of autistic children, but available evidence suggests that siblings are at risk for specific social and communicative deficits. These deficits are strikingly similar to those reported in HFA individuals.

Much of the current research on genetic etiologies of autism focuses on families having more than one autistic family member. Interviews with family members as well as statistical and laboratory procedures are used to determine patterns of inheritance, what is inherited, and the location and action of the genes that may cause autism. Researchers suspect that autism is a complex genetic disorder caused by an interaction of numerous genes and, possibly, environmental variables (e.g., intrauterine viruses). The rapid increase in statistical and laboratory technology as well as rapid advances in the fields of genetics and neuroscience are likely to result in substantial progress in our understanding of the causes of autism and beneficial interventions.

CONCLUSION

Pragmatic functioning is a critical part of everyday functioning. Success in social communication has an impact on an individual's adaptive functioning and overall well-being. Although individuals with autism and AS exhibit pragmatic impairment, they have many strengths that should be recognized. Not all aspects of pragmatic behavior are abnormal all the time. Methods are available for assessing and treating pragmatic disorders for individuals of all ages. With ongoing research, our ever-growing understanding of brain function in individuals with HFA and AS sets the stage for earlier diagnosis and more appropriate intervention.

REFERENCES

American Psychiatric Association. (1994). *Diagnostic and statistical manual of mental disorders* (4th ed). Washington, DC: Author.

Andreasen, N. (1979). Thought, language, and communication disorders 1: Clinical assessment, definition of terms, and evaluation of their reliability. *Archives of General Psychiatry, 36,* 1315–1321.

Asperger, H. (1944). Die "Autistischen psychopathen" im Kindesalter. *Archiv für Psychiatrie und Nervenkrankheiten, 117,* 76–136.

Austin, J. (1962). *How to do things with work.* Cambridge, MA: Harvard University Press.

Bailey, A., Le Couteur, A., Gottesman, I., & Bolton, P. (1995). Autism as a strongly genetic disorder: Evidence from a British twin study. *Psychological Medicine, 25,* 63–77.

Baltaxe, C. A. M. (1977). Pragmatic deficits in the language of autistic adolescents. *Journal of Pediatric Psychology, 2,* 176–180.

Baltaxe, C. A. M., & D'Angiola, N. (1992). Cohesion in the discourse interaction of autistic, specifically language-impaired, and normal children. *Journal of Autism and Developmental Disorders, 22,* 1–21.

Baltaxe, C. A. M., & Simmons, J. Q. (1977). Language patterns of German and English autistic adolescents. In P. Mittler (Ed.), *Proceedings of the International Association for the Scientific Study of Mental Deficiency* (pp. 267–278). New York: University Park Press.

Baltaxe, C. A. M., & Simmons, J. Q. (1985). Prosodic development in normal and autistic children. In E. Schopler & G. B. Mesibov (Eds.), *Communication problems in autism* (pp. 95–126). New York: Plenum.

Baron-Cohen, S. (1987). Autism and symbolic play. *British Journal of Developmental Psychology, 5,* 139–148.

Baron-Cohen, S. (1988). Social and pragmatic deficits in autism: Cognitive or affective? *Journal of Autism and Developmental Disabilities, 18,* 379–402.

Bates, E. (1976). *Language in context.* New York: Academic Press.

Bates, E., & MacWhinney, B. (1987). Competition, variation, and language learning. In B. MacWhinney (Ed.), *Mechanisms on language acquisition.* Hillsdale, NJ: Erlbaum.

Bates, E., O'Connell, B., & Shore, C. (1987). Language and communication in infancy. In J. Osofsky (Ed.), *Handbook of infant development* (2nd ed., pp. 149–203). New York: Wiley.

Bennetto, L., Pennington, B. F., & Rogers, S. J. (1994). *Working memory in autism.* Poster presented at the 22nd meeting of the International Neuropsychological Society, Cincinnati.

Bloom, A., Russell, A., & Wassenberg, K. (1987). Turn-taking affects the quality of infant vocalizations. *Journal of Child Language, 14,* 211–227.

Boucher, J. (1988). Word fluency in high-functioning autistic children. *Journal of Autism and Developmental Disorders, 18,* 637–646.

Bruner, J. (1978). The role of dialogue in language acquisition. In A. Sinclair, R. J. Jarvella, & W. J. M. Levelt (Eds.), *The child's conception of language* (pp. 241–256). Berlin: Springer-Verlag.

Caparulo, B., & Cohen, D. (1977). Cognitive structures, language, and emerging social competence in autistic and aphasic children. *Journal of the Academy of Child Psychiatry, 15,* 620–644.

Chomsky, N. (1968). *Language and mind.* New York: Harcourt Brace Jovanovich.

Courchesne, E., Lincoln, A. J., Kilman, B. A., & Galambos, R. (1985). Event-related brain potential correlates of the processing of novel visual and auditory information in autism. *Journal of Autism and Developmental Disorders, 15,* 55, 75.

Dalrymple, N. J. (1995). Environmental supports to develop flexibility and independence. In K. A. Quill (Ed.), *Teaching children with autism: Strategies to enhance communication and socialization* (pp. 243–264). New York: Delmar.

Dewey, M., & Everard, P. (1974). The near normal autistic adolescent. *Journal of Autism and Childhood Schizophrenia, 4,* 348–356.

Dore, J. (1977). Children's illocutionary acts. In R. O. Freedle (Ed.), *Discourse production and comprehension* (pp. 227–244). Norwood, NJ: Ablex.

Dykens, E., Volkmar, F., & Glick, M. (1991). Thought disorder in high-functioning autistic adults. *Journal of Autism and Developmental Disorders, 21,* 291–301.

Ervin-Tripp, S. (1977). Wait for me, Roller Skate! In S. Ervin-Tripp & C. Mitchell-Kernan (Eds.), *Child discourse* (pp. 165–188). New York: Academic Press.

Ervin-Tripp, S. (1979). Children's verbal turn-taking. In E. Ochs & B. B. Schieffelin (Eds.), *Developmental pragmatics* (pp. 391–429). New York: Academic Press.

Fay, W. H., & Schuler, A. L. (1980). *Emerging language in autistic children.* Baltimore: University Park Press.

Fine, J., Bartolucci, G., Ginsberg, G., & Szatmari, P. (1991). The use of intonation to communicate in subjects with pervasive developmental disorders. *Journal of Child Psychology and Psychiatry, 32,* 771–882.

Fine, J., Bartolucci, G., Szatmari, P., & Ginsberg, G. (1994). Cohesive discourse in pervasive developmental disorders. *Journal of Autism and Developmental Disorders, 14,* 315–329.

Flavell, J., Botkin, P. T., Fry, C. C., Wright, J. W., & Jarvis, P. E. (1968). *The development of role-taking and communication skills in children.* New York: Wiley.

Folstein, S., & Rutter, M. (1977). Infantile autism: A genetic study of 21 twin pairs. *Journal of Child Psychology and Psychiatry, 18,* 297–321.

Folstein, S., & Rutter, M. (1988). Autism: Familial aggregation and genetic implications. *Journal of Autism and Developmental Disorders, 18,* 3–30.

Foster, S. (1981). The emergence of topic type in children under 2:6: A chicken and egg problem. *Papers and Reports on Child Language Development, 20,* 52–60.

Foster, S. (1986). Learning discourse topic management in the preschool years. *Journal of Child Language, 13,* 231–250.

Gallagher, T. (1977). Revision behaviors in the speech of developing children. *Journal of Speech and Hearing Research, 20,* 303–318.

Ghaziuddin, M., Leininger, L., & Tsai, L. Y. (1995). Brief report: Thought disorder in

Asperger syndrome: Comparison with high-functioning autism. *Journal of Autism and Developmental Disorders, 25,* 311–317.

Gray, C., & Garand, J. (1993). Social stories: Improving responses of students with autism with accurate social information. *Focus on Autistic Behavior, 8,* 1–10.

Grice, H. P. (1975). Logic and conversation. In P. Cole & J. Morgan (Eds.), *Syntax and semantics: Speech acts* (pp. 41–58). New York: Academic Press.

Halliday, M. A. K., & Hassan, R. (1976). *Cohesion in English.* London: Longman.

Hobson, R. P. (1989). Beyond cognition: A theory of autism. In G. Dawson (Ed.), *Autism: Nature, diagnosis, and treatment* (pp. 22–48). New York: Guilford Press.

Kanner, L. (1943). Autistic disturbances of affective content. *Nervous Child, 2,* 227–250.

Kanner, L., & Eisenberg, L. (1957). *Early infantile autism, 1945–1955* (psychiatric report). Washington, DC: American Psychiatric Association.

Landa, R., Folstein, S. E., & Isaacs, C. (1991). Spontaneous narrative-discourse performance of parents of autistic children. *Journal of Speech and Hearing Research, 34,* 1339–1345.

Landa, R., Martin, M., Minshew, N., & Goldstein, G. (1995). *Discourse and abstract language ability in non-retarded individuals with autism.* Paper presented at the Society for Research in Child Development, Indianapolis.

Landa, R., Piven, J., Wzorek, M. M., Gayle, J. O., Cloud, D., Chase, G. A., & Folstein, S. (1990). Social language use in parents of autistic children. *Psychological Medicine, 22,* 245–254.

Landry, S. H., & Loveland, K. A. (1988). Communication behaviors in autism and developmental language delay. *Journal of Child Psychology and Psychiatry, 29,* 621–634.

Langdell, T. (1980, September). *Pragmatic aspects of autism: Or why is "I" a normal word.* Unpublished paper presented at the BPS Developmental Psychology Conference, Edinburgh.

Lewis, V., & Boucher, J. (1995a). Generativity in the play of young people with autism. *Journal of Autism and Developmental Disorders, 25,* 105–121.

Lewis, V., & Boucher, J. (1995b). Spontaneous, instructed, and elicited play in relatively able autistic children. *British Journal of Developmental Psychology, 6,* 325–339.

Liles, B. Z., Coelho, C. A., Duffy, R. J., & Zalagens, M. R. (1989). Effects of elicitation procedures on the narratives of normal and closed head-injured adults. *Journal of Speech and Hearing Disorders, 54,* 356–366.

Loveland, K. A., & Landry, S. H. (1986). Joint attention and communication in autism and language delay. *Journal of Autism and Developmental Disorders, 16,* 335–349.

Loveland, K. A., McEvoy, R. E., Kelley, M. L., & Tunali, B. (1990). Narrative storytelling in Autism and Down's syndrome. *British Journal of Developmental Psychology, 8,* 923.

Loveland, K. A., & Tunali, B. (1991). Social scripts for conversational interactions in autism and Down's syndrome. *Journal of Autism and Developmental Disorders, 21,* 177–186.

Macdonald, H., Rutter, M., Howlin, P., Rios, P., Le Couteur, A., Evered, C., & Folstein, S. (1989). Recognition and expression of emotional cues by autistic and normal adults. *Journal of Child Psychology and Psychiatry, 30,* 865–877.

Matson, J. L., & Swiezy, N. (1994). Social skills training with autistic children. In J. L. Matson (Ed.), *Autism in children and adults: Etiology, assessment and intervention* (pp. 241–260). Pacific Grove, CA: Brooks/Cole.

Menyuk, P., & Quill, K. (1985). Semantic problems in autistic children. In E. Schopler & G.

B. Mesibov (Eds.), *Communication problems in autism* (pp. 257–279). New York: Plenum.

Mesibov, G. B. (1984). Social skills training with verbal autistic adolescents and adults: A program model. *Journal of Autism and Developmental Disorders, 14,* 395–404.

Minshew, N. J., & Goldstein, G. (1993). Is autism an amnestic disorder: Evidence from the California Verbal Learning Test. *Neuropsychology, 7,* 209–216.

Minshew, N. J., Goldstein, G., & Siegel, D. J. (1995). Speech and language in high-functioning autistic individuals. *Neuropsychology, 9,* 255–261.

Mundy, P., & Sigman, M. (1989). The theoretical implications of joint attention deficits in autism. *Development and Psychopathology, 1,* 173–183.

Mundy, P., Sigman, M., Ungerer, J. A., & Sherman, T. (1986). Defining the social deficits in autism: The contribution of non-verbal communication measures. *Journal of Child Psychology and Psychiatry, 27,* 658–669.

Ninio, A., & Bruner, J. S. (1978). The achievement and antecedents of labelling. *Journal of Child Language, 5,* 1–15.

Ozonoff, S., & Miller, J. (1995). Teaching theory of mind: A new approach to social skills training for individuals with autism. *Journal of Autism and Developmental Disorders, 25,* 415–433.

Ozonoff, S., & Miller, J. (1996). An exploration of right hemisphere contributions to the pragmatic impairments of autism. *Brain and Language, 52,* 411–434.

Ozonoff, S., Rogers, S. J., & Pennington, B. F. (1991). Asperger's syndrome: Evidence of an empirical distinction from high-functioning autism. *Journal of Child Psychology and Psychiatry, 32,* 1107–1122.

Palkowitz, R. W., & Wiesenfeld, A. R. (1980). Differential autonomic responses of autistic and normal children. *Journal of Autism and Developmental Disorders 10,* 347–360.

Phelps-Terasaki, D., & Phelps-Gunn, T. (1992). *Test of Pragmatic Language.* Austin, TX: ProEd.

Piven, J., Landa, R., Wzorek, M. M., & Folstein, S. (1990). A family history study of neuropsychiatric disorders in the adult siblings of autistic individuals. *Journal of the American Academy of Child and Adolescent Psychiatry, 29,* 177–183.

Piven, J., Wzorek, M., Landa, R., Lainhart, J., Bolton, P., Chase, G., & Folstein, S. (1994). Personality characteristics of the parents of autistic individuals: A preliminary report. *Psychological Medicine, 24,* 783–795.

Prizant, B. M., & Wetherby, A. (1987). Communicative intent: A framework for understanding social-communicative behavior in autism. *Journal of the American Academy of Children and Adolescent Psychiatry, 26,* 472–479.

Quill, K. A. (1995). *Teaching children with autism: Strategies to enhance communication and socialization.* New York: Delmar.

Ricks, D., & Wing, L. (1975). Language, communication, and the use of symbols in normal and autistic children. *Journal of Autism and Childhood Schizophrenia, 5,* 191–221.

Ritvo, E. R., Freeman, B. J., Pingree, C., Mason-Brothers, A., Jorde, L., Jenson, W., McMahon, W. M., Peterson, B., Mo, A., & Ritvo, A. (1989). The UCLA–University of Utah epidemiologic survey of autism: Prevalence. *American Journal of Psychiatry, 146,* 194–199.

Rumsey, J., Andreasen, N. C., & Rapoport, J. (1986). Thought, language, communication, and affective flattening in autistic adults. *Archives of General Psychiatry, 43,* 771–777.

Rumsey, J., & Hanahan, A. P. (1990). Getting it "right": Performance of high-functioning autistic adults on a right hemisphere battery. *Journal of Clinical and Experimental Neuropsychology, 12,* 81.

Rutter, M., Macdonald, H., Le Couteur, A., Harrington, R., Bolton, P., & Bailey, A. (1990). Genetic factors in child psychiatric disorders—II. Empirical findings. *Journal of Child Psychology and Psychiatry, 31,* 39–83.

Scaife, M., & Bruner, J. S. (1975). The capacity for joint visual attention. *Nature, 253,* 265–266.

Schaffer, H. R., Collis, G. M., & Parsons, G. (1977). Vocal interchange and visual regard in verbal and preverbal children. In H. R. Schaffer (Ed.), *Studies in mother–infant interaction* (pp. 291–324). New York: Academic Press.

Searle, J. R. (1975). A taxonomy of illocutionary acts. In K. Gunderson (Ed.), *Minnesota studies in the philosophy of language* (pp. 344–396). Minneapolis: University of Minnesota Press.

Shatz, M., & Gelman, R. (1973). The development of communication skills: Modifications in the speech of young children as a function of the listener. *Monographs of the Society for Research in Child Development* (5, Serial No, 152).

Shulman, B. (1985). *Test of Pragmatic Skills.* Tucson, AZ: Communication Skills Builders.

Siebert, J. M., Hogan, A. E., & Mundy, P. C. (1982). Assessing interactional competencies: The Early Social-Communication Scales. *Infant Mental Health Journal, 3,* 244–245.

Sigman, M. D., Yirmiya, N., & Capps, L. (1995). Social and cognitive understanding in high-functioning children with autism. In E. Schopler & G. Mesibov (Eds.), *Learning and cognition in autism* (pp. 159–176). New York: Plenum.

Simmons, J. Q., & Baltaxe, C. (1975). Language patterns of adolescent autistics. *Journal of Autism and Childhood Schizophrenia, 5,* 333–351.

Smalley, S. L., & Asamow, R. F. (1990). Brief report: Cognitive sub-clinical markers in autism. *Journal of Autism and Developmental Disorders, 20,* 271–278.

Stein, N. L., & Glenn, C. G. (1979). An analysis of story comprehension in elementary school children. In R. O. Freedle (Ed.), *New directions in discourse processing* (pp. 53–120). Norwood, NJ: Ablex.

Stern, D. N. (1974). Mother and infant at play: The dyadic interaction involving facial, vocal and gaze behaviours. In M. Lewis & L. A. Rosenblum (Eds.), *The effect of the infant on its caregiver* (pp. 187–213). New York: Wiley.

Tager-Flusberg, H. B. (1981). On the nature of linguistic functioning in early infantile autism. *Journal of Autism and Developmental Disorders, 11,* 45–56.

Tager-Flusberg, H. B., Baron-Cohen, S., & Cohen, D. (1993). An introduction to the debate. In S. Baron-Cohen & H. B. Tager-Flusberg (Eds.), *Understanding other minds* (pp. 1–9). New York: Oxford University Press.

Turner, M. (1995, March). *Repetitive behavior and generation of ideas in high-functioning individuals with autism: Is there a link?* Paper presented at the Society for Research in Child Development, Indianapolis.

Ungerer, J., & Sigman, M. (1981). Symbolic play and language comprehension in autistic children. *Journal of the American Academy of Child and Adolescent Psychiatry, 20,* 318–337.

Van Bourgondien, M. E., & Mesibov, G. B. (1987). Humor in high-functioning autistic adults. *Journal of Autism and Developmental Disorder, 17,* 417–424.

Volkmar, F. R., Sparrow, S. S., Goudrequ, D., Cicchetti, D. V., Paul, R., & Cohen, D. J. (1987). Social deficits in autism: An operational approach using the Vineland Adaptive Behavior Scales. *Journal of the Academy of Child and Adolescent Psychiatry, 26,* 155–161.

Wetherby, A. M., & Prizant, B. M. (1993). *Manual of Communication and Symbolic Behavior Scales*. Chicago: Riverside Press.

Wetherby, A. M., & Prutting, C. A. (1984). Profiles of communicative and cognitive–social abilities in autistic children. *Journal of Speech and Hearing, 27,* 364–377.

Wiig, E. (1982). *Let's talk: Developing prosocial communication skills*. Columbus, OH: Charles E. Merrill.

Wiig, E. H., & Secord, W. (1989). *Test of Language Competence—Expanded edition*. San Antonio, TX: Psychological Corporation.

Williams, T. I. (1989). A social skills group for autistic children. *Journal of Autism and Developmental Disorders, 19,* 143–155.

Wing, L., & Attwood, A. (1987). Syndromes of autism and atypical development. In D. J. Cohen & A. M. Donnellan (Eds.), *Handbook of autism and pervasive developmental disorders* (pp. 3–19). New York: Wiley.

Wolff, S., Narayan, S., & Moyes, B. (1988). Personality characteristics of parents of autistic children. *Journal of Child Psychology and Psychiatry, 29,* 177–183.

World Health Organization. (1993). *International classification of diseases: Tenth revision*. Chapter V. Mental and behavioral disorders (including disorders of psychological development). Diagnostic criteria for research. Geneva: Author.

Zachman, L., Huisingh, R., Barrett, M., Orman, J., & LoGiudia, C. (1994). *Test of Problem Solving—Revised elementary version*. East Moline, IL: Linguisystems.

II

Family Genetics
and Neurobiological Aspects

5

Does Asperger Syndrome Aggregate in Families?

SUSAN E. FOLSTEIN
SUSAN L. SANTANGELO

If we wish to discover if and how Asperger syndrome (AS) aggregates in families, it is necessary to be clear about what we mean by AS. First, how is AS to be distinguished from autism on the one hand and from the broader autism phenotype on the other? The diagnostic criteria for autism are clear, having changed little in concept since Kanner's (1943) original description. However, these concepts have been operationalized in various ways, producing uncertainty as to how to include cases with very low IQs at one extreme and with mild symptoms, usually with normal IQ, at the other extreme. Are these mild cases to be called autism or AS?

In his paper describing fathers of autistic children, Leon Eisenberg (1957), described even milder symptoms that are reminiscent of autism. These autistic-like (or Asperger-like) traits seen in parents of autistic children include a preference for solitary activities (Piven et al., 1994), having few friends (Santangelo & Folstein, 1995), rigidity, a preference for sameness and resistance to change (Piven et al., 1997), abnormalities of social (Landa et al., 1992) and narrative language (Landa, Folstein, & Isaacs, 1991), and mild deficits in executive function (Ozonoff et al., 1993). Collectively, these features have been called broader autism phenotype (BAP) (Bailey et al., 1995; Bolton et al., 1994; Piven et al., 1997; Piven, Palmer, Jacobi, Childress, & Arndt, 1997). Although AS blends into autism on one side and into the BAP on the other, it can, for the most part, be distinguished phenomenologically from both of them (Szatmari, Bartolucci, & Bremner, 1989). Children with AS do not meet criteria for autism because of their normal language development (Kerbeshian, Burd, & Fisher, 1990) and milder cognitive deficits (Ozonoff, Rogers, & Pennington, 1991), although the boundaries of high-functioning autism overlap with those of AS (Szatmari, Bremner, & Nagy, 1989). Family members with BAP do not meet criteria for AS because their social deficits are not pervasive enough to interfere with marriage and the ability to hold jobs and advance their careers. Thus, in families ascertained through an autistic proband, it is possible to discern approximately which family members have AS and which have BAP. Nevertheless, because the boundaries of these three conditions are indistinct and (we will argue) occur in the same families, we hypothesize that they are genetically related.

More serious problems of definition arise if one wishes to ascertain cases of AS in the community, as would be necessary to study what disorders or traits aggregate in families of probands with AS. The similarity between AS and schizoid personality disorder and, perhaps, schizotypal personality disorder (SPD) makes it difficult to define probands clearly as AS, schizoid, or SPD (see Chapter 10, this volume, for a discussion of SPD in childhood). The latter is a condition virtually defined by its occurrence in families with schizophrenia, which is etiologically unrelated to autism. Whereas the *Diagnostic and Statistical Manual of Mental Disorders*, fourth edition (DSM-IV; American Psychiatric Association, 1994) emphasizes such features as magical thinking and illusions, the specific signs and symptoms of SPD that best distinguish the family members of schizophrenics from family members of several comparison groups in the Roscommon Family Study (Kendler, McGuire, Gruenberg, & Walsh, 1995) are the same ones that define AS: odd speech, social dysfunction, avoidant symptoms, and "negative schizotypy," which includes poor rapport, aloofness, guardedness, and odd behavior. Therefore, it may be difficult to distinguish AS from schizophrenia-related SPD in a community survey. If it is true, as stated in DSM-IV, that SPD begins later in life, then age at onset may be a basis on which to distinguish between the two. However, this later age at onset requires verification.

To demonstrate that AS aggregates in families, or that autism and AS aggregate in the same families, and to assess the strength of that association, it is necessary to have an estimate of the population prevalence of AS. One study by Ehlers and Gillberg (1993) estimated the prevalence of AS in schoolchildren at 3 to 7 per 1,000; we are unaware of any published reports of estimates of the population prevalence of AS in adults. It is possible that Ehlers and Gillberg's epidemiologically obtained AS sample contains some children with schizotypal disorder. Similarly, it is possible that some of the Roscommon County schizotypal probands (Kendler et al., 1993) had AS. We cannot know the prevalence of AS or SPD until we directly compare those cases found in families of autistic and schizophrenic probands, respectively, and determine whether they are clinically distinguishable, either as adults or as children.

Parallel arguments could be made about AS and schizoid personality.

The diagnostic criteria for these two conditions are similar, and we know of no studies that have compared them directly. Likewise, the relationship between AS and Nonverbal Learning Disability (see Chapter 8, this volume) or semantic–pragmatic disorder (see Chapter 9, this volume) has yet to be directly assessed. Thus, a whole series of studies is needed to assess how all these conditions are related phenomenologically and genetically.

Despite all these caveats, a few studies exist from which we can begin to address AS from a genetic perspective. In this chapter, we review these data as well as suggest hypotheses for testing in future research.

CO-OCCURRENCE IN FAMILIES OF AUTISM, ASPERGER SYNDROME, AND THE BROADER AUTISM PHENOTYPE

As often as possible in this discussion, we use the DSM-IV definitions of autism and AS. However, not all the published studies have followed these criteria, particularly in requiring at least superficially normal language development in persons diagnosed with AS. Some of the reported cases of AS seem to us to be indistinguishable from autistic individuals with normal intelligence, cases in which symptom severity usually lessens with maturity. These inconsistencies are noted as they occur.

Although different research groups have developed empirical definitions based on family study data, there is no official definition of BAP. As noted earlier, this term has been used to describe a set of personal attributes and behaviors that are found more frequently in the parents and siblings of autistic children than in relatives of controls. In concept, BAP is similar to both autism and AS, but the traits and behaviors are not usually severe and sometimes have adaptive value; it usually does not come to clinical attention. Individuals with BAP generally lack the markedly restricted interests or striking difficulties getting along in the workplace that plague individuals with AS.

If, as we hypothesize, these three conditions (autism, AS, and BAP) are genetically related, they should co-occur in families more often than expected based on their prevalence in the population. For the purposes of this review, we have assumed a population prevalence of autism of 4 per 10,000. Our prevalence estimate of AS is based on the Swedish survey of all children ages 7–16 residing in Torslanda, a "typical Swedish middle-class area," in March 1991. Ehlers and Gillberg screened 1,519 children who attended five normal schools in the area. They estimated the rate of AS to be between 3.6 and 7.1 per 1,000, depending on their confidence in the diagnosis; we use 4 per 1,000. For the population prevalence of BAP, we assume a rate of about 4 per 100, based on estimates of 4% from 40 control families in Baltimore (Folstein & Santangelo, 1998) and 3% from 30 control families in Iowa (Piven, personal communication, 1998), all of whom were ascertained through a proband with Down syndrome.

Prevalence of Asperger Syndrome in Families Ascertained through a Proband with Asperger Syndrome

Before considering the co-occurrence of AS with autism and BAP, we should ask whether AS is itself familial. Several case reports suggest that it is familial. Burgoine and Wing (1983) reported a set of monozygotic triplets, all of whom they diagnosed as having AS, although they pointed out that at least one of them may be more appropriately called autistic. Each triplet had some speech delay, but no mention was made of echolalia or other typical early features of autistic speech.

Kracke (1994) reported a well-documented case with AS who came to her attention because of the individual's difficulty in obtaining a job, and whom she later discovered to have prosopagnosia (the inability to recognize faces). Both parents were scientists and thought to have AS-like features, although milder than the proband. By description, the parents were probably affected with BAP.

Of the four cases of AS being followed by one of us (SF), who were not ascertained through an autistic proband, none of the parents has AS, but two fathers would qualify for BAP. One has two autistic cousins.

A few more systematic papers have reported information about families of individuals with AS. In the process of a statewide survey of autism, Kerbeshian and colleagues found six individuals who did not meet criteria for autism but did meet criteria for AS (Kerbeshian & Burd, 1986). Using the family history method, the authors found at least one individual who "had similar problems" in three of the six families (p. 732).

Gillberg has reported on the family history of 23 individuals with AS who, he took pains to report, were ascertained without reference to autism in the family (Gillberg, 1989). Again, by the family history method, one father had definite AS (1/46 parents, or about 2%). Another 10 fathers and 2 mothers had milder but similar symptoms, perhaps qualifying for BAP. From the text, we calculated a rate of 26%, which is similar to the rate of BAP we found in autism families (see later). No siblings with AS were mentioned; one AS proband had a sibling with autism, and another AS proband had an aunt with autism. These authors found more AS/BAP in the families with an AS proband than they did in a comparison group of families ascertained through a proband with autism.

A study of 100 families with an Asperger syndrome proband is currently under way at Yale (Volkmar et al., 1998),in which family members are being directly interviewed. When completed, this study will provide more detailed information about disorders in family members of individuals diagnosed with AS (however, see earlier caveats on the uncertainties of diagnosing AS outside an autism family). Preliminary family history data from that study suggest that at least 14% of fathers and 4% of mothers had AS, and that a much larger number had isolated features of BAP. Autism was diagnosed in 3.5% of siblings, the same rate in which it occurs in families ascertained through an autistic proband.

It is not clear in any of these cases or studies that the family members who were said to have AS actually met criteria, except possibly one father in the Gillberg study. There were certainly odd individuals, but from the descriptions it seems likely that many may have had the milder BAP. The rate of autism in the Yale study, 3.5%, was probably accurate because that diagnosis is more easily detected. These limited observations support the hypothesis that all three conditions tend to co-occur in families, but it has not yet been demonstrated, using systematic, direct assessments of family members, that AS itself is more common in family members of AS probands.

Prevalence of Asperger Syndrome in Families Ascertained through a Proband with Autism

If AS is etiologically related to autism, it should occur more frequently than by chance in families of autistic probands. The issue might be addressed by the study of twins, siblings, parents, and other relatives.

Monozygotic Co-Twins

There are three published population-based twin studies of autism. Although autistic-like deficits have been found in the nonautistic monozygotic co-twins, none of these studies has specifically reported whether any of the nonautistic co-twins met criteria for AS. An examination of the original interview data from the first twin study (Folstein & Rutter, 1977) suggests that none of the nonautistic co-twins had AS. One of the dizygotic co-twins (pair 13) was quite peculiar, but his mother (who was also eccentric) claimed that his early social development was normal.

Siblings

In one family history study of autistic probands (Piven et al., 1990), the parents of adult autistic probands were interviewed in some detail, mainly by telephone, about their nonautistic children. Parents described behaviors in three of their nonautistic children (4.4%) that seem likely to represent AS, although we did not label it as such in the publication. These three individuals were extremely eccentric in their habits, were socially isolated, and had restricted and unusual interests. All had normal intelligence and normal early language development and were never thought, as children, to have autism. Piven et al. (1990) describe these three individuals.

In the Baltimore Family Study of autism, all adolescent and adult siblings of 90 autistic probands were directly interviewed and tested on measures of social language, personality, and cognition. Two of the 48 siblings (both brothers) who were old enough for all these examinations met criteria for AS. This rate of 4% is over 10 times the expected rate, based on our estimated population prevalence of 4/1,000. Two other younger siblings in other families had social deficits and normal intelligence but were not old enough to fully participate in the tests and interviews by which we made our diagnosis.

Parents

In the Baltimore Family Study, the parents of the 90 unselected autistic probands were also studied directly, in the same way as the adult siblings. Based on the direct interview data, four parents, 2.2% (three fathers and one mother) met criteria for AS (Folstein & Santangelo, 1998). This rate is more than five times greater than expected.

The only publication known to us that describes family members with AS in autism families is a family history study by DeLong (DeLong & Dwyer, 1988), who diagnosed AS in 5% of first-degree relatives of autism families and said that it was more frequent in relatives of high-IQ probands. However, the relatives were not directly interviewed, and it is not clear what method was used to elicit the symptoms of AS or what criteria were used for the diagnosis. If all these individuals were to meet DSM-IV criteria for AS, the rate of 5% would be more than 10 times greater than expected from our estimated prevalence rate.

Thus, the available evidence, although scant, supports the hypothesis that AS is probably genetically related to autism: In the autism families that were directly assessed as part of the Baltimore Family Study, about 2% of parents and 4% of siblings appear likely to have met criteria for AS. However, much more work needs to be done to confirm this very preliminary estimate.

Prevalence of Autism in Families Ascertained through a Proband with Asperger Syndrome

A more difficult test of the hypothesis that autism and AS are genetically related would be to find an excess of autism in the families of AS probands. Given the population prevalence of autism of only 4/10,000, a very large sample of AS probands would be required to demonstrate that autism was *not* more common. Two papers give some information on the topic: the 23 AS families reported by Gillberg (1989), where one sibling was autistic, and the 100 families reported by the Yale group where the rate was 3.5%. No autistic relatives were reported in the six AS families reported by Kerbeshian (Kerbeshian & Burd, 1986). In the four AS families known to the author (SF), who were not ascertained through an autistic proband, none have autistic siblings or parents, but one has two autistic cousins. Thus, it seems highly likely that the rate of autism is increased in AS families, and that it is somewhere near the prevalence of autism in autism families.

Table 5.1 summarizes the scant data from published studies. Such as they are, and we caution the reader to view them skeptically, they support the hypothesis that autism, AS, and BAP are clustered in the same families and appear to be genetically related conditions. However, the population frequency of AS is uncertain. The family data are severely limited by the lack of systematic interviews to diagnose AS and BAP in relatives of AS probands in the Gillberg and Kerbeshian studies. Although the Baltimore Family Study on autism was not designed to diagnose AS, diagnoses were based on extensive examination of signs and symptoms obtained by systematic, structured, and semistructured interviews of both parents and siblings.

OTHER DISORDERS REPORTED IN ASPERGER FAMILIES

That AS may be genetically related to autism and BAP is conceptually coherent since their defining features are so similar in type although very different in severity. However, a few other conditions that seem less obviously related to AS (from a phenomenological perspective) have been reported to occur in these families. These may represent comorbid states and are described here to encourage clinicians and investigators to explore these associations more fully.

TABLE 5.1. Family History Studies

	AS probands		Autism probands
Relatives	Gillberg (1989) (*n* = 23)	Volkmar et al. (1998) (*n* = 99)	Baltimore (*n* = 90)
Autism			
In parents	0%	0%	0%
In sibs	one case (number of sibs not reported)	3.5%	2% (prevalence in sibs)
Asperger			
In parents	2%	11%	2%
In sibs	not reported	not reported	4%
Broader phenotype			
In parents	21%	46% of *families* had at least one affected first-degree relative	25%
In sibs	not reported		unknown

Major Affective Disorder

Major affective disorder has been noted both in individuals with AS and in their families. The presence of mood disorders in AS patients has been reported by Gillberg (1985) and in a clinical review by Szatmari, Bremner, and Nagy (1989). Three of the four AS patients under the care of one of us (SF) have a mood disorder. The mother of one case and the sister of another have bipolar disorder. We have not seen this reported elsewhere, but in his studies, DeLong has consistently reported bipolar disorder among the family members of high-functioning autistic probands, a population in which the distinction between autism and AS may sometimes be arbitrary (DeLong & Dwyer, 1988).

Selective Mutism

Selective mutism has been reported in a sister of a proband diagnosed with AS (Saliba & Griffiths, 1990). From the case description, however, the proband may be more properly considered to have autism. Gillberg (1989) mentions two cases of selective mutism in relatives of 23 AS cases in his study. Selective mutism has also been reported to co-occur with AS in another study (Cunningham, Cataldo, Mallion, & Keyes, 1983). One of the individuals with AS under the care of one of us (SF) came to attention because of selective mutism, and one of his parents suffers from social phobia. Szatmari (1991) mentions that selective mutism occurs in early school years in individuals with AS. He does not give a reference, so we presume that he speaks from clinical experience. In the same article, Szatmari remarked about phobias of public speaking and other social phobias among AS family members.

Tourette Syndrome

Several authors have remarked on the association between AS and Tourette syndrome (TS). In one report, a patient with AS developed signs of TS after stopping neuroleptics (Littlejohns, Clarke, & Corbett, 1990). This may have been difficult to distinguish from tardive dyskinesia. The mother was said to have schizophrenia.

Kerbeshian and Burd (1986) reported an association between AS and TS; three of the six AS cases found in their statewide survey were also diagnosed as having TS. Only one case was reported in detail, and the description of TS is not entirely convincing. The only vocal tic was "uhm" between words, and the motor tics might also have been interpreted as autistic mannerisms.

Berthier, Bayes, and Tolosa (1993) carried out an MRI study on nine cases ascertained for TS who also met criteria for AS. These cases were found among 100 consecutive TS patients. Again, these cases are not described in detail.

POSSIBLE GENETIC MECHANISMS

It appears, based on the limited evidence from case reports and case series, that AS is seen in the same families with autism and BAP, and that the severity of AS falls between the two.

Although autism is a genetically complex disorder, we believe the most plausible and parsimonious genetic model for idiopathic autism (about 95% of the cases) is one in which three or four genes interact with one another to produce the autism phenotype. In a latent-class analysis of a British family history study of autism, Pickles et al. (1995) rejected a single-locus model and heterogeneity models in favor of a multilocus epistatic model involving anywhere from 2 to 10 loci, with 3 loci being most plausible. This analysis examined rates of autism/pervasive developmental disorder, as well as both narrow and broad definitions of BAP, in first-, second-, and third-degree relatives of autistic probands. In a second analysis, applying a graphical analytical method (Craddock, Khodel, Van Eerdewegh, & Reich, 1995) to examine the Baltimore Family Study data, a single-locus model as well as heterogeneity models were also rejected in favor of a model with three to six epistatic loci (Van Eerdewegh, unpublished analysis, 1996). This analysis was based on the population prevalence of classical autism, as well as the recurrence risk for autism in siblings of autistic probands, and the rate in MZ co-twins. Although it is not clear that all idiopathic autism shares the same mode of genetic transmission, presently the most compelling hypothesis for the genetic transmission of autism is a model involving three or four interacting genes.

This oligogenic model is consistent with the finding of a broad range of conceptually similar phenotypes—autism, AS, and BAP—in the same families. Parents with the broader phenotype seldom have more than one or two of the traits that make up the broader phenotype. For example, a parent may be socially interactive but have dysfluent or abnormal pragmatic language; another may be socially reticent and rigid but be verbally fluent and articulate. Often both parents have one or more traits. This suggests that each of the BAP traits may be the phenotypic manifestation of one or more of the genes that are hypothesized to interact to cause autism. AS may occur when a slightly different combination of genes occurs.

Empirical support for this way of conceptualizing the problem comes from a recent linkage study of dyslexia (Grigorenko et al., 1997). Two earlier linkage studies, in which individuals meeting full criteria for dyslexia were considered affected, identified two possible genetic loci for dyslexia on chromosomes 6 and 15, but the evidence for linkage was weak and had not been replicated. Instead of the unitary construct of dyslexia, five theoretically derived phenotypes were used in the linkage analysis by Grigorenko et al. (1997): phonological awareness, phonological decoding, rapid automatized naming, single-word reading, and discrepancy between intelligence and reading performance. This analysis provided significant evidence for linkage to the two loci identified in earlier studies, each of which was linked to a different reading-related trait. Phonological awareness was linked to the locus on chromosome 6 and single-word reading was linked to the locus on chromosome 15.

GENETIC COUNSELING

Clearly, we do not know enough about the genetics of AS to provide genetic counseling to parents who have one child with AS. When counseling parents who have an autistic child however, it may be appropriate to say that over and above the 6–8% recurrence risk for autism, there may be an additional risk for a milder autism-related phenotype, such as AS, in the range of 4–5%. This opinion is based only on our own work described previously, not all of which has yet been peer reviewed; more studies are needed. In the Baltimore Family Study, 4.2% (2/48) of the adult siblings of autistic probands met criteria for AS (Folstein & Santangelo, 1998). In a family history study (Piven et al., 1990), 4.4% (3/67) of siblings of autistic probands met criteria for AS.

SUGGESTIONS FOR FURTHER WORK

If we are to understand the genetics of AS outside the context of autistic families, it will first be necessary to determine whether AS can be clinically distinguished from, and thus ascertained in the community separately from, SPD and several other syndromes that appear to have similar diagnostic criteria, such as schizoid personality disorder, Nonverbal Learning Disabilities, and semantic–pragmatic disorder. This would probably require some collaboration among investigators whose work is "autism based," "schizophrenia based," and "neuropsychology based," similar in concept to the U.S.–U.K. study of psychosis that took place in the 1960s to assess the reasons for the differential rates of diagnosis of schizophrenia and affective psychosis between the United States and Britain. Using a common set of interviews and tests, interviews with schizotypal persons from schizophrenia families, persons with AS from autism families, and neuropsychologically defined cases of Nonverbal Learning Disabilities would be videotaped and rated, blind to ascertainment source. If it could be established that the phenomenology of some or all of these conditions is distinct, it might be feasible to ascertain families through probands with AS for genetic studies of AS.

However, the importance of a family study of AS could be debated in terms of its utility in finding genes. It is not likely to be the most efficient method of finding genes for autism. Moreover, once genes are found that contribute to autism, studies of the occurrence of those genes in cases of AS and other phenomenologically similar conditions would immediately follow. If genes related to autism were not found in AS (which seems highly unlikely given the phenomenology and aggregation in autism families), a separate search for AS genes might then be warranted.

CONCLUSIONS

Although they are scant and weak, the available data suggest that AS, autism, and BAP may co-segregate and may be genetically related to one another. However, well-designed family studies of AS and its association with autism, BAP, and other phenomenologically similar disorders such as SPD, schizoid personality disorder, Nonverbal Learning Disabilities, and semantic–pragmatic disorder are sorely needed, both to establish diagnostic boundaries and to determine which disorders co-segregate and which are transmitted independently. Unless and until the genes involved in the etiologies of autism and schizophrenia are discovered, the process of "reverse genetics" is not likely to be helpful in further elucidating the etiology of AS or distinguishing it genetically from schizophrenia-related phenotypes.

REFERENCES

American Psychiatric Association. (1994). *Diagnostic and statistical manual of mental disorders* (4th ed.). Washington, DC: Author.

Bailey, A., Le Couteur, A., Gottesman, I., Bolton, P., Simonoff, E., Yuzda, E., & Rutter, M. (1995). Autism as a strongly genetic disorder: Evidence from a British twin study. *Psychological Medicine, 25*(1), 63–77.

Berthier, M. L., Bayes, A., & Tolosa, E. S. (1993). Magnetic resonance imaging in patients with concurrent Tourette's disorder and Asperger's syndrome. *Journal of the American Academy of Child and Adolescent Psychiatry, 32*(3), 633–639.

Bolton, P., Macdonald, H., Pickles, A., Rios, P., Goode, S., Crowson, M., Bailey, A., & Rutter, M. (1994). A case-control family history study of autism. *Journal of Child Psychology and Psychiatry, 35*(5), 877–900.

Burgoine, E., & Wing, L. (1983). Identical triplets with Asperger's syndrome. *British Journal of Psychiatry, 143*, 261–265.

Craddock, N., Khodel, V., Van Eerdewegh, P., & Reich, T. (1995). Mathematical limits of multilocus models: The genetic transmission of bipolar disorder. *American Journal of Human Genetics, 57*(3), 690–702.

Cunningham, C. E., Cataldo, M. F., Mallion, C., & Keyes, J. B. (1983). Review and controlled single case evaluation of behavioural approaches to the management of elective mutism. *Child and Family Behavior Therapy, 5*, 25–49.

DeLong, G. R., & Dwyer, J. T. (1988). Correlation of family history with specific autistic subgroups: Asperger's syndrome and bipolar affective disease. *Journal of Autism and Developmental Disorders, 18*(4), 593–600.

Ehlers, S., & Gillberg, C. (1993). The epidemiology of Asperger syndrome. A total population study. *Journal of Child Psychology and Psychiatry, 34*(8), 1327–1350.

Eisenberg, L. (1957). The fathers of autistic children. *American Journal of Orthopsychiatry, 127,* 715–724.

Folstein, S., & Rutter, M. (1977). Infantile autism: A genetic study of 21 twin pairs. *Journal of Child Psychology and Psychiatry and Allied Disciplines, 18*(4), 297–321.

Folstein, S., & Santangelo, S. L. (1998). Unpublished raw data.

Gillberg, C. (1985). Asperger's syndrome and recurrent psychosis—A case study. *Journal of Autism and Developmental Disorders, 15*(4), 389–397.

Gillberg, C. (1989). Asperger syndrome in 23 Swedish children [Review]. *Developmental Medicine and Child Neurology, 31*(4), 520–531.

Grigorenko, E. L., Wood, F. B., Meyers, M. S., Hart, L. A., Speed, W. C., Shuster, A., & Pauls, D. L. (1997). Susceptibility loci for distinct components of developmental dyslexia on chromosomes 6 and 15. *American Journal of Human Genetics, 60*(1), 27–39.

Kanner, L. (1943). Autistic disturbances of affective contact. *Nervous Child, 2,* 217–250.

Kendler, K. S., McGuire, M., Gruenberg, A. M., Spellman, M., O'Hare, A., & Walsh, D. (1993). The Roscommon Family Study. II. The risk of nonschizophrenic nonaffective psychoses in relatives. *Archives of General Psychiatry, 50*(8), 645–652.

Kendler, K. S., McGuire, M., Gruenberg, A. M., & Walsh, D. (1995). Schizotypal symptoms and signs in the Roscommon Family Study. Their factor structure and familial relationship with psychotic and affective disorders. *Archives of General Psychiatry, 52*(4), 296–303.

Kerbeshian, J., & Burd, L. (1986). Asperger's syndrome and Tourette syndrome: The case of the pinball wizard. *British Journal of Psychiatry, 148,* 731–736.

Kerbeshian, J., Burd, L., & Fisher, W. (1990). Asperger's syndrome: To be or not to be? *British Journal of Psychiatry, 156,* 721–725.

Kracke, I. (1994). Developmental prosopagnosia in Asperger syndrome: Presentation and discussion of an individual case. *Developmental Medicine and Child Neurology, 36*(10), 873–886.

Landa, R., Folstein, S. E., & Isaacs, C. (1991). Spontaneous narrative-discourse performance of parents of autistic individuals. *Journal of Speech and Hearing Research, 34*(6), 1339–1345.

Landa, R., Piven, J., Wzorek, M. M., Gayle, J. O., Chase, G. A., & Folstein, S. E. (1992). Social language use in parents of autistic individuals. *Psychological Medicine, 22*(1), 245–254.

Littlejohns, C. S., Clarke, D. J., & Corbett, J. A. (1990). Tourette-like disorder in Asperger's syndrome. *British Journal of Psychiatry, 156,* 430–433.

Ozonoff, S., Rogers, S. J., Farnham, J. M., Pennington, B. F., Garofalo, G., Ragusa, R. M., Argiolas, A., Scavuzzo, C., Spina, E., & Barletta, C. (1993). Can standard measures identify subclinical markers of autism? Evidence of chromosomal fragile sites in schizophrenic patients. *Journal of Autism and Developmental Disorders, 23*(3), 132–135.

Ozonoff, S., Rogers, S. J., & Pennington, B. F. (1991). Asperger's syndrome: Evidence of an empirical distinction from high-functioning autism. *Journal of Child Psychology and Psychiatry, 32*(7), 1107–1122.

Pickles, A., Bolton, P., Macdonald, H., Bailey, A., Le Couteur, A., Sim, C. H., & Rutter, M. (1995). Latent-class analysis of recurrence risks for complex phenotypes with selection and measurement error: A twin and family history study of autism. *American Journal of Human Genetics, 57*(3), 717–726.

Piven, J., Gayle, J., Chase, G. A., Fink, B., Landa, R., Wzorek, M. M., & Folstein, S. E. (1990). A family history study of neuropsychiatric disorders in the adult siblings of autistic individuals. *Journal of the American Academy of Child and Adolescent Psychiatry, 29*(2), 177–183.

Piven, J., Palmer, P., Landa, R., Santangelo, S., Jacobi, D., & Childress, D. (1997). Personality and language characteristics in parents from multiple-incidence autism families. *American Journal of Medical Genetics (Neuropsychiatric Genetics), 74*, 398–411.

Piven, J., Palmer, P., Jacobi, D., Childress, D., & Arndt, S. (1997). The broader autism phenotype: Evidence from a family study of multiple-incidence autism families. *American Journal of Psychiatry, 154*, 185–190.

Piven, J., Wzorek, M., Landa, R., Lainhart, J., Bolton, P., Chase, G. A., & Folstein, S. (1994). Personality characteristics of the parents of autistic individuals. *Psychological Medicine, 24*(3), 783–795.

Saliba, J. R., & Griffiths, M. (1990). Brief report: Autism of the Asperger type associated with an autosomal fragile site. *Journal of Autism and Developmental Disorders, 20*(4), 569–575.

Santangelo, S. L., & Folstein, S. E. (1995). Social deficits in the families of autistic probands. *American Journal of Human Genetics, 57*(4), 89.

Szatmari, P. (1991). Asperger's syndrome: Diagnosis, treatment, and outcome. *Psychiatric Clinics of North America, 14*(1), 81–93.

Szatmari, P., Bartolucci, G., & Bremner, R. (1989). Asperger's syndrome and autism: Comparison of early history and outcome. *Developmental Medicine and Child Neurology, 31*(6), 709–720.

Szatmari, P., Bremner, R., & Nagy, J. (1989). Asperger's syndrome: A review of clinical features. *Canadian Journal of Psychiatry, 34*(6), 554–560.

Van Eerdewegh, P. (1996). Unpublished analysis.

Volkmar, F. R., Klin, A., & Pauls, D. (1998). Nosological and genetic aspects of Asperger syndrome. *Journal of Autism and Developmental Disorders, 28*(5), 457–463.

6

Neurofunctional Models of Autistic Disorder and Asperger Syndrome
Clues from Neuroimaging

ROBERT T. SCHULTZ
LIZABETH M. ROMANSKI
KATHERINE D. TSATSANIS

Asperger syndrome (AS) is a pervasive developmental disorder affecting social functioning and behavioral interests and activities that likely has a strong genetic component (Volkmar, Klin, & Pauls, 1998). The commonly described clinical features of AS include troubles forming friendships; difficulties with social cognition (e.g., naive, inappropriate, one-sided social interactions), diminished capacity for empathy, and poor nonverbal communication (including pedantic and monotonic speech and deficits in face perception) (Wing, 1981). In addition to these disturbances in social functioning, individuals with AS also display restricted, repetitive patterns of interests, and behavior (American Psychiatric Association, 1994) and frequently have an intense absorption in circumscribed topics (e.g., facts about maps, train schedules, or other narrowly defined topics) (Wing, 1981). Hans Asperger (1944/1991) first described the syndrome, shortly after Leo Kanner's (1943) seminal paper on autism. Asperger described the boys he saw as "little professors," who often learned to talk before they walked. Contemporary understanding of AS continues to emphasize intact language skills and motor clumsiness, both of which are important clues to the functional organization of the brain in AS. Although Kanner and Asperger were apparently unaware of each other's work, each described children with many similarities, particularly disturbance in the arena of social functioning. Social deficits continue to be seen as the hallmark of these disorders.

For nearly 40 years AS was essentially unrecognized in the Western literature. Interest in AS greatly increased after an influential review by Lorna Wing in 1981, culminating a little more than a decade later in AS being recognized as a discrete diagnostic category in both of the major diagnostic classification systems for psychiatric disorders (World Health Organization, 1993; American Psychiatric Association, 1994). Official sanctioning has caused an acceleration in research on the disorder, and there is now a sufficient data base from which some tentative conclusions can be drawn about the primary features and developmental course. However, in many areas there are few direct data on AS, and we are forced to extrapolate from work done on autistic disorder (AD). This is especially true for more complex research endeavors such as those involving postmortem examinations of the brain and *in vivo* neuroimaging, where work specific to AS has been sparse or nonexistent. Given the paucity of neurobiological data on AS, a developing understanding of the pathobiology of AS must at present be based primarily on what has been learned about AD. The phenotypical overlap between AS and AD is substantial, making it likely that many of the fundamental mechanisms will also be similar for the two conditions. Indeed, the relationship between AS and AD is bidirectional, and some of what we believe to be specific to AD probably has been influenced by AS. Many individuals who currently receive an AS diagnosis undoubtedly received autism spectrum diagnoses in years prior, and therefore cases of AS must populate the research samples in studies of "autism" before 1994 (Volkmar & Klin, Chapter 1, this volume).

It is valuable to borrow from the AD literature to construct heuristic models of brain functioning in AS, but it is important also to define ways in which AS is unique from AD. If AS overlaps too extensively with AD, there may be little value in retaining it as a distinct diagnostic entity. This argument can be extended to the larger domain of autism spectrum disorders and their relationship to individual differences in the general population. The behavior and functions central to all the pervasive developmental disorders might form one extreme tail of the larger normal population, with no clear "point of rarity" separating the distributions of the two populations; that is, there may be no evidence for a bimodal distribution across any phenotypic, genetic, or neurobiological variable. Until such evidence is accumulated, it is wise to bear in mind that the whole notion of distinct categories of social disability remains only a theoretical possibility that should be used only if a clear rationale for doing so exists. Although categorical classification has many important functions (Blashfield, 1984; Hempel, 1961), often it is more powerful to make continuous measurements of the phenotype of interest and to examine potential correlations to continuous measurements made of the underlying neurobiology.

Be that as it may, it is certainly true that the external validity of AS vis-à-vis AD is at present uncertain (Ozonoff & Griffith, Chapter 2, this volume). In fact, current diagnostic systems describe the phenomenology of AS as completely overlapping with AD. A developmental history of impaired language in AD but not AS is the major distinguishing feature according to the fourth edition of the *Diagnostic and Statistical Manual of Mental Disorders* (DSM-IV; American Psychiatric Association, 1994). Aside from this, AS and AD both involve impairments in social interactions, and restrictive, repetitive stereotyped behaviors ("repetitive behaviors" for short). These then are the two broad classes of phenomena we wish to explain through a model of brain functioning, and from which our understanding might benefit by extrapolation from the AD literature.

The intent of this chapter is to develop a framework that can begin to explain the social deficits and repetitive behaviors seen in AS. We need models of AS that can be tested through experimentation. In doing so, it is likely that information relevant to issues of classification will be generated. There are undoubtedly separate neural systems mediating specific aspects of repetitive behavior and social functioning, but there is as of yet no comprehensive understanding of what those neural systems are. Much work remains to be done at the phenotypic level. In fact, brain-imaging studies are dependent on good descriptive working models of these systems. We cannot, for example, begin to use a technique such as functional magnetic resonance imaging (fMRI) without social cognitive and neuropsychological models of the functions we wish to map in the brain. It needs to be a collaborative endeavor with neuroimaging results informing the questions to be addressed by social and neurocognitive studies, and vice versa, with each iteration further refining the model and resulting in more specific hypotheses. Our investigation of AS and AD is also critically dependent on understanding the systems that normally mediate social functions and regulate repetitive behaviors and patterns of interest. Although rapidly progressing, especially since the advent of fMRI, our knowledge of normative processes is still in its infancy. It would be premature to investigate instances of psychopathology without some knowledge of the normative processes governing the defining features of the disorder. Fortunately for social and emotional processes, there is now good data emerging on some of the brain systems that mediate these processes. Much less, however, is known about the neural systems that might mediate restricted, repetitive patterns of interests, and behavior.

This chapter first briefly reviews some of the neuropsychological studies on AS and AD in order to better describe and specify the neural systems that should be studied with neuroimaging techniques. Several models of neuropsychological functioning already exist, and these can now be directly tested and revised as need be to accommodate neuroimaging findings. Following this, we review the neuroimaging literature in AS. Because this literature is so small, we augment our review by discussing the major neurobio-

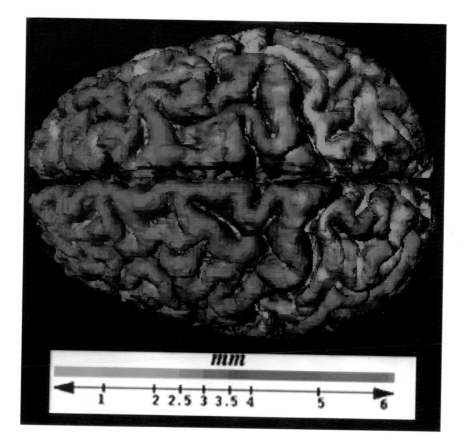

PLATE 6.1. A color-coded display of cortical thickness generated from a novel algorithm that captures and represents the inner (gray–white) and outer (gray–CSF) cortical surfaces and calculates the shortest distance between them for every pixel (see Zeng et al., in press, for a complete description of these methods). Preliminary work on normal control participants consistently shows areas of relative thinness in the postcentral gyrus (the somatosensory strip) and the lateral surfaces of the occipital lobe, confirming postmortem data on cortical thickness (Pakkenberg & Gundersen, 1997). This approach is being used to test for developmental abnormalities in cortical thickness in AS and AD.

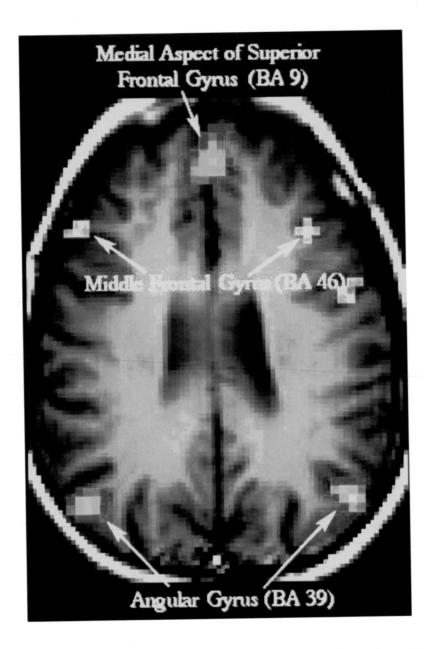

PLATE 6.2. Functional MRI (fMRI) activation map for a 20-year-old normal control male participant from our studies on social attribution (Schultz, Klin, van der Gaag, Skudlarski, Herrington, & Gore, 1999). The process of assessing social motives and intentions strongly engages a large area of the medial prefrontal cortex (shown in red and yellow), centered around Brodmann's area (BA) 9. Bilateral engagement of the angular gyrus can also be seen in this subject. The visuospatial control task engaged bilateral areas of middle frontal gyrus, a region that has been linked to visuospatial processing, especially on-line representations of the visuospatial data in working memory (Goldman-Rakic, 1987; McCarthy et al., 1996).

logical findings in autism. Our developing ideas about the pathobiology of both AS and AD center on the role of the amygdala and the relationship between the amygdala and particular systems in the temporal and frontal cortices. Limbic system abnormalities are hypothesized to cause early affective impairments that lead to social deficits and problems with repetitive behaviors. We propose that amygdala–frontal and amygdala–temporal systems serve key roles in the development of AS and AD.

NEUROPSYCHOLOGICAL SYSTEMS AFFECTED IN AUTISTIC DISORDER AND ASPERGER SYNDROME

Neuropsychological studies of AS and AD have suggested substantial overlap in many areas of functioning (e.g., Szatmari, Tuff, Finlayson, & Bartolucci, 1990). Nevertheless, two areas of functioning—motor skills and visuospatial functioning—have emerged as leading candidates for differentiating these two disorders. Beginning with Asperger's original work (Asperger, 1944/1991), motor deficits have been consistently described in AS (e.g., Wing, 1981) even though official diagnostic criteria consider these as only associated features that are not necessarily observed in all cases (American Psychiatric Association, 1994; World Health Organization, 1993). The research literature provides substantial evidence suggesting that motor deficits are frequent in AS, but there is mixed evidence in support of these deficits distinguishing AS from AD (see Ozonoff & Griffith, Chapter 2, this volume; Smith, Chapter 3, this volume, for comprehensive reviews). Neuroimaging studies of the frontal lobe and related motor centers in the basal ganglia and cerebellum would help to clarify the nature of the motor system abnormalities and the degree of overlap between AS and AD. In addition, there is currently much interest in executive function (EF) deficits in AS and AD. EF is sometimes conceptualized as a cognitive outgrowth or extension of the motor system. Both are concerned with the organization and execution of behavior, and both are mediated by frontal–striatal systems. Deficits in one often predict deficits in the other, a phenomenon known as a "neighborhood" sign. Thus, EF studies ought to be linked to careful study of motor systems (Rogers & Pennington, 1991) in order to dissect the functional similarities and overlap in neighboring brain regions that may stem from a core etiological factor central to the pathobiology of both AS and AD.

Despite the enthusiasm with which studies of EF are embraced, EF remains a poorly delineated construct (Parkin, 1998; Pennington, 1991). EF is often described as including functions such as planning, sustained attention, rule governed behavior, self regulation, working memory, cognitive flexibility (set shifting), and inhibitory control. However, there is not yet a good taxonomy of EF that specifies the relationships between these different EFs, making some subordinate to others by identifying core and auxiliary EF components (Pennington, 1991). The study of EF is often linked to specific tests. One of the oldest and most commonly used test of EF is the Wisconsin Card Sorting Test (WCST). A growing number of studies using the WCST and other tests of EF (e.g., the Tower of Hanoi) show performance deficits among persons with AD and AS (Bennetto, Pennington, & Rogers, 1996; Ozonoff & McEvoy, 1994; Ozonoff, Rogers, & Pennington, 1991; Rumsey, 1985; Rumsey & Hamburger, 1990; Szatmari et al., 1990). Two components of EF—inhibition of prepotent responses, and shifting response set—have been examined more closely to better account for the poor performance of individuals with AD on the WCST (Ozonoff & Strayer, 1997; Ozonoff, Strayer, McMahon, & Filloux, 1994). Results suggest that poor performance on the WCST, at least in high-functioning children with AD, is better accounted for by deficits in flexibility versus inhibition. Ozonoff (1995) argues for the primacy of EF deficits, and by analogy frontal–striatal dysfunction, in understanding the range of impairments in AD. In this model, EF deficits are related more generally to an inability to disengage from immediate environmental cues and to be guided by internal rules or mental representations (Ozonoff, 1995). Although there is growing neuroimaging evidence for general involvement of the frontal lobes in autism spectrum disorders (reviewed later), it is critical to delineate functioning in subregions of this very large territory. Particularly relevant regions include the dorsolateral, orbital and medial prefrontal cortices. Dorsolateral prefrontal cortex (PFC) is most strongly linked to working memory and other high-level cognitive functions (Goldman-Rakic, 1987; Mesulam, 1998; Sarazin et al., 1998). Orbital and medial prefrontal regions are more strongly associated with social and affective behavior (Damasio, 1985, 1996; Dias, Robbins, & Roberts, 1996; Sarazin et al., 1998).

Some data suggest that visuospatial functions may be specifically impaired in AS (see Ozonoff & Griffith, Chapter 2, this volume, for a complete review), and this is likely related to the finding of greater verbal IQ (VIQ) than performance IQ (PIQ) scores in AS (Klin, Volkmar, Sparrow, Cicchetti, & Rourke, 1995; Lincoln, Courchesne, Allen, Hanson, & Ene, 1998). Findings of greater VIQ than PIQ in AS is especially noteworthy because visuospatial skills have been consistently shown to be an area of strength in AD (Green, Fein, Joy, & Waterhouse, 1995; Shah & Frith, 1993), and thus this domain may enable tests of the external validity of AS. Lincoln and colleagues recently reviewed seven studies that compared AS (total n = 117) and AD (total n = 157) and found evidence for VIQ–PIQ profile differences in these two disorders (Lincoln et al., 1998). Computation of the n-weighted mean VIQ–PIQ difference in the AS sample yielded a VIQ advantage of 6 points, whereas in AD there was a mean PIQ advantage of 10 points. This latter figure compares favorably with an n-weighted average PIQ advantage of about 10 points from a larger series of AD studies with a combined sample of 333 described in the same review (Lincoln et al., 1998). The mean AS profile, however, was driven by two of the seven studies (mean VIQ advantage =

22.9) whereas the other five studies found VIQ and PIQ scores that differed by 5 points or less in either direction. Moreover, the Full Scale IQs (FSIQ) of the persons with AS in these seven studies averaged about 12 points higher than the AD subjects (93 vs. 81), suggesting not only a performance profile difference but an overall level of functioning difference, perhaps mediated by the superior verbal abilities in the AS group. The cause of the variability in findings across studies is unclear, but one factor may be that some studies were conducted prior to the establishment of formal diagnostic criteria (World Health Organization, 1993; American Psychiatric Association, 1994). It is also possible that this line of investigation is in part an artifact of diagnostic criteria used to define AS. The simple fact that a history of language disturbance is not permitted for a diagnosis of AS stacks the deck in favor of finding more persons with relative nonverbal deficits.

In consideration of these kinds of findings, it is popular to lateralize brain functions and to hypothesize about lateralized dysfunction in specific psychiatric disorders; for example, the role of left-hemisphere dysfunction has been emphasized in AD (Fein, Humes, Kaplan, Lucci, & Waterhouse, 1984). In contrast, it is frequently proposed that AS is a disorder specifically of the right hemisphere (Ellis, Ellis, Fraser, & Deb, 1994; McKelvey, Lambert, Mottron, & Shevell, 1995). A wide range of evidence supports the special role of the right hemisphere for visuospatial and social–emotional processes (Kolb & Whishaw, 1996). Several groups have proposed that AS can be understood by analogy to developmental disabilities of the right hemisphere and nonverbal learning disabilities (Klin et al., 1995; Rourke, 1989; Voeller, 1986; Weintraub & Mesulam, 1983). The Nonverbal Learning Disabilities (NLD) syndrome (Rourke, 1989) refers to a profile of neuropsychological strengths and weaknesses that includes relative preservation of some verbal skills, in the context of deficits in visual–spatial skill and gestural communication. Associated problems of individuals with NLD include poor pragmatics and prosody in speech and significant deficits in social perception, social judgment, and social interaction skills. Rourke draws from the neurodevelopmental model of Goldberg and Costa (1981) in describing persons with NLD as being poor at analysis and synthesis of information and better at serial information processing and rote aspects of learning. Rourke (1989) suggests that the common pathogenic mechanism in the NLD syndrome is a disturbance of the integrity of the white matter fibers, particularly those in the right hemisphere. This hypothesis remains largely untested, but it may be a heuristic guide to brain imaging studies on AS.

NEUROIMAGING RESEARCH IN ASPERGER SYNDROME

Keeping in mind the major findings on the neuropsychology of AS, we now turn to a discussion of neuroimaging data. In contrast to the relatively large number of neuroimaging studies in AD, there have been few studies of individuals with AS. An early case study of AS by Ozbayrak, Kapucu, Erdem, and Aras (1991) found left occipital hypoperfusion. Subsequently, a small study of three persons with AS by McKelvey and colleagues revealed consistent evidence of abnormal right-hemisphere dysfunction with single photon emission computed tomography (SPECT) (McKelvey et al., 1995). Hypoperfusion was observed in all cases, but it was not localized to a particular area in the right hemisphere. We recently reported MRI findings for a father and son who both have AS (Volkmar et al., 1996). Impressively, both relatives had nearly identical areas of dysmorphology of the dorsolateral prefrontal cortex in both hemispheres (see Figure 6.1). There was a region measuring 1 to 2 cm^3 of missing tissue in each hemisphere at the point at which the middle frontal gyrus normally intersects with the precentral sulcus. Moreover, this cortical abnormality was associated with regional changes in the orientation of adjacent gyri. The son, who was more severely affected, also had an area of dysmorphology in the left anterior–mesial temporal lobe, abutting the amygdala. As described in more detail later in this chapter, the amygdala appears to be a central structure in the pathobiology of AD and AS, with early lesions leading to dysfunction in other areas to which it is closely connected (Bertolino et al., 1997; Saunders, Kolachana, Bachevalier, & Weinberger, 1998).

Berthier, Bayes, and Tolosa (1993) compared MRIs of seven patients with concurrent Tourette syndrome (TS) and AS to those of nine patients with TS only. Dependent variables were qualitative assessments of gross structural abnormalities, not quantified measurement of regional size. Five of the seven AS patients had cortical brain abnormalities, compared to only one of the subjects with TS alone. Moreover, four of these cases involved abnormalities of cortical morphology. This is interesting because cortical malformations have also been reported in two studies of AD (Piven et al., 1990; Schifter et al., 1994). Cortical abnormalities are likely caused during specific periods of prenatal brain development (Caviness, Takahashi, & Nowakowski, 1995). Therefore, evidence of malformation may help specify critical developmental epochs during which the neural bases of AS are laid. These studies, however, do not provide data that are consistent with respect to localization of the cortical abnormalities in AS and AD. In a follow-up report, Berthier (1994) found specific thinning of the posterior corpus callosum (CC) in three of the original seven subjects with concurrent TS and AS. Interestingly, all three of these patients and no others showed parietal lobe abnormalities. These data are consistent with two studies in AD. Egass, Courchesne, and Saitoh (1995) measured cross-sectional area of the CC in 51 autistic subjects (3–42 years of age) and 51 age- and gender-matched normal subjects. They found significant reductions in total cross-sectional area of the CC in persons with AD. Analyses of subregions showed that it was only the posterior two-fifths that were significantly thinner. This has now been confirmed in a second study by Piven, Bailey, Ranson, and Arndt (1997). Af-

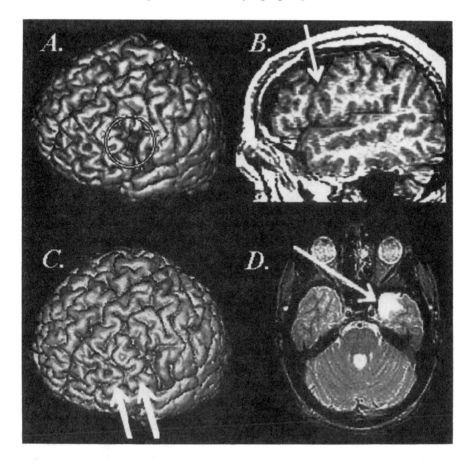

FIGURE 6.1. Magnetic resonance images (MRIs) of a father (A, C) and his 14-year-old son (B, D) both with Asperger syndrome. Both father and son showed an identical abnormality of the dorsolateral prefrontal cortex (A, B), which for both individuals was present in the same position in both hemispheres. The cortical abnormality entails focal areas of hypoplasia, presumably of a developmental origin. In addition, the neighboring cortical morphology appears perturbed, with an altered orientation (C). These gyri usually run in an anterior to posterior direction, but in both of these cases the gyri are turned 90 degrees and are oriented in an inferior to superior manner. The son had an additional abnormality (D), involving an area of hypoplasia in the anterior–mesial left temporal lobe that has been filled by cerebrospinal fluid (CSF) on this T2–weighted MR image. Its proximity to the amygdala is believed to be of particular significance (see text). Adapted from Volkmar et al. (1996).

ter controlling for total brain volume, gender, and PIQ, they found that the posterior two-thirds of the CC was thinner in a group of 35 adolescents and adults with AD compared to an age-matched group of 36 controls.

More recently, Lincoln et al. (1998) measured the area of subdivisions of the midsagittal cerebellar vermis and CC, and the cross-sectional area of the hippocampal body in seven persons with AS. This group was compared to larger groups of persons with AD and normal controls. The AD group had significantly smaller vermian lobules VI and VII compared to controls and persons with AS. The corpus callosum and the cross-sectional area of the hippocampus were measured in many of these same subjects. No differences were observed between the AS and controls on total cross-sectional area of the CC, regional fifth measurements of the CC or the cross-sectional measure of the hippocampal body. There were, however, some findings for AD versus the other two groups. Although not directly stated, the implication was that many of participants with AD had appeared in prior published studies by their laboratory. The groups were chosen to be similar in age, but the authors did not describe the gender distribution of the three groups. Moreover, they reported the IQ scores for the seven AS cases but did not report any IQ data for the comparison groups or make mention of whether the groups were matched on this important variable. Without controlling for such factors, it is difficult to interpret these findings (Piven et al., 1992; Schultz et al., 1994).

In the recent past, the cerebellum and brainstem were the focal point for much research in AD. Such neuroimaging studies were bolstered by postmortem studies of a small number of persons with AD that revealed a range of abnormalities, including a significant decrease in the number of Purkinje cells and a variable decrease in granule cells throughout the cerebellar hemispheres (Arin, Bauman, & Kemper, 1991; Bauman & Kemper, 1985, 1994). At about the same time that Bauman and colleagues were describing the neuropathology of the cerebellum in AD, Courchesne and colleagues published several reports on hypoplasia of the cerebellar vermis (Courchesne, Yeung-Courchesne, Press, Hesselink, & Jernigan, 1988; Courchesne, Saitoh, et al., 1994; Courchesne, Townsend, & Saitoh, 1994; Murakami, Courchesne, Press, Yeung-Courchesne, & Hesselink, 1989). The presence of two independent findings implicating the cerebellum strengthened the argument for a central role of this structure in the pathobiology of the AD. However, the postmortem comparisons showed that the reduction in Purkinje cell numbers was confined to the cerebellar hemispheres and was not observed in the vermis (Bauman & Kemper, 1996). Moreover, MRI studies in favor of vermal hypoplasia in AD have been criticized for a consistent failure to match subject samples for age and IQ, both of which have a reliable correlation with overall size of the brain and its subdivisions (e.g., Andreasen et al., 1993; Schultz et al., 1994; Willerman, Schultz, Rutledge, & Bigler, 1991), including area measurements of the vermis (e.g., Courchesne, Saitoh, et al., 1994;

Courchesne, Townsend, et al., 1994; Filipek et al., 1992, 1995; Piven & Arndt, 1995; Piven et al., 1992). Vermal findings have not been replicated in appropriately controlled studies using similar measurement protocols (Filipek et al., 1992; Holttum, Minshew, Saunders, & Phillips, 1992; Kleiman, Neff, & Rosman, 1992; Piven et al., 1992; Ritvo & Garber, 1988). In fact, the only research group besides that of Courchesne and colleagues to find decreased size of vermal lobules VI–VII or brain stem regions also employed control groups that were substantially higher functioning than the autistic group (Hashimoto, Tayama, Miyazaki, Murakawa, & Kuroda, 1993; Hashimoto et al., 1995).

Recently, we completed an MRI study on the volume of the brainstem and cerebellum and the cross-sectional area of the cerebellar vermis and its subdivisions in samples of 15 persons with AD (age = 22 ± 10), 22 persons with AS (age = 19 ± 12), 12 persons with pervasive developmental disorder not otherwise specified (PDD-NOS) (age = 15 ± 11), and 39 matched controls (age = 22 ± 10) (Lee, Schultz, Win, Rambo, & Staib, 1999; Schultz, Lee, Klin, Win, Rambo, Volkmar, & Staib, 1999). This study was the first of its kind in AS and PDD-NOS and it was conducted to determine whether better subtyping of autism spectrum disorders might further shed light on the inconsistencies that mark this area of study. All subjects were male, and FSIQ ranged from 56 to 141, with no significant differences between groups (group averages were between 95 and 105). Comparisons of the volume of the cerebellum, midbrain, pons, and medulla and area measurements of the cerebellar vermis and its conventional subdivisions (lobules I–V, VI–VII, and VIII–X) failed to reveal any significant group differences. We explored other compound variables as well (e.g., ratio of vermal lobule VI–VII to the entire cross-sectional area of the vermis) and conducted various covariate analyses (covarying whole brain volume and cerebellum volume) and found no significant effects. Correlational analyses between vermal lobule VI–VII and FSIQ showed a modest positive correlation and demonstrated that vermal hypoplasia previously reported in AD could be an artifact of lower IQ among persons with AD compared to controls.

Our results for the posterior fossa suggest that gross morphology of these regions is not related to the pathobiology of AS. However, other recent studies in AD have begun to provide consistent evidence for the pathobiology of this condition (e.g., Bauman & Kemper, 1994; Piven, Arndt, Bailey, & Andreasen, et al., 1996), and it is quite likely that these clues are important for the study of AS. The three findings with the most support and promise for helping unravel the neurobiological mechanisms in autism spectrum conditions include evidence for abnormalities in the temporal lobe/limbic system, abnormalities in frontal lobe functioning, and widespread abnormalities in neural growth and cell migration resulting in globally increased brain size and malformations in the cerebral cortex. This evidence is reviewed briefly before devoting more attention to the functions of the amygdala and the role that it might play as a central mediator of temporal and frontal lobe systems as they participate in processes critical to social functioning.

REVIEW OF NEUROBIOLOGICAL RESEARCH RELEVANT TO THE PATHOBIOLOGY OF ASPERGER SYNDROME AND AUTISTIC DISORDER

Abnormalities of Brain Size and of Cortical Morphology

Several studies of AD provide evidence for megalencephaly (whole brain enlargement) (Bailey et al., 1993; Filipek et al., 1992; Piven et al., 1992; Piven et al., 1995) and for increased head circumference (Bailey et al., 1995; Lainhart et al., 1997; Steg & Rapoport, 1975; Walker, 1977; see also Fombonne, Roge, Claverie, Courty, & Fremolle, 1999, for evidence of macro- and microcephaly in AD). The nature of this enlargement has yet to be carefully studied, and of possible significance is that the increase in brain enlargement reported by Piven et al. (1996) occurred only for males and not females with AD. In addition, Piven et al. (1996) found a selective enlargement of occipital, parietal, and temporal lobes but, importantly, not frontal cortex. The sparing of the frontal lobe is particularly interesting and may indicate a unique role for the frontal lobe in the pathobiology of AD and related conditions. As of yet, there are no studies of brain size in AS.

There may be a direct relationship between the thinning of the posterior CC that has been found in both AS and AD (described earlier), and findings of whole brain enlargement. There are physical constraints on how large the brain can grow while still maintaining adequate levels of connectedness. The rate of connectivity (i.e., the proportion of neurons to which a single neuron is directly connected) is a negative function of brain size across species (Ringo, 1991). This makes sense, as high connectivity means that adding a single neuron would leave no room in the skull for anything other than its connections. That everything is not connected to everything else is what enables neural and psychological subsystems to be studied in relative isolation. In fact, there appears to be an evolutionary trend toward greater specialization—more modularity with increasing brain size (Ringo, 1991).

There is also evidence within humans that larger brains are more specialized. For example, adjusting for body size, males have larger brains than do females (Ankney, 1992) and males tend to be more strongly lateralized for functions than females (e.g., for language, Kimura, 1987). In this example, greater lateralization of function in males is taken to be a reflection of increased modularity and decreased interconnectedness that is dictated by the physical constraints imposed by their larger brains. There is also evidence that males have a thinner CC than do females, especially in posterior areas (e.g., Allen, Richey, Chai, & Gorski, 1991). It may be that AS and AD involve an extreme form of this difference, with a bigger brain and less interconnectedness. One consequence of a larger brain in persons with an autism spectrum condition would be increased modularity of function, with less overlap and integration of functions (perhaps resulting in the lack of "central coherence" that is posited in Frith's theory, 1989). This hypothesis takes the form of a continuum, with females at one extreme and persons with AD or AS at the other extreme. This hypothesis would be consistent with evidence for a female advantage in such things as face and emotion recognition (Burton & Levy, 1989; Goldstein & Chance, 1970; Orozco & Ehlers, 1998) and with the much lower rates of AD (Volkmar, Szatmari, & Sparrow, 1993). Although appealing, many details need to be resolved, such as the concern that not all big-brained males are autistic. Perhaps large brain size confers a risk that in the context of other vulnerabilities can produce autistic symptomatology.

Some studies on AD suggest that the growth abnormality is postnatal (Lainhart et al., 1997; but see Woodhouse et al., 1996). Defining a restricted developmental period during which the growth abnormality occurs is very important because there are different mechanisms during pre- versus postnatal neurodevelopment responsible for volumetric expansion. The identification of a critical period has direct implications for the nature of the causal mechanisms involved in AS and AD. There are several possible mechanisms to account for an increase rate of growth in the first years after birth, including excess proliferation of glial cells and neuronal synapses (or inadequate pruning) in the cortex. The most potent influence on overall brain size, however, occurs very early in embryogenesis. During the first weeks of embryogenesis, the progenitors of eventual neurons, the stem cells, multiply rapidly through the process of symmetric mitotic division (Rakic, 1988, 1995; Kornack & Rakic, 1995). After about the first 6 weeks of fetal developmental, there is a gradual shift to asymmetric cell division (Caviness et al., 1995; Kornack & Rakic, 1998), a process that directly produces individual neurons. The number of founder progenitors, supplied by symmetric divisions, affects the final number of cortical columns and thus has the greatest impact on eventual brain volume (Rakic, 1995). Interference with asymmetric division eventuates in fewer neurons per column (Kornack & Rakic, 1995), with direct impact on cortical thickness and general morphology. In addition, apoptosis, or programmed cell death (occurring primarily during the third trimester) also has a substantial influence on cortical thickness and brain volume, with one estimate indicating that 70% of all neurons are intentionally pruned before birth (Rabinowicz, de Courten-Myers Petetot, Xi, & de los Reyes, 1996). This discussion is relevant because a recent postmortem study in AD found increased cortical thickness in two of the six subjects studied (Bailey et al., 1998). New image-analytical techniques (Zeng, Staib, Schultz, & Duncan, in press) now allow for measurement of cortical thickness from MRI (see Plate 6.1., opposite page 174). These will allow more detailed *in vivo* examination of cortical thickness and morphology than has been possible to date. Moreover, abnormalities in cortical morphology have been seen with MRI in both AD (Piven et al., 1990; Schifter et al., 1994; Bailey et al., 1998) and AS (Berthier et al., 1993; Volkmar et al., 1996). Future studies need to focus on possible developmental epochs and mechanisms responsible for observed abnormalities in gross brain size and regional cortical aberrations.

Temporal Lobe

Bauman and Kemper (1985, 1994) studied postmortem brain tissue from individuals with AD and found abnormalities in size and density of neurons in the mesial temporal lobe and limbic system, including the amygdala, hippocampus, and entorhinal cortex. These neuropathological abnormalities make sense with respect to some of the major symptoms of AD, because the limbic–temporal lobe system is known to have a principal role in mediating social–emotional functioning (Adolphs, Tranel, Damasio, & Damasio, 1994; Adolphs, Damasio, Tranel, & Damasio, 1996; Bachevalier, 1994; Hamann et al., 1996; Kling & Brothers, 1992). Limbic system structures have dense reciprocal interconnections with secondary and tertiary association areas of the temporal lobe (Amaral & Price, 1984; Turner, Mishkin, & Knapp, 1980), thereby forming an integrated system (Figure 6.2). Other evidence implicating this system in AD includes (1) case studies of patients with temporal lobe lesions and autistic-like sequelae (Gillberg, 1986, 1991; Hoon & Reiss, 1992), (2) a significant and specific association between temporal lobe lesions from tuberous sclerosis and AD (Bolton & Griffiths, 1997), (3) a volumetric decrease in the amygdala in AD (Aylward et al., in press), (4) reduced functional activity on SPECT scans in the temporal lobes in AD (Mountz, Lelland, Lill, Katholi, & Liu, 1995), (5) animal models of AD based on early lesions to mesial temporal lobe structures (Bachevalier, 1994), and (6) evidence from our own fMRI studies of autism spectrum conditions documenting ventral temporal lobe dysfunction during face recognition tasks (Schultz, 1998; Schultz et al., in press) and lateral temporal lobe dysfunction during facial expression discrimination (Schultz, 1999).

Temporal lobe findings in autism spectrum disorders are of particular interest in light of the literature on face recognition and emotion recognition deficits in both AD and AS. Numerous studies have reported that children with AD are impaired on measures of emotion perception and comprehension (Fein, Lucci, Braverman, & Waterhouse, 1992; Hobson, 1986a, 1986b; Hobson & Lee, 1989; Hobson, Ouston, & Lee, 1988a, 1988b; Macdonald et al., 1989). High-functioning individuals with AD have been found to perform more poorly on labeling and explaining the emotions of children in a videotaped vignette (Yirmiya, Sigman, Kasari, & Mundy, 1992), explaining their own emotions (Capps, Yirmiya, & Sigman, 1992), and relating their emotions to goal-oriented and social situations (Jaedicke, Storoschuk, & Lord,

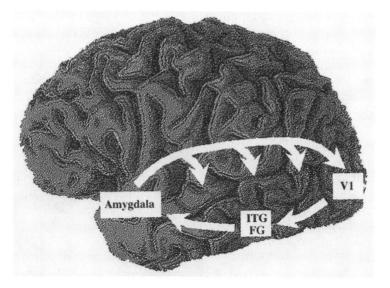

FIGURE 6.2. Schematic of the dense reciprocal connections between the amygdala and all regions of the temporal lobes, especially association cortices, including the fusiform gyrus (FG) and the inferior temporal gyrus (ITG). This system allows for feed-forward and feed-back communications and presumably would be critical during social–emotional development, including the development of face and affect recognition systems. Redrawn from Toveé (1995).

1994). In addition, limitations are observed in affective displays, including imitating expression of emotion (Macdonald et al., 1989) and expression and integration of affect in interactions with others (Dawson, Hill, Spencer, Galpert, & Watson, 1990; McGee, Feldman, & Chernin, 1991; Snow, Hertzig, & Shapiro, 1987; Yirmiya, Kasari, Sigman, & Mundy, 1989).

Related and perhaps more fundamental is that both AD and AS show deficits in neutral face perception in the context of person identity tasks (Boucher & Lewis, 1992; Braverman, Fein, Lucci, & Waterhouse, 1989; Davies, Bishop, Manstead, & Tantam, 1994; Hobson, 1986a, 1986b; Hobson et al., 1988a; Langdell, 1978; Macdonald et al., 1989; Szatmari et al., 1990; Tantam, Monaghan, Nicholson, & Stirling, 1989; Weeks & Hobson, 1987). Recognition of individual faces is an integral part of interpersonal interactions and successful functioning within a social group. Face perception is normally a holistic process, reliant on the configuration of major features (Farah, 1996). Object perception, on the other hand, is more reliant on feature analysis (Bartlett & Searcy, 1993; Tanaka & Farah, 1993). Distorting the configuration of the major features of the face (e.g., inverting the face) has a larger impact on task accuracy and reaction time (RT) than distorting major feature configuration in objects (Moscovitch, Winocur, & Behrmann, 1997; Valentine, 1988). Development of visual expertise is associated with a transition from feature-based to configural processing and an increase in the magnitude of the inversion effect (Diamond & Carey, 1986; Gauthier & Tarr, 1997). These normative processes are important to describe because persons with AD and related conditions appear to rely more on individual pieces of the face for identification (e.g., the lower face and mouth area) rather than the overall configuration (Hobson et al., 1988a; Langdell, 1978). Consistent with this, several studies have found that individuals with autism spectrum disorders show better object perception than expected based on their ability with faces (Boucher & Lewis, 1992; Davies et al., 1994; Hauck, Fein, Maltby, Waterhouse, & Feinstein, 1998; Hobson et al., 1988a; Tantam et al., 1989). These results suggest that individuals with AD may be performing perceptual processes on faces as if they were objects, perhaps because of their early deficits in "affiliative drive" and the consequent failure to develop configural processing capabilities characteristic of "face experts."

We recently studied the role of temporal cortices in face and object recognition in AD and AS with fMRI. The function of ventral temporal cortices (especially the fusiform gyrus) in face perception is well documented (Gauthier, Tarr, Anderson, Skudlarski, & Gore, 1999; Haxby et al., 1999; Kanwisher, McDermott, & Chun, 1997; McCarthy, Puce, Gore, & Allison, 1997; Sergent, Ohta, & Macdonald, 1992). Results from our study showed significant functional abnormalities in a group of persons with AD or AS during a person discrimination task using neutral/nonexpressive pictures of the human face (Schultz, 1998; Schultz et al., in press). Subgroup analyses revealed no differences between AS and AD, suggesting that face perception abnormalities are shared at a biological level. The combined AS/AD group showed significantly less fusiform gyrus (FG) and more inferior temporal gyrus (ITG) activity when performing person identity tasks. The ITG is the region that showed the greatest activity when normal controls performed the object discrimination task. Thus, autism spectrum subjects appeared to be using "object regions" for processing faces.

There are several possible interpretations for this finding. First, persons with AS or AD may rely more on piecemeal feature analyses and less on configural strategies for processing faces. Second, these data could be supportive of theories that posit a general information processing disturbance in AD (as opposed to face-specific difficulties), such as the "weak central coherence" theory of Frith (1989). A third possible explanation is that AD and AS involve an abnormality specific to the FG, such that it fails to function properly and adjacent regions subsume its normal activities. In our study, careful qualitative analyses of the FG by two independent neuroradiologists did not reveal any morphometric abnormalities among participants with AD or AS. We are now in the midst of attempting to confirm this impression with more rigorous quantitative analyses. Fourth, the abnormal pattern of face-related activity may relate to a lack of interest in faces. If faces are not emotionally salient or relevant, less attention would be paid to them, and across time there would be many missed opportunities for learning both about faces and about social interactions. In this way, the social detachment and lack of affiliative drive characteristic of autism could curtail the development of visuoperceptual expertise for faces, and, as a consequence, the FG would be less engaged during face discrimination. We favor this type of developmental hypothesis, involving a primary dysfunction in the limbic system. Our findings may be likened to a "shadow on the wall," or more specifically a limbic shadow on the cortex cast after some years of developmental experience in a world populated more with objects than with people.

In a related fMRI study of facial expression discrimination, we have preliminary evidence for significantly reduced activity in the middle temporal gyrus in patients with AS or AD as compared to matched controls (Schultz, 1999). While the ventral temporal cortices are mostly involved in neutral face recognition, a region in the superior temporal sulcus and the middle temporal gyrus appears specific to evaluating facial expressions and/or direction of eye gaze (Eacott, Heywood, Gross, & Cowey, 1993; Heywood & Cowey, 1992; Puce, Allison, Bentin, Gore, & McCarthy, 1998; Schultz et al., 1997). These temporal regions have direct reciprocal inputs to the amygdala (Amaral & Price, 1984; Turner et al., 1980), suggesting that there is a larger system important for reading emotional displays. Thus, abnormalities in the amygdala and functionally related temporal cortices may cause difficulties in processing social stimuli and in acquiring or communicating emotional responses to these stimuli. Given the central relevance of the amygdala to the interpretation of our fMRI studies of AD and AS, we now turn to a more detailed discussion of its structure, connectivity, and functions in order to elaborate on its potential role in the pathobiology of autism spectrum conditions.

Amygdala

Several decades of research have led to the notion that the amygdala plays a critical role in emotional arousal, assigning behavioral significance to environmental stimuli, and attaching emotional valence to stimuli (Geschwind, 1965; Kluver & Bucy, 1937; LeDoux, 1996). Deficits in normal social and emotional behavior result when the amygdala is lesioned (Kling & Brothers, 1992). For example, bilateral ablation of the amygdala plus surrounding entorhinal cortex alters vocalizations in juvenile rhesus monkeys (Newman & Bachevalier, 1997). The changes in vocal structure consist of a flattening of the vocal waveform and a perceived decrease in affective tone to the monkey's calls. This finding is of considerable interest to the study of AD and AS because it links a communication symptom (abnormalities in prosody) with social/affective difficulties following amygdalar lesions.

The amygdaloid complex is a small, almond-shaped structure located in the medial temporal lobe. Although previously conceptualized as a singular entity, it is actually a complex anatomical structure composed of more than a dozen nuclei, each with a different set of afferent and efferent connections, neurochemical makeup and cytoarchitecture (Amaral, Price, Pitkanen,

& Carmichael, 1992; Amaral & Price, 1984). Afferents to the amygdala include frontal, cingulate, insular, and temporal neocortex as well as subcortical regions of the thalamus. These terminate specifically in the lateral nucleus of the amygdala, making the lateral nucleus the "sensory interface" of the amygdala (Amaral et al., 1992; LeDoux, Cicchetti, Xagoraris, & Romanski, 1990; Romanski & LeDoux, 1993; Turner et al., 1980). The cortical targets of amygdala include almost every visual processing region in the temporal and occipital lobes (Amaral & Price, 1984), and multiple regions of the prefrontal cortex, most notably the orbital prefrontal cortex, and the medial wall of the prefrontal cortex, including the anterior cingulate (Carmichael & Price, 1995; Mufson, Mesulam, & Pandya, 1981; Price, Carmichael, & Drevets, 1996). Thus, the amygdala has a reciprocal set of connections with the temporal cortex (see Figure 6.2) and orbital and medial prefrontal cortex. Not surprisingly, both of these amygdalar–cortical systems appear to have special relevance to social–emotional functions, and disturbance in these systems may form the primary basis for autism spectrum conditions.

Within the amygdaloid nuclei, there is a high density of benzodiazepine/GABA-A receptors (Niehoff & Kuhar, 1983) suggesting that the anxiolytic effects of benzodiazepines may be mediated by the amygdala. This is of special interest to the pathobiology of autism spectrum disorders because of the high rates of anxiety and difficulty with arousal regulation in these conditions (e.g., Martin, Scahill, Klin, & Volkmar, 1999; Ornitz, 1985). Connections between various nuclei within the amygdala provide paths for incoming information to be processed before making a relay back to the cortex (Pitkanen, Savander, & LeDoux, 1997; Pitkanen & Amaral, 1991). Information can pass into the lateral nucleus, over to the basal and accessory basal nuclei, and then either out to the cortex for further processing or over to the central nucleus and onward to "fight-or-flight" regions of the brainstem and hypothalamus via intra-amygdaloid connections. Studies in animals indicate that damage to any part of this circuitry disrupts normal emotional learning or produces problems in producing autonomic reactions to emotional stimuli.

The amygdala appears to be the central structure mediating visual-reward association or "emotional" learning (Gaffan, Gaffan, & Harrison, 1988) and in signaling the emotional salience of social events and behaviors. Most of what has been learned about these processes comes from the animal studies of LeDoux and colleagues. LeDoux (1996) and others have concentrated on determining the role of the amygdala in emotional processing using the model of classically conditioned fear. In this model, a rat is conditioned to associate an auditory tone and an aversive electrical shock. After such training, animals show emotional reactions to the tone including an increase in heart rate, an increase in blood pressure, ultrasonic vocalizations and "freezing" behavior. Whereas lesions of the auditory cortex do not disrupt the fear response (LeDoux, Sakaguchi, & Reis, 1984; LeDoux & Farb, 1991; Romanski & LeDoux, 1992a, 1992b), lesions of the amygdala do. Finer analyses have demonstrated that lesions of just the lateral nucleus of the amygdala are needed to block classically conditioned emotional reactions, presumably because these lesions prevent incoming sensory information from becoming emotionally salient. Lesions of the central nucleus of the amygdala, on the other hand, have a greater impact on the production of emotional expressions than on emotional learning. Both of these functions seem impaired in AD and AS, suggesting multiple foci of dysfunction within the amygdala.

Recordings from the lateral nucleus of the amygdala have shown that emotional learning modifies the responses in the amygdala by increasing their magnitude, modifying cell coupling within the amygdala, and even converting previously nonresponsive cells to responsive cells (Quirk, Repa, & LeDoux, 1995). The lateral nucleus, therefore, is a critical structure for assigning emotional valence to events and for emotional learning. Electrophysiological recordings of the amygdala demonstrate extremely low spontaneous rates of firing (Bordi & LeDoux, 1992; Romanski, Clugnet, Bordi, & LeDoux, 1993). This has been attributed to the presence of GABA-ergic interneurons providing inhibition to intra-amygdaloid projection neurons (LeDoux, 1996). To overcome this inhibition, temporal convergence of a neutral stimulus with an emotionally salient stimulus is necessary for the neutral stimulus to be "pushed" through the amygdala and out to the cortex, brainstem, and hypothalamus for evaluation and emotional reaction (Bordi & LeDoux, 1992; LeDoux, 1996; Romanski et al., 1993).

This process of temporal convergence in the lateral nucleus provides a mechanism by which stimuli can be assigned an emotional valence, and it may be key to understanding the failure of normal emotional learning during early development in persons with AD and AS. Such cross-modal associations form the basis for the developing infant to form relationships to caretakers, and they establish associations between face representations received from the temporal lobe and information about primary reinforcers, such as food and physical comfort (Rolls, 1995). This begins the process of selective attunement toward people rather than other elements of the environment and creates a focus of attention that permits the acquisition of much more complex and subtle learning about the function of other people and the effect of one's own actions on social transactions.

Role of Amygdalar Dysfunction in Asperger Syndrome and Autistic Disorder

Some of the most compelling evidence for the role of amygdalar dysfunction in AS and AD comes from the postmortem studies of Bauman and Kemper (1985, 1994), showing an increase in the packing density and a decrease in neuron size in many regions of the limbic system, including the amygdala. This type of abnormality may represent a curtailment of neurodevelopment and a state of relative functional immaturity. A functionally abnormal amygdala would be a severe developmental handicap, because, as already noted, the amygdala is the key structure for the formation of stimulus reward associations and for signaling the emotional salience of events (Gaffan et al., 1988; LeDoux, 1996; Rolls, 1995). The amygdala's role in the development of face recognition skill may be to signal the salience and emotional relevance of the human face and to bind face percepts with the neural correlates of emotional experience as a secondary reinforcer (Ono, Nishijo, & Uwano, 1995). Without normally functioning limbic structures, persons with autism spectrum disorders would fail to take special notice of faces and emotions expressed on faces and across early development they would be deprived of critical social learning opportunities. These earliest experiences may be necessary precursors for achieving later developmental milestones, including the emergence of a theory of mind, empathy, and the emotional reactions to others which fuel the use of a theory of mind (Klin, Schultz, & Cohen, 1999). In addition, failure of the amygdala to transmit social–emotional information to cognitive and motor output centers of the frontal lobe would result in abnormal responses to social stimuli, such as faces, and difficulties conveying social emotional information (e.g., prosody). Thus, early emotional learning failures could cause a cascade of neurodevelopmental events, including the emergence of profoundly disturbed social relatedness.

The animal model of autism put forth by Bachevalier (1994) provides a second piece of important information. This research indicates that bilateral damage to the amygdala, hippocampus, and adjacent cortical areas (e.g., entorhinal cortex) in infant monkeys can produce patterns of behavior that are similar to autism. As they matured, these animals displayed little eye contact, withdrew from social situations, failed to initiate social contact, had expressionless faces, and engaged in motor stereotypies. These deficits were not observed in monkeys with early damage to the hippocampal formation alone and were expressed mildly in monkeys with early damage confined to the amygdaloid complex. Although all monkeys received early postnatal lesions in as similar a manner as possible, there was nevertheless considerable variability in subsequent social–emotional dysfunction. This is of significance, as it suggests that heterogeneity in autistic symptomatology across individuals does not necessarily involve a heterogeneous pathophysiology. Moreover, monkeys with early postnatal lesions to the amygdala do not immediately show signs characteristic of autism spectrum disorders (Bachevalier, 1994; Thompson, 1981); that is, the animals "grow into" their autistic-like deficits. This implies an important role for emotional learning in the development of normal social capacities, and that by contrast a simple global loss of affective behavior cannot accurately model AD and AS.

More recently Bachevalier and colleagues demonstrated that early lesions to the medial temporal cortex affect the integrity (Bertolino et al., 1997) and functioning of the prefrontal cortex later in adulthood (Saunders et al., 1998). Monkeys with neonatal lesions to the amygdala and surrounding cortex showed frontal dysregulation of striatal dopamine activity. Most interesting was the finding that when the animals were stressed socially, they exhibited motor stereotypies. Saunders and colleagues' data, therefore, provide a mechanism that could account for the co-occurrence of social dysfunction and motor stereotypies in persons with AD or AS. If these findings can be replicated, they will provide the first solid leads on the core neurofunctional mechanisms in the pathobiology of autism spectrum conditions.

Frontal Lobe

In addition to the studies on the role of the limbic–temporal lobe system in autism spectrum disorders, there is a growing body of data implicating the frontal lobes in the cognitive and social–emotional aspects of AD and related conditions. As reviewed earlier, indirect evidence comes from neuropsychological studies of executive and motor dysfunction in AD and AS. Interest in possible frontal–subcortical abnormalities in AD is not new. Damasio and Maurer (1978) theorized that AD and related disorders result from dysfunction of mesial frontal and mesolimbic cortex, and the basal ganglia. Neuroimaging studies provide additional, direct evidence of the role of the frontal lobes in the pathobiology of AD. For example, decreased frontal lobe perfusion has been suggested by two SPECT studies (George, Costa, Houris, Rang, & Ell, 1992; Zilbovicus et al., 1995).

The frontal lobe can be partitioned into different functional systems, including (1) a motor region just anterior to the central sulcus; (2) the dorsolateral PFC, which has a specific role in cognitive and EF (as does the cingulate gyrus); and (3) the orbital–medial PFC which appears to be more involved in social–emotional functioning (Damasio, 1996; Goldman-Rakic, 1987; Rolls, 1995; Stuss & Benson, 1986). Different features of AD and AS might preferentially map onto separate divisions (e.g., EF deficits to the dorsolateral PFC and socio–emotional deficits to the orbital–medial PFC). Moreover, some neuroimaging evidence specifically implicates the dorsolateral PFC in AD. For example, a P31 MR spectroscopy study found alterations in phospholipid metabolism as well as enhanced membrane degradation in the dorsal PFC of individuals with AD (Minshew, Goldstein, Dombrowski, Panchalingam, & Pettegrew, 1993). Orbital and medial prefrontal cortices have a key role in social and emotional functioning (Bechara, Tranel, Damasio, & Damasio, 1996; Brothers, Ring, & Kling, 1990; Damasio, 1996; Devinsky, Morrell, & Vogt, 1995; Goel, Grafman, Sadato, & Hallett, 1995; Lane, Reiman, Ahern, Schwartz, & Davidson, 1997; Lane, Reiman,

Bradley, et al., 1997; Lane, Fink, Chau, & Dolan, 1997). The orbital and medial PFC have dense reciprocal connections with medial temporal areas, forming a system for regulating emotional processes (Carmichael & Price, 1995; Price et al., 1996). Nonhuman primate studies have documented abnormal social responsivity and loss of social position within the group following lesions to orbital and medial prefrontal cortices (Butter, McDonald & Snyder, 1969; Bachevalier & Mishkin, 1986). The relative importance of the orbital and medial PFC to AD is suggested by a recent neuropsychological study that revealed deficits in both dorsolateral PFC and in medial temporal/orbital PFC, but only the latter correlated with AD symptom severity (Dawson, Meltzoff, Osterling, & Rinaldi, 1998).

The neuroimaging literature directly implicates the orbital and medial sections of the PFC in social abilities and cognitive–emotional integration (Klin et al., 1999). Medial prefrontal dopaminergic activity as measured by [^{18}F] fluorodopa positron emission tomography (PET) has been found to be significantly reduced in AD (Ernst, Zametkin, Matochik, Pascualvaca, & Cohen, 1997). In addition, reduced glucose metabolism has been reported in a subdivision of the anterior cingulate gyrus (right Brodmann area [BA] 24′) among persons with AD engaged in a verbal memory test (Haznedar et al., 1997). There were also alterations in brain morphology in the anterior cingulate, with BA 25 larger bilaterally and BA 24′ smaller in the right hemisphere. This underscores the importance of studies that specifically address structure–function relationships. PET studies have also examined systems that are specifically engaged by social cognition using a theory-of-mind (ToM) paradigm. Fletcher et al. (1995) studied six male volunteers while they read stories and answered questions that entailed either mental attributions of another's beliefs or attributions of physical causality. "Mentalism" was associated with specific engagement of left medial prefrontal cortex (centered on the border between BA 8 and 9) and of the posterior cingulate gyrus. Happé et al. (1996) compared these control subjects to a group of five males with AS. Although the subjects with AS showed ToM specific engagement of the medial PFC, the center of activation was displaced 2 cm below and 8 mm more anterior compared to the controls, in a transitional region between BA 9 and 10. Another PET study (Goel et al., 1995) requiring reasoning about the beliefs and intentions of others revealed prominent activation of the left temporal lobe and left medial frontal lobe (primarily BA 9) that overlapped with the medial PFC area found by Fletcher and colleagues. An earlier SPECT study of healthy controls suggested that areas of the right orbital frontal cortex were involved in processing mental state terms (Baron-Cohen et al., 1994). More superior areas within the medial PFC were not explored. Involvement of orbital and medial PFC in social cognition is also consistent with findings of ToM task deficits among neurological patients with bilateral orbital and medial PFC lesions (Stone, Baron-Cohen, & Knight, 1998).

Contribution of Prefrontal Cortex to Social–Emotional Processing

We recently completed an fMRI study on the neurofunctional components of the process by which individuals make social inferences (Schultz et al., 1999), using a novel animation task developed by our group—the Social Attribution Task (SAT; Klin et al., 1999). The SAT is based on a classic study by Heider and Simmel (1944) using a silent film in which moving geometric shapes (a circle, a small triangle, and a larger triangle) interacted with each other. The movements of the shapes are contingent upon one another; that is, they move in synchrony, against one another, or as a result of the action of one another. In our pilot studies (Klin, 1999; see also Klin et al., 1999) of several dozen typically developing children and adults outside the MR machine, nearly all persons automatically labeled the events as social. In contrast, persons with AS or AD frequently failed to make social attributions, instead describing the scene only in terms of the actual physical properties of the characters and the movements. Use of simple shapes to display human social interactions strips the social event down to the essential elements needed to convey the social meanings. We hypothesize that children normally develop a social template to decode and understand social situations. The template is engaged automatically and with little effort in daily social interactions, and during the initially ambiguous scene established by the SAT. The propensity to search for social meaning is so strong that we usually impose social structure on ambiguous situations as a matter of course. For example, witness the normal childhood play activity of finding faces in the clouds and inventing social stories using these precepts. In autism and related conditions, the propensity to interpret ambiguous scenes through a social lens seems to be missing.

Given the sensitivity of this measure to the core social deficits in AS and AD, we have now completed our first fMRI studies using the SAT in two groups of eight healthy young adults in order to identify brain regions involved in the process of attributing social meaning to events (Schultz, Klin, van der Gaag, Skudlarski, Herrington, & Gore, 1999). The study contrasted brain activity during the SAT with a visuospatial control task. Both tasks involved moving geometric shapes. The control task required participants to determine whether one or more than one of the three shapes was moving in a trajectory identical to its geometric shape (i.e., in a circular or triangular path). During the experimental task, participants observed contingent interactions between these same shapes and were required to infer whether or not the characters were "friends" or "not friends." An effort was made to equate the two tasks with respect to image complexity, and movement quantity and location, so that the comparison between the two tasks would isolate the variable of social ideation. The results were surprisingly strong, with significant selective brain activation for the social reasoning task in a fairly large area of the medial PFC (see Plate 6.2, opposite page 175). Statistical analyses revealed that the major area of activation, however, was circumscribed to Brodmann's area 9. As already described, this is in the same general brain region that has been shown to be involved in ToM tasks (Fletcher et al., 1995). Thus, there is now a convergence of data suggesting that the orbital and medial PFC are critical to social functioning and to the pathobiology of autism spectrum conditions.

A related series of functional imaging studies has linked orbital–medial PFC to affective processing in healthy controls (Lane, Reiman, Ahern, et al., 1997; Lane, Reiman, Bradley, et al., 1997; Lane, Fink, et al., 1997; Reiman et al., 1997). The orbital and medial PFC may have a specific role in integrating affective with cognitive processes (e.g., Bechara et al., 1996; Damasio, 1996; Hornak, Rolls, & Wade, 1996). Studies of the orbital cortex in patients (Damasio, Tranel, & Damasio, 1990; Hornak et al., 1996) and nonhuman primates (Dias et al., 1996) suggest that it participates in integrating information about rewards and punishments to bias future behavior. The integration of social and emotional information is critically important vis-á-vis the primary deficits found in AD and AS. Because the orbital and medial PFC are densely interconnected with limbic areas, especially the amygdala (Carmichael & Price, 1995), it may be more appropriate to conceptualize a limbic–frontal system as critical to AD symptomatology, as opposed to isolated regions in one or the other. This pattern of connections would allow the amygdala to transmit information about emotional significance to prefrontal regions involved in guiding behaviors such as social interactions and related social cognitive processes. Disconnection of the amygdala from orbital and medial prefrontal cortical processing regions could result in the failure to transmit information about stimulus valence and also a more general dysregulation of emotional responsivity. In this scenario, social stimuli would not acquire their normal valence, causing social processing difficulties similar to the insensitivity to consequences displayed by patients with acute ventromedial prefrontal lesions (Bechara et al., 1996).

In addition to the possible effects of amygdalar dysfunction on the functioning of the PFC, dysfunction of the orbital–medial PFC might also have an important impact on amygdalar functions. For example, when lesions of the medial PFC are made just prior to fear conditioning, animals show normal acquisition of the emotional learning; that is, they show typical autonomic changes and freezing behavior when the conditioned stimulus (an auditory cue) is turned on. However, these animals do not show the normal rate of extinction. The animals continue to show fear responses when the auditory tone is repeatedly presented without the foot shock (Morgan, Romanski, & LeDoux, 1993). These results indicate that the medial PFC may be essential in "turning off" the amygdalar fear systems when they are no longer necessary. The uninformed amygdala continues to send out its cry of alarm because it has not received the safety signal from the PFC that the situation is no longer fearful. When the medial prefrontal systems are damaged it is as if the amygdala is "stuck on" and unable to disengage from the fear response (LeDoux, 1996). If a ventromedial prefrontal lesion is present from birth, learning about social stimuli, such as facial expressions, gestures, and prosody, might be impaired. A faulty connection between ventromedial PFC and the amygdala could explain the lack of appropriate emotional and social behavior that is seen with autism.

The high levels of anxiety that many patients with AS and AD experience (Martin et al., 1999), and the avoidance of eye contact to reduce anxiety and arousal (Hutt & Ounsted, 1966) may be related to the amygdala-medial PFC circuit. If the amygdala is "stuck on" because of inadequate medial prefrontal input, a continuous tonic, anxiety-producing output from the central nucleus of the amygdala directly to autonomic centers of the hypothalamus will result. In this state, although arousal and general anxiety may be elevated, the individual is unable to mount a normal emotional response to fear and other emotional stimuli because the circuit may be already nearly fully activated (LeDoux, Sakaguchi, & Reis, 1982). This model would explain the inability of the affected individual to appreciate and respond to new social–emotional events.

CONCLUSIONS AND FUTURE DIRECTIONS

At present, an understanding of the neurobiology of AS remains limited. We have argued that heuristic models of AS should be built on our understanding of the neurobiology of AD, especially as the diagnostic validity of AS apart from AD remains fully in doubt. Our model has highlighted the central role that the amygdala plays in social–emotional functions. Assuming that AS is an independent and valid biological entity, a working model of the disorder would include dysfunction of diverse frontal and temporal cortical systems, perhaps with some bias toward right-hemisphere dysfunction. Although it is true that there is modularity in brain function, with different regions assuming responsibility for different cognitive, perceptual, emotional, and motor functions, it is perhaps a stumbling block in our thinking to become too enamored with the localization of function. In isolation, brain modules never do much of anything of practical significance. That is, although we might localize regions of the dorsolateral PFC as critical to particular cognitive functions such as working memory, or the FG on the ventral side of the temporal lobe to face perception, it is important to recognize that these regions operate in cooperation with many other regions, and they are merely one node in a distributed network. In this chapter we have attempted to account for these difficulties, by specifying parallel frontal and temporal loops through the amygdala, necessary for productive and receptive elements of social–emotional functioning. Future work with the powerful new imaging technique of fMRI will help define more precisely the roles of these loops in social–emotional functions. As argued at the outset of this chapter, much work needs to be done on typically developing and developed individuals to map those systems that participate in the functions disturbed in AS and AD. In addition, neuroimaging work needs to proceed in tandem with neurobehavioral studies, for neither is very powerful without the other.

Any attempt to devise neurofunctional models of AS must be inclusive of the two domains affected—social interactions and restricted, repetitive patterns of interests, and behavior. From a neuropsychological perspective it is rather odd that these two domains that seemingly share little in common should co-occur with such frequency so as to be syndromic (for the sake of argument, we assume that the individual signs and symptoms within each domain represent unitary constructs). The pervasive developmental delay that characterizes both AD and AS would suggest that a rather diverse and spatially disparate set of neural processing centers has been affected. However, widespread dysfunction does not preclude developmental events that were at one point very localized. In this chapter, we have emphasized the point that early mesial temporal lobe dysfunction can result in autistic-like sequelae, with social dysfunction directly mediated by developmental dysfunction of the amygdalar–cortical systems. Significantly, there is now evidence in nonhuman primates that the motor stereotypies characteristic of both AS and AD can also result from mesial temporal lobe lesions, but that the effect is mediated by developmental influences on the integrity and functioning of distant cortical sites in the frontal lobes (Bertolino et al., 1997; Saunders et al., 1998).

These animal data give us a developmental model of how initial damage in a circumscribed subcortical system can have wider implications for function in cortical regions. This type of model is powerful and offers great promise for eventually understanding the pervasive developmental difficulties present in both AD and AS. This does not discount the possibility that AS and AD are genetic disorders with multiple independent manifestations, but it does indicate that we need not have multiple initial insults to later have multiple areas of brain dysfunction and multiple areas of behavioral and social disability. Because analogous damage during adulthood does not have the same effect, it will be of critical importance to conduct developmental animal and neuroimaging studies. However, developmental neural network phenomena are difficult to study with imaging methods. Techniques such as PET and fMRI are exceptionally good at localizing potential problem areas in the brain, but in current practice they are not good at defining networks that collaborate in creating behavioral phenotypes. Neuroimaging techniques allow one to have a glimpse at a particular system at a particular time. These techniques are less well suited to the real task of integrating information across time and across diverse brain regions. Thus, it will be important to conduct longitudinal neuroimaging studies, and to continue to draw on animal studies where it is possible to have much greater control in studying developmental effects of early lesions.

Although we have emphasized the potential role of the amygdala in the pathobiology of AD and AS, the premise that the integrity and functioning of subcortical structures early in development will affect higher cortical processes applies to other structures as well. One structure in particular—the thalamus—is especially well positioned by virtue of its anatomical connections to have a pervasive influence on brain functioning. The thalamus receives input from and projects to virtually every major region of the brain, making it a primary source of extracortical activation for the cortex as well as corticocortical communication (Carpenter, 1991; Guillery, 1995; Kandel, Schwartz, & Jessell, 1991; Newman, 1995). Further, a current perspective of the thalamus indicates that it is involved in multiple processes that permit the transmission, tuning, modification, and integrated processing of information in the brain (Baars, 1995; Barth & MacDonald, 1996; Bogen, 1995; Carpenter, 1991; Castro-Alamancos & Connors, 1996; Jones, 1997; Guillery, 1996; Kandel et al., 1991; Newman, 1995; Singer, 1993; Steriade, McCormick, & Sejnowski, 1993). These observations alone make the thalamus an attractive target for future investigations in AD and AS. There is also evidence to suggest that the thalamus is critically involved in the organization of connections in the developing cortex (Bolz, Kossel, & Bagnard, 1995; Ghosh, 1995; Molnár & Blakemore, 1995; O'Leary, Borngasser, Fox, & Schlaggar, 1995). Thus, like the amygdala, early dysfunction of the thalamus could have significant effects on the structure and function of higher cortical centers. Importantly, both of these structures, through their extensive connections, are also central to the major neural systems implicated in AD and AS. The pulvinar nucleus of the thalamus may be of particular importance for the pathobiology of AD and AS. Nonhuman primate studies implicate the pulvinar in signaling the salience of visual inputs (Robinson, 1993). Moreover, a recent PET study in human subjects found increased right pulvinar activity with experimentally manipulated changes in the salience of visual stimuli (emotionally expressive faces) (Morris, Friston, & Dolan, 1997). The pulvinar activity was correlated with activity in the right amygdala, suggesting that both structures participate in signaling the emotional salience of visual stimuli. We speculate that disturbance of this system may be involved in AD and AS and may have special relevance to our fMRI results on face perception. Thus, it will be important to systematically study and characterize the role of the thalamus in autism spectrum disorders.

At present, however, the existing data argue strongly for a role of the amygdala and its collaborating cortical systems in the pathobiology of autism spectrum conditions. Even though it is premature to attempt a comprehensive neurofunctional model based on one structure alone, we have provided evidence to show that it would be highly unlikely for the amygdalar–cortical systems described in this chapter to have no or only a limited role in the pathobiology of AD and AS. Although any approach that places faith in the explanatory power of a single construct is normally highly suspect, the unifying power of a centrally located and developmentally well-positioned structure such as the amygdala is striking.

REFERENCES

Adolphs, R., Damasio, H., Tranel, D., & Damasio, A. R. (1996). Cortical systems for the recognition of emotion in facial expressions. *Journal of Neuroscience, 16*(23), 7678–7687.

Adolphs, R., Tranel, D., Damasio, H., & Damasio, A. (1994). Impaired recognition of emotion in facial expressions following bilateral damage to the human amygdala. *Nature, 372,* 669–672.

Allen, L. S., Richey, M. F., Chai, Y. M., & Gorski, R. A. (1991). Sex differences in the corpus callosum of the living human being. *Journal of Neuroscience, 11,* 933–942.

Amaral, D. G., & Price, J. L. (1984). Amygdalo–cortical projections in the monkey (Macaca fascicularis). *Journal of Comparative Neurology, 230,* 465–496.

Amaral, D. G., Price, J. L., Pitkanen, A., & Carmichael, S. T. (1992). Anatomical organization of the primate amygdaloid complex. In J. Aggleton (Ed.), *The amygdala: Neurobiological aspects of emotion, memory and mental dysfunction* (pp. 1–66). New York: Wiley-Liss.

American Psychiatric Association. (1994). *Diagnostic and statistical manual of mental disorders* (4th ed.). Washington, DC: Author.

Andreasen, N. C., Flaum, M., Swayze, V., O'Leary, D. S., Alliger, R., Cohen, G., Ehrhardt, J., & Yuh, W. T. C. (1993). Intelligence and brain structure in normal individuals. *American Journal of Psychiatry, 150,* 130–134.

Ankney, C. D. (1992). Sex differences in relative brain size: The mismeasure of women, too? *Intelligence, 16,* 329–336.

Arin, D. M., Bauman, M. L., & Kemper, T. L. (1991). The distribution of Purkinje cell loss in the cerebellum in autism. *Neurology, 41,* 307.

Asperger, H. (1991). Autistic psychopathy in childhood. In U. Frith (Ed.), *Autism and Asperger syndrome.* Cambridge, UK: Cambridge University Press. (Original work published 1944)

Aylward, E. H., Minshew, N. J., Goldstein, G., Honeycutt, N. A., Augustine, A. M., Yates, K. O., Barta, P. E., & Pearlson, G. D. (in press). MRI volumes of amygdala and hippocampus in non-mentally retarded autistic adolescents and adults. *Neurology.*

Baars, B. J. (1995). Tutorial commentary: Surprisingly small subcortical structures are needed for the *state* of waking consciousness, while cortical projection areas seem to provide perceptual *contents* of consciousness. *Consciousness and Cognition, 4,* 159–162.

Bachevalier, J. (1994). Medial temporal lobe structures and autism: A review of clinical and experimental findings. *Neuropsychologia, 32,* 627–648.

Bachevalier, J., & Mishkin, M. (1986). Visual recognition impairment follows ventromedial but not dorsolateral prefrontal lesions in monkeys. *Behavioural Brain Research, 20*(3), 249–261.

Bailey, A., Le Couteur, A., Gottesman, I., Bolton, P., Simonoff, E., Yuzda, E., & Rutter, M. (1995). Autism as a strongly genetic disorder: Evidence from a British twin study. *Psychological Medicine, 25,* 63–77.

Bailey, A., Luthert, P., Bolton, P., Le Couteur, A., Rutter, M., & Harding, B. (1993). Autism and megalencephaly. *Lancet, 341,* 1225–1226.

Bailey, A., Luthert, P., Dean, A., Harding, B., Janota, I., Montgomery, M., Rutter, M., & Lantos, P. (1998). A clinicopathological study of autism. *Brain, 121,* 889–905.

Baron-Cohen, S., Ring, H., Moriarty, J., Schmidt, B., Costa, D., & Ell, P. (1994). Recognition of mental state terms: Clinical findings in children with autism and a functional neuroimaging study of normal adults. *British Journal of Psychiatry, 165,* 640–649.

Barth, D. S., & MacDonald, K. D. (1996). Thalamic modulation of high-frequency oscillating potentials in auditory cortex. *Nature, 383,* 78–81.

Bartlett, J. C., & Searcy, J. (1993). Inversion and configuration of faces. *Cognitive Psychology, 25,* 281–316.

Bauman, M. L., & Kemper, T. L. (1985). Neuroanatomic observations of the brain in early infantile autism. *Neurology, 35,* 866–874.

Bauman, M. L., & Kemper, T. L. (1994). Neuroanatomic observations of the brain in autism. In M. L. Bauman & T. L. Kemper (Eds.), *The neurobiology of autism* (pp. 119–145). Baltimore: Johns Hopkins University Press.

Bauman, M. L., & Kemper, T. L. (1996). Observations on the Purkinje cells in the cerebellar vermis in autism. *Journal of Neuropathology and Experimental Neurology, 55,* 613.

Bechara, A., Tranel, D., Damasio, H., & Damasio, A. R. (1996). Failure to respond autonomically to anticipated future outcomes following damage to prefrontal cortex. *Cerebral Cortex, 6,* 215–225.

Bennetto, L., Pennington, B. F., & Rogers, S. J. (1996). Intact and impaired memory functions in autism. *Child Development, 67,* 1816–1835.

Berthier, M. L. (1994). Corticocallosal anomalies in Asperger's syndrome. *American Journal of Roentgenology, 162,* 236–237.

Berthier, M. L., Bayes, A., & Tolosa, E. S. (1993). Magnetic resonance imaging in patients with concurrent Tourette's disorder and Asperger's syndrome. *Journal of the American Academy of Child and Adolescent Psychiatry, 32,* 633–639.

Bertolino, A., Saunders, R. C., Mattay, V. S., Bachevalier, J., Frank, J. A., & Weinberger, D. R. (1997). Altered development of prefrontal neurons in rhesus monkeys with neonatal mesial temporo-limbic lesions: A proton magnetic resonance spectroscopic imaging study. *Cerebral Cortex, 7*(8), 740–748.

Blashfield, R. K. (1984). *The classification of psychopathology: Neo-Kraepelinian and quantitative approaches.* New York: Plenum.

Bogen, J. E. (1995). On the neurophysiology of consciousness: I. An overview. *Consciousness and Cognition, 4,* 52–62.

Bolton, P. F., & Griffiths, P. D. (1997). Association of tuberous sclerosis of temporal lobes with autism and atypical autism. *Lancet, 349*(9049), 392–395.

Bolz, J., Kossel, A., & Bagnard, D. (1995). The specificity of interactions between the cortex and the thalamus. *Ciba Foundation Symposium: The Development of the Cerebral Cortex, 193,* 173–191.

Bordi, F., & LeDoux, J. E. (1992). Sensory tuning beyond the sensory system: An initial analysis of auditory response properties of neurons in the lateral nucleus of the amygdala and overlying areas of the striatum. *Journal of Neuroscience, 12,* 2493–2503.

Boucher, J., & Lewis, V. (1992). Unfamiliar face recognition in relatively able autistic children. *Journal of Child Psychology and Psychiatry, 33*(5), 843–859.

Braverman, M., Fein, D., Lucci, D., & Waterhouse, L. (1989). Affect comprehension in children with pervasive developmental disorders. *Journal of Autism and Developmental Disorders, 19,* 301–316.

Brothers, L., Ring, B., & Kling, A. (1990). Response of neurons in the macaque amygdala to complex social stimuli. *Behavioural Brain Research, 41,* 199–213.

Burton, L. A., & Levy, J. (1989). Sex differences in the lateralized processing of facial emotion. *Brain and Cognition, 11,* 210–228.

Butter, C. M., McDonald, J. A., & Snyder, D. R. . (1969). Orality, preference behavior, and reinforcement value of nonfood object in monkeys with orbital frontal lesions. *Science, 164(885)*, 1306–1307.

Capps, L., Yirmiya, N., & Sigman, M. (1992). Understanding of simple and complex emotions in nonretarded children with autism. *Journal of Child Psychology and Psychiatry, 33*, 1169–1182.

Carmichael, S. T., & Price, J. L. (1995). Limbic connections of the orbital and medial prefrontal cortex in macaque monkeys. *Journal of Comparative Neurology, 363*, 615–641.

Carpenter, M. B. (1991). *Core text of neuroanatomy: Fourth edition.* Baltimore: Williams & Wilkins.

Castro-Alamancos, M. A., & Connors, B. W. (1996). Short-term plasticity of a thalamocortical pathway dynamically modulated by behavioral state. *Science, 272*, 274–277.

Caviness, V. S., Jr., Takahashi, T., & Nowakowski, R. S. (1995). Numbers, time, neocortical neuronogenesis: A general developmental and evolutionary model. *Trends in Neurosciences, 18*, 379–383.

Courchesne, E., Saitoh, O., Yeung-Courchesne, R., Press, G. A., Lincoln, A. J., Haas, R. H., & Schreibman, L. (1994). Abnormality of cerebellar vermian lobules VI and VII in patients with infantile autism: Identification of hypoplastic and hyperplastic subgroups with MR imaging. *American Journal of Roentgenology, 162*, 123–130.

Courchesne, E., Townsend, J., & Saitoh, O. (1994). The brain in infantile autism: Posterior fossa structures are abnormal. *Neurology, 44*, 214–223.

Courchesne, E., Yeung-Courchesne, R., Press, G. A., Hesselink, J. R., & Jernigan, T. L. (1988). Hypoplasia of cerebellar vermal lobules VI and VII in autism. *New England Journal of Medicine, 318*, 1349–1354.

Damasio, A. R. (1985). The frontal lobes. In K. M. Heilman & E. Valenstein (Eds.), *Clinical neuropsychology* (2nd ed., pp. 339–375). New York: Oxford University Press.

Damasio, A. R. (1996). The somatic marker hypothesis and the possible functions of the prefrontal cortex. *Philosophical Transactions of the Royal Society of London—Series B: Biological Sciences, 351*, 1413–20

Damasio, A. R., & Maurer, R. G. (1978). A neurological model of childhood autism. *Archives of Neurology, 35*, 777–786.

Damasio, A. R., Tranel, D., & Damasio, H. (1990). Face agnosia and the neural substrates of memory. *Annual Review of Neuroscience, 13*, 89–109.

Davies, S., Bishop, D., Manstead, A. S. R., & Tantam, D. (1994). Face perception in children with autism and Asperger's syndrome. *Journal of Child Psychology and Psychiatry, 35(6)*, 1033–1057.

Dawson, G., Hill, D., Spencer, A., Galpert, L., & Watson, L. (1990). Affective exchanges between young autistic children and their mothers. *Journal of Abnormal Child Psychology, 18*, 335–345.

Dawson, G., Meltzoff, A. N., Osterling, J., & Rinaldi, J. (1998). Neuropsychological correlates of early symptoms of autism. *Child Development, 69(5)*, 1276–1285.

Devinsky, O., Morrell, M. J., & Vogt, B. A. (1995). Contributions of anterior cingulate cortex to behavior. *Brain, 118*, 279–306.

Diamond, R., & Carey, S. (1986). Why faces are and are not special: An effect of expertise. *Journal of Experimental Psychology: General, 115*, 107–117.

Dias, R., Robbins, T. W., & Roberts, A. C. (1996). Dissociation in prefrontal cortex of affective and attentional shifts. *Nature, 380*, 69–72.

Eacott, M. J., Heywood, C. A., Gross, C. G., & Cowey, A. (1993). Visual discrimination impairments following lesions of the superior temporal sulcus are not specific for facial stimuli. *Neuropsychologia, 31*(6), 609–619.

Egaas, B., Courchesne, E., & Saitoh, O. (1995). Reduced size of corpus callosum in autism. *Archives of Neurology, 52*, 794–801.

Ellis, H. D., Ellis, D. M., Fraser, W., & Deb, S. (1994). A preliminary study of right hemisphere cognitive deficits and impaired social judgments among young people with Asperger syndrome. *European Child and Adolescent Psychiatry, 3*(4), 255–266.

Ernst, M., Zametkin, A. J., Matochik, J. A., Pascualvaca, D., & Cohen, R. M. (1997). Reduced medial prefrontal dopaminergic activity in autistic children. *Lancet, 350*, 638.

Farah, M. J. (1996). Is face recognition "special"? Evidence from neuropsychology. *Behavioural Brain Research, 76*, 181–189.

Fein, D., Humes, M., Kaplan, E., Lucci, D., & Waterhouse, L. (1984). The question of left hemisphere dysfunction in infantile autism. *Psychological Bulletin, 95*, 258–281.

Fein, D., Lucci, D., Braverman, M., & Waterhouse, L. (1992). Comprehension of affect in context in children with pervasive developmental disorders. *Journal of Child Psychology and Psychiatry, 33*, 1157–1167.

Filipek, P. A., Richelme, C., Kennedy, D. N., Rademacher, J., Pitcher, D. A., Zidel, S., & Caviness, V. S. (1992). Morphometric analysis of the brain in developmental language disorders and autism. *Annals of Neurology, 32*, 475.

Fletcher, P. C., Happé, F., Frith, U., Baker, S. C., Dolan, R. J., Frackowiak, R. S., & Frith, C. D. (1995). Other minds in the brain: A functional imaging study of "theory of mind" in story comprehension. *Cognition, 57*(2), 109–128.

Fombonne, E., Roge, B., Claverie, J., Courty, S., & Fremolle, J. (1999). Microcephaly and Macrocephaly in Autism. *Journal of Autism and Developmental Disorders, 29*(2), 113–119.

Frith U. (1989). *Autism: Explaining the enigma*. Oxford: Blackwell.

Gaffan, E. A., Gaffan, D., & Harrison, S. (1988). Disconnection of the amygdala from visual association cortex impairs visual-reward association learning in monkeys. *Journal of Neuroscience, 8*, 3144–3150.

Gauthier, I., & Tarr, M. J. (1997). Becoming a "Greeble" expert: Exploring mechanisms for face recognition. *Vision Research, 37*, 1673–1681.

Gauthier, I., Tarr, M., Anderson, A., Skudlarski, P., & Gore, J. (1999). Activation of the middle fusiform "face area" increases with expertise in recognizing novel objects. *Nature Neuroscience, 2*, 568–573.

George, M. S., Costa, D. C., Houris, K., Rang, H. A., & Ell, P. J. (1992). Cerebral blood flow abnormalities in adults with infantile autism. *Journal of Nervous and Mental Disease, 180*, 413–417.

Geschwind, N. (1965). The disconnexion syndromes in animals and man. Part I. *Brain, 88*, 237–294.

Ghosh, A. (1995). Subplate neurons and the patterning of thalamocortical connections. *Ciba Foundation Symposium: The Development of the Cerebral Cortex, 193*, 150–172.

Gillberg, C. (1986). Brief report: Onset at age 14 of a typical autistic syndrome. A case report of a girl with herpes simplex encephalitis. *Journal of Autism and Developmental Disorders, 16*, 369–375.

Gillberg, I. C. (1991). Autistic syndrome with onset at age 31 years: Herpes encephalitis as a possible model for childhood autism. *Developmental Medicine and Child Neurology, 33*, 912–929.

Goel, V., Grafman, J., Sadato, N., & Hallett, M. (1995). Modeling other minds. *Neuroreport, 6*(13), 1741–1746.

Goldberg, E., & Costa, L. (1981). Hemispheric differences in the acquisition and use of descriptive systems. *Brain and Language, 14*, 144–173.

Goldman-Rakic, P. S. (1987). Circuitry of the primate prefrontal cortex and regulation of behavior by representational memory. In F. Plum, V. Mountcastle, & S. Geiger (Eds.), *Handbook of physiology: The nervous system* (pp. 373–416). Bethesda, MD: American Physiological Society.

Goldstein, A. G., & Chance, J. E. (1970). Visual recognition memory for complex configurations. *Perception and Psychophysics, 9*(2B), 237–241.

Green, L. A., Fein, D., Joy, S., & Waterhouse, L. (1995). Cognitive functioning in autism: An overview. In E. Schopler, & G. B. Mesibov (Eds.), *Learning and cognition in autism* (pp. 13–31). New York: Plenum.

Guillery, R. W. (1995). Anatomical evidence concerning the role of the thalamus in corticocortical communication: A brief review. *Journal of Anatomy, 187*, 583–592.

Hamann, S. B., Stefanacci, L., Squire, L. R., Adolphs, R., Tranel, D., Damasio, H., & Damasio, A. (1996). Recognizing facial emotion. *Nature, 379*, 497.

Happé, F., Ehlers, S., Fletcher, P., Frith, U., Johansson, M., Gillberg, C., Dolan, R., Frackowiak, R., & Frith, C. (1996). "Theory of mind" in the brain: Evidence from a PET scan study of Asperger syndrome. *Neuroreport, 8*(1), 197–201.

Hashimoto, T., Tayama, M., Miyazaki, M., Murakawa, M., & Kuroda, Y. (1993). Brainstem and cerebellar vermis involvement in autistic children. *Journal of Child Neurology, 8*, 149–153.

Hashimoto, T., Tayama, M., Murakawa, M., Yoshimoto, T., Miyazaki, M., Harada, M., & Kuroda, Y. (1995). Development of the brainstem and cerebellum in autistic patients. *Journal of Autism and Developmental Disorders, 25*, 1–18.

Hauck, M., Fein, D., Maltby, N., Waterhouse, L., & Feinstein, C. (1998). Memory for faces in children with autism. *Child Neuropsychology, 4*, 187–198.

Haxby, J. V., Ungerleider, L. G., Clark, V. P., Schouten, J. L., Hoffman, E. A., & Martin, A. (1999). The effect of face inversion on activity in human neural systems for face and object perception. *Neuron, 22*(1), 189–199.

Haznedar, M. M., Buchsbaum, M. S., Metzger, M., Solimando, A., Spiegel-Cohen, J., & Hollander, E. (1997). Anterior cingulate gyrus volume and glucose metabolism in autistic disorder. *American Journal of Psychiatry, 154*(8), 1047–1050.

Heider, F., & Simmel, M. (1944). An experimental study of apparent behavior. *The American Journal of Psychology, 57*(2), 243–259.

Hempel, C. G. (1961). Introduction to problems of taxonomy. In J. Zubin (Ed.), *Field studies in the mental disorders* (pp. 3–22). New York: Grune & Stratton.

Heywood, C. A., & Cowey, A. (1992). The role of the "face-cell" area in the discrimination and recognition of faces by monkeys. *Philosophical Transactions of the Royal Society of London—Series B: Biological Sciences, 335*(1273), 31–38.

Hobson, R. P. (1986a). The autistic child's appraisal of expressions of emotion: A further study. *Journal of Child Psychology and Psychiatry, 2*, 671–680.

Hobson, R. P. (1986b). The autistic child's appraisal of expressions of emotion. *Journal of Child Psychology and Psychiatry, 27*, 321–342.

Hobson, R. P., & Lee, A. (1989). Emotion-related and abstract concepts in autistic people: Evidence from the British Picture Vocabulary Scale. *Journal of Autism and Developmental Disorders, 19,* 601–623.

Hobson, R. P., Ouston, J., & Lee, A. (1988a). What's in a face? The case of autism. *British Journal of Psychology, 79,* 441–453.

Hobson, R. P., Ouston, J., & Lee, A. (1988b). Emotion recognition in autism: Coordinating faces and voices. *Psychological Medicine, 18,* 911–923.

Holttum, J. R., Minshew, N. J., Sanders, R. S., & Phillips, N. E. (1992). Magnetic resonance imaging of the posterior fossa in autism. *Biological Psychiatry, 32,* 1091–1101.

Hoon, A. H., & Reiss, A. L. (1992). The mesial–temporal lobe and autism: Case report and review. *Developmental Medicine and Child Neurology, 34,* 252–259.

Hornak, J., Rolls, E. T., & Wade, D. (1996). Face and voice expression identification in patients with emotional and behavioural changes following ventral frontal lobe damage. *Neuropsychologia, 34*(4), 247–261.

Hutt, C., & Ounsted, C. (1966). The biological significance of gaze aversion with particular reference to the syndrome of infantile autism. *Behavioral Science, 11*(5), 346–356.

Jaedicke, S., Storoschuk, S., & Lord, C. (1994). Subjective experience and causes of affect in high-functioning children and adolescents with autism. *Development and Psychopathology, 6,* 273–284.

Jones, E. G. (1997). Cortical development and thalamic pathology in schizophrenia. *Schizophrenia Bulletin, 23,* 483–501.

Kandel, E. R., Schwartz, J. H., & Jessell, T. M. (1991). *Principles of neural science: Third edition.* New York: Elsevier.

Kanner, L. (1943). Autistic disturbances of affective contact. *Nervous Child, 2,* 217–250.

Kanwisher, N., McDermott, J., & Chun, M. M. (1997). The Fusiform face area: A module in human extrastriate cortex specialized for face perception. *The Journal of Neuroscience, 17,* 4302–4311.

Kimura, D. (1987). Are men's and women's brains really different? *Canadian Psychology, 28*(2), 133–147.

Klin, A. (1999). *Attributing social meaning to ambiguous visual stimuli in higher functioning autism and Asperger syndrome: The social attribution task.* Manuscript submitted for publication.

Kleiman, M. D., Neff, S., & Rosman, N. P. (1992). The brain in infantile autism: Are posterior fossa structures abnormal? *Neurology, 42,* 753–760.

Klin, A., Schultz, R. T., & Cohen, D. J. (1999). The need for a theory of theory of mind in action: Developmental and neurofunctional perspectives on social cognition. In S. Baron-Cohen, H. Tager-Flusberg, & D. Cohen (Eds.), *Understanding other minds* (2nd ed., pp. 362–393). Oxford, UK: Oxford University Press.

Klin, A., Volkmar, F. R., Sparrow, S. S., Cicchetti, D. V., & Rourke, B. P. (1995). Validity and neuropsychological characterization of Asperger syndrome. *Journal of Child Psychology and Psychiatry, 36*(7), 1127–1140.

Kling, A. S., & Brothers, L. A. (1992). The amygdala and social behavior. In J. P. Aggelton (Ed.), *The amygdala: Neurobiological aspects of emotion, memory, and mental dysfunction* (pp. 353–377). New York: Wiley-Liss.

Kluver, H., & Bucy, P. C. (1937). "Psychic blindness" and other symptoms following bilateral temporal lobectomy in rhesus monkeys. *American Journal of Physiology, 119,* 352–353.

Kolb, B., & Whishaw, I. Q. (1996). *Fundamentals of human neuropsychology* (4th ed.). New York: Freeman.

Kornack, D. R., & Rakic, P. (1995). Radial and horizontal deployment of clonally related cells in the primate neocortex: Relationship to distinct mitotic lineages. *Neuron, 15,* 311–321.

Kornack, D. R., & Rakic, P. (1998). Changes in cell-cycle kinetics during the development and evolution of primate neocortex. *Proceedings from the National Academy of Science (USA), 95,* 1242–1246.

Lainhart, J. E., Piven, J., Wzorek, M., Landa, R., Santangelo, S. L., Coon, H., & Folstein, S. E. (1997). Macrocephaly in children and adults with autism. *Journal of the American Academy of Child and Adolescent Psychiatry, 36,* 282–290.

Lane, R. D., Fink, G. R., Chau, P. M., & Dolan, R. J. (1997). Neural activation during selective attention to subjective emotional responses. *Neuroreport, 8*(18), 3969–3972.

Lane, R. D., Reiman, E. M., Ahern, G. L., Schwartz, G. E., & Davidson, R. J. (1997). Neuroanatomical correlates of happiness, sadness, and disgust. *American Journal of Psychiatry, 154*(7), 926–933.

Lane, R. D., Reiman, E. M., Bradley, M. M., Lang, P. J., Ahern, G. L., Davidson, R. J., & Schwartz, G. E. (1997). Neuroanatomical correlates of pleasant and unpleasant emotion. *Neuropsychologia, 35*(11), 1437–1444.

LeDoux, J. E. (1996). *The emotional brain: The mysterious underpinnings of emotional life.* New York: Simon & Schuster.

LeDoux, J. E., Cicchetti, P., Xagoraris, A., & Romanski, L. M. (1990). The lateral amygdaloid nucleus: Sensory interface of the amygdala in fear conditioning. *Journal of Neuroscience, 10,* 1062–1069.

LeDoux, J. E., & Farb, C. R. (1991). Neurons of the acoustic thalamus that project to the amygdala contain glutamate. *Neuroscience Letters, 134,* 145–149.

LeDoux, J. E., Sakaguchi, J., & Reis, D. J. (1982). Behaviorally-selective cardiovascular hyperreactivity in spontaneously hypertensive rats: Evidence for hypoemotionality and enhanced appetitive motivation. *Hypertension, 4,* 853–863.

LeDoux, J. E., Sakaguchi, A., & Reis, D. J. (1984). Subcortical efferent projections of the medial geniculate nucleus mediate emotional responses conditioned by acoustic stimuli. *Journal of Neuroscience, 4*(3), 683–698.

Lee, S. J., Schultz, R. T., Win, L., Rambo, J., & Staib, L. H. (1999, May 15–20). *Cerebellum and brainstem in autism spectrum disorders: Comparison of Asperger's syndrome, autism and pervasive developmental disorders NOS.* Poster presented at the 152nd annual meeting of American Psychiatric Association, Washington, DC.

Lincoln, A., Courchesne, E., Allen, M., Hanson, E., & Ene, M. (1998). Neurobiology of Asperger syndrome: Seven case studies and quantitative magnetic resonance imaging findings. In E. Schopler, G. B. Mesibov, & L. J. Kunce (Eds.), *Asperger syndrome or high-functioning autism? Current issues in autism* (pp. 145–163). New York: Plenum.

Macdonald, H., Rutter, M., Howlin, P., Rios, P., Le Couteur, A., Evered, C., & Folstein, S. (1989). Recognition and expression of emotional cues by autistic and normal adults. *Journal of Child Psychology and Psychiatry, 30,* 865–877.

Martin, A., Scahill, L., Klin, A., & Volkmar, F. R. (1999). Higher-functioning pervasive developmental disorders: rates and patterns of psychotropic drug use. *Journal of Child and Adolescent Psychiatry, 38*(7), 923–931.

McCarthy, G., Puce, A., Constable, R. T., Krystal, J. H., Gore, J. C., & Goldman-Rakic, P. (1996). Activation of human prefrontal cortex during spatial and nonspatial working memory tasks measured by functional MRI. *Cerebral Cortex, 6,* 600–611.

McCarthy, G., Puce, A., Gore, J. C., & Allison, T. (1997). Face-specific processing in the human fuisform gyrus. *Journal of Cognitive Neuroscience, 9,* 605–610.

McGee, G. G., Feldman, R. S., & Chernin, L. (1991). A comparison of emotional facial display by children with autism and typical preschoolers. *Journal of Early Intervention, 15,* 237–245.

McKelvey, J. R., Lambert, R., Mottron, L., & Shevell, M. (1995). Right hemisphere dysfunction in Asperger's syndrome. *Journal of Child Neurology, 10*(4), 310–314.

Mesulam, M. M. (1998). From sensation to cognition. *Brain, 121,* 1013–1052.

Minshew, N. J., Goldstein, G., Dombrowski, S. M., Panchalingam, K., & Pettegrew, J. W. (1993). A preliminary 31P MRS study of autism: Evidence for undersynthesis and increased degradation of brain membranes. *Biological Psychiatry, 33,* 762–773.

Molnár, Z., & Blakemore, C. (1995). Guidance of thalamocortical innervation. *Ciba Foundation Symposium: The Development of the Cerebral Cortex, 193,* 127–149.

Morgan, M. A., Romanski, L. M., & LeDoux, J. E. (1993). Extinction of emotional learning: Contribution of medial prefrontal cortex. *Neuroscience Letters, 163,* 109–113.

Morris, J. S., Friston, K. J., & Dolan, R. J. (1997). Neural responses to salient visual stimuli. *Proceedings of the Royal Society of London — Series B: Biological Sciences, 264*(1382), 769–775.

Moscovitch, M., Winocur, G., & Behrmann, M. (1997). What is special about face recognition? Nineteen experiments on a person with visual object agnosia and dyslexia but normal face recognition. *Journal of Cognitive Neuroscience, 9,* 555–604.

Mountz, J. M., Lelland, C. T., Lill, D. W., Katholi, C. R., & Liu, H. (1995). Functional deficits in autistic disorder: Characterization by Technetium-99m-HMPAO and SPECT. *Journal of Nuclear Medicine, 36,* 1156–1162.

Mufson, E. J., Mesulam, M. M., & Pandya, D. N. (1981). Insular interconnections with the amygdala in the rhesus monkey. *Neuroscience, 6,* 1231–1248.

Murakami, J. W., Courchesne, E., Press, G. A., Yeung-Courchesne, R., & Hesselink, J. R. (1989). Reduced cerebellar hemisphere size and its relationship to vermal hypoplasia in autism. *Archives of Neurology, 46,* 689–694.

Newman, J. (1995). Review: Thalamic contributions to attention and consciousness. *Consciousness and Cognition, 4,* 172–193.

Newman, J. D., & Bachevalier, J. (1997). Neonatal ablations of the amygdala and inferior temporal cortex alter the vocal response to social separation in rhesus macaques. *Brain Research, 758*(1–2), 180–186.

Niehoff, D. L., & Kuhar, M. J. (1983). Benzodiazepine receptors: Localization in rat amygdala. *Journal of Neuroscience, 3,* 2091–2097.

O'Leary, D. D., Borngasser, D. J., Fox, K., & Schlagger, B. L. (1995). Plasticity in the development of neocortical areas. *Ciba Foundation Symposium, 193,* 214–230.

Ono, T., Nishijo, H., & Uwano, T. (1995). Amygdala role in associative learning. *Progress in Neurobiology, 46,* 401–422.

Ornitz, E. M. (1985). Neurophysiology of infantile autism. *Journal of the American Academy of Child Psychiatry, 24*(3), 251–262.

Orozco, S., & Ehlers, C. L. (1998). Gender differences in electrophysiological responses to facial stimuli. *Biological Psychiatry, 44,* 281–289.

Ozbayrak, K. R., Kapucu, O., Erdem, E., & Aras, T. (1991). Left occipital hypoperfusion in a case with the Asperger syndrome. *Brain and Development, 13*(6), 454–456.

Ozonoff, S. (1995). Executive functions in autism. In E. Schopler & G. B. Mesibov (Eds.), *Learning and cognition in autism* (pp. 199–219). New York: Plenum.

Ozonoff, S., & McEvoy, R. E. (1994). A longitudinal study of executive function and theory of mind development in autism. *Development and Psychopathology, 6,* 415–431.

Ozonoff, S., Rogers, S. J., & Pennington, B. F. (1991). Asperger's syndrome: Evidence of an empirical distinction from high-functioning autism. *Journal of Child Psychology and Psychiatry, 32,* 1107–1122.

Ozonoff, S., & Strayer, D. L. (1997). Inhibitory function in nonretarded children with autism. *Journal of Autism and Developmental Disorders, 27,* 59–77.

Ozonoff, S., Strayer, D. L., McMahon, W. M., & Filloux F. (1994). Executive function abilities in autism and Tourette syndrome: An information processing approach. *Journal of Child Psychology and Psychiatry and Allied Disciplines, 35*(6), 1015–1032.

Pakkenberg, B., & Gundersen, H. J. (1997). Neocortical neuron number in humans: Effect of sex and age. *Journal of Comparative Neurology, 384,* 312–320.

Parkin, A. J. (1998). The central executive does not exist. *Journal of the International Neuropsychological Society, 4,* 518–522.

Pennington, B. F. (1991). *Diagnosing learning disorders: A neuropsychological framework.* New York: Guilford Press.

Pitkanen, A., & Amaral, D. G. (1991). Demonstration of projections from the lateral nucleus to the basal nucleus of the amygdala: A PHA-L study in the monkey. *Experimental Brain Research, 83,* 465–470.

Pitkanen, A., Savander, V., & LeDoux, J. E. (1997). Organization of intra-amygdaloid circuitries in the rat: An emerging framework for understanding functions of the amygdala. *Trends in Neurosciences, 20,* 517–523.

Piven, J., & Arndt, S. (1995). The cerebellum and autism. *Neurology, 45*(2), 398–402.

Piven, J., Arndt, S., Bailey, J., & Andreasen, N. (1996). Regional brain enlargement in autism: A magnetic resonance imaging study. *Journal of the American Academy of Child and Adolescent Psychiatry, 35*(4), 530–536.

Piven, J., Arndt, S., Bailey, J., Havercamp, S., Andreasen, N., & Palmer, P. (1995). An MRI study of brain size in autism. *American Journal of Psychiatry, 152,* 1145–1149.

Piven, J., Bailey, J., Ranson, B. J., & Arndt, S. (1997). An MRI study of the corpus callosum in autism. *American Journal of Psychiatry, 154*(8), 1051–1056.

Piven, J., Berthier, M. L., Starkstein, S. E., Nehme, E., Pearlson, G., & Folstein, S. (1990). Magnetic resonance imaging in autism: Evidence for a defect of cerebral cortical development in autism. *American Journal of Psychiatry, 147,* 734–739.

Piven, J., Nehme, E., Simon, J., Barta, P., Pearlson, G., & Folstein, S. E. (1992). Magnetic resonance imaging in autism: Measurement of the cerebellum, pons, and fourth ventricle. *Biological Psychiatry, 31,* 491–504.

Price, J. L., Carmichael, S. T., & Drevets, W. C. (1996). Networks related to the orbital and medial prefrontal cortex; a substrate for emotional behavior? *Progress in Brain Research, 107,* 523–536.

Puce, A., Allison, T., Bentin, S., Gore, J. C., & McCarthy, G. (1998). Temporal cortex activation in humans viewing eye and mouth movements. *Journal of Neuroscience, 18*(6), 2188–2199.

Quirk, G. J., Repa, C., & LeDoux, J. E. (1995). Fear conditioning enhances short-latency auditory responses of lateral amygdala neurons: Parallel recordings in the freely behaving rat. *Neuron, 15,* 1029–1039.

Rabinowicz, T., de Courten-Myers, G. M., Petetot, J. M., Xi, G., & de los Reyes, E. (1996).

Human cortex development: Estimates of neuronal numbers indicate major loss late during gestation. *Journal of Neuropathology and Experimental Neurology, 55*(3), 320–328.

Rakic, P. (1988). Specification of cerebral cortical areas. *Science, 241,* 170–176.

Rakic, P. (1995). A small step for the cell, a giant leap for mankind: A hypothesis of the neocortical expansion during evolution. *Trends in Neurosciences, 18,* 383–388.

Reiman, E. M., Lane, R. D., Ahern, G. L., Schwartz, G. E., Davidson, R. J., Friston, K. J., Yun, L. S., & Chen, K. (1997). Neuroanatomical correlates of externally and internally generated human emotion. *American Journal of Psychiatry, 154*(7), 918–925.

Ringo, J. L. (1991). Neuronal interconnection as a function of brain size. *Brain, Behavior, and Evolution, 38,* 1–6.

Ritvo, E. R., & Garber, J. H. (1988). Cerebellar hypoplasia and autism. *New England Journal of Medicine, 319,* 1152.

Robinson, D. L. (1993). Functional contributions of the primate pulvinar. *Progress in Brain Research, 95,* 371–380.

Rogers, S., & Pennington, B. F. (1991). A theoretical approach to the deficits in infantile autism. *Developmental Psychopathology, 3,* 137–162.

Rolls, E. T. (1995). A theory of emotion and consciousness, and its application to understanding the neural basis of emotion. In M. S. Gazzaniga (Ed.), *The cognitive neurosciences* (pp. 1091–1106). Cambridge, MA: MIT Press.

Romanski, L. M., Clugnet, M. C., Bordi, F., & LeDoux, J. E. (1993). Somatosensory and auditory convergence in the lateral nucleus of the amygdala. *Behavioral Neuroscience, 107,* 444–450.

Romanski, L. M., & LeDoux, J. E. (1992a). Equipotentiality of thalamo–amygdala and thalamo–cortico–amygdala circuits in auditory fear conditioning. *Journal of Neuroscience, 12,* 4501–4509.

Romanski, L. M., & LeDoux, J. E. (1992b). Bilateral destruction of neocortical and perirhinal projection targets of the acoustic thalamus does not disrupt auditory fear conditioning. *Neuroscience Letters, 142,* 228–232.

Romanski, L. M., & LeDoux, J. E. (1993). Information cascade from primary auditory cortex to the amygdala: Corticocortical and corticoamygdaloid projections of temporal cortex in the rat. *Cerebral Cortex, 3,* 515–532.

Rourke, B. P. (1989). *Nonverbal Learning Disabilities: The syndrome and the model.* New York: Guilford Press.

Rumsey, J. M. (1985). Conceptual problem-solving in highly verbal, nonretarded autistic men. *Journal of Autism and Developmental Disorders, 15,* 23–36.

Rumsey, J. M., & Hamburger, S. D. (1990). Neuropsychological divergence of high-level autism and severe dyslexia. *Journal of Autism and Developmental Disorders, 20,* 155–168.

Sarazin, M., Pillon, B., Giannakopoulos, P., Rancurel, G., Samson, Y., & Dubois, B. (1998). Clinicometabolic dissociation of cognitive functions and social behavior in frontal lobe lesions. *Neurology, 51,* 142–148.

Saunders, R. C., Kolachana, B. S., Bachevalier, J., & Weinberger, D. R. (1998). Neonatal lesions of the medial temporal lobe disrupt prefrontal cortical regulation of striatal dopamine. *Nature, 393,* 169–171.

Schifter, T., Hoffman, J. M., Hatten, H. P., Jr., Hanson, M. W., Coleman, R. E., & DeLong, G. R. (1994). Neuroimaging in infantile autism. *Journal of Child Neurology, 9*(2), 155–161.

Schultz, R. T. (1998, May 26–30). *Neuroimaging studies in autism.* Abstracts of the annual meeting of Biological Psychiatry, Toronto, Canada.

Schultz, R. T. (1999, June 17–19). *Perception of faces and facial expressions in autism spectrum disorders: fMRI studies.* Paper presented at the annual TENNET meeting of Theoretical and Experimental Neuropsychology, Montreal, Canada.

Schultz, R. T., Cho, N. K., Staib, L. H., Kier, L. E., Fletcher, J. M., Shaywitz, S. E., Shankweiler, D. P., Katz, L., Gore, J. C., Duncan, J. S., & Shaywitz, B. (1994). Brain morphology in normal and dyslexic children: The influence of sex and age. *Annals of Neurology, 35,* 732–742.

Schultz, R. T., Gauthier, I., Fulbright, R., Anderson, A. W., Lacadie, C., Skudlarski, P., Tarr, M. J., Cohen, D. J., & Gore, J. C. (1997, May 17–22). *Are face identity and emotion processed automatically?* Abstracts of the Third International Conference on Functional Mapping of the Human Brain Mapping, Coppenhagen, Denmark.

Schultz, R. T., Gauthier, I., Klin, A., Fulbright, R., Anderson, A., Volkmar, F., Skudlarski, P., Lacadie, C., Cohen, D. J., & Gore, J. C. (in press). Abnormal ventral temporal cortical activity among individuals with autism and Asperger syndrome during face discrimination. *Archives of General Psychology.*

Schultz, R. T., Klin, A., van der Gaag, C., Skudlarski, P., Herrington, J., & Gore, J. C. (19xx). *Medial prefrontal involvement in the process of social attribution: An fMRI study.* Manuscript submitted for publication.

Schultz, R. T., Lee, S. J., Klin, A., Win, L., Rambo, J., Volkmar, F., & Staib, L. H. (1999). *Cerebellum and brainstem in autism spectrum disorders: Comparison of Asperger's syndrome, autism and pervasive developmental disorders NOS.* Manuscript submitted for publication.

Sergent, J., Ohta, S., & Macdonald, B. (1992). Functional neuroanatomy of face and object processing. *Brain, 115,* 15–36.

Shah, A., & Frith, U. (1993). Why do autistic individuals show superior performance on the block design task? *Journal of Child Psychology and Psychiatry and Allied Disciplines, 34(8),* 1351–1364.

Singer, W. (1993). Synchronization of cortical activity and its putative role in information processing and learning. *Annual Review of Physiology, 55,* 349–374.

Snow, M. E., Hertzig, M. E., & Shapiro, T. (1987). Expression of emotion in young autistic children. *Journal of the American Academy of Child and Adolescent Psychiatry, 26,* 836–838.

Steg, J. P., & Rapoport, J. L. (1975). Minor physical anomalies in normal, neurotic, learning disabled, and severely disturbed children. *Journal of Autism and Childhood Schizophrenia, 5,* 299–307.

Steriade, M., McCormick, D. A., & Sejnowski, T. J. (1993). Thalamocortical oscillations in the sleeping and aroused brain. *Science, 262,* 679–685.

Stone, V. E., Baron-Cohen, S., & Knight, R. T. (1998). Frontal lobe contributions to theory of mind. *Journal of Cognitive Neuroscience, 10(5),* 640–656.

Stuss, D. T., & Benson, D. (1986). *The frontal lobes.* New York: Raven Press.

Szatmari, P., Tuff, L., Finlayson, M. A. J., & Bartolucci, G. (1990). Asperger's syndrome and autism: Neurocognitive aspects. *Journal of the American Academy of Child and Adolescent Psychiatry, 29,* 130–136.

Tanaka, J. W., & Farah, M. J. (1993). Parts and wholes in face recognition. *Quarterly Journal of Experimental Psychology, 46A,* 225–245.

Tantam, D., Monaghan, L., Nicholson, H., & Stirling, J. (1989). Autistic children's ability to interpret faces: A research note. *Journal of Child Psychology and Psychiatry, 30,* 623–630.

Thompson, C. I. (1981). Long-term behavioral development of rhesus monkeys after amygdalectomy in infancy. In Y. Ben-Ari (Ed.), *The amygdaloid complex. INSERM Symposium No. 20* (pp. 259–270). Amsterdam: Elsevier.

Tovee, M. J. (1995). Face recognition. What are faces for? *Current Biology, 5*(5), 480–482.

Turner, B. H., Mishkin, M., & Knapp, M. (1980). Organization of the amygdalopetal projections from modality-specific cortical association areas in the monkey. *Journal of Comparative Neurology, 191*, 515–543.

Valentine, T. (1988). Upside-down faces: A review of the effect of inversion upon face recognition. *British Journal of Psychology, 79*, 471–491.

Voeller, K. K. S. (1986). Right-hemisphere deficit syndrome in children. *American Journal of Psychiatry, 143*, 1004–1009.

Volkmar, F. R., Klin, A., & Pauls, D. (1998). Nosological and genetic aspects of Asperger syndrome. *Journal of Autism and Developmental Disorders, 28*(5), 457–463.

Volkmar, F. R., Klin, A., Schultz, R. T., Bronen, R., Marans, W., Sparrow, S., & Cohen, D. J. (1996). Grand rounds: Asperger's syndrome. *Journal of the American Academy of Child and Adolescent Psychiatry, 35*, 118–123.

Volkmar, F. R., Szatmari, P., & Sparrow, S. S. (1993). Sex differences in pervasive developmental disorders *Journal of Autism and Developmental Disorders, 23*, 579–591.

Walker, H. A. (1977). Incidence of minor physical anomaly in autism. *Journal of Autism and Child Schizophrenia, 7*, 165–176.

Weeks, S. J., & Hobson, R. P. (1987). The salience of facial expression for autistic children. *Journal of Child Psychology and Psychiatry, 28*, 137–151.

Weintraub, S., & Mesulam, M. M. (1983). Developmental learning disabilities of the right hemisphere: Emotional, interpersonal, and cognitive components. *Archives of Neurology, 40*(8), 463–468.

Willerman, L., Schultz, R., Rutledge, N., & Bigler, E. (1991). In vivo brain size and intelligence. *Intelligence, 15*, 223–228.

Wing, L. (1981). Asperger's syndrome: A clinical account. *Psychological Medicine, 11*, 115–130.

Woodhouse, W., Bailey, A., Rutter, M., Bolton, P., Bard, G., & Le Couteur, A. (1996). Head circumference and other pervasive developmental disorders. *Journal of Child Psychology and Psychiatry and Allied Disciplines, 37*, 665–671.

World Health Organization. (1993). *International classification of diseases: Tenth revision.* Chapter V. Mental and behavioral disorders (including disorders of psychological development). Diagnostic criteria for research. Geneva: Author.

Yirmiya, N., Kasari, C., Sigman, M. D., & Mundy, P. (1989). Facial expressions of affect in autistic, mentally retarded, and normal children. *Journal of Child Psychology and Psychiatry, 30*, 725–735.

Yirmiya, N., Sigman, M. D., Kasari, C., & Mundy, P. (1992). Empathy and cognition in high-functioning children with autism. *Child Development, 63*, 150–160.

Zeng, X., Staib, L., Schultz, R. T., & Duncan, J. (in press). Segmentation and measurement of the cortex from 3D MR images using coupled surfaces propagation. *IEEE Transactions on Medical Imaging.*

Zilbovicius, M., Garreau, B., Samson, Y., Remy, P., Barthelemy, C., Syrota, A., & Lelord, G. (1995). Delayed maturation of the frontal cortex in childhood autism. *American Journal of Psychiatry, 152*, 248–252.

7

Psychopharmacological Treatment of Higher-Functioning Pervasive Developmental Disorders

ANDRÉS MARTIN
DAVID K. PATZER
FRED R. VOLKMAR

This chapter examines the role of psychopharmacology in the treatment of individuals with higher-functioning pervasive developmental disorders (HFPDDs), including Asperger syndrome (AS) and other pervasive developmental disorders (PDDs) not accompanied by mental retardation. To that effect, it first reviews the small available literature on the topic, pointing out some methodological and ascertainment limitations. Second, it describes a recently conducted naturalistic study on the psychotropic medication use patterns in a sample of over 100 subjects with AS and related conditions, highlighting the schism between available research and usual standards of clinical practice. Finally, the chapter sets forth recommendations for future research directions. In particular, it underscores the role for consortium-wide collaborative efforts for the field, as specifically exemplified in the recently National Institute of Mental Health (NIMH)-funded Research Units in Pediatric Psychopharmacology (RUPPs) focused on the study of autism and related conditions.

BACKGROUND

Although educational and behavioral interventions are generally the mainstay for the management of individuals with PDDs, psychotropic medications can be an important component of an individually tailored treatment plan (McDougle, 1997). A wide range of psychotropic agents has been used in the treatment of the PDDs, and a growing body of literature has described the short-term efficacy of medications generally acting through serotonin and dopamine neural pathways in the treatment of children, adolescents, and adults with these disorders (for reviews, see Cook & Leventhal, 1995; McDougle, 1997). Medications have usually been directed at symptoms of aggression, impulsivity, stereotypies, or self-injurious behaviors. Given such target symptoms, it is not surprising that most subjects with PDDs involved in pharmacological studies have been severely impaired and generally functioning in the mentally retarded range. By contrast, the higher-functioning and overall less severely affected individuals with PDDs have routinely been excluded from pharmacological studies. In this way, HFPDDs in general, and AS in particular, have become "orphan disorders" within psychopharmacology research. Given that 15–20% of individuals with autism have IQs above the mental retardation cutoff range (Schopler & Mesibov, 1992), and that the proportion of individuals with nonautistic PDDs with normative IQs is larger still, it is apparent that a sizable portion of the PDD population has not routinely been included in psychopharmacological studies, thus failing to benefit from research efforts in this area. This situation is regrettable inasmuch as symptoms of anxiety and depression, while not being at the core of the social disability paradigmatic of these disorders, are often quite debilitating and can be some of the most amenable to intervention with psychotropic agents.

Despite the increasingly common resort to pharmacotherapy in the clinical management of individuals with AS and related conditions, there is a paucity of empirical data on which to support such practice. In fact, a computerized search of the literature for clinical trials, drug surveys, psychotropic medication prevalence, or patterns of medication use specifically conducted for subjects with AS or higher-functioning autism (HFA) found no scientific reports other than a few letters to the editor (Szabo & Bracken, 1994; Damore, Stein, & Brody, 1998), or small, open-label trials in autism that included some subjects diagnosed with AS (Brodkin, McDougle, Naylor, Cohen, & Price, 1997; McDougle et al., 1998; McDougle, Holmes, et al., 1997; McDougle et al., 1998). What scant information is available has generally been incorporated from studies of subjects with autism, or from pharmacological trials in conditions (such as obsessive–compulsive disorder) that have symptomatic similarities—and perhaps phenomenological continuity, or clinical comorbidity—with AS.

For example, phenomenological similarities and differences in repetitive thoughts and actions between adults with obsessive–compulsive disorder and autistic disorder have been described by McDougle, Kresch, et al. (1995). Discriminant function analysis of Yale–Brown Obsessive Compulsive Scale Symptom checklist variables indicated that adults with autistic disorder and obsessive–compulsive disorder can be distinguished on the basis of their repetitive thoughts and actions. Two obsession variables (aggression and symmetry) and five compulsion variables (checking; counting; hoarding; need to touch, tap, or rub; and self-damaging or self-mutilating behaviors) served to maximally separate the two groups. Such studies have partly supported the rationale behind the use of antiobsessional agents in the treatment of the PDDs (as reviewed in McDougle, 1998).

Given the general lack of controlled clinical trials or empirical data available, large-scale community sampling studies have sought to document the prevalence and patterns of medication use in the PDD population. In the largest survey to date specifically involving subjects with autism (Aman, Van Bourgondien, Wolford, & Sarphare, 1995), 838 care providers reported that 30.5% of affected subjects were taking one or more psychotropic medications. Nearly 80% of the subjects included in that survey had some degree of mental retardation. When counting the use of anticonvulsants for seizure control (and not for mood regulation), the proportion of medicated subjects rose to 50%. Neuroleptics were the most frequently used psychotropic medications (used in 12% of subjects), and second only to the anticonvulsants (in 13.2%). Increasing age and housing away from family were associated with greater drug use. Moderate to profound mental retardation was associated with neuroleptic and anticonvulsant use, the latter reflecting the higher incidence of seizure disorders among the more cognitively impaired individuals with autism (Volkmar & Nelson, 1990).

Two surveys from our group have found widespread use of psychotropic medications in separate samples of more than 100 individuals who were awaiting screening and evaluation for AS. In the first survey, over 75% of subjects had received stimulants at some point in their lives; over one-third had received selective serotonin reuptake inhibitors (SSRIs), and fewer than 10 had received neuroleptics (Klin & Volkmar, 1997). Overall, lifetime psychotropic drug use was common, with agents often used in combinations and not necessarily following a clearly articulated rationale. Results from the second survey (Martin, Scahill, Klin, & Volkmar, 1999) are discussed in more detail later in the chapter.

MEDICATION USE PATTERNS

We recently completed a naturalistic study designed to (1) document the rate and characteristics of psychotropic drug use among a representative sample of individuals with HFPDDs, (2) evaluate the demographic and clinical correlates associated with the use of psychotropic drugs in this population, and (3) identify target symptom clusters and possible prescription patterns associated with psychotropic drug use in this clinical sample.

The subjects selected were drawn from a pool of 125 children, adolescents, and adults consecutively seeking enrollment during a 6-month period (July–December, 1997) in the Yale Child Study Center's Project on Social Learning Disabilities that has been described elsewhere (Klin, Volkmar, Schultz, Pauls, & Cohen, 1997). Most subjects referred had been previously diagnosed with autism, AS, or pervasive developmental disorder not otherwise specified (PDD-NOS). The project includes phenomenological, neuropsychological, neuroimaging, genetic, and psychopharmacological studies of individuals with autism and related conditions.

Three subjects with a Full Scale IQ of 69 or lower were excluded from analysis. An additional 13 subjects were excluded because they were not previously diagnosed with a HFPDD (defined as AS, autism, or PDD-NOS in the context of a Full Scale IQ ≥ 70). In this group of 13 excluded subjects, previous diagnoses had included obsessive–compulsive disorder ($n = 3$), learning disabilities + social–emotional problems ($n = 3$), no clear diagnosis ($n = 3$), and depression, sensory integration problems, schizophrenia, learning disabilities + attention-deficit/hyperactivity disorder (ADHD), and bipolar illness, each in one case. The resulting study sample consisted of 109 subjects.

Survey questionnaires were mailed to subjects' families. Data collected included (1) demographic information such as age, gender, ethnicity, living arrangements, and educational level of both parents; (2) clinical information, including reports of previous assessments, as well as developmental, behavioral, and educational inventories, such as the Autism Behavior Checklist (ABC; Krug, Arick, & Almond, 1980); and (3) a medication survey that elicited all current psychotropic medications taken regularly, the target symptoms they were intended to treat, what practitioner had prescribed the medication, and the dose and duration of treatment. In addition, similar information was elicited about past psychotropic drug use.

Subjects were referred from 26 states across the United States and one province in Canada. The mean age of the sample was 13.9 years ($SD = 6.9$; range = 4 to 43): 20 subjects (18.3%) were children up to 9 years of age, 28 (25.7%) were preadolescents between 9 and 12 years old, 40 (36.7%) were adolescents 12 to 16 years of age, and 21 (19.3%) were adolescents and adults, 16 years or older. There were 90 males (82.6%) and 19 females (17.4%). Most subjects were Caucasian (104, 95.4%) and lived with their families of origin (88, 80.7%). Three subjects (2.7%) were African American, 2 were Hispanic (1.8%), 5 (4.8%) were adopted, and 21 (19.3%) lived in residential or sheltered living arrangements.

Subjects had received a variety of diagnoses during prior evaluations, including AS in 94 subjects (86.2%), autism in 32 (29.4%), and PDD-NOS in 14 (12.9%). 37 subjects (39.4%) had simultaneously received diagnoses of AS *and* either HFA *or* PDD-NOS. Based on the ABC, 46 subjects (42.2%) were considered *unlikely* to have autism, 20 (18.3%) were considered *questionably* autistic, and 43 (39.4%) *probably* autistic. Intellectual functioning had been previously assessed in all respondents and was distributed in the following ranges: *gifted* (Full Scale IQ > 130), 23 (21.1%); *high average* (Full Scale IQ 115–129), 19 (17.4%); *average* (Full Scale IQ 86–114), 55 (50.5%); and *low average* (Full Scale IQ 70–85), 12 (11%).

Of the 109 respondents, 21 subjects (19.3%) had completed our full diagnostic and neuropsychological protocol at the time of this writing. Of 15 subjects within this group referred with a previous diagnosis of AS, 10 received a project diagnosis of AS, 2 of autism, and 3 of PDD-NOS. Of the remaining 6 subjects referred with other HFPDD diagnoses, 5 were diagnosed with autism and 1 with PDD-NOS. Results from this study are reported elsewhere.

Table 7.1 lists the number and percentage among respondents reporting psychotropic medication use. The figures listed in the table do not necessarily sum to 100% because some subjects were simultaneously taking more than one agent. The most frequently prescribed medications were antidepressants (32.1%), stimulants (20.2%), and neuroleptics (16.5%). Valproate and carbamazepine were included as mood stabilizers when not primarily used to treat a seizure disorder. Beta-blockers and alpha-2 agonists were included among the antihypertensives. Overall, 60 subjects (55%) were taking

TABLE 7.1. Subjects Taking Psychotropic Medications on Date of Survey

Drug type	No.	%
Any antidepressant	35	32.1
SSRI	29	26.6
Stimulant	22	20.2
Any neuroleptic	18	16.5
Atypical neuroleptic	14	12.8
Mood stabilizer	10	9.2
Anxiolytic	7	6.4
Antihypertensive	7	6.4
Tricyclic antidepressant	7	6.4
Traditional neuroleptic	5	4.6
Any psychotropic (current)	60	55.0
One drug	28	25.7
Two drugs	25	22.9
Three drugs	5	4.6
Four drugs	2	1.8
Any psychotropic (lifetime)	75	68.8

Note. n = 109. From Martin, Scahill, Klin, and Volkmar (1999). Copyright 1999 by Lippincott Williams & Wilkins. Reprinted by permission.

psychotropic medications. Among these, 32 (53.3%) were taking two or more drugs simultaneously. The most common medication combination was an atypical neuroleptic with an SSRI ($n = 9$). Nineteen subjects not currently taking psychotropic medications had done so at some past point in time, raising the total number of subjects with *lifetime* use of psychotropics to 75 (68.8% of the total sample).

The most common drugs within each class were as follows: (1) SSRIs: fluoxetine ($n = 17$), sertraline ($n = 6$), and fluvoxamine ($n = 6$); (2) stimulants: methylphenidate ($n = 17$), and dextroamphetamine ($n = 5$); (3) atypical neuroleptics: risperidone ($n = 12$), and olanzapine ($n = 2$); (4) mood stabilizers: valproate ($n = 7$), lithium ($n = 2$), and carbamazepine ($n = 1$); (5) anxiolytics: buspirone ($n = 4$), and clonazepam ($n = 3$); (6) antihypertensives: clonidine ($n = 5$), and propranolol ($n = 2$); (7) tricyclic antidepressants: imipramine ($n = 4$), and nortriptyline ($n = 3$); and (8) traditional neuroleptics: thioridazine ($n = 3$), and haloperidol ($n = 2$).

Medications had been prescribed by general psychiatrists in 35/60 (58.3%) of subjects, by child psychiatrists in 26.7%, by pediatric neurologists in 15%, and by neurologists or pediatricians in 3 subjects (5%) each. There were no differences in prescription patterns by specialty. Table 7.2 lists the number and percentage of target symptom clusters endorsed among subjects taking psychotropic medications ($n = 60$). The figures listed in the table do not necessarily sum to 100% because subjects commonly endorsed more than one target symptom cluster.

The use of each medication class was compared across gender, age range, IQ, and associated target symptoms. Considering the substantial overlap in clinical diagnoses given to subjects, an analysis of medication type by diagnosis could not be meaningfully conducted. No significant dif-

TABLE 7.2. Target Symptoms Identified among Subjects Taking Psychotropic Medications on Date of Survey

Target symptom	No.	%
Any anxiety symptom	39	65.0
Inattention/distractibility/hyperactivity	50.0	30
Generalized anxiety	27	45.0
Disruptive/violent/self-injurious behaviors	26	43.3
Obsessions–compulsions/repetitive behaviors	24	40.0
Depression	19	31.7
Social–relational difficulties	17	28.3
Delusions/hallucinations	11	18.3
Sleep problems	8	0.13
Tics	3	0.05
Seizures	1	0.02

Note. $n = 60$. From Martin, Scahill, Klin, and Volkmar (1999). Copyright 1999 by Lippincott Williams & Wilkins. Reprinted by permission.

ferences were evident when comparing medication or target symptom patterns between the 21 subjects with a finalized project diagnosis (AS = 15, autism = 5, PDD-NOS = 1). In another effort to assess medication type by diagnostic category, comparisons were made among groups defined by ABC scores. Table 7.3 summarizes significant findings in the comparison of drug classes by target symptom clusters, demographic characteristics, and diagnostic ratings.

TABLE 7.3. Percentage of Medication Use for Related Demographic and Clinical Variables

Agent variables	Level 1	Level 2	Level 3	Level 4
Any medication				
Age range[a]	25.0	42.9	60.0	90.5
SSRIs				
Age range[a]	0.0	17.2	34.5	48.3
Depression[b]	34.1	78.9	—	—
OC symptoms[b]	33.3	70.8	—	—
Anxiety[b]	23.8	61.5	—	—
Inattention[b]	63.3	33.3	—	—
Gender[c]	40.8	81.8	—	—
Stimulants				
Inattention[b]	2.5	66.7	—	—
Atypical neuroleptics				
SIB[b]	4.8	38.5	—	—
Age range[a]	10.0	7.1	7.5	33.3
OC Symptoms[b]	5.9	37.5	—	—
Antihypertensives				
ABC[d]	0.0	5.0	14.0	—
Anxiety[b]	21.2	0.0	—	—
TCAs				
Anxiety[b]	1.4	15.4	—	—
Anxiolytics				
Age range[a]	0.0	3.6	0.0	28.6
Mood stabilizers				
Age range[a]	5.0	0.0	10.0	23.8

Note. All figures are percentages for the respective levels of the variable concerned. The variable levels were as follows: [a]0–9 years, 9–12 years, 12–16 years, 16+ years; [b]target symptom cluster absent, present; [c]male, female; [d]Autism Behavior Checklist: "unlikely autistic," "questionably autistic," "probably autistic." SSRIs, selective serotonin reuptake inhibitors; SIB, self-injurious behavior; OC, obsessive–compulsive; ABC, Autism Behavior Checklist; TCAs, tricyclic antidepressants. From Martin, Scahill, Klin, and Volkmar (1999). Copyright 1999 by Lippincott Williams & Wilkins. Reprinted by permission.

IMPLICATIONS FOR CLINICAL ASSESSMENT AND PHARMACOLOGICAL TREATMENT

Medication Prevalence and Patterns of Medication Use

Apart from the preliminary findings previously reported by members of our group (Klin & Volkmar, 1997), ours is, to the best of our knowledge, the first survey to address the prevalence and patterns of psychotropic medication use among subjects with AS and HFA. With over half of our subject sample taking psychotropic medications at the time of survey, it is clear that individuals diagnosed with HFPDDs are overall a heavily medicated clinical population. Nearly 70% of subjects had received psychotropics at some point in their lives, and over half of those currently on medication took two or more agents simultaneously. By way of comparison, in the large-scale survey of subjects with autism (Aman, Singh, Stewart, & Field, 1995), a more modest 30.5% of subjects were taking psychotropic drugs. Considering that there have been *no* psychotropic medication studies specifically designed for individuals with HFPDDs, these elevated rates are all the more significant and indicate the need for further psychopharmacological investigation of this subject population.

In terms of specific agents, SSRIs were the most widely used medications. This finding is in keeping with extensive research on serotonin pathway dysregulation in autism (for review, see Potenza & McDougle, 1997), and particularly of the serotonin transporter as a candidate gene for the disorder (Cook et al., 1997). SSRIs have been investigated in the treatment of autism, starting with clomipramine (Gordon, State, Nelson, Hamburger, & Rapoport, 1993; McDougle et al., 1992; Sanchez et al., 1996), and more recently by open studies with fluoxetine (Cook, Rowlett, Jaselskis, & Leventhal, 1992), sertraline (McDougle et al., 1998), and fluvoxamine (McDougle et al., 1996). These agents have been found beneficial in most studies, and generally through their effects on repetitive or compulsive behaviors (McDougle, 1998), although their direct antidepressant and anxiolytic effects may also be quite relevant.

Lest these encouraging findings be prematurely generalized to the HFPDD population (as the high rates of SSRI use in this study would suggest), a caveat warrants mention. The encouraging results with fluvoxamine have not been replicated in the treatment of children with PDDs (McDougle, personal communication, 1998), and adults with AS did not respond to open-label sertraline, as had those with autism (McDougle et al., 1998). Together with the fact that fluvoxamine and sertraline have both been found effective in the treatment of children and adolescents with obsessive–compulsive disorder, these findings point to potential age- and disorder-specific differences that give generalizations limited clinical utility. Finally, it is worth noting that over the last decade there has been an overall exponential increase in the prescription of SSRIs, particularly for individuals under 18 years of age (Olfson et al., 1998). The high rates of SSRI use in our study population may thus reflect this broader change in prescription practices. These changes are in turn likely related to the limited side effects and perceived "benign" nature associated with the SSRIs, leading to a lower threshold to prescribe, despite a lack of long-term safety data, especially for children.

The stimulants were the second most frequently prescribed medication class in our sample. This finding is in contrast to general clinical lore and older literature suggesting that the stimulants are of limited use in the PDDs, and that they may contribute to the exacerbation of stereotypies and irritability, particularly in "classically" autistic children. Although other reports (Birmaher, Quintana, & Greenhill, 1988) have revisited the role of the stimulants in the treatment of autism, there has to date been no controlled study to more definitively resolve the controversy. Although there were no age-related differences in the use of stimulants in our sample, higher rates among younger children have been previously reported by our group (Klin & Volkmar, 1997). Such a pattern of stimulant use may reflect the fact that initial complaints concerning individuals with these conditions usually have to do with difficulties in effectively participating in classroom activities, problems that for the majority of children are conceptualized as attentional in nature. Individuals with higher-functioning social disabilities, given that their social and communicative dysfunctions are less obvious, are often first diagnosed with ADHD. Alternatively, ADHD may be a discrete comorbid condition.

The atypical neuroleptics were the third most commonly used medication class. Their association with disruptive, aggressive, and self-injurious behaviors is consistent with the growing literature on the use of atypical neuroleptics in the treatment of these symptom clusters in autism (McDougle, 1997). It was surprising to find that such symptoms were endorsed in 40% of our high-functioning survey respondents taking medications. The fact that there was no association between ABC scores and atypical neuroleptic use suggests that "autistic-like behaviors" (which include aggression and self-injury) were not the only or main target symptom for the use of these agents. Given that in 9 of 14 instances these medications were used in combination with SSRIs, and that their use was significantly associated with obsessive–compulsive target symptoms, it is likely that they may be used in this population as treatment for obsessive–compulsive disorder or for obsessive–compulsive features. This use would be consistent with the practice of augmenting SSRIs with atypical neuroleptics in the management of treatment-refractory obsessive–compulsive disorder (McDougle, Fleischmann, et al., 1995). Our study had a preponderance of atypical neuroleptic use, in distinct contrast to the quoted medication survey in subjects with autism (Aman et al., 1995), where *all* subjects on neuroleptics were taking traditional agents. This prescription shift in the short interval between both studies points to clinicians' predilection for the newer agents. The preference may be based on the more benign perception of the atypical agents (e.g., lower incidence of tardive dyskinesia), as well as on the pharmacological properties of the medications themselves (i.e., effects on both serotonin and dopamine pathways).

The remaining medication classes were reported among few enough subjects (< 10), that interpretation of their use need be especially cautious and tentative, even when found to be statistically significant. The mood stabilizers, for example, were used in 10 respondents, but there was no observed association with a particular target symptom cluster, suggesting that their use may be nonspecific.

Target Symptoms, Clinical Heterogeneity, and Patterns of Comorbidity

Although most of the pharmacological literature on autism has focused on target symptoms of aggression, irritability, or self-injurious behavior, or of repetitive and stereotyped behaviors, our findings suggest that other target symptoms may also be operative among individuals with HFPDDs. The clinical heterogeneity of our sample was remarkable, with many symptoms unrelated to diagnostic criteria and not generally associated with the PDDs leading to pharmacological intervention. Symptoms of anxiety were especially common, and endorsed in over half of the subjects in our sample. The present study was not specifically designed to address the comorbidity of AS and HFA, or even to do a comprehensive analysis of all clinically relevant symptoms, but rather to identify potentially medication-sensitive target symptoms associated with the use of psychotropics.

Most studies of comorbidity in AS have been based on case reports or cases series (Gillberg & Ehlers, 1998). The observation of high rates of affective disorder in AS is of interest in light of the finding of neuropsychological profiles convergent with the Nonverbal Learning Disabilities (NLD) syndrome (Klin, Volkmar, Sparrow, Cicchetti, & Rourke, 1995), as individuals with NLD appear to be at markedly increased risk for depression and suicidality (Rourke, Young, & Leenaars, 1989). Preliminary data on a sample of 99 individuals with AS (Klin & Volkmar, 1997) suggested that frequently associated conditions included ADHD (28% of cases), obsessive–compulsive disorder (19%), and depression (15%). In that case series the importance of developmental and maturational changes was noted, as ADHD was more apparent in younger children, whereas mood disorders were more frequent in older individuals.

Given the absence of drugs which clearly and specifically target the social deficit of AS, it is not surprising that most of the available literature on drug treatments has focused on associated conditions which may be more amenable to pharmacological interventions. However, two major factors limit our knowledge in the area. First, there are significant issues relative to comorbid diagnoses, namely, whether they are truly independent disorders or just one aspect of AS. Second, most available information is based on case reports or, less frequently, on case series. In addition, the psychopharmacology literature in the PDDs has been plagued by diagnostic ambiguity and a lack in the use of standardized diagnostic instruments such as the Autism Diagnostic Observation Schedule (Lord et al., 1989) and the Autism Diagnostic Inventory—Revised (Lord, Rutter, & Le Couteur, 1994). Such ambiguity has been particularly keen in the study of the HFPDDs, where ongoing controversies in taxonomy persist, and where different investigators may at times not coincide in assigning diagnostic labels. In the absence of controlled drug studies, it remains unclear to what extent results may be replicated in more rigorous double-blind and placebo-controlled studies. However, even with all these caveats, it is clear that many individuals with AS are treated with psychotropic medications both before and after the diagnosis of AS is made.

Early interest in AS was based, in part, on the impression that the condition might be associated with psychosis in general or with schizophrenia in particular (Clarke, Littlejohns, Corbett, & Joseph, 1989; Tantam, 1988a; Tantam, 1988b; Taiminen, 1994). In this regard, it appeared that AS might be a "bridge" between autism and schizophrenia (see Wolff, 1995). Several reports have noted potential comorbidity with other psychotic conditions, including major depression and bipolar disorder (Berthier, 1995; Fujikawa, Kobayashi, Koga, & Murata, 1987; Gillberg, 1985). Definitive information on the frequency of psychosis in individuals with AS is generally lacking. At least two case series (Tantam, 1991; Nagy & Szatmari, 1986) have reported such cases as well. And yet, the tendency of patients with AS to verbalize their thoughts may lead to an overready, and inappropriate, attribution of thought disorder or schizophrenia. Bejerot and Duvner (1995) and Taiminen (1994) have noted the difficulties in differential diagnosis of AS and schizophrenia. Consistent with this view, Ghaziuddin, Leininger, and Tsai (1995) reported no differences between patients with HFA and AS in overall levels of thought disorder. There is some evidence that individuals with schizoid personality disorder may be at increased risk for early-onset schizophrenia (Werry, 1992), although the issue of the extent to which schizoid personality disorder overlaps with AS is problematic. As was true for autism (Rutter, 1972), it is possible that schizophrenia is no more common than would be expected based on chance alone (see Volkmar & Cohen, 1991). There is also the suggestion (Ryan, 1992) that AS may be misdiagnosed as chronic, treatment-resistant mental illness.

Other reports have suggested associations of AS with other conditions, including Tourette syndrome (Kerbeshian & Burd, 1986; Littlejohns, Clarke, & Corbett, 1990), obsessive–compulsive disorder (Thomsen, 1994), and affective disorders (Berthier, 1995; Fujikawa et al., 1987; Gillberg, 1985; Ellis, Ellis, Fraser, & Deb, 1994).

FUTURE GUIDELINES FOR PSYCHOPHARMACOLOGICAL TREATMENT AND DIRECTIONS FOR FUTURE RESEARCH

In summary, the use of psychotropic medications among subjects with HFPDDs is widespread yet based on limited scientific grounds. Indeed, there is a lack of controlled studies on the use of psychotropic medications among individuals with AS and HFA. Based on our naturalistic study and on ongoing clinical experience and early implementation phases of pharmacological trials specific to this population, several clinical conclusions can be drawn, with research implications discussed for each. Table 7.4 also summarizes these guidelines.

Diagnostic Clarification

Available studies on the psychopharmacological treatment of the HFPDDs have generally been limited by poor diagnostic assessments. In some instances, and based on the descriptions provided or diagnostic instruments used, it is not even clear whether some of the included subjects had *any* PDD diagnosis. This is unfortunate given the excellent instruments currently available and well studied for the diagnosis of the PDDs (Autism Diagnostic Observation Schedule, Lord et al., 1989; Autism Diagnostic Interview, Le Couteur et al., 1989).

Although taxonomic differences between AS and HFA are unlikely to be resolved any time soon, our survey indirectly suggests that these distinctions may be less critical in terms of psychopharmacological treatment and research than those between the higher- and lower-functioning PDDs, or among groups with different target symptom clusters. Target symptom clusters and medication types used appear to be similar across the HFPDD subtypes (where antidepressant use predominates) but quite different from those in lower-functioning subjects (where neuroleptic use is the norm). The pharmacological study of HFA and AS as separate entities may prove to be too restrictive and logistically difficult and may ultimately reveal few significant differences. Our findings suggest that future psychopharmacology research will likely benefit more from having lower- and higher-functioning PDD groups studied separately than in trying to "lump" all cases together, or in having more narrowly defined and separate trials for AS and for HFA.

Comorbidity and Target Symptomatology

Individuals diagnosed with AS or HFA can demonstrate wide-ranging psychiatric symptomatology. Heterogeneity in clinical presentation is the norm and often associated with psychotropic medication use. It is presently unclear which of these symptoms is an integral part of the syndromes themselves, and which may represent psychiatric comorbid conditions, particu-

TABLE 7.4 Guidelines for Psychopharmacologic Treatment and Suggested Directions for Future Research

Diagnostic clarification

- Need for standardized diagnostic assessment in clinical trials (e.g., Autism Diagnostic Interview and Autism Diagnostic Observation Schedule)
- Documentation of intellectual functioning, neuropsychological profile and adaptive functioning using standardized, replicable instruments (e.g., Wechsler Intelligence Scale for Children, third edition, and Vineland scales)
- Higher- versus lower-functioning PDD, or symptom-based distinctions may be more relevant to pharmacological trials than diagnostic subcategorization within the HFPDDs (e.g., AS versus HFA)

Comorbidity and target symptomatology

- Distinction of "core" PDD symptomatology versus presence of comorbid psychiatric conditions
- Determination of comorbid conditions using standardized instruments (e.g., Children's Schedule for Affective Disorders and Schizophrenia, Present and Lifetime Version)

Instrumentation for the measurement of change

- Instruments available for diagnostic purposes are generally more adequate than those for the measurement of baseline severity and clinical change
- Negative findings in studies to date may have had to do with inability to measure change, rather than with lack of change
- A promising starting point may be in adapting available instruments used in pharmacologic trials in childhood anxiety disorders (e.g., SCARED and CARS), as well as developing and piloting new instruments
- Need for concurrent patient-, caregiver-, and clinician-based ratings

Pharmacologic intervention

- Limitations of "extension" studies
  - Age-related differences (e.g., pre- vs. post-pubertal efficacy and tolerability)
  - Behavioral activation and dose-sensitivity seemingly more likely in HFPDD than in obsessive–compulsive disorder and major depressive disorder
- Limitations of traditional, short-term, safety and efficacy pharmacological studies for the treatment of chronic conditions
- Confounders of premature discontinuation and resort to polypharmacy

Therapeutic agents available

- Nonspecificity of all available agents
  - SSRI antidepressants most widely used and likely to be studied in near future
  - Stimulants widely used
  - Atypical neuroleptics increasingly resorted to—concerns with long-term side effects (cognitive blunting, weight gain and obesity, tardive dyskinesia)
- Promising new agents under development: substance P and corticotropin releasing hormone (CRH) antagonists

larly as there have been limited studies of comorbidity in the HFPDDs. Systematic analysis of patterns of comorbidity in these conditions using structured instruments (e.g., Children's Schedule for Affective Disorders and Schizophrenia, Present and Lifetime Version, Kaufman et al., 1997) are lacking. Such studies could provide important guidelines to tailor more adequate psychopharmacology interventions for this population.

Instrumentation for the Measurement of Change

Available instruments used for the assessment of symptom severity and change in the HFPDD population are lacking and not nearly as robust as those available for establishing diagnoses. Moreover, medication-sensitive target symptoms in the treatment of autism (such as aggression or self-injury, which are more adequately ascertained in instruments such as the Aberrant Behavior Checklist (Aman et al., 1985) may not adequately address the clinical needs of the HFPDD group, in which anxiety and depression are especially common. At least one study (McDougle et al., 1998) has reported AS to be less responsive to psychopharmacological intervention than autism. Although there may be neurobiological reasons to explain the discrepancy, it is more likely that an inability to *detect or measure* change, rather than a lack of change, was responsible for that particular negative finding. Future pharmacological research in the HFPDDs will require the development and implementation of change measures specifically addressing depression and anxiety—social anxiety in particular. Adapting measures currently used in the pharmacological study of social anxiety may, for example, be a promising starting point (e.g., Screen for Child Anxiety-Related Disorders [SCARED], Birmaher et al., 1997). Particularly in light of limited insight, difficulties in the articulation of internal emotional states and of discrepant views commonly reported between affected individuals and other observers, it is critical that patient-, caregiver-, and clinician-based ratings be concurrently utilized in the determination of change or response to treatment interventions.

Pharmacologic Intervention

There are important age-related differences in the frequency and type of medication use among subjects with AS and HFA. Target symptoms are likely to change substantially over time, with attentional problems giving way with age to anxiety and depressive symptoms. Together with preliminary evidence that there may be age-related differences in response to medication, and that behavioral activation and dose-sensitivity may be heightened in the HFPDDs, these data point to the importance of considering developmental and diagnostic factors in designing medication studies. In particular, simple "extension" from available studies in other age- or diagnostic groups may provide limited useful information. Ongoing trials comparing pre- and postpubertal target symptoms and medication response in carefully ascertained HFPDD individuals may be particularly fruitful.

Traditional short-term pharmacologic trials assessing safety and efficacy have a definite, if limited, role in the evaluation of medication strategies for the treatment of chronic conditions such as the PDDs. Longer-term studies relying on survival analysis and alternative analytic strategies as well as careful naturalistic studies are likely to provide much valuable information. The common confounders of premature drug discontinuation or addition (leading to the commonly seen practice of polypharmacy) are to be especially considered in such studies.

Therapeutic Agents Available

All the pharmacological agents available and studied to date are nonspecific to the PDDs and indeed extensively used for the treatment of other neuropsychiatric conditions of childhood. It is likely that this trend will continue until the more specific biologic underpinnings of these conditions are discovered and specific drug strategies are designed in rational response.

The SSRI antidepressants have been the most extensively used agents and are likely to be the better studied drugs in the near future. Promising antidepressant agents currently in early and middle phases of development may prove beneficial to the treatment of the anxiety and depression symptom clusters of the HFPDDs. Such agents include substance P and corticotropin releasing hormone (CRH) antagonists, which are likely to become clinically available in upcoming years. Finally, it is worth mentioning that in response to the general paucity of available data on pediatric psychopharmacology, the NIMH has funded within the last 3 years the RUPP network. The area of autism and other PDDs has been identified as a high priority, and large-scale, multisite collaborative efforts are under way. The RUPPs will be uniquely placed to make contributions to the pharmacology of autism in general, and to the orphan HFPDDs more particularly. Such programmatic efforts will be able to address other longstanding difficulties in research in the field, such as limits in subject recruitment, and shortening the lag between marketing of medications and their systematic study.

ACKNOWLEDGMENT

Portions of this chapter have been adapted, and Tables 7.1–7.3 reprinted, from Martin, Scahill, Klin, and Volkmar (1999). Copyright 1999 by Lippincott Williams & Wilkins. Adapted and reprinted by permission.

REFERENCES

Aman, M. G., Singh, N. N., Stewart, A. W., & Field, C. J. (1985). The Aberrant Behavior Checklist: A behavior rating scale for the assessment of treatment effects. *American Journal of Mental Deficiency, 89,* 485–491.

Aman, M. G., Van Bourgondien, M. E., Wolford, P. L., & Sarphare, G. (1995). Psychotropic and anticonvulsant drugs in subjects with autism: Prevalence and patterns of use. *Journal of the American Academy of Child and Adolescent Psychiatry, 34,* 1672–1681.

Bejerot, S., & Duvner, T. (1995). Asperger's syndrome or schizophrenia? *Nordic Journal of Psychiatry, 49*(2), 145.

Berthier, M. (1995). Hypomania following bereavement in Asperger's syndrome: A case study. *Neuropsychiatry, Neuropsychology, and Behavioral Neurology, 8*(3), 222–228.

Birmaher, B., Quintana, H., & Greenhill, L. L. (1988). Methylphenidate treatment of hyperactive autistic children. *Journal of the American Academy of Child and Adolescent Psychiatry, 27*, 248–251.

Birmaher, B., Khetarpal, S., Brent, D., Cully, M., Balach, L., Kaufman, J., & Neer, J. M. (1997). The Screen for Child Anxiety Related Emotional Disorders (SCARED): Scale construction and psychometric characteristics. *Journal of the American Academy of Child and Adolescent Psychiatry, 36*, 545–553.

Brodkin, E. S., McDougle, C. J., Naylor, S. T., Cohen, D. J., & Price, L. H. (1997). Clomipramine in adults with pervasive developmental disorders: A prospective open-label investigation. *Journal of Child and Adolescent Psychopharmacology, 7*, 109–121.

Clarke, D. J., Littlejohns, C. S., Corbett, J. A., & Joseph, S. (1989). Pervasive developmental disorders and psychoses in adult life. *British Journal of Psychiatry, 155*, 692–699.

Cook, E. H., Courchesne, R., Lord, C., Cox, N. J., Yan, S., Lincoln, A., Haas, R., Courchesne, E., & Leventhal, B. L. (1997). Evidence of linkage between the serotonin transporter and autistic disorder. *Molecular Psychiatry, 2*, 247–250.

Cook, E. H., & Leventhal, B. L. (1995). Autistic disorder and other pervasive developmental disorders. *Child and Adolescent Psychiatric Clinics of North America, 4*, 381–400.

Cook, E. H., Jr., Rowlett, R., Jaselskis, C., & Leventhal, B. L. (1992). Fluoxetine treatment of children and adults with autistic disorder and mental retardation. *Journal of the American Academy of Child and Adolescent Psychiatry, 31*, 739–745.

Damore, J., Stine, J., & Brody, L. (1998). Medication-induced hypomania in Asperger's disorder [letter]. *Journal of the American Academy of Child and Adolescent Psychiatry, 37*, 248–249.

Ellis, H. D., Ellis, D. M., Fraser, W., & Deb, S. (1994). A preliminary study of right hemisphere cognitive deficits and impaired social judgments among young people with Asperger syndrome. *European Child and Adolescent Psychiatry, 3*(4), 255–266.

Fujikawa, H., Kobayashi, R., Koga, Y., & Murata, T. (1987). A case of Asperger's syndrome in a nineteen-year-old who showed psychotic breakdown with depressive state and attempted suicide after entering university. *Japanese Journal of Child and Adolescent Psychiatry, 28*(4), 217–225.

Ghaziuddin, M., Leininger, L., & Tsai, L. Y. (1995). Brief report: Thought disorder in Asperger syndrome: Comparison with high-functioning autism. *Journal of Autism and Development Disorders, 25*, 311–317.

Gillberg, C. (1985). Asperger's syndrome and recurrent psychosis: A case study. *Journal of Autism and Developmental Disorders, 15*(4), 389–397.

Gillberg, C., & Ehlers, S. (1998). High-functioning people with autism and Asperger syndrome: A literature review. In E. Schopler, G. B. Mesibov, & L. J. Kunce (Eds.), *Asperger syndrome or high-functioning autism?* (pp. 79–106). New York: Plenum.

Gordon, C. T., State, R. C., Nelson, J. E., Hamburger, S. D., & Rapoport, J. L. (1993). A double-blind comparison of clomipramine, desipramine, and placebo in the treatment of autistic disorder. *Archives of General Psychiatry, 50*, 441–447.

Kaufman, J., Birmaher, B., Brent, D., Rao, U., Flynn, C., Moreci, P., Williamson, D., & Ryan, N. (1997). Schedule for Affective Disorders and Schizophrenia for School-Age

Children—Present and Lifetime version (K-SADS-PL): Initial reliability and validity data. *Journal of the American Academy of Child and Adolescent Psychiatry, 36,* 980–988.

Kerbeshian, J., & Burd, L. (1986). Asperger's syndrome and Tourette syndrome: The case of the pinball wizard. *British Journal of Psychiatry, 148,* 731–736.

Klin, A., & Volkmar, F. R. (1997). Asperger's syndrome. In D. J. Cohen & F. R. Volkmar (Eds.), *Handbook of autism and pervasive developmental disorders* (2nd ed., pp. 94–112). New York: Wiley.

Klin, A., Volkmar, F. R., Schultz, R., Pauls, D., & Cohen, D. J. (1997, October 16). *Asperger's syndrome: Phenomenology, neuropsychology, and neurobiology.* Paper presented at the 44th annual meeting of the American Academy of Child and Adolescent Psychiatry, Toronto, Ontario.

Klin, A., Volkmar, F. R., Sparrow, S. S., Cicchetti, D. V., & Rourke, B. P. (1995). Validity and neuropsychological characterization of Asperger syndrome: Convergence with nonverbal learning disabilities syndrome. *Journal of Child Psychology and Psychiatry, 36,* 1127–1140.

Krug, D. A., Arick, J., & Almond, P. (1980). Behavior checklist for identifying severely handicapped individuals with high levels of autistic behavior. *Journal of Child Psychology and Psychiatry, 21,* 221–229.

Le Couteur, A., Rutter, M., Lord, C., Rios, P., Robertson, S., Holdgrafer, M., & McLennan, J. (1989). Autism Diagnostic Interview: A semistructured interview for parents and caregivers of autistic persons. *Journal of Autism and Developmental Disorders, 19,* 363–387.

Littlejohns, C. S., Clarke, D. J., & Corbett, J. A. (1990). Tourette-like disorder in Asperger's syndrome. *British Journal of Psychiatry, 156,* 430–433.

Lord, C., Rutter, M., Goode, S., Heemsbergen, J., Jordan, H., Mawhood, L., & Schopler, E. (1989). Autism Diagnostic Observation Schedule: A standardized observation of communicative and social behavior. *Journal of Autism and Developmental Disorders, 19*(2), 185–212.

Lord, C., Rutter, M., & Le Couteur, A. (1994). Autism Diagnostic Interview—Revised: A revised version of a diagnostic interview for caregivers of individuals with possible pervasive developmental disorders. *Journal of Autism and Developmental Disorders, 24,* 659–685.

Martin, A., Scahill, L., Klin, A., & Volkmar, F. R. (1999). Higher-functioning pervasive developmental disorders: Rates and patterns of psychotropic drug use. *Journal of the American Academy of Child and Adolescent Psychiatry, 38*(9), 923–931.

McDougle, C. J. (1997). Psychopharmacology. In D. J. Cohen & F. R. Volkmar (Eds.), *Handbook of autism and pervasive developmental disorders* (2nd ed., pp. 707–729). New York, Wiley.

McDougle, C. J. (1998). Repetitive thoughts and behavior in pervasive developmental disorders: Phenomenology and pharmacotherapy. In E. Schopler, G. B. Mesibov, & L. J. Kunce (Eds.), *Asperger syndrome or high functioning autism?* (pp. 293–316). New York: Plenum.

McDougle, C. J., Brodkin, E. S., Naylor, S. T., Carlson, D. C., Cohen, D. J., & Price, L. H. (1998). Sertraline in adults with pervasive developmental disorders: A prospective open-label investigation. *Journal of Clinical Psychopharmacology, 18,* 62–66.

McDougle, C. J., Fleischmann, R. L., Epperson, C. N., Wasylink, S., Leckman, J. F., & Price, L. H. (1995). Risperidone addition in fluvoxamine-refractory obsessive–compulsive disorder: Three cases. *Journal of Clinical Psychiatry, 56,* 526–528.

McDougle, C. J., Holmes, J. P., Bronson, M. R., Anderson, G. M., Volkmar, F. R., Price, L. H., & Cohen, D. J. (1997). Risperidone treatment of children and adolescents with pervasive developmental disorders: A prospective open-label study. *Journal of the American Academy of Child and Adolescent Psychiatry, 36,* 685–693.

McDougle, C. J., Kresch, L. E., Goodman, W. K., Naylor, S. T., Volkmar, F. R., Cohen, D. J., Price, L. H. (1995b). A case-controlled study of repetitive thoughts and behavior in adults with autistic disorder and obsessive–compulsive disorder. *American Journal of Psychiatry, 152*(5), 772–777.

McDougle, C. J., Naylor, S. T., Cohen, D. J., Volkmar, F. R., Heninger, G. R., & Price, L. H. (1996). A double-blind, placebo-controlled study of fluvoxamine in adults with autistic disorder. *Archives of General Psychiatry, 53,* 1001–1008.

McDougle, C. J., Price, L. H., Volkmar, F. R., Goodman, W. K., Ward, O. B. D., Nielsen, J., Bregman, J., & Cohen, D. J. (1992). Clomipramine in autism: Preliminary evidence of efficacy. *Journal of the American Academy of Child and Adolescent Psychiatry, 31*(4), 746–750.

Nagy, J., & Szatmari, P. (1986). A chart review of schizotypal personality disorders in children. *Journal of Autism and Developmental Disorders, 16*(3), 351–367.

Olfson, M., Marcus, S. C., Pincus, H. A., Zito, J. M., Thompson, J. W., & Zarin, D. A. (1998). Antidepressant prescribing practices of outpatient psychiatrists. *Archives of General Psychiatry, 55,* 310–316.

Potenza, M. N., & McDougle, C. J. (1997). The role of serotonin in autistic-spectrum disorders. *CNS Spectrums, 2,* 25–42.

Rourke, B., Young, G. C., & Leenaars, A. A. (1989). A childhood learning disability that predisposes those afflicted to adolescent and adult depression and suicide risk. *Journal of Learning Disabilities, 22,* 169–185.

Rutter, M. L. (1972). Relationships between child and adult psychiatric disorders: Some research considerations. *Acta Psychiatrica Scandinavica, 48,* 3–21.

Ryan, R. M. (1992). Treatment-resistant chronic mental illness: Is it Asperger's syndrome? *Hospital Community Psychiatry, 43,* 807–811.

Sanchez, L. E., Campbell, M., Small, A. M., Cueva, J. E., Armenteros, J. L., & Adams, P. B. (1996). A pilot study of clomipramine in young autistic children. *Journal of the American Academy of Child and Adolescent Psychiatry, 35,* 537–544.

Schopler, E., & Mesibov, G. B. (1992). *High-functioning individuals with autism.* New York: Plenum.

Szabo, C. P., & Bracken, C. (1994). Imipramine and Asperger's [letter]. *Journal of the American Academy of Child and Adolescent Psychiatry, 33,* 431–432.

Taiminen, T. (1994). Asperger's syndrome or schizophrenia: Is differential diagnosis necessary for adult patients? *Nordic Journal of Psychiatry, 48*(5), 325–328.

Tantam, D. (1988a). Asperger's syndrome. *Journal of Child Psychology and Psychiatry, 29,* 245–255.

Tantam, D. (1988b). Lifelong eccentricity and social isolation. II: Asperger's syndrome or schizoid personality disorder? *British Journal of Psychiatry, 153,* 783–791.

Tantam, D. (1991). Asperger's syndrome in adulthood. In U. Frith (Ed.), *Autism and Asperger syndrome* (pp. 147–183). Cambridge: Cambridge University Press.

Thomsen, P. H. (1994). Obsessive–compulsive disorder in children and adolescents: A 6–22-year follow-up study: Clinical descriptions of the course and continuity of obsessive–compulsive symptomatology. *European Child and Adolescent Psychiatry, 3*(2), 82–96.

Volkmar, F. R., & Cohen, D. J. (1991). Comorbid association of autism and schizophrenia. *American Journal of Psychiatry, 148,* 1705–1707.

Volkmar, F. R., & Nelson, D. S. (1990). Seizure disorders in autism. *Journal of the American Academy of Child and Adolescent Psychiatry, 29,* 127–129.

Werry, J. S. (1992). Child and adolescent (early onset) schizophrenia: A review in light of DSM-III-R. *Journal of Autism and Developmental Disorders, 22,* 601–624.

Wolff, S. (1995). *Loners: The life path of unusual children.* London: Routledge.

III

Related Diagnostic Constructs

8

Nonverbal Learning Disabilities and Asperger Syndrome

BYRON P. ROURKE
KATHERINE D. TSATSANIS

The objective of this chapter is to present an overview of the Nonverbal Learning Disabilities (NLD) syndrome and to consider its relationship to Asperger syndrome (AS). In pursuing an understanding of the NLD syndrome, our aim has been to develop and refine a comprehensive theoretical model of the brain–behavior relationships that might underlie its developmental course. In the first sections of this chapter, we review the background and content of the investigative effort that has been expended in our laboratory with respect to NLD. This review is followed by a description of the model developed to explain the syndrome's dynamics. In part, the purpose of this presentation is to consider whether and to what extent these formulations might also apply to an understanding of AS. Following these sections, we next present a comparison of the two disorders, with evidence to suggest a correspondence in the clinical manifestation of NLD and AS. Further, we propose that the processes involved in integrative and adaptive activity, that are central to the dynamics of NLD, may also be especially relevant to a consideration of AS.

BACKGROUND

Several descriptions of children with learning disabilities characterized by chronic difficulties in social and emotional functioning have appeared in the literature. In these descriptions, an association between a lack of ability to make sense of and to navigate the social environment and deficits in visual–spatial and mathematical skills is consistently noted. Although these basic features are shared, researchers have approached this type of learning disability from different perspectives, which is reflected in the varied nomenclature. Terms include "minimal brain dysfunction," "nonverbal learning disability," "developmental learning disability of the right hemisphere," "social and emotional learning disability," and "developmental right-hemisphere syndrome" (Denckla, 1983; Gross-Tsur, Shalev, Manor, & Amir, 1995; Myklebust, 1975; Tranel, Hall, Olson, & Tranel, 1987; Weintraub & Mesulam, 1983; Voeller, 1986). This literature consists largely of clinical studies of groups of individuals with apparently similar learning difficulties selected out of a larger clinical population. The similarities are striking, but an understanding of why these particular difficulties should fall together is more limited. At minimum, this learning disability subtype has been commonly understood in the context of right-hemisphere dysfunction.

In this chapter, we present a systematic approach to the identification of this type of learning disability—NLD—and propose a coherent conceptual model by which to understand its manifestations. Since 1971, research efforts in our laboratory have been largely devoted to the delineation of learning disability subtypes in children. We have engaged in the intensive investigation of two subtypes of learning disability in particular (see Rourke, 1975, 1978, 1982, 1987, 1988a, 1989, 1993; Rourke & Finlayson, 1978; Rourke & Fisk, 1992; Rourke & Fuerst, 1992; Rourke & Strang, 1978, 1983; Strang & Rourke, 1983, 1985a, 1985b). As a result of our clinical observations and empirical investigations, we are able to state with considerable confidence the characteristics (content validity) of the two subtypes, which we describe briefly in the following sections.

BASIC PHONOLOGICAL PROCESSING DISORDER

One group of children, Group R-S (Reading–Spelling), demonstrates many relatively deficient psycholinguistic skills in conjunction with very well-developed abilities in visual–spatial organizational, tactile–perceptual, psychomotor, and nonverbal problem-solving skills. These children also exhibit poor reading and spelling skills and significantly better, although still impaired, mechanical arithmetic competence. Their outstanding problem is in the area of phonological awareness and processing, and we have since referred to this subtype of learning disability as a basic phonological processing disorder (BPPD).

Figure 8.1 outlines in schematic form the characteristics and developmental dynamics that we have developed to encompass these observations and research findings.

In this model, the patterns of academic deficits experienced by individ-

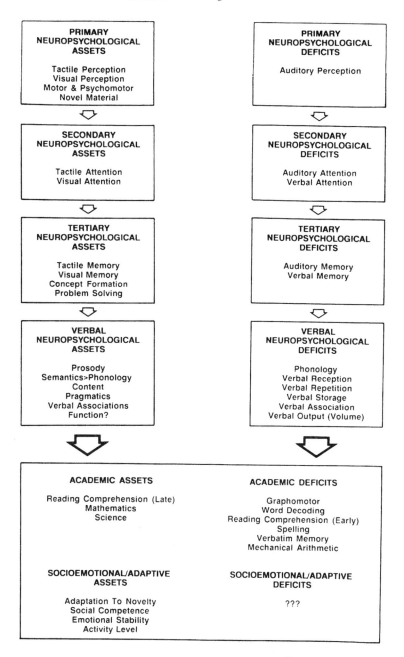

FIGURE 8.1. Content and dynamics of basic phonological processing disorder.

uals who exhibit this learning disability are viewed as the *direct* result of the interaction of a common set of neuropsychological assets and deficits. The primary, secondary, tertiary, and linguistic neuropsychological assets and deficits that are outlined in Figure 8.1 can be understood within the context of a set of cause-and-effect relationships. For example, considering the hypothesized "deficit" stream, the primary neuropsychological deficits experienced by the child with BPPD are seen to have their roots in aspects of auditory perception. Specifically, these deficits relate especially to phonemic awareness and processing (e.g., discrimination, segmentation, and blending). Such deficits are expected to eventuate in disordered or diminished attention to auditory–verbal input; in turn, problems in memory for verbal material delivered through the auditory modality would be expected to ensue. This set of deficits is considered to eventuate in the particular constellation of linguistic deficiencies outlined in Figure 8.1.

The academic, psychosocial, and adaptive deficiencies listed are the expected sequelae of these neuropsychological deficits. It is especially important to note that this set of deficits is not thought to lead in a necessary way to any particular configuration of problems in psychosocial/adaptive behavior either within or outside the academic situation (Rourke, 1988a, 1989; Rourke & Fuerst, 1992). Specifically, there is nothing intrinsic to the deficits exhibited by children of this subtype that would necessarily result in problems in social perception, social judgment, and the like. This outcome can be contrasted to that of the second subtype. For a more extensive description of BPPD, interested readers are referred to Rourke (1989).

NONVERBAL LEARNING DISABILITIES

Children comprising the second subtype present with a different pattern of performance. These children exhibit outstanding neuropsychological deficits in visual–spatial–organizational, tactile–perceptual, psychomotor, and nonverbal problem-solving and concept-formation skills, within a context of clear neuropsychological assets in psycholinguistic skills such as rote verbal learning, regular phoneme–grapheme matching, amount of verbal output, and verbal classification. On measures of achievement, we found major learning difficulties in mechanical arithmetic but advanced levels of word recognition and spelling. In addition, we identified a particular pattern of psychosocial disturbance that is marked by a failure to appreciate the nonverbal aspects of communication. Myklebust (1975) originally coined the term for this subtype of learning disability, NLD.

Both subtypes have been the subject of much clinical and scientific inquiry in our laboratory (see earlier discussion), and have been subjected to clinical, empirical, and theoretical scrutiny by others (e.g., Bieliauskas, 1991; Fletcher, 1985; Sparrow, 1991; Torgeson, 1993; van der Vlugt, 1991; van der

Vlugt & Satz, 1985). In the context of a discussion of AS, NLD distinguishes itself as a particularly useful syndrome and model. By way of contrast, the content and dynamics of the neuropsychological assets and deficits displayed by children with BPPD are in no way similar to those exhibited by persons with AS. This is especially the case when one considers the following dimensions of BPPD: (1) Phonologically loaded linguistic skills are relatively impaired and represent the primary area of deficit, (2) virtually all other neuropsychological skills and abilities fall within average limits, and (3) psychosocial functioning is expected to be normal unless resulting from factors not indigenous to the disorder itself. Whereas the profile of assets and deficits in BPPD is in some respects the opposite of that in AS, it is apparent that NLD involves dimensions that are very much akin to the disorder. These dimensions are characterized in greater detail next.

Characteristics of the NLD Syndrome

The principal clinical manifestations (content) of the NLD syndrome, that we identified through a process of intensive clinical examination, are as follows:

1. Bilateral tactile–perceptual deficits, usually more marked on the left side of the body. Evidence of simple tactile imperception and suppression tends to subside with age, but problems in dealing with complex tactile input tend to persist.

2. Bilateral psychomotor coordination deficiencies, often more marked on the left side of the body. Relatively simple motor skills, such as finger tapping and static steadiness, tend to normalize with advancing years. Complex psychomotor skills, especially when required within a novel framework, tend to worsen relative to age-based norms.

3. Outstanding deficiencies in visual–spatial–organizational abilities. Simple visual discrimination, especially for material that can be verbalized, usually approaches normal levels with age. Complex visual–spatial–organizational skills, especially when required within a novel framework, tend to worsen relative to age-based norms.

4. Extreme difficulty in adapting to novel and otherwise complex situations. An overreliance on prosaic, rote (and, in consequence, frequently inappropriate) behaviors in such situations. Capacity to deal with novel experiences often remains poor, or even worsens, with age.

5. Marked deficits in nonverbal problem solving, concept formation, hypothesis testing, and the capacity to benefit from positive and negative informational feedback in novel or otherwise complex situations. Included are significant difficulties in dealing with cause–effect relationships and marked deficiencies in the appreciation of incongruities (e.g., age-appropriate sensitivity to humor). Such deficiencies tend to persist, and even worsen, with age.

6. Distorted sense of time. This distortion is reflected in poor esti- mation of elapsed time during common activities and poor estimation of time of day. (This deficit may not appear spontaneously; it usually requires a direct attempt to elicit it.)

7. Well-developed rote verbal capacities, including extremely well- developed rote verbal memory skills. "Memory" for complex verbal mate- rial is usually poor, probably as a result of poor initial comprehension of such material.

8. Much verbosity of a repetitive, straightforward, rote nature. Con- tent disorders of language and poor psycholinguistic pragmatics. Little or no speech prosody, except on an imitative basis. Excessive reliance on lan- guage as the principal means for social relating, information gathering, and relief from anxiety.

9. Outstanding relative deficiencies in mechanical arithmetic as com- pared to proficiencies in reading (word recognition) and spelling. Misspell- ings are almost exclusively of the phonetically accurate variety. Comprehen- sion of, as opposed to rote memory for, complex text may continue to be poor with advancing age.

10. Significant deficits in social perception, social judgment, and so- cial interaction skills. During preschool and early school years, the child is often seen as "hyperactive." However, there is a marked tendency toward hypoactivity as age increases, often including social withdrawal and even social isolation. There is considerable risk for the development of psycho- social disturbance, especially "internalized" forms of psychopathology, in older childhood and adolescence.

In addition to explaining an extensively detailed clinical characteriza- tion of the syndrome of NLD, we have also endeavored to understand why this particular constellation of difficulties should emerge over the course of development. The next section presents our formulation of the dynamics of the syndrome. With this model, we offer unique consideration to the devel- opmental manifestations and brain–behavior relationships that would be expected to give rise to NLD. Further, we advance a conceptual framework that may promote new avenues of research, particularly with regard to an understanding of AS.

Dynamics of the NLD Syndrome

An especially salient feature of NLD, one that differentiates it from other learning disabilities, is the extent of associated psychosocial and adaptive difficulties. Moreover, the particular pattern of academic, psychosocial, and adaptive abilities and deficiencies is the expected sequelae of the pattern of neuropsychological assets and deficits displayed by persons with NLD (Rourke, 1989, 1995). In this model, the principal or primary dimensions of the NLD syndrome are deficits in visual–perceptual–organizational abilities, complex psychomotor skills, and tactile perception, as well as difficulties in dealing with novelty. Primary assets include proficiency in most rote verbal and some simple motor and psychomotor skills. These formulations were arrived at on the basis of clinical observations by ourselves and other practitioners. Confirmation of these dimensions as primary arises from the results of recent studies (e.g., Casey, Rourke, & Picard, 1991; Harnadek & Rourke, 1994). It should be emphasized that in the Rourke models, the patterns of academic and psychosocial deficits experienced by individuals who exhibit NLD are viewed as the *direct* result of the interaction of the primary, secondary, tertiary, and linguistic neuropsychological assets and deficits that are outlined schematically in Figure 8.2.

For example, considering the hypothesized "deficit" stream, the primary neuropsychological deficits experienced by the child with NLD are seen as having to do with aspects of tactile and visual perception, complex psychomotor skills, and the capacity to deal adaptively with novel material. Such deficits are expected to eventuate in disordered tactile and visual attention and stunted exploratory behavior; in turn, problems in memory for material delivered through the tactile and visual modalities as well as deficits in concept formation and problem solving would be expected to ensue. This set of deficits is considered to eventuate in the particular linguistic deficiencies outlined in Figure 8.2 (see Rourke & Tsatsanis, 1996, for a more extensive explanation of these linguistic deficits).

It is especially important to note that this set of neuropsychological deficits is expected to lead, in a necessary way, to a particular configuration of problems in psychosocial/adaptive behavior both within and without the academic situation (Rourke, 1988a, 1989, 1995; Rourke & Fuerst, 1992). The notion that a particular pattern of neuropsychological assets and deficits (resulting in a particular subtype of learning disability) can lead to both a particular pattern of academic assets and deficits and to a particular pattern of psychosocial disturbance is well-illustrated by the NLD syndrome. In a series of investigations (Casey et al., 1991; Harnadek & Rourke, 1994; Rourke & Fuerst, 1991, for a summary of several studies), we have been able to demonstrate the concurrent and predictive validity of these formulations relating to the academic and psychosocial consequences of NLD. Also, it has been possible to demonstrate that particular patterns of academic assets and deficits are reliably related to particular patterns of psychosocial dysfunction across the age span of interest (Fuerst & Rourke, 1993; Tsatsanis, Rourke, & Fuerst, 1997). The precise dynamics of NLD have been discussed in detail elsewhere (Rourke, 1989, especially pp. 80–100 and 142–149) and are presented in brief here where they pertain to a discussion of AS.

In addition to describing the content and dynamics of the NLD syndrome, a model to explain the syndrome's dynamics has been proposed (Rourke, 1987, 1988b, 1989, 1995). The model involves an integration of

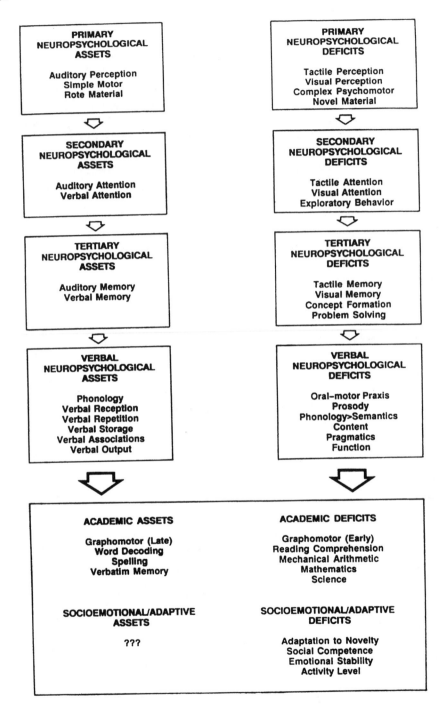

FIGURE 8.2. Content and dynamics of the syndrome of nonverbal learning disabilities.

Piagetian developmental theory and a concept of brain development that extends the theoretical tenets of Goldberg and Costa (1981). An approach is advanced in which the manifestation of this syndrome is viewed in terms of the complex and complementary interaction of cognitive, brain maturational, and experiential factors.

COGNITIVE–DEVELOPMENTAL PERSPECTIVE

A considered account of the dynamics of NLD emphasizes Piaget's (1954; Piaget & Inhelder, 1969) emphasis on sensorimotor functioning as one of the early developmental features upon which formal operational thought is founded (Casey & Rourke, 1992; Strang & Rourke, 1985a). From this perspective, development is characterized as a continuing process of organization, integration, and consolidation of one's experiences engendered by newly emerging capacities. At the earliest stages, the interaction between self and environment is organized through the body (sensory processes) and action (Piaget, 1954). The external world is known to the young child principally through touch, vision, and movement. In addition, early learning takes place in the context of goal-directed behavior, which is outwardly manifested in action or active experimentation (Piaget, 1954). Motivated exploration and manipulation of the environment furnish the child with the necessary information to begin forming mental schemata. This early activity is thought to yield the development of higher-order mental processes, such as an understanding of cause-and-effect relationships, hypothesis testing, nonverbal concept formation, and reasoning abilities.

In this regard, Piaget (1954) maintained that the adequacy of children's sensorimotor experience is related in a direct way to their cognitive development. The primary deficits of NLD—tactile perception, psychomotor coordination, and visual perception—are precisely those domains identified as essential to early learning. Furthermore, children with NLD have considerable difficulty adapting to novel stimuli and are unlikely to explore their environment or seek out stimulation. It may be argued that there is little organized interaction between children with NLD and the external world, and that there is, as a result, a fundamental inability to make sense of complex and novel stimuli.

At the same time, it is clear that children with NLD can exhibit some areas of adequate language development. Language is transmitted to the child in ready-made and compulsory form (Piaget & Inhelder, 1969). Young children receive structured auditory input and highly directed speech in their "conversations" with caregivers. In addition, some language skills (e.g., verbal output, syntax and grammar, word knowledge, and word decoding) are readily routinized behaviors that are governed by explicit rules. In contrast, children are, for the most part, left to their own devices to make sense of and lend order to, for example, the visual–spatial, tactile, and social worlds. Play may be considered the predominant childhood arena for practicing social skills, developing relationships, exercising new capacities, and permitting a mode of self-expression (Piaget, 1951). Children with NLD demonstrate a disproportionate reliance on language (compared to play-based activity) as the principal means of social relating, information gathering, and relief from anxiety. In addition, these children appear to excel at the rule-governed aspects of language (e.g., language form) but struggle with the semantic and pragmatic dimensions.

A similar distinction may be drawn between areas of mathematics that are learned in a formulaic manner and those that are acquired through reasoning. Number facts are taught explicitly and achieved largely through a process of rote memorization, a relative strength for children with NLD. However, in addition to the formal mathematics instruction that takes place, children must also develop an appreciation for number concepts. That is, they must develop an idea of what is meant by "number," "more and less," "greater than and less than," "fraction," "conservation of quantity," and so on. An understanding of these mathematical constructs is built on principles that derive from physical experience. The concepts are revealed in children's ability to think about and mentally represent the relations between objects and their experiences of them (Piaget & Inhelder, 1969). Higher-level mathematics further draws on spatial visualization and representation, a relative area of deficit for children with NLD.

A pervasive difficulty in making sense of and adapting to external events is also expected to affect the ability to interact socially. In Piagetian terms, schemata are developed and applied to the social experience (Piaget, 1954). This process depends on a capacity to draw out the common and more general features of interpersonal events. In this regard, the pattern of neuropsychological assets and deficits exhibited by persons with NLD is expected to eventuate in compromised social development. Social interaction involves the perception, evaluation, and application of nonverbal cues, all of which have been shown to be defective in children with NLD. Deficits in visual–perceptual–organizational skills are considered to give rise to their problems in deciphering the meaning of various facial expressions, gestures, and other forms of paralinguistic information important for effective human communication. Furthermore, clumsiness and poor psychomotor skills (e.g., speeded eye–hand coordination) also make it likely that individuals with NLD will be perceived as socially awkward.

More basic problems in intermodal integration, reasoning, and concept formation are thought to contribute to their deficits in social judgment and interaction (Rourke, 1993; Strang & Rourke, 1983). Specifically, limitations in the capacities of persons with NLD within the realm of intermodal integration are expected to give rise to the following adaptive difficulties: (1) problems in the assessment of another's emotional state, which depends on the analysis and synthesis (integration) of information gleaned from facial expressions, tone of voice, posture, psychomotor patterns, and the like; (2) impaired assessment of social cause-and-effect relationships, which arises because of a failure to integrate data from a number of sources, as is often necessary to generate reasonable hypotheses regarding the chain of events in social intercourse; (3) failure to appreciate humor because of the complex intermodal judgments required for assessing the juxtaposition of the incongruous; and (4) misinterpretation of the behavior of others, such as attributing unreasonable or oversimplified causes for their behavior, and making such attributions in situations that would often lead to embarrassment for these people.

Social competence also requires adaptability to novel interpersonal situations and a constantly shifting pattern of exchange. A basic deficit identified in persons with NLD is coping with novelty, which is exacerbated by poor problem-solving and hypothesis-testing skills. This constellation of difficulties conspires to render a smooth adaptation to the constantly changing milieu of social interactions all but impossible for the child or adult with NLD. Although some social rules may be learned, a formulaic descriptive system is not likely to eventuate in the spontaneous give-and-take of a social exchange. Despite an initial desire to interact with others, the totality of these problems usually creates an unrewarding social experience for the child with NLD. With increasing age and social pressures, they tend to be ostracized or ridiculed. These experiences are expected to lead to an increased likelihood of social withdrawal, isolation, and depression on the part of the person with NLD. Indeed, evidence suggests that depression and suicide attempts are greater than average in individuals who exhibit this syndrome (Bigler, 1989; Fletcher, 1989; Rourke, Young, & Leenaars, 1989).

WHITE MATTER MODEL

A central theoretical hypothesis of the NLD model is that perturbations of white matter (long myelinated fiber) development or damage to white matter are the cause of the phenotypical manifestations of NLD. From this perspective, the role of neural pathways (i.e., axonal or "white matter" connections) in flexibly processing information and responding to changes in functional demands is seen as crucial. This can be contrasted to strict localizationist theory because the outcome is conceptualized more broadly in terms of the functional organization of systems within the brain. In particular, three principal axes of neurodevelopment are considered for their role in the integrative action of the brain. A brief account is presented next. For a full description of the syndrome and the "white matter" model, interested readers are referred to Rourke (1989, 1995) and Tsatsanis and Rourke (1995).

Neurodevelopmental Factors

Critical events in the developing brain include neuronal proliferation and migration, cell differentiation, axon and dendrite growth, axon guidance and target recognition, and synaptic formation. The modification of cortical connections is further associated with processes such as nerve cell death and the formation and elimination of excess axonal connections and synapses. Cell proliferation and migration occur early in development and are complete at birth. However, relatively few fiber tracts are completely myelinated at birth. Indeed, the most rapid period of myelination occurs within the first 2 years of life (Dietrich & Bradley, 1988; Rourke, Bakker, Fisk, & Strang, 1983). In addition, postnatal growth spurts in the brain are reported to occur without a concurrent increase in neuronal proliferation; rather, it is the growth of dendritic processes, synapses, and myelination that are thought to account for these postnatal increases in brain weight (Kolb & Fantie, 1989). As noted, an important event in postnatal development is the excess production and eventual elimination of neurons, dendrites, and synapses (Huttenlocher, 1984, 1994). These findings indicate that the development of axonal connections (white matter pathways) and the process of myelination are far from complete in the brain of the very young child. Moreover, the integrity of these systems is expected to bear on the child's ability to adapt to increasing environmental demands.

A description of these events also underscores the notion that brain development involves a dynamic interplay between two main processes— differentiation and integration. The brain evolves to greater complexity through the integrative action of neuronal growth and differentiation and associated organization of these component parts to yield more refined neural systems (Majovski, 1989). Similarly, the mark of higher-order processing is both the activation of specialized subsystems and the capacity to integrate them toward an identified goal. In the current white matter model, functions that involve inter- rather than intramodal processing are expected to be more likely to be affected by white matter perturbations. It follows that white matter disturbances will have a more profound effect on neural systems that are characterized by a high degree of interregional connectivity. In their capacity to deal with novel and complex information, it is expected that both the right hemisphere and frontal systems display greater interregional connectivity (e.g., Damasio, 1990; Tulving, Markowitsch, Kapur, Habib, & Houle, 1994).

The pattern of development displayed by children with NLD has been interpreted by Rourke (1982, 1987, 1989), on the basis of formulations of the Goldberg and Costa (1981) model, to involve right-hemisphere dysfunction. Through an analysis of differences in the neuroanatomical organization of the right and left hemispheres, Goldberg and Costa identified distinct roles for the cerebral hemispheres in the acquisition, integration, and application of descriptive systems. Their examination suggested that the right hemisphere has a crucial role in the initial stages of the acquisition of descriptive systems, whereas the left hemisphere is superior at deploying these codes in a routinized manner once they have been assembled. Hence, it is hypothesized that systems within the right hemisphere are highly efficient at processing novel information for which the individual has no preexisting code. In contrast, left-hemispheral systems are thought to be superior at processing that takes advantage of these fully formed codes—that is, the storage and application of multiple overlearned descriptive systems. The specific pattern of neuropsychological assets and deficits displayed by children with NLD is expected to develop under conditions that compromise the functioning of, or accessibility to, right-hemispheral systems in particular.

This perspective is supported by recent findings using quantified electroencephelogram (EEG) or EEG coherence analyses obtained over the lifespan (Thatcher, 1994, 1997). These studies reveal a *left–right* hemisphere pole of development, involving complementary sequences of predominantly left-hemisphere growth spurts followed by predominantly right-hemisphere growth spurts. Furthermore, cycles within the left hemisphere exhibit a developmental sequence involving a progressive lengthening or expansion of intracortical connections—that is, short distance intracortical growth spurts followed by growth spurts in longer-distance connection systems. In contrast, cycles in the right hemisphere consisted of a sequential consolidation of intracortical connections—that is, a progression from growth spurts in long-distance connections to shorter distance subsystems over time. These results were interpreted to suggest a developmental sequence of functional integration of differentiated subsystems in the left hemisphere, and the convergence of distributed systems to form specialized subsystems in the right hemisphere. In brief, Thatcher (1997) described these developmental processes as "integrating differentiation" in the left hemisphere and "differentiating integration" in the right hemisphere. Consistent with Goldberg and Costa's (1981) formulation, the left hemisphere is found to predominate in the integration of systems that are fully formed, whereas the right hemisphere is involved in the assembly of new systems.

Thatcher's (1994, 1997) work also points to a frontal-to-caudal dominance of changes in intracortical connections. A role for frontal systems in higher-level cognitive functioning has been well documented (Stuss, 1992; Damasio & Anderson, 1993). In particular, frontal systems are thought to play an integral role in executive control of novel responses (i.e., in directing, planning, and organizing lower-level systems toward a selected goal). EEG coherence measures examining the development of intracortical connections offer support for this role. The results of these investigations indicate that postnatal cerebral maturation is characterized by the expansion of reciprocal connections between regions of the frontal lobes and posterior, central, and temporal cortical regions (Case, 1992; Thatcher, 1994, 1997). The finding of an anterior–posterior gradient of development in the formation of these connections has been interpreted to suggest a mechanism of integration by frontal systems of elemental sensorimotor units to form higher-level abstractions and systems of abstraction (Thatcher, 1994).

The third dimension of interest would appear to be the long fibers projecting from subcortical and limbic system structures to cortical areas, particularly frontal regions. Evidence suggests that reciprocal connections between these regions influence information processing at higher levels. Such roles include the assignment of affective meaning to external events, formation of novelty encoding networks, and synchronization and desynchronization of cortical activity (Barth & MacDonald, 1996; Damasio & Anderson, 1993; Mega, Cummings, Salloway, & Malloy, 1997; Steriade, McCormick, & Sejnowski, 1993; Tulving et al., 1994). Developmentally, a perturbation in these pathways would be expected to result in diminished subcortical–limbic influences on refinement and organization of the cortex, thereby affecting regulation and coordination of higher-order mental activity.

CORRESPONDENCE OF THE NLD SYNDROME AND ASPERGER SYNDROME

Content

The clinical features of NLD and AS reveal a strikingly similar pattern of behavior and adaptive functioning. In the initial series of case reports by Wing (1981), the most typical features of AS are described. These include (1) pedantic one-sided and lengthy discourse; (2) limited appreciation of humor; (3) poor apprehension and application of the nonverbal aspects of communication, including facial expression, gestures, and prosody; (4) limited ability to understand and use the rules governing social behavior, reflected in a difficulty maintaining reciprocal interaction and forming friendships; (5) motor incoordination; and (6) a circumscribed area of all-absorbing interest or extensive factual knowledge. School years may be marked by teasing and increasing isolation of the affected individual; depression and anxiety may manifest at later ages.

Wing (1981) also makes reference to a cluster of cognitive assets and deficits in children with AS. These children are noted to begin to speak early and have no difficulty acquiring grammar. Prominent features include marked verbosity and excellent rote memories; however, visual–spatial abilities may be considerably inferior to expressive language skills. Subsequent accounts presenting detailed clinical descriptions have supported these observations (e.g., Nass & Gutman, 1997; Volkmar et al., 1996).

In addition, the results of a study conducted by Ehlers et al. (1997) are suggestive of this pattern of better verbal relative to poorer perceptual organizational skills. This investigation was directed at determining the ability of the Wechsler Intelligence Scale for Children—Revised to discriminate between three diagnostic groups—autism, AS, and a disorder of attention, motor control, and perception (DAMP). The researchers examined 120 children, diagnosed according to criteria previously published by one of the authors as well as criteria according to the third edition, revised, of the *Diagnostic and Statistical Manual of Mental Disorders* (DSM-III-R; American Psychiatric Association, 1987). Overall, the mean Verbal (VIQ), Performance (PIQ), and Full Scale IQ (FSIQ) scores of the Asperger group were greater than for the autism group. Notably, however, there was a 13-point difference in the mean VIQ and PIQ scores of the individuals with AS, favoring VIQ, whereas no such discrepancy was exhibited by the individuals with autism. Intragroup analyses indicated that the Asperger group obtained significantly higher scores on Information, Similarities, Comprehension, and Vocabulary. Significantly lower results were obtained on Arithmetic, Object Assembly, and Coding. The highest score for the autism group was obtained on Block Design.

A more extensive investigation comparing the neuropsychological profiles of well-characterized individuals with AS and high-functioning autism (HFA) offers strong support for a relationship between AS and NLD (Klin, Volkmar, Sparrow, Cicchetti, & Rourke, 1995). The sample in this study consisted of 19 individuals with HFA and 21 individuals with AS, diagnosed using stringent criteria according to the *International Classification of Diseases, Tenth revision* (ICD-10; World Health Organization, 1992). The neuropsychological records of each subject were reviewed and rated according to 22 items—7 assets and 15 deficits considered to be the defining criteria of NLD. An overwhelming concordance between AS and NLD was obtained ($n = 18$), whereas there was virtually no overlap between HFA and NLD ($n = 1$). Furthermore, 11 of the 22 NLD items were found to discriminate between AS and HFA, of which 9 appeared to be independent of diagnostic criteria. A detailed analysis of the individual criteria revealed that six criteria were predictive of AS and another five criteria were predictive of "not AS." Deficits that were predictive of AS were fine motor skills, visual motor integration, visual–spatial perception, nonverbal concept formation, gross motor skills, and visual memory. Deficits that were identified as not predictive of AS included articulation, verbal output, auditory perception, vocabulary, and verbal memory. This finding was reflected more generally in the pattern of IQ scores in the two groups, consistent with the findings by Ehlers et al. (1997). The Asperger group showed a significant and unusually large Verbal–Performance discrepancy (higher VIQ compared to PIQ score), whereas no such discrepancy was exhibited by the HFA group.

The descriptive accounts of individuals with AS show considerable overlap with the clinical manifestations of the NLD syndrome. In addition to the same basic difficulties in social interaction, particularly the nonverbal dimensions, it is notable that both groups of individuals show an overreliance on language to learn about themselves and the external world. Language is an ideal medium to deal with categorical information, but it is less effective at conveying direct experience (e.g., sensory and affective components of experience). This can be seen in the kinds of formulaic exchanges that often take place in the interpersonal interactions of persons with AS or NLD. It has also been observed that the function of verbal thought is to know or state truths (Piaget, 1954), which is reminiscent of the accumulation of factual knowledge that so characterizes individuals with AS.

Finally, it is of note that there is convincing preliminary evidence to indicate a correspondence in the neuropsychological profiles of the two groups. The pattern of neuropsychological assets and deficits that is manifest in NLD seems also characteristic of AS, pointing to a potential basis for the distinction between the latter disorder and HFA.

Dynamics

In previous reports, it has been observed that the pattern of impairment in AS is suggestive of dysfunction in the right hemisphere (Brumback, Harper, & Weinberg, 1996; Molina, Ruata, & Soler, 1986; Nass & Gutman, 1997). Most recently, Ellis and Gunter (1999) have supported the thesis that AS can be accounted for by a deficit that primarily affects right-hemisphere function and is centered on incomplete or dysfunctional white matter. Preliminary support for this idea is revealed in the case report of three individuals with AS who presented with right-hemisphere abnormalities on CT, MRI, and SPECT (McKelvey, Lambert, Mottron, & Shevell, 1995). In addition, right-hemisphere abnormalities were reported in an MRI study of seven males with concurrent AS and Tourette syndrome (Berthier, Bayes, & Tolosa, 1993). More generally, the association is drawn in the context of a long line of research on patients with brain damage that identifies selected functions most strongly mediated by systems within the right hemisphere.

From the current perspective, an emphasis is also placed on the role of right-hemispheral systems in the expression of NLD and AS but is applied more broadly. The central point of consideration is directed toward fundamental processes of both cognitive development and brain maturation that promote integrative and adaptive activity. These processes are thought to be integral to an understanding of both NLD and AS.

Development is defined in terms of change that takes place to make sense of and adapt to environmental complexity. An understanding of cognitive maturation parallels developments in the brain in this regard. In Piaget's framework, intelligence is understood to be governed by two interrelated and invariant processes—organization and adaptation (Piaget, 1963). It is suggested that "intelligence organizes the world by organizing itself" (Piaget, 1954, p. 355). This is thought to begin at the level of the sensorimotor experience. Higher-order mental activity is thought to emerge from the integration of more basic sensory and motor elements. Adaptation is proposed to consist of two components—assimilation and accommodation. The reciprocal activity of these processes is thought to organize the interaction between self and environment. Schemata are constructed and applied to give structure and meaning to one's experiences.

Related processes are also emphasized in understanding the natural adaptation of the brain. A central dimension of this development lies in the dynamic interplay between integration and differentiation, which can be observed in early brain processes. Thatcher's (1994, 1997) work also points to a cyclical reorganization and reintegration of intracortical connections over time, through which elemental units yield functionally more specialized or higher-order systems.

In this connection, it is important to note that postnatal spurts in brain growth have also been found to overlap with Piaget's main stages of intellectual development (Kolb & Fantie, 1989). Further evidence is suggested from EEG coherence studies that indicate that brain maturation progresses in a discontinuous manner and, more specifically, that the cycles in brain maturation are consistent with Piagetian theory (Case, 1992; Hudspeth & Pribram, 1990, 1992; Thatcher, 1994, 1997). Intracortical connections are noted to demonstrate growth spurts and plateaus that coincide with developments in cognitive functioning described by Piaget.

Distinct roles for systems within the right and left hemispheres have also been proposed (Goldberg & Costa, 1981). These are reminiscent of Piaget's conception of assimilation and accommodation. The right hemisphere is thought to be responsible for assembling descriptive systems (accommodation), whereas the left hemisphere is equipped for integrating and applying these well-formed descriptive systems (assimilation). This mechanism is further considered to embody the dichotomy between the processing of events that are novel or unexpected and the processing of highly predictable, expected, or routine events. A third dimension of interest is revealed in descriptions of the activity intrinsic to accommodation and assimilation (Piaget, 1954). Accommodation is involved in seeking regularities in one's experiences, which are established through experimentation (i.e., through inductive reasoning processes). In contrast, assimilation incorporates one's experiences into a preexisting system of relationships; that is, assimilation operates through the deductive construction of previously developed schemata.

The preceding discussion emphasized three principal axes of neurodevelopment for their role in the integrative action of the brain. One outcome of a perturbation in these neural systems may be reflected in the inability of the child with NLD or AS to form mental schemata or representations of his or her world; that is, to form the adaptive descriptive systems that entail both coding and representing novel experiences, and to apply those systems effectively and efficiently. From this it can also be expected that these children will gravitate toward the rule-governed aspects of learning and show a limited capacity for abstraction and generalization. Similarly, it may be predicted that there will be a greater reliance on poorly developed and limited deductive versus inductive reasoning processes when coping with new information.

DIRECTIONS FOR FUTURE RESEARCH

The NLD syndrome is manifest most clearly on a "developmental" basis and persists into adulthood (Rourke & Fisk, 1988, 1992). However, it is also seen in the clinical presentation of persons suffering from a wide variety of types of neurological and neuroendocrine disease, disorder, and dysfunction. These include significant tissue destruction within the right cerebral hemisphere (Rourke et al., 1983) and some types of hydrocephalus (Fletcher, Brookshire, Bohan, Brandt, & Davidson, 1995), callosal agenesis (Smith & Rourke, 1995), congenital hypothyroidism (Rovet, 1995), and other pathological processes that have as one of their results significant perturbations of neuronal white matter (long myelinated fibers). Some other examples include persons with Williams syndrome (Anderson & Rourke, 1995; MacDonald & Roy, 1988; Udwin & Yule, 1991) and AS (Klin, Sparrow, Volkmar, Cicchetti, & Rourke, 1995). It is because of this that we refer to the NLD phenotype as the "final common pathway" for a variety of neurological disorders. It also why we maintain that significant right-hemisphere damage or dysfunction is sufficient to cause the NLD syndrome, but it is not necessary (Rourke, 1995).

In addition, whereas there is evidence to suggest that these disorders share the neurocognitive profile evident in NLD, there are observable differences in terms of the manifestation of social disabilities in these groups. There are many individuals with NLD and no associated disorder whose social disability is not as severe as that seen in AS. An especially interesting direction for future research will be to examine the relationship between the NLD neuropsychological profile and the manifestation of social disability. In this regard, we have presented an account of the dynamics of the NLD syndrome from which testable hypotheses can be developed and studied. Predictions have also been made based on our knowledge of brain development. Advances in neuroimaging provide the opportunity to explore further the brain maturational factors that are thought to be involved in NLD. (For an up-to-date account of the diseases and disorders of childhood wherein the NLD syndrome is manifest, readers should consult Rourke, 1995).

CONCLUSIONS

There is strong evidence to suggest that individuals with AS present with virtually all the characteristics of NLD. Most important, this neuropsychological phenotype may offer a basis from which to draw a distinction between AS and HFA. Relative differences in their neuropsychological profiles may be indicative of a differential pathway of expression. The research on AS is at a relatively early stage, and this is especially the case here with respect to understanding its pathogenesis. Given the similar phenomenology of NLD and AS, it is also expected that the developmental manifestations of NLD can offer an understanding of AS.

A model has been proposed to explain the dynamics of the NLD syndrome from both a cognitive–developmental and brain maturation perspective, and it is hoped that this discussion points to new avenues of investigation. In our continuing studies, we also expect to shed some further light on the similarities between the AS and the NLD phenotype as well as on the possible brain abnormalities that underlie their expression.

REFERENCES

American Psychiatric Association. (1987). *Diagnostic and statistical manual of mental disorders* (3rd ed., rev.). Washington, DC: Author.

Anderson, P. E., & Rourke, B. P. (1995). Williams syndrome. In B. P. Rourke (Ed.), *Syndrome of nonverbal learning disabilities: Neurodevelopmental manifestations* (pp. 138–170). New York: Guilford Press.

Barth, D. S., & MacDonald, K. D. (1996). Thalamic modulation of high-frequency oscillating potentials in auditory cortex. *Nature, 383,* 78–81.

Berthier, M. L., Bayes, A., & Tolosa, E. S. (1993). Magnetic resonance imaging in patients with concurrent Tourette's disorder and Asperger's syndrome. *Journal of the American Academy of Child and Adolescent Psychiatry, 32,* 633–639.

Bieliauskas, L. A. (1991). Case studies of adults with nonverbal learning disabilities. In B. P. Rourke (Ed.), *Neuropsychological validation of learning disability subtypes* (pp. 370–376). New York: Guilford Press.

Bigler, E. D. (1989). On the neuropsychology of suicide. *Journal of Learning Disabilities, 22,* 180–185.

Brumback, R. A., Harper, C. R., & Weinberg, W. A. (1996). Nonverbal learning disabilities, Asperger's syndrome, pervasive developmental disorder—Should we care? *Journal of Child Neurology, 11,* 427–429.

Case, R. (1992). The role of the frontal lobes in regulation of cognitive development. *Brain and Cognition, 20,* 51–73.

Casey, J. E., & Rourke, B. P. (1992). Disorders of somatosensory perception in children. In I. Rapin & S. J. Segalowitz (Eds.), *Handbook of neuropsychology, Vol. 6: Child neuropsychology* (pp. 477–494). Amsterdam: Elsevier.

Casey, J. E., Rourke, B. P., & Picard, E. M. (1991). Syndrome of nonverbal learning disabilities: Age differences in neuropsychological, academic, and socioemotional functioning. *Development and Psychopathology, 3,* 329–345.

Damasio, A. R. (1990). Synchronous activation in multiple cortical regions: A mechanism for recall. *Seminars in Neuroscience, 2,* 287–296.

Damasio, A. R., & Anderson, S. W. (1993). The frontal lobes. In K. M. Heilman & E.

Valenstein (Eds.), *Clinical neuropsychology* (3rd ed., pp. 409–460). New York: Oxford University Press.

Denckla, M. B. (1983). The neuropsychology of social–emotional learning disabilities. *Archives of Neurology, 40,* 461–462.

Dietrich, R. B., & Bradley, W. G. (1988). Normal and abnormal white matter maturation. *Seminars in Ultrasound, CT, and MR, 9,* 192–200.

Ehlers, S., Nyden, A., Gillberg, C., Dahlgren-Sandberg, A., Dahlgren, S. -O., Hjelmquist, E., & Oden, A. (1997). Asperger syndrome, autism, and attention disorders: A comparative study of the cognitive profiles of 120 children. *Journal of Child Psychology and Psychiatry, 38,* 207–217.

Ellis, H. D., & Gunter, H. L. (1999). Asperger syndrome: A simple matter of white matter? *Trends in Cognitive Sciences, 3,* 192–200.

Fletcher, J. M. (1985). External validation of learning disability typologies. In B. P. Rourke (Ed.), *Neuropsychology of learning disabilities: Essentials of subtype analysis* (pp. 187–211). New York: Guilford Press.

Fletcher, J. M. (1989). Nonverbal learning disabilities and suicide: Classification leads to prevention. *Journal of Learning Disabilities, 22,* 176, 179.

Fletcher, J. M., Brookshire, B. L., Bohan, T. P., Brandt, M. E., & Davidson, K. C. (1995). Early hydrocephalus. In B. P. Rourke (Ed.), *Syndrome of nonverbal learning disabilities: Neurodevelopmental manifestations* (pp. 206–238). New York: Guilford Press.

Fuerst, D. R., & Rourke, B. P. (1993). Psychosocial functioning of children: Relations between personality subtypes and academic achievement. *Journal of Abnormal Child Psychology, 21,* 597–607.

Goldberg, E., & Costa, L. D. (1981). Hemisphere differences in the acquisition and use of descriptive systems. *Brain and Language, 14,* 144–173.

Gross-Tsur, V., Shalev, R. S., Manor, O., & Amir, N. (1995). Developmental right-hemisphere syndrome: Clinical spectrum of the nonverbal learning disability. *Journal of Learning Disabilities, 28,* 80–86.

Harnadek, M. C. S., & Rourke, B. P. (1994). Principal identifying features of the syndrome of nonverbal learning disabilities in children. *Journal of Learning Disabilities, 27,* 144–154.

Hudspeth, W. J., & Pribram, K. H. (1990). Stages of brain and cognitive maturation. *Journal of Educational Psychology, 82,* 881–884.

Hudspeth, W. J., & Pribram, K. H. (1992). Psychological indices of cerebral maturation. *International Journal of Psychophysiology, 12,* 19–29.

Huttenlocher, P. R. (1984). Synapse elimination and plasticity in developing human cerebral cortex. *American Journal of Mental Deficiency, 88,* 488–496.

Huttenlocher, P. R. (1994). Synaptogenesis in human cerebral cortex. In G. Dawson & K. W. Fischer (Eds.), *Human behavior and the developing brain* (pp. 137–152). New York: Guilford Press.

Klin, A., Sparrow, S. S., Volkmar, F. R., Cicchetti, D. V., & Rourke, B. P. (1995). Asperger syndrome. In B. P. Rourke (Ed.), *Syndrome of nonverbal learning disabilities: Neurodevelopmental manifestations* (pp. 93–118). New York: Guilford Press.

Klin, A., Volkmar, F. R., Sparrow, S. S., Cicchetti, D. V., & Rourke, B. P. (1995). Validity and neuropsychological characterization of Asperger syndrome: Convergence with Nonverbal Learning Disabilities syndrome. *Journal of Child Psychology and Psychiatry, 36,* 1127–1140.

Kolb, B., & Fantie, B. (1989). Development of the child's brain and behavior. In C.

Reynolds & E. Fletcher-Janzen (Eds.), *Handbook of clinical child neuropsychology.* New York: Plenum.

MacDonald, G. W., & Roy, D. L. (1988). Williams syndrome: A neuropsychological profile. *Journal of Clinical and Experimental Neuropsychology, 10,* 125–131.

Majovski, L. V. (1989). Higher cortical functions in children: A developmental perspective. In C. Reynolds & E. Fletcher-Janzen (Eds.), *Handbook of clinical child neuropsychology.* New York: Plenum.

McKelvey, J. R., Lambert, R., Mottron, L., & Shevell, M. I. (1995). Right-hemisphere dysfunction in Asperger's syndrome. *Journal of Child Neurology, 10,* 310–314.

Mega, M. S., Cummings, J. L., Salloway, S., & Malloy, P. (1997). The limbic system: An anatomic, phylogenetic, and clinical perspective. *Journal of Neuropsychiatry and Clinical Neurosciences, 9,* 315–330.

Molina, J. L., Ruata, J. M., & Soler, E. P. (1986). Is there a right-hemisphere dysfunction in Asperger's syndrome? *British Journal of Psychiatry, 148,* 745–746.

Myklebust, H. R. (1975). Nonverbal learning disabilities: Assessment and intervention. In H. R. Myklebust (Ed.), *Progress in learning disabilities* (Vol. 3, pp. 85–121). New York: Grune & Stratton.

Nass, R., & Gutman, R. (1997). Boys with Asperger's disorder, exceptional verbal intelligence, tics, and clumsiness. *Developmental Medicine and Child Neurology, 39,* 691–695.

Piaget, J. (1951). *Play, dreams, and imitation in childhood.* New York: Norton.

Piaget, J. P. (1954). *The construction of reality in the child.* New York: Basic Books.

Piaget, J. P. (1963). *The origins of intelligence in children.* New York: Norton.

Piaget, J. P., & Inhelder, B. (1969). *The psychology of the child.* London: Routledge & Kegan Paul.

Rourke, B. P. (1975). Brain–behavior relationships in children with learning disabilities. *American Psychologist, 30,* 911–920.

Rourke, B. P. (1978). Reading, spelling, arithmetic disabilities: A neuropsychologic perspective. In H. R. Myklebust (Ed.), *Progress in learning disabilities* (Vol. 4, pp. 97–120). New York: Grune & Stratton.

Rourke, B. P. (1982). Central processing deficiencies in children: Toward a developmental neuropsychological model. *Journal of Clinical Neuropsychology, 4,* 10–18.

Rourke, B. P. (1987). Syndrome of nonverbal learning disabilities: The final common pathway of white-matter disease/dysfunction? *The Clinical Neuropsychologist, 1,* 209–234.

Rourke, B. P. (1988a). Socioemotional disturbances of learning disabled children. *Journal of Consulting and Clinical Psychology, 56,* 801–810.

Rourke, B. P. (1988b). The syndrome of nonverbal learning disabilities: Developmental manifestations in neurological disease, disorder, and dysfunction. *The Clinical Neuropsychologist, 2,* 293–330.

Rourke, B. P. (1989). *Nonverbal learning disabilities: The syndrome and the model.* New York: Guilford Press.

Rourke, B. P. (1993). Arithmetic disabilities, specific and otherwise: A neuropsychological perspective. *Journal of Learning Disabilities, 26,* 214–226.

Rourke, B. P. (Ed.). (1995). *Syndrome of nonverbal learning disabilities: Neurodevelopmental manifestations.* New York: Guilford Press.

Rourke, B. P., Bakker, D. J., Fisk, J. L., & Strang, J. D. (1983). *Child neuropsychology: An introduction to theory, research, and clinical practice.* New York: Guilford Press.

Rourke, B. P., & Finlayson, M. A. J. (1978). Neuropsychological significance of variations in patterns of academic performance: Verbal and visual–spatial abilities. *Journal of Abnormal Child Psychology, 6,* 121–133.

Rourke, B. P., & Fisk, J. L. (1988). Subtypes of learning-disabled children: Implications for a neurodevelopmental model of differential hemispheric processing. In D. L. Molfese & S. J. Segalowitz (Eds.), *Brain lateralization in children: Developmental implications* (pp. 547–565). New York: Guilford Press.

Rourke, B. P., & Fisk, J. L. (1992). Adult presentations of learning disabilities. In R. F. White (Ed.), *Clinical syndromes in adult neuropsychology: The practitioner's handbook* (pp. 451–473). Amsterdam: Elsevier.

Rourke, B. P., & Fuerst, D. R. (1991). *Learning disabilities and psychosocial functioning: A Neuropsychological perspective.* New York: Guilford Press.

Rourke, B. P., & Fuerst, D. R. (1992). Psychosocial dimensions of learning disability subtypes: Neuropsychological studies in the Windsor Laboratory. *School Psychology Review, 21,* 360–373.

Rourke, B. P., & Strang, J. D. (1978). Neuropsychological significance of variations in patterns of academic performance: Motor, psychomotor, and tactile–perceptual abilities. *Journal of Pediatric Psychology, 3,* 62–66.

Rourke, B. P., & Strang, J. D. (1983). Subtypes of reading and arithmetical disabilities: A neuropsychological analysis. In M. Rutter (Ed.), *Developmental neuropsychiatry* (pp. 473–488). New York: Guilford Press.

Rourke, B. P., & Tsatsanis, K. D. (1996). Syndrome of nonverbal learning disabilities: Psycholinguistic assets and deficits. *Topics in Language Disorders, 16,* 30–44.

Rourke, B. P., Young, G. C., & Leenaars, A. A. (1989). A childhood learning disability that predisposes those afflicted to adolescent and adult depression and suicide risk. *Journal of Learning Disabilities, 21,* 169–175.

Rovet, J. (1995). Congenital hypothyroidism. In B. P. Rourke (Ed.), *Syndrome of nonverbal learning disabilities: Neurodevelopmental manifestations* (pp. 255–281). New York: Guilford Press.

Smith, L. A., & Rourke, B. P. (1995). Callosal agenesis. In B. P. Rourke (Ed.), *Syndrome of nonverbal learning disabilities: Neurodevelopmental manifestations* (pp. 45–92). New York: Guilford Press.

Sparrow, S. S. (1991). Case studies of children with nonverbal learning disabilities. In B. P. Rourke (Ed.), *Neuropsychological validation of learning disability subtypes* (pp. 349–355). New York: Guilford Press.

Steriade, M., McCormick, D. A., & Sejnowski, T. J. (1993). Thalamocortical oscillations in the sleeping and aroused brain. *Science, 262,* 679–685.

Strang, J. D., & Rourke, B. P. (1983). Concept-formation/non-verbal reasoning abilities of children who exhibit specific academic problems with arithmetic. *Journal of Clinical Child Psychology, 12,* 33–39.

Strang, J. D., & Rourke, B. P. (1985a). Adaptive behavior of children who exhibit specific arithmetic disabilities and associated neuropsychological abilities and deficits. In B. P. Rourke (Ed.), *Neuropsychology of learning disabilities: Essentials of subtype analysis* (pp. 302–328). New York: Guilford Press.

Strang, J. D., & Rourke, B. P. (1985b). Arithmetic disability subtypes: The neuropsychological significance of specific arithmetical impairment in childhood. In B. P. Rourke (Ed.), *Neuropsychology of learning disabilities: Essentials of subtype analysis* (pp. 167–183). New York: Guilford Press.

Stuss, D. T. (1992). Biological and psychological development of executive functions. *Brain and Cognition, 20,* 8–23.

Thatcher, R. W. (1994). Cyclic cortical reorganization: Origins of human cognitive development. In G. Dawson & K. W. Fischer (Eds.), *Human behavior and the developing brain* (pp. 232–266). New York: Guilford Press.

Thatcher, R. W. (1997). Neuroimaging of cyclic cortical reorganization during human development. In R. W. Thatcher (Ed.), *Developmental neuroimaging: Mapping the development of brain and behavior* (pp. 91–106). San Diego: Academic Press.

Torgeson, J. K. (1993). Variations on theory in learning disabilities. In G. R. Lyon, D. B. Gray, J. F. Kavanagh, & N. A. Krasnegor (Eds.), *Better understanding learning disabilities: New views from research and their implications for education and public policies* (pp. 153–170). Baltimore: Paul H. Brookes.

Tranel, D., Hall, L. E., Olson, S., & Tranel, N. N. (1987). Evidence for a right hemisphere developmental learning disability. *Developmental Neuropsychology, 3,* 113–120.

Tsatsanis, K. D., Fuerst, D. R., & Rourke, B. P. (1997). Psychosocial dimensions of learning disabilities: External validation and relationship with age and academic functioning. *Journal of Learning Disabilities, 30,* 490–502.

Tsatsanis, K. D., & Rourke, B. P. (1995). Conclusions and future directions. In B. P. Rourke (Ed.), *Syndrome of nonverbal learning disabilities: Neurodevelopmental manifestations* (pp. 476–496). New York: Guilford Press.

Tulving, E., Markowitsch, H. J., Kapur, S., Habib, R., & Houle, S. (1994). Novelty encoding networks in the human brain: positron emission tomography data. *NeuroReport, 5,* 2525–2528.

Udwin, O., & Yule, W. (1991). A cognitive and behavioral phenotype in Williams syndrome. *Journal of Clinical and Experimental Neuropsychology, 13,* 232–244.

van der Vlugt, H. (1991). Neuropsychological validation studies of learning disability subtypes: Verbal, visual–spatial, and psychomotor abilities. In B. P. Rourke (Ed.), *Neuropsychological validation of learning disability subtypes* (pp. 140–159). New York: Guilford Press.

van der Vlugt, H., & Satz, P. (1985). Subgroups and subtypes of learning-disabled and normal children: A cross-cultural replication. In B. P. Rourke (Ed.), *Neuropsychology of learning disabilities: Essentials of subtype analysis* (pp. 212–227). New York: Guilford Press.

Voeller, K. K. S. (1986). Right-hemisphere deficit syndrome in children. *American Journal of Psychiatry, 143,* 1004–1009.

Volkmar, F. R., Klin, A., Schultz, R., Bronen, R., Marans, W. D., Sparrow, S., & Cohen, D. J. (1996). Asperger's syndrome. *Journal of the American Academy of Child and Adolescent Psychiatry, 35,* 118–123.

Weintraub, S., & Mesulam, M.-M. (1983). Developmental learning disabilities of the right hemisphere: Emotional, interpersonal, and cognitive *components. Archives of Neurology, 40,* 463–469.

Wing, L. (1981). Asperger's syndrome: A clinical account. *Psychological Medicine, 11,* 115–130.

World Health Organization. (1992). *International classification of diseases: Tenth revision.* Chapter V. Mental and behavioral disorders (including disorders of psychological development). Diagnostic criteria for research. Geneva: Author.

9

What's So Special about Asperger Syndrome?
The Need for Further Exploration of the Borderlands of Autism

D. V. M. BISHOP

Readers may be surprised to find that this volume contains a contribution by an expert on childhood language disorders, as according to the fourth edition of the *Diagnostic and Statistical Manual of Mental Disorders* (DSM-IV; American Psychiatric Association, 1994) definition of Asperger syndrome (AS) the diagnosis requires that there is no clinically significant language delay. The aim of this chapter is to provide a counterbalance to the weight of research that is concerned with whether there is a continuum between AS and autistic disorder. I argue that, by concentrating on these two conditions, researchers have created the impression that there is a single continuum, with autistic disorder at one end and AS at the other. This impression has led many people to suppose that AS is the appropriate diagnosis for any child who falls within the autistic spectrum, is of normal intelligence, but who does not meet full criteria for autistic disorder. In this chapter, I present evidence against this view. My argument is that there are many children whose deficits resemble mild forms of autism but who do *not* have the constellation of features characterizing AS. Some of these children occupy a position intermediate between autistic disorder and developmental language disorder. The diagnostic boundaries between pervasive and specific developmental disorders are, according to this view, much less clear-cut than the textbooks seem to imply.

A second point is that the judgment of whether or not a child has normal language development depends critically on which aspects of language we consider. In particular, there are children whose ability to use language appropriately in communicative contexts is extremely poor, despite good or even superior knowledge of grammar and phonology (speech sounds). Questions about the relationship between language disorder and autistic spectrum disorders have been clouded by a failure to draw a distinction between formal knowledge of language structure and ability to use language to communicate effectively.

The structure of the chapter is as follows. First, I review the way in which autistic disorder and specific language impairment (SLI) have been conceptualized over the past 18 years. I then consider the evidence for children who fall between conventional diagnostic boundaries, moving on to focus specifically on children whose symptom profile overlaps with both autism and SLI. The category of "semantic–pragmatic disorder" has been proposed for such cases but has been difficult to validate because we lack suitable measures to quantify the relevant symptoms. I present some checklist data from a pilot study that was designed to tackle this issue. These checklist data confirm that there are significant numbers of language-impaired children who do have disproportionate difficulty with language content and use, and that they tend to have associated autistic features. However, there is substantial variation in symptom profile from child to child, and such children do not typically have distinctive semantic impairments. It is proposed that rather than subsuming such children under the umbrella category of pervasive developmental disorder not otherwise specified (PDD-NOS), they should be referred to as cases of pragmatic language impairment. It should be recognized that these children have some symptomatic overlap with *both* SLI *and* autistic disorder, rather than forcing them into one category or the other. Finally, I conclude by pointing out that the emphasis on differential diagnosis between AS and autistic disorder has diverted attention from other conditions which may be regarded as falling in the autistic spectrum, and which are clinically important but have attracted little research attention.

RELATIONSHIP BETWEEN LANGUAGE DISORDER AND AUTISTIC SPECTRUM: EVOLVING DIAGNOSTIC CONCEPTS IN DSM

DSM-III (American Psychiatric Association, 1980) drew a theoretical distinction between the *specific* developmental disorders and *pervasive* developmental disorders as follows:

Pervasive Developmental Disorders differ from the Specific Developmental Disorders in two basic ways. First, only a single specific function is affected in each Specific Developmental Disorder, whereas in Pervasive Developmental Disorders multiple functions are always affected. Second, in Specific Developmental Disorder the children behave as if they are passing through an earlier normal developmental stage, because the disturbance is a *delay* in development, whereas children with Pervasive Developmental Disorders display severe qualitative abnormalities that are not normal for any stage of development, because the disturbance is a *distortion* in development. (p. 86).

At the time that DSM-III appeared, most children who were thought to merit a diagnosis of pervasive developmental disorder (PDD) were cases of infantile autism, plus a smattering of cases with rarer forms where there was onset in childhood or an atypical presentation. Developmental language disorder was regarded as a prototypical *specific* developmental disorder (see Figure 9.1). An early study by Bartak, Rutter, and Cox (1975), comparing children with autism and children with receptive developmental language disorder (then termed "developmental dysphasia"), offered some validation of this view: Children in the autistic group had a much broader range of impairments, affecting nonverbal as well as verbal communication, and they had a number of features that did not seem to correspond to any normal stage of development, and so could reasonably be described as distortions (see Figure 9.2).

A problem with the DSM-III scheme was that clinicians soon found that there were many children whose pattern of impairments did not correspond to clear-cut cases of either autism or developmental language disorder. In

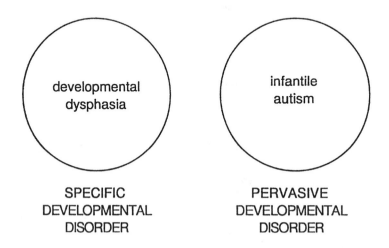

FIGURE 9.1. Diagnostic distinction between specific and pervasive developmental disorders as specified in DSM-III.

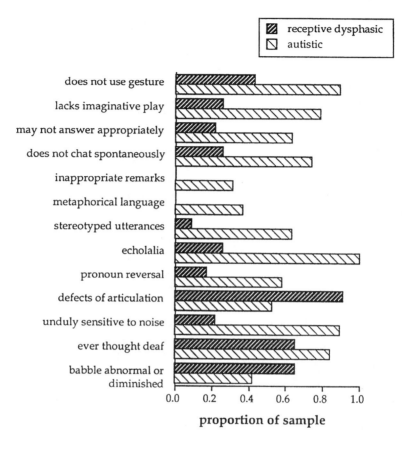

FIGURE 9.2. Summary of findings from Bartak et al. (1975), comparing 19 autistic children with 23 children with developmental receptive dysphasia. Most characteristics were scored positive if the child had ever shown that behavior, regardless of whether it was still present at the time of assessment.

1981, Wing published a paper drawing attention to Asperger's descriptions of children who appeared to have no difficulty in learning the intricacies of language but who had unusual interests and impairments of social behavior. Most clinicians welcomed the term "AS," which provided a diagnostic label for a group of children who had hitherto been difficult to categorize.

The limitations of the DSM-III scheme were addressed to some extent in later revisions, so that by DSM-IV, three modifications were in place:

1. The diagnostic criteria for what was now referred to as "autistic disorder" were refined. The language impairments of autistic children

were described in more detail, stressing that the abnormalities affected both verbal and nonverbal communication.

2. The category of AS was added (with diagnostic criteria as described in Chapter 2, this volume). Although the diagnostic criteria specify that "there are no clinically significant delays in language," this is defined in relation to mastery of language milestones and in terms of sentence length and complexity rather than to how language is used.

3. The category of PDD-NOS was added to provide a diagnosis for cases in which there is a "severe and pervasive impairment in the development of reciprocal social interaction, verbal and nonverbal communication skills or the development of stereotyped behaviour, interests and activities," including cases where there is late age at onset, or "atypical" or "subthreshold" symptomatology (pp. 77–78).

Figure 9.3 illustrates this framework.

A categorical diagnostic label implies that a cluster of symptoms tends to co-occur, and that individuals in the particular part of three-dimensional space corresponding to that cluster will be more numerous than those in surrounding regions. This is reflected in DSM-IV, where PDD-NOS merits eight lines of description, compared with just over two pages for AS, and five and a half pages for autistic disorder. The message is clear: PDD-NOS is thought of as a default diagnosis, to be applied only to rare children for whom other diagnoses are inappropriate. Accordingly, PDD-NOS is not a focus of clinical or research interest, and there is little published information about the nature, correlates, prognosis, and treatment of children with this diagnosis.

HOW COMMON ARE CHILDREN WHO FALL BETWEEN DIAGNOSTIC BOUNDARIES?

The existence of children who fall in the unlabeled areas of Figure 9.3 cannot be doubted, but it is difficult to establish is how rare they are. Quite simply, children who do not meet diagnostic criteria for autistic disorder, AS, or SLI tend not to be included in research studies. However, Klin (personal communication, 1996) reported that a diagnosis of PDD-NOS was *more* common than either AS or autism in children referred to the Yale Child Study Center.

Further evidence for "intermediate" or "subclinical" cases comes from a study of relatives of individuals affected with autistic disorder. Bolton et al. (1994) used a standardized interview to assess functioning in the domains of language, social interaction, and stereotyped behavior and reported that although few relatives met criteria for autistic disorder, many of them had impairments in just one or two of these domains.

Turning the question on its head, we may also consider how common

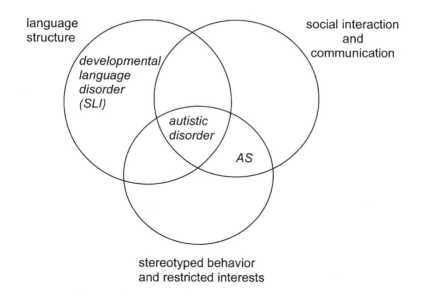

FIGURE 9.3. Set diagram representation of the diagnostic possibilities offered by DSM-IV. Each set shows impairment in one domain of functioning: "Language structure" refers to mastery of grammar and speech sounds, as reflected in age at passing language milestones, and complexity and clarity of spoken language. "Social interaction and communication" refers to use of language and nonverbal means to communicate with others. "Stereotyped behavior and restricted interests" refers to diversity of interests and creativity as well as repetitive behaviors. The default category PDD-NOS would be applied to children who had impairments in one or two of the three areas of functioning but who fell outside the boundaries of one of the other categories (i.e., those areas that are unlabeled in the figure).

are social impairments in children with language difficulties. It is commonly assumed that any social limitations in language-impaired children are just a secondary consequence of their communicative problems (see Bishop, 1997, for a review). However, it is difficult to reconcile this view with work by Paul, Spangle-Looney, and Dahm (1991), who reported that in a sample of children with expressive language delay at 2 years of age, 48% were impaired on the socialization scale of the Vineland Adaptive Behavior Scales at 3 years of age, even when items with a verbal component were excluded from consideration. Receptive language delay in 3-year-olds was virtually *always* accompanied by socialization problems.

Taken together, these pieces of evidence indicate that there is no necessary association between the three domains of impairment that characterize autism: They can be dissociated, especially in higher-functioning individuals. "Subthreshold symptomatology," or impairments affecting only two of the three domains shown in Figure 9.3, are not uncommon. Many children whose predominant presenting problems are with spoken language are found to have broader limitations of socialization when properly assessed. In practice, such individuals may be labeled PDD-NOS, or, if their language problems are particularly striking, they may be included as cases of developmental language disorder. My own studies suggest that the latter situation commonly arises, and that the population of children diagnosed as having developmental language disorder contains a substantial minority who have abnormalities in the use of nonverbal as well as verbal communication, and some who have restricted or peculiar interests similar to those in AS.

HOW SHARP IS THE BOUNDARY BETWEEN AUTISM AND DEVELOPMENTAL LANGUAGE DISORDER?

The pioneering study by Bartak et al. (1975), comparing cases of infantile autism and developmental receptive dysphasia, is typically cited as evidence for a qualitative distinction between these two disorders. However, this study did include five cases which, at the outset, were recognized as having both a language disorder and some autistic features: These cases were termed the "mixed group." Furthermore, as the children have been followed up into adolescence and adulthood, clearer evidence has emerged of more pervasive impairments of social interaction and abnormal interests in some of the original dysphasic group (Mawhood, 1995), and the separation of the two groups by a discriminant function analysis has proved much less efficient. The following vignettes from Mawhood illustrate that individuals initially classified as cases of developmental receptive dysphasia had abnormalities in the areas of social behavior and interests in adulthood, although these typically were far less severe than those seen in adults with autism.

> (participant DLD8, age 22 years)
>
> In all aspects of self-care he was entirely independent and he could use a telephone and manage his finances himself. Most of his spare time was spent pursuing his preoccupation with trains and his less intense interest in CB radio. He spent a lot of time hanging around railway stations, going on train rides when he could afford it, and looking at train magazines. His social overtures were somewhat limited and he would speak if spoken to but would not make the first move. There were two friends that he visited regularly; one shared his interest in trains, the other was interested in CB radio. These relationships were clearly selective, did involve some apparent pleasure in each other's company, and some sharing of confidences, but there was still nonetheless a slightly odd quality to them because of their restricted range of interests. He did not appear to be lonely. (p. 384)

(participant DLD9, age 25 years)

[At 9 years of age] the quality of his peer relationships was said to be slightly abnormal. He showed some evidence of ritualistic behaviour and marked quasi-obsessive activities and attachments to odd objects. When followed-up . . . he was living independently in a flat belonging to an organisation that specialised in providing accommodation for disabled people. . . . He looked after himself entirely independently. . . . He was able to cope with most things provided he had come across them before but had difficulty with the unexpected, e.g., his cooker started to smoke and he didn't know what to do. . . . He did voluntary work cleaning a local monument twice a week, but other than this filled his time with doing his domestic chores, weight training at a local health club and looking after his extensive collection of model aeroplanes. He was very interested in this collection, but not really preoccupied. . . . His speech was now fairly well developed and his grammar was largely correct with occasional errors. . . . He could follow a fairly simple plot but would get lost if the story became too complex. If he gave an account of events he would pay attention to minute detail, and he could converse well although he would tend to talk about things he was interested in. . . . He could make acquaintances but sometimes started conversations in slightly inappropriate ways, e.g., by talking about the *Encyclopedia Britannica* and saying "Did you know that . . . ?" He did not appear to want any close friends although he met up with the curate at his church every couple of weeks for a chat and a meal, and seemed to enjoy his company. . . . He showed some understanding of how other people were feeling and his mother said he would show appropriate concern if someone was not feeling happy. Girls were of absolutely no interest to him. He could only see the difficulties involved rather than any of the positive emotional aspects and said "girls are just trouble." (pp. 385–386)

These cases suggest that far from being separate conditions, receptive language disorder and autism might lie on a single continuum. Yet this view is radically different from conventional wisdom as embodied in our textbooks and depicted in Figure 9.1. How are we to resolve this paradox?

THE CONCEPT OF A "SEMANTIC–PRAGMATIC" SUBTYPE OF DEVELOPMENTAL LANGUAGE DISORDER

Light was thrown on this question with the publication of a nosology of developmental dysphasia by Rapin and Allen (1983). Rather than adopting traditional distinctions between "expressive" and "receptive" forms of language disorder, Rapin and Allen drew attention to the different ways in which expressive and receptive language could be impaired. Of particular interest was their delineation of a category of "semantic–pragmatic deficit syndrome," in which children had relatively good mastery of language form (i.e., grammar and phonology) but abnormal content and poor use of language. Rapin (1982) gave the following account of semantic–pragmatic syndrome[1]:

> Children with this syndrome have no difficulty decoding phonology or producing well formed sentences. Their deficit affects comprehension and use of language. They have trouble understanding discourse. . . . The children usually have an intact or superior auditory memory and are fluent. They may repeat whole sentences verbatim or recite TV commercials. While they often have no difficulty retrieving verbal labels for objects or pictures, they nonetheless have an anomia in spontaneous speech. As a result, some of their words miss the mark despite the fact that they belong to the appropriate semantic field. This gives their speech a loose, tangential, or somewhat inappropriate quality. Their train of thought appears illogical and difficult to follow. . . . The children's comprehension deficit is likely to be overlooked or underestimated because their spontaneous speech is so fluent and because they understand single words and simple phrases and are sociable. (p. 145)

In their nosology, Rapin and Allen were not concerned with differential diagnosis from autism or AS: They regarded the characterization of a child's language disorder as orthogonal to a psychiatric diagnosis, and they noted that semantic–pragmatic disorder is commonly seen in children with autism (although other language profiles are also found). However, importantly, they noted that the same type of language difficulties could be observed in children who did not have autism, a point reiterated in a recent review by Rapin (1996).

In a study of *nonautistic* children receiving special educational facilities for those with specific developmental language disorders, Bishop and Adams (1989) described a number of distinctive communicative characteristics of children who met the clinical picture of semantic–pragmatic disorder (see Table 9.1). Similarities with observations of communicative behavior in children with AS are evident, but the children studied by Bishop and Adams had severe delays in passing early language milestones as well.

Bishop and Rosenbloom (1987) noted that children who are diagnosed as having semantic–pragmatic disorder seemed to differ qualitatively from other language-impaired children: They tended to have associated social and behavioral abnormalities similar to those seen in autism. These similarities have led some authors to argue that semantic–pragmatic disorder

---

[1]Rapin and Allen (1987) refer to "semantic–pragmatic deficit syndrome," and Bishop and Rosenbloom (1987) to "semantic–pragmatic disorder." The latter term is used henceforth in this chapter.

TABLE 9.1. Conversational Characteristics of Language-Impaired Children with Semantic–Pragmatic Disorder

The following examples of conversational extracts are taken from children ages 8 to 12 years who fit the clinical picture of semantic–pragmatic disorder (Bishop & Adams, 1989). "C" denotes child, "A" denotes adult. Categories marked "*" are those in which children with semantic–pragmatic disorder differed not just from age-matched controls but also from younger control children aged 4 to 5 years.

Expressive problems in semantics/syntax*

Example 1
C: We went on a bus because Lee was sick out of the window. [Use of term that is overspecific in meaning, e.g., "because" or "but" when "and" is required]
Example 2
A: Why did you have to go to the doctor?
C: I used to have a headache. [Wrong verb tense/aspect]

Failure of literal comprehension

Example 3
A: Where did you go on holiday?
C: In September.

Failure to use context in comprehension (overliteral interpretation)

Example 4
A: (*after long session of work*) Can you stand to do some more?
C: (*Stands up.*)
Example 5
A: Are there any other times when you have parties?
C: No.
A: What about at Christmas?
C: It snows.

Too little information*

Example 6
C: (*talking about a jeweler's shop*) when you take the ring off it ones both of them are crowns. [Unestablished referent: unclear what "them" refers to]
Example 7
C: My brother was feeling sick on Monday.
A: Right.
C: And I took my trouser off.
A: Uhuh. Why did you take your trousers off?
C: He was sick on my trouser. [Logical step omitted, critical information provided only when A asked for clarification]

Too much information*

Example 8
A: Where have you been on a boat?
C: Where have I been? Haven't sailed a cruiser, you know. [Unnecessary denial of something that A had not assumed]
Example 9
A: Is that a good place to break down? (*referring to photograph of stranded motorist*)
C: The answer whether it's a good place to break down is no, because if see if anybody broke down, cos there's no telephone to telephone, there's no telephone for the breakdown. [Excessive elaboration]

(*continued*)

TABLE 9.1. (*cont.*)

Unusual content*

Example 10
A: What's going on there? (*referring to photo of birthday party*)
C: It's someone's birthday. Something could be dangerous, you know, like a fire from the candles. [Topic drift: child connects to previous utterances but steers conversation to a favored topic]

Example 11
A: Have you ever been to the doctor?
C: I had an apple a day. [Stereotyped language: no evidence that child was attempting to be humorous]

Example 12
C: Do you like candyfloss?
A: No.
C: Do you hate it?
A: I think it's all horrible and sticky.
C: Why? [Remorseless questioning by child]

is just another term for autism (Lister Brook & Bowler, 1992). There are two ways of interpreting this. It could mean that semantic–pragmatic disorder is simply a more acceptable label for children who actually would meet criteria for autistic disorder according to DSM-IV or *International Classification of Diseases* (World Health Organization, 1992). To accept this conclusion, not only would one have to assume a high rate of misdiagnosis among children attending special schools for those with language impairment, but one would also be left with the problem of how to classify the "intermediate" cases described in research studies that applied diagnostic criteria very carefully, such as that by Bartak et al. (1975) and Bolton et al. (1994).

A more reasonable hypothesis is that there are continuities between autistic disorder and semantic–pragmatic disorder, either in terms of underlying causes or in terms of symptomatology (Bishop, 1989). If this is the case, then semantic–pragmatic disorder would belong more properly in the autistic spectrum, corresponding to a subtype of PDD-NOS, rather than be seen as a subtype of specific developmental disorder. Tantalizing evidence suggesting etiological similarities comes from Woodhouse et al. (1996), who found that children with semantic–pragmatic disorder, like those with autism, had unusually large heads, whereas those with other kinds of developmental language disorder did not. In my own studies, I have been interested in trying to devise better methods for documenting the communicative and related impairments that characterize semantic–pragmatic disorder in order to assess the validity of the concept and to provide a means for comparing and contrasting children with this diagnosis and those with unambiguous diagnoses of autism or AS.

THE CHECKLIST FOR LANGUAGE-IMPAIRED CHILDREN: A PILOT STUDY[2]

A major difficulty confronting anyone wishing to study subtypes of language disorder is that we lack suitable instruments for the objective assessment of the behaviors that characterize semantic–pragmatic disorder. Most language tests measure complexity of expressive language form, verbal memory, or comprehension of vocabulary or sentences of increasing length and complexity. The impairments that are seen as typifying semantic–pragmatic disorder, such as verbosity, overliteral responding to questions, or problems in understanding connected discourse, are not identified on such measures. These behaviors are not only difficult to assess using contemporary measures but probably also more variable than other aspects of language behavior. Thus a child who appears "verbose" in some situations might be silent in others. For these reasons, it seemed worthwhile developing a checklist to obtain ratings from people who know the child well and have therefore had an opportunity to observe the child's behavior over time and in a range of situations. The disadvantages of ratings are well-known: Raters may differ in how they interpret questions, and they may use different criteria for deciding that a behavior applies. For this reason, a rating scale is only useful if one can demonstrate reasonable agreement between two independent raters. The study described here represents a preliminary attempt to devise a rating scale that would provide data that were both reliable and valid in distinguishing children with semantic–pragmatic disorder from other language-impaired children.

Design of the Checklist

After obtaining feedback from teachers and therapists on pilot versions of questions, a Checklist for Language-Impaired Children (CLIC) was devised.

As shown in Table 9.2, the checklist represented a range of communicative behaviors. Most of these items were selected with the aim of including behaviors that were highlighted in clinical classifications of language impairment but were not readily assessed on standardized tests. Additional items were included to assess nonverbal communication and behaviors that have been described as associated with PDD (i.e., social interaction, interests, attention, and gross motor skills).

Each CLIC item had five possible responses. In general, these were de-

---

[2]This section was written prior to the publication of an update on the empirical validation of Dr. Bishop's instrument. For this update, the reader is referred to Bishop (1998).

TABLE 9.2. Areas Covered by Checklist

Intelligibility (F)	Conversational responsiveness (C)
Expressive phonology (F)	Conversational assertiveness (C)
Grammar (F)	Conversational coherence (C)
Morphosyntax (F)	Use of context in comprehension (C)
Vocabulary (C)	Echolalia (past or present) (A)
Literal comprehension	Jargon (past or present) (A)
Narrative skills (C)	Eye contact (A)
Speech rate	Peer relations (A)
Fluency	Relations with adults (A)
Speech volume (C)	Interests (A)
Intonational melody (C)	Attention
	Gross motor skills

Note. Items coded F, C, or A contributed to composite scales (see text).

signed to fall on an ordinal scale, with one pole of the scale corresponding to the most normal response and the other to the most abnormal. However, for some behaviors it was difficult to devise items of this kind, because departures from normal behavior could take different forms, and for some items both poles represented abnormality, with more typical behavior corresponding to the mid-point of the scale. Table 9.3 shows a sample item. Raters were asked to check the item that was *most like* the child. If they felt that the child's behavior fell between two adjacent options, they were asked to check both options. Such dual responses were assigned a score intermediate between the two responses.

Sample

Head teachers from three residential schools were approached, and all agreed to take part, although the amount of data provided by each school depended on the willingness of individual staff members to participate. Each of the schools specialized in the education of children with specific language disorders and had stringent entry requirements, excluding children with mental handicap or serious behavioral problems. The aim was to obtain independent ratings for each pupil from two members of staff, one a teacher and one a speech–language therapist, each of whom had known the child for at least 3 months. A total of 17 teachers and 27 speech–language therapists participated in data collection. School head teachers were also sent a "diagnostic checklist" for each child, which included questions about whether the child had ever had a diagnosis of definite or possible semantic–pragmatic disorder, autistic disorder, autistic features, AS, or "clumsiness"/ coordination disorder. It was explained that these categories were not mutually exclusive, and the respondent was encouraged to check as many diagnoses as seemed to apply. Information was also gathered about any other

TABLE 9.3. Sample Item from CLIC

CLIC Item 10

How responsive is the child to conversational overtures from a familiar person?

- Frequently ignores conversational overtures from others (e.g., if asked "What are you making?" the child just continues working as if nothing had happened).
- Sometimes ignores conversational overtures from others.
- May not always give a verbal response to a conversational overture but will almost always respond nonverbally; by demonstration, gesture, nodding or shaking the head, smiling, etc. (e.g., if asked "What are you making?" the child will hold up or point to the thing that he is making and respond by looking or smiling).
- Usually gives an appropriate verbal response to a conversational overture but does not elaborate beyond the minimum response that is required (e.g., if asked "What are you making?" will reply "A boat").
- Typically gives a full and appropriate response that goes beyond the minimum required (e.g., if asked "What are you making?" will reply "A boat; we're going to sail it on the lake when it's finished").

Note. The full checklist is not shown here, because a new version is under evaluation. Readers interested in using CLIC should contact the author for details of the most recent version.

physical or sensory deficits. Only those who were diagnosed as having a developmental language disorder were included, and any children with a diagnosis of possible or definite autism were excluded. Table 9.4 shows the sample composition. Two checklists were completed by independent raters for the majority of pupils, but there was a subset of children for whom only one rating was available. Mean age for the whole sample was 11.07 years, with a range from 5 to 16 years.

Combination of Items into Language Dimensions

Each checklist item was recoded on a 5-point scale, such that maximum deficit corresponded to a score of –3, average performance to a score of 0, and

TABLE 9.4. Constitution of Sample for Checklist Study

Diagnostic information obtained from school	Checklist completed by therapist and teacher	Checklist completed by therapist only	Checklist completed by teacher only
Has developmental language disorder: not diagnosed as semantic–pragmatic disorder	71	28	3
Has developmental language disorder: diagnosed as possible or definite semantic–pragmatic disorder	26	5	0

superior performance to a score of 1. (For bipolar items, where the middle of
the scale represented normality, both poles might be given the same negative score.) After excluding individual items with low interrater reliability
(those assessing literal comprehension, speech rate, and fluency), scores
were combined into three scales (see Table 9.2): The first (F-scale) was composed of items assessing language *form* and the second (C-scale) measured
language *content and use*. A third scale, (A-scale) assessed presence of *autistic
features*, including several nonverbal behaviors.

Composite scale scores are reported only for those checklists in which
all items constituting the scales had been completed by both raters ($n = 83$).
For this sample size, a correlation of .22 is significant at the 5% level, and a
correlation of .28 at the 1% level. The F-scale (language form) had a possible
range of -12 to $+4$, and gave interrater agreement (r_i) of .848. The C-scale
(language content and use) had a possible range of scores from -22 to $+6$.
Interrater agreement on this scale was $r_i = .468$. The A-scale (autistic features) had a possible range from -12 to 0, with $r_i = .777$. Ratings on the
C-scale and A-scale were unrelated to age ($r < |.22|$). Scores on the F-scale
showed a statistically significant correlation with age (for teachers' ratings, $r
= .256$; for therapists' ratings, $r = .447$, $p < .05$).

The correlation between the F-scale and A-scale was nonsignificant for
teachers ($r = .016$), but a weak *negative* association was seen in ratings by
therapists ($r = -.237$), with better scores on language form being associated
with more autistic features. There was a positive association between the
C-scale and A-scale for both teachers ($r = .469$) and therapists ($r = .406$).

Distribution of Scores on Two Dimensions

Because more data were available from therapists than from teachers, the
therapists' data were used to explore relationships between the scales. Analyses were based just on the subset of children who had no missing data.

Figure 9.4 shows the scatterplot of data on the two language scales,
with children subdivided according to whether or not they had a school diagnosis of semantic–pragmatic disorder. It is evident from inspection that
children with such a diagnosis tend to cluster in the lower-right-hand side of
the figure, as would be expected if the diagnosis were being used for children with a relative strength in language form and weakness in content/
use.

One noteworthy aspect of Figure 9.4 is that it illustrates that there are
several children with marked impairments on both the C-scale and the
F-scale. Indeed, overall, there was a modest but significant correlation between scores on F- and C-scales ($r = .289$). Thus, there are children who had
problems in both domains, as well as others who have problems predominantly on just one scale.

A further analysis was done to see whether the degree of *mismatch* be-

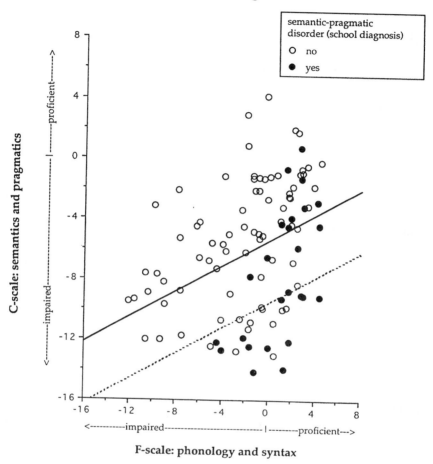

FIGURE 9.4. Scatterplot showing distribution of F-scale and C-scale scores in relation to school diagnostic categorization as definite or possible semantic–pragmatic disorder ("yes" or "no"). The two subgroups differed significantly on the F-scale (mean for "yes" = 1.01; SD = 2.34; mean for "no" = –2.3; SD = 4.19; $t(114)$ = 4.05; $p < .001$), on the C-scale (mean for "yes" = –7.52, SD = 4.47; mean for "no" = –5.54, SD = 4.32; $t(114)$ = 2.11; $p < .05$). (Data were missing for two children in the "yes" group and three in the "no" group.) The bold line is the regression line for predicting C-scale scores from F-scale scores. The SP deficit score corresponds to the shortest distance between a point and the bold line, with those below the line being negative, and above the line positive. Points below the dotted line are cases where C-scale scores are more than 1 *SD* below the level predicted from F-scale scores.

tween C- and F-scales may be better at differentiating groups than the absolute level of impairment on either scale. This can be quantified using the regression equation for predicting C-scores from F-scores to compute residuals which reflect the extent to which C-scale scores were discrepant with F-scale scores. In effect, these scores, which will be referred to as *SP deficit scores*, measure how far away from the bold line a child's score falls.

These SP deficit scores clearly differentiated children who did and did not have a school diagnosis of semantic–pragmatic disorder ("no" group mean = 0.24; $SD = .936$; $n = 84$; "yes" group mean = -0.59; $SD = .99$; $n = 28$; $t(110) = 4.00$, $p < .001$), and also had acceptable interrater reliability ($r_i = .548$; $n = 65$).

Item Analysis and Individual Variation

Although the analyses presented so far offer support to the notion of a subgroup of children with semantic–pragmatic disorder within the language-impaired population, there are aspects of the data that caution us against regarding this as a "syndrome." An item analysis comparing the pattern of responses seen in children who had a school diagnosis of semantic–pragmatic disorder and those who did not was used to find those response options (i.e., from all five possibilities offered for each item) that most clearly discriminated groups. Table 9.5 shows these response profiles. It is noteworthy that four of these items (lack of eye contact, poor peer relations, poor rapport with adults, obsessional interests) came from the Autistic Features scale. However, as can be seen from that table, different patterns of deficit characterize different children in the semantic–pragmatic group. Table 9.5 also shows which children had school diagnoses of "autistic features," AS, or developmental clumsiness (the latter category being of interest because of a possible association with Asperger's disorder). The only child thought to have a definite diagnosis of AS (shown as + in the table) had significant language delay and would not have met DSM-IV criteria for this disorder. Although several of the children with semantic–pragmatic disorder were regarded as clumsy, this was not a discriminating item on the checklist: Clumsiness was fairly common throughout the sample.

Pragmatic Language Impairments and Pervasive Developmental Disorder

As we have seen, the original definition of PDD requires two conditions be met: The child's disorder involves several areas of development, and the impairments correspond to distortions rather than delays in development.

The CLIC study offers some support to the view that there is a subset of children in the language-impaired population who meet both these requirements. First, there was a clear link between impairments on the Content and Use language scale and the Autistic Features scale but no relation between

TABLE 9.5. Response Profiles of Individual Children with Diagnosis of "Semantic–Pragmatic Disorder"

Age (yr)	6	6	8	8	9	9	9	10	10	11	11	11	12	13	13	13	13	14	14	14	14	14	15	15	15	15	16
Sex	F	F	M	F	M	M	M	M	M	M	M	F	M	M	M	F	M	F	M	M	M	M	M	M	M	M	M
Autistic features[a]	?	·	—	—	—	?	?	—	—	—	·	?	?	?	?	—	?	·	—	—	·	—	?	?	·	—	—
Asperger syndrome[a]	—	·	—	—	—	?	?	—	—	+	·	?	?	?	—	—	—	—	·	—	—	—	?	·	+	?	—
Clumsiness[a]	+	·	+	+	+	—	—	+	+	+	+	?	?	?	—	?	—	·	—	?	—	·	?	—	+	·	—
Intelligibility (excellent)	—	—	—	—	—	+	+	+	+	+	+	+	+	+	+	+	+	+	+	+	+	+	+	+	+	+	+
Expressive phonology (all sounds correct)	—	—	—	+	+	—	+	+	—	+	+	+	+	+	+	+	+	+	+	+	+	+	+	+	+	+	—
Intonation (expressive but stereotyped)	+	+	+	+	+	+	+	+	+	—	—	+	+	—	—	+	—	+	+	+	+	—	—	·	—	·	—
Grammar (complex, adult-like)	—	—	—	—	—	+	—	—	—	+	+	+	+	+	+	+	—	+	+	+	+	—	+	+	+	+	+
Morphosyntax (occasional errors only)	+	+	+	+	+	+	+	+	+	+	+	+	+	+	+	+	+	+	+	+	+	+	+	+	+	+	·
Conversational responsiveness (sometimes ignores overtures)	—	—	—	—	+	+	+	+	+	—	—	—	—	+	—	—	+	+	+	+	+	+	+	+	+	—	—
Conversational assertiveness (tends not to initiate conversation)	—	—	+	+	+	+	—	+	—	—	—	—	—	—	+	—	+	+	—	+	+	—	+	+	+	+	+
Conversational coherence (controls or abruptly changes topic)	—	+	+	+	—	—	+	+	+	+	+	+	+	+	+	+	+	+	+	+	+	+	+	+	+	·	+
Use of context (overliteral comprehension)	—	+	+	+	+	+	+	+	+	+	+	+	+	—	—	+	—	+	+	+	+	+	+	+	+	—	—
Eye contact (seldom/never)	—	—	—	+	+	—	—	—	—	—	+	—	—	—	—	—	—	—	—	—	—	—	+	+	+	·	—
Peer relations (avoided/neglected by others)	—	—	—	+	+	+	—	+	—	—	—	·	—	+	+	—	—	·	+	+	—	+	—	+	—	·	—
Adult relations (hard to establish rapport)	—	—	+	+	—	—	+	—	—	—	—	—	+	+	—	—	+	+	—	—	—	—	—	+	—	·	—
Interests (obsessional)	—	—	+	+	—	—	+	+	+	+	+	+	+	+	+	+	+	+	+	+	+	+	+	+	+	+	—

Note. + Indicates presence; — indicates absence; ? indicates possible or previous; · indicates missing data.

[a]Information from school diagnostic checklist.

271

autistic features and impairments on the Language Form scale. Second, most children with a clinical diagnosis of semantic–pragmatic disorder did have ratings indicating impairment on one or more of the nonverbal behaviors from the A-scale (see Table 9.5). Third, whereas items assessing language form showed clear developmental trends, those assessing content and use did not. This is tentative evidence for the view that these items correspond to distortions rather than delays in development. However, this finding could reflect the relatively low reliability of the Content and Use scale and the selected nature of the cross-sectional sample used here; a proper test would involve longitudinal assessment using more reliable measures.

One limitation of the CLIC study was that we did not use a standard diagnostic assessment but relied on diagnostic information in children's records to exclude those with possible or definite diagnoses of autistic disorder. The checklist provides a useful first step toward reliably identifying pragmatic communicative deficits in children: This approach now needs to be combined with more systematic diagnostic studies, using observational and interview methods such as the Autism Diagnostic Observation Schedule (Lord et al., 1989) or the Autism Diagnostic Interview—Revised (Lord, Rutter, & Le Couteur, 1994), which will enable us to quantify autistic behaviors in the same children. This would make it possible to confirm that the diagnostic information provided by the school was accurate in stating that these children did not meet criteria for autistic disorder.

If we accept that significant impairments of language content and use are seen in children who do not meet criteria for autistic disorder, how should we interpret such findings? Should we adopt the concept of semantic–pragmatic disorder, or would it be more proper to abandon the term and simply diagnose such children as cases of PDD-NOS? There are problems with both solutions. The term "semantic–pragmatic disorder" implies a clear-cut diagnostic entity, yet the CLIC study showed fairly wide variation in the particular constellation of reported abnormalities. Although the low reliability of items could contribute to this variable picture, this is unlikely to be the whole story. In other studies I am conducting, which involve fine-grained analysis of conversational behavior of children with semantic–pragmatic disorder, individual differences in behavior are the rule rather than the exception. Thus there are some children with marked limitations in use of eye contact and others who make excellent use of gaze and facial expression; some children have clear evidence of returning to favored topics in conversation and others have no special subjects that they prefer. Some have marked peculiarities of prosody; others do not. Such observations suggest that a categorical label such as semantic–pragmatic disorder may be misleading in implying sharper diagnostic boundaries and greater uniformity of problems than is the case. Another problem with the term "semantic–pragmatic disorder" is that it implies semantic and pragmatic difficulties go hand in hand, whereas the CLIC study gave little support to this view. Table 9.5 shows those items that best discriminated children with a diagnosis of semantic–pragmatic disorder from the remainder: None of these included items assessing semantic abilities, although such items had been included in the checklist. Semantic difficulties tended to characterize all language-impaired children but did not discriminate between subtypes.

What of the alternative, which would be to abandon the term "semantic–pragmatic disorder" altogether for PDD-NOS or "autistic spectrum"? The difficulty with this solution is that both PDD-NOS and autistic spectrum are vaguely defined, catch-all terms which encompass a huge variety of children (see, e.g., Towbin, 1997, for an account of PDD-NOS). Klin, Mayes, Volkmar, and Cohen (1995) argue that the use of PDD-NOS "adds little more than a demarcation of uncharted territory of clinical complexity" (p. S7). Clinically, these labels are unhelpful in specifying either the kind of educational provision the child requires or the severity of the problems. Also, by emphasizing the continuity with autism and related disorders, they draw attention to the social and behavioral impairments and give less prominence to children's structural language difficulties, which are also important, especially in younger children. In common with Conti-Ramsden, Crutchley, and Botting (1997), I recommend that the term "pragmatic language impairment" (PLI) be used to refer to children who occupy an intermediate position between core autistic disorder and specific language impairment (see Figure 9.5). As the diagram illustrates, however, there are no

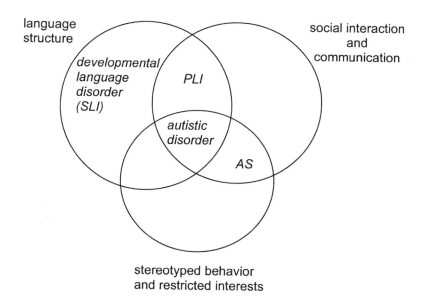

FIGURE 9.5. Set diagram showing how pragmatic language impairment relates to typical SLI and autistic disorder.

sharp boundaries between disorders, and this categorical label should be seen as a shorthand to describe children who occupy a particular region of a multidimensional space, rather than implying that there is a discrete syndrome.

If these children do fall between classic autistic disorder and SLI, why do so few of them attract an autism-related diagnosis? Further research is needed on this point, but I can offer some speculations, based on personal observations. First, the pragmatic difficulties themselves are relatively subtle. In the early study by Bishop and Adams (1989), children with a diagnosis of semantic–pragmatic disorder had higher levels of conversational inappropriacy than did other language-impaired children, but it was nevertheless the case that the majority of their conversational contributions were deemed appropriate. Second, the *social* limitations of children with a diagnosis of semantic–pragmatic disorder are typically milder than those seen in core autistic disorder. These children are usually outgoing and sociable, although the quality of their interaction may be odd or deficient. Finally, the language profile of these children can change radically over time. I have seen children whose early language milestones were seriously delayed (e.g., still using single words at 4 years of age) yet who were talking fluently in long, complex sentences by middle childhood. The combination of serious delays in acquiring formal language skills, coupled with an outgoing social manner, may lead professionals to assume that the language difficulties are the primary problem, with any social limitations being secondary to poor language comprehension or expression. It is only when the child grows older and starts to speak intelligibly that it becomes apparent that there are oddities of social interaction that cannot be attributed to linguistic limitations.

BEYOND ASPERGER SYNDROME

The CLIC study has been used to illustrate the fact that children who fall between diagnostic boundaries for AS, autistic disorder, and developmental language disorder are not uncommon: The region marked as PLI in Figure 9.5 is not as sparsely populated as the textbooks suggest. Furthermore, children inhabiting that region are fairly diverse. My emphasis has been on children who are receiving special educational provision for language difficulties; I suspect that even greater variability might have been seen had checklist data been gathered from a broader range of settings. Indeed, when relatively high-functioning children present with subtle deficits affecting a range of different behaviors, one has the impression that the particular diagnosis, and consequently the type of intervention received, may be more a function of the discipline of the specialist who is the point of first referral than of the particular symptom profile. The same child might receive a diagnosis of PDD-NOS or atypical autism from a psychiatrist, of developmental language disorder (semantic–pragmatic type) from a speech–language therapist, or right-hemisphere learning disability from a neuropsychologist (see Shields, 1991; Klin, Volkmar, et al., 1995).

What does this diversity represent and how should we respond to it? The question boils down to whether the different patterns of impairment represent different manifestations of a common underlying disorder or a group of distinct disorders. The answer depends partly on the level of description we choose to adopt. There is mounting evidence that if we are interested in uncovering biological causal factors, it can be misleading to focus on a stringently defined disorder; a broader phenotype gives a more coherent picture of heritability (see, e.g., Bailey et al., 1995). However, even if the ultimate genetic or other neurodevelopmental cause is similar for the whole range of PDD, there might be variability in the brain regions affected, and this could be one reason why such a wide range of patterns of neuropsychological deficit is observed. For the neuroscientist interested in brain–behavior relationships it might make sense to focus on much more tightly defined groups of children with similar patterns of symptoms, as this would provide the best opportunity for uncovering a common site of brain dysfunction. For instance, the specific behavioral profile characterizing AS seems to reflect right-hemisphere involvement, whereas high-functioning autism does not (Klin, Volkmar, et al., 1995). For the psychologist interested in exploring the cognitive and social processes that underpin a child's deficits, a focus on a single domain of functioning might be appropriate, and the emphasis would be on children who show selective impairments in just one area, because such children allow us to study a deficit in a relatively pure form, in the absence of other deficits that might cloud interpretation. Thus, for instance, in considering whether a "theory of mind" deficit can explain abnormalities of social behavior, it could make sense to focus on those rare children in the PDD spectrum with a relatively pure impairment of social behavior and relatively good formal language skills. Finally, for those interested in planning appropriate intervention, it is necessary to concentrate on assessing the individual child's pattern of strengths and weaknesses, so categorical labels become much less important, especially if they fail to capture the full range of variation seen clinically.

The category of AS has its uses. There are certain research questions that are best approached by focusing on one tightly defined subgroup of children, and the potential domain of PDD is so broad that it can make sense to start with a tightly defined condition and then expand outward, rather than trying to uncover order in PDD as a whole. However, I would recommend that such highly focused research should be complemented by studies that start with a more broadly defined group of PDD, attempt to measure the salient dimensions of variation, and look for correlates of these dimensions and natural clusterings of behaviors. An exclusive focus on narrow categories such as AS has led us to behave as if there are sharp boundaries when these are probably artificial. It has also produced a disproportionate focus of research effort on a small subset of children who seem seriously underrepresentative of the range of cases seen in clinical practice. Not only will a complementary approach adopting a broader perspective redress this imbalance, but it may also help throw light on the puzzling deficits seen in AS by revealing similar difficulties in children with other profiles of impairment.

ACKNOWLEDGMENT

Thanks are due to the staff at John Horniman School, Worthing; Moor House School, Oxted; and Dawn House School, Mansfield, for their willing participation in the CLIC study, and their helpful feedback. I would also like to thank Pat Wright for advice on checklist design.

REFERENCES

American Psychiatric Association. (1980). *Diagnostic and statistical manual of mental disorders* (3rd ed.). Washington, DC: Author.

American Psychiatric Association. (1994). *Diagnostic and statistical manual of mental disorders* (4th ed.). Washington, DC: Author.

Bailey, A., Le Couteur, A., Gottesman, I., Bolton, P., Simonoff, E., Yuzda, E., & Rutter, M. (1995). Autism as a strongly genetic disorder: Evidence from a British twin study. *Psychological Medicine, 25,* 63–77.

Bartak, L., Rutter, M., & Cox, A. (1975). A comparative study of infantile autism and specific developmental language disorder. *British Journal of Psychiatry, 126,* 127–145.

Bishop, D. V. M. (1989). Autism, Asperger's syndrome and semantic–pragmatic disorder: Where are the boundaries? *British Journal of Disorders of Communication, 24,* 107–121.

Bishop, D. V. M. (1997). *Uncommon understanding: Development and disorders of language comprehension in children.* Hove, UK: Psychology Press.

Bishop, D. V. M. (1998). Development of the Children's Communication Checklist (CCC): A method for assessing qualitative aspects of communicative impairment in children. *Journal of Child Psychology and Psychiatry, 39*(6), 879–891.

Bishop, D. V. M., & Adams, C. (1989). Conversational characteristics of children with semantic–pragmatic disorder. II. What features lead to a judgement of inappropriacy? *British Journal of Disorders of Communication, 24,* 241–263.

Bishop, D. V. M., & Rosenbloom, L. (1987). Classification of childhood language disorders. In W. Yule & M. Rutter (Eds.), *Language development and disorders* (pp. 16–41). London: Mac Keith Press.

Bolton, P., MacDonald, H., Pickles, A., Rios, P., Goode, S., Crowson, M., Bailey, A., & Rutter, M. (1994). A case-control family history study of autism. *Journal of Child Psychology and Psychiatry, 35,* 877–900.

Conti-Ramsden, G., Crutchley, A., & Botting, N. (1997). The extent to which psychometric tests differentiate subgroups of children with SLI. *Journal of Speech, Language, and Hearing Research, 40,* 765–666.

Klin, A., Mayes, L. C., Volkmar, F. R., & Cohen, D. J. (1995). Multiplex developmental disorder. *Developmental and Behavioral Pediatrics, 16,* S7–S11.

Klin, A., Volkmar, F. R., Sparrow, S. S., Cicchetti, D. V., & Rourke, B. P. (1995). Validity and neuropsychological characterization of Asperger syndrome: Convergence with nonverbal learning disabilities syndrome. *Journal of Child Psychology and Psychiatry, 36,* 1127–1140.

Lister Brook, S., & Bowler, D. (1992). Autism by another name? Semantic and pragmatic impairments in children. *Journal of Autism and Developmental Disorders, 22,* 61–82.

Lord, C., Rutter, M., Goode, S., Heemsbergen, J., Jordan, H., Mawhood, L., & Schopler, E. (1989). Autism Diagnostic Observation Schedule: A standardized observation of communicative and social behavior. *Journal of Autism and Developmental Disorders, 19,* 185–212.

Lord, C., Rutter, M., & Le Couteur, A. (1994). Autism Diagnostic Interview—Revised: A revised version of a diagnostic interview for caregivers of individuals with possible pervasive developmental disorders. *Journal of Autism and Developmental Disorders, 24,* 659–685.

Mawhood, L. (1995). *Autism and developmental language disorder: Implications from a follow-up in early adult life.* Unpublished doctoral dissertation, University of London.

Paul, R., Spangle-Looney, S., & Dahm, P. (1991). Communication and socialization skills at ages two and three in "late-talking" young children. *Journal of Speech and Hearing Research, 34,* 858–865.

Rapin, I. (1982). *Children with brain dysfunction.* New York: Raven Press.

Rapin, I. (1996). Developmental language disorders: A clinical update. *Journal of Child Psychology and Psychiatry, 37,* 643–655.

Rapin, I., & Allen, D. (1983). Developmental language disorders: nosologic considerations. In U. Kirk (Ed.), *Neuropsychology of language, reading and spelling* (pp. 155–184). New York: Academic Press.

Shields, J. (1991). Semantic–pragmatic disorder: A right hemisphere syndrome? *British Journal of Disorders of Communication, 26,* 383–392.

Towbin, K. E. (1997). Pervasive developmental disorder not otherwise specified. In D. J. Cohen, & F. R. Volkmar (Eds.), *Pervasive developmental disorders* (2nd edition, pp. 123–147). New York: Wiley.

Wing, L. (1981). Asperger's syndrome: A clinical account. *Psychological Medicine, 11,* 115–129.

Woodhouse, W., Bailey, A., Rutter, M., Bolton, P., Baird, G., & Le Couteur, A. (1996). Head circumference in autism and other pervasive developmental disorders. *Journal of Child Psychology and Psychiatry, 37,* 665–671.

World Health Organization. (1992). *International classification of diseases: Tenth revision.* Chapter V. Mental and behavioral disorders (including disorders of psychological development). Diagnostic criteria for research. Geneva: Author.

Editors' Note: The present chapter was written prior to the publication of a comprehensive description and empirical validation of the instrument described by Dr. Bishop in *The Children's Communication Checklist.* For an update of the empirical work described in this chapter, the reader is referred to Bishop, D. V. M. (1998). Development of the Children's Communication Checklist (CCC): A method for assessing qualitative aspects of communicative impairment in children. *Journal of Child Psychology and Psychiatry, 39*(6), 879–891.

10

Schizoid Personality in Childhood and Asperger Syndrome

SULA WOLFF

This chapter focuses on the clinical picture of a group of children, seen in child psychiatric practice since the 1960s, who were followed up into adult life. They were diagnosed as having a schizoid personality disorder because they resembled descriptions of this disorder in the psychiatric literature (Kraepelin, 1919; Kretschmer, 1925; Nannarello, 1953; E. Bleuler, 1950; M. Bleuler, 1954) and in the ninth edition of *International Classification of Disease* (ICD-9; World Health Organization, 1978), at a time when this label was used for disorders now comprising the Type A personality disorders of the fourth edition of the *Diagnostic and Statistical Manual of Mental Disorders* (DSM-IV; American Psychiatric Association, 1994). As soon as Asperger's seminal paper on "autistic psychopathy of childhood" (Asperger, 1944; translated by Frith, 1991) became known to English readers, it was clear that our schizoid children were like the children he described, except that we found the condition to affect girls also. More recently, an even older case report of six boys with a similar condition diagnosed as "schizoid psychopathy of childhood" has surfaced (Ssucharewa, 1926; Wolff, 1996). We need to be clear that in German, "psychopathy" means personality disorder. Our children also resembled children given a diagnosis of schizotypal personality disorder by Nagy and Szatmari (1986), and described in the older literature under a variety of different diagnostic terms (Wolff & Chick, 1980).

As we shall see, our schizoid young people were, as a group, much less impaired socially both in childhood and adult life, than groups of patients described more recently as having Asperger syndrome (AS) (Wing, 1981, 1992; Tantam, 1986, 1991). And they did not fully meet the diagnostic criteria for this condition in ICD-10 (World Health Organization, 1992, 1993) and DSM-IV (American Psychiatric Association, 1994).

In clinical practice it is important to recognize such more mildly affected children and to distinguish them from children with the more common conduct and mixed conduct and emotional disorders, which are often associated and which may obscure the diagnosis. The treatment needs of children with schizoid personality are different from those of children with reactive psychiatric disorders, and their prognosis is different too.

This chapter begins with an account of the childhood picture, followed by a description of two prognostic validation studies. Some changes in diagnostic nomenclature over the years are then discussed, as well as the relationships between schizoid personality in childhood, as we have used the term, and pervasive developmental disorders of childhood, including AS, pervasive developmental disorder not otherwise specified (PDD-NOS), and multiplex developmental disorder. The results of two records surveys follow, exploring the association of schizoid personality in childhood with psychiatric morbidity, including schizophrenia, in later life; and with adult criminality. A section on helpful treatment interventions is followed by a discussion of schizoid personality in relation to the justice system. The chapter ends with speculations about the genetic causes of the syndrome, in particular a possible link between schizoid personality traits and childhood autism on the one hand, schizophrenia on the other.

THE CHILDHOOD PICTURE

Matthew was referred when he was 10 because he had run away from his boarding school. His parents described him as a nonconformist, insensitive to the needs of others, oppositional, impulsive, and obstructive. He was a poor mixer, impertinent to older boys at school, and a bully with the younger ones. He had grandiose ideas, a vivid imagination and was fearless. Once, in a temper, he lay down in the middle of the road waiting to be run over. He was of very superior intelligence, rather better at verbal than visuomotor tasks, and his arithmetical skills were poor. His father was an able professional man who thought Matthew was like himself in personality. The mother had a deteriorating illness and this was why the two children of the family were sent to boarding school. Tragically, both parents were killed in a car crash when Matthew was 13 and his sister 15.

The research follow-up interview took place when Matthew was 34. He had had a university education and was now in a secure job he enjoyed as a health and safety inspector. Part of his work was to interview victims of factory accidents. He was happily married to a former nurse and had a very gregarious son age 3.

He said his mother's chronic illness had had no impact on him. While his sister had burst into tears on hearing about the parents' death, "it didn't

really hit me at all. I was independent or had a hard shell. It sank in slowly
... I used to go to the telephone and then I'd remember they were no
more." He had looked up the details of the accident in a library newspaper.
An aunt and uncle offered to make a home for the children and Matthew
settled down and remains in close touch with them. His schoolwork and social adjustment improved after he joined this family. But his sister could not
accept a new family, failed her school exams, took a menial job and went
into lodgings. She too later undertook a professional training and, after an
unsuccessful first marriage, is now once again and more happily married.

At the end of his interview, Matthew asked what I had thought of him
as a boy. I described his childhood personality and introduced the word
"loner." This, he said, "fitted" and a lot of things "fell into place." He had
never been popular at school ("the boys cheered when they were told I was
leaving"); at university he had had a small circle of friends and spent his
spare time going for long, solitary walks. He said, "I'm trying to be more
considerate now. I'm not a very considerate person. I'm quite self-centered;
I can filter things out." He had left his first job after "a personality clash
with the chief engineer." In fact he believes he has changed jobs more than
was good for his financial advancement. But he always lands on his feet.

His special interests are the stage and photography. He took 2,000 photographs of a drama group he once belonged to and used the slides for fund
raising. He was also the photographer at a recent family wedding. He said:
"I have a theory that the shyer the photographer, the longer the telephoto
lens and the further the photographer from his subject ... [but] I'm getting
better. The lens is shorter!" He also said: "I'm still a cynic."

Among children referred to a general child psychiatric department,
some 4% and more boys than girls (a sex ratio of around 3.5:1; Wolff &
McGuire, 1995), were found to present in middle childhood, often with common child psychiatric symptoms but without the background of adversity
that usually explains such symptoms. Individual and family explorations of
possible psychopathology failed to shed light on the difficulties, and the
children did not respond to psychotherapeutic interventions. More than half
were outgoing, but some were withdrawn and uncommunicative, and occasionally they had elective mutism. They often caused enormous difficulties
for parents and teachers because they could not conform to social demands,
especially at school, reacting with outbursts of weeping, rage, or aggression
if pressed to do so (Wolff, 1995). The children had often had an unusual development during the preschool years but rarely to a worrying degree. The
data here are anecdotal only, except for the frequency of specific developmental delays (see later) and the absence of evidence of significant rates of
obstetric difficulties or evidence of cerebral dysfunction. Some parents described their children's difficulty in adjusting to new circumstances, obsti-
nacy and ritualistic behavior, emotional remoteness, and a "lack of feeling."
Some children had adjusted quite well in their preschool nursery. It was
school entry that usually revealed the children's difficulty in relating to their
peers and adapting to the demands for conformity in the classroom.

The following five core features characterized the children, although not all were found in every case: (1) solitariness; (2) lack of empathy and emotional detachment; (3) increased sensitivity, at times with paranoid ideas; (4) rigidity of mental set, especially the single-minded pursuit of special interests; and (5) unusual or odd styles of communication (such as over- or undercommunicativeness, vagueness, and odd use of metaphor). Our later studies found the children to have one further characteristic, described also by Asperger (1944): (6) an unusual fantasy life. Parents often shared their children's personality traits.

It needs to be made clear that solitariness (e.g., having no close friends), was not at variance with being "outgoing." This feature consisted of superficial sociability, verbosity, and often tactless verbal communications with little regard to the needs and interests of the other person, in contrast to the verbal uncommunicativeness and apparent shyness that characterized others of our children.

We operationalized the five postulated core features for the purpose of our follow-up studies (see later) (Chick, 1978; Wolff & Chick, 1980), and for each child diagnosed schizoid, we identified as a control, another clinic attender, matched as well as possible for sex, age, occupational background, IQ, and year of referral.

A retrospective case note analysis was undertaken for 32 matched pairs of schizoid and control boys who had been followed up (out of a total cohort of 109 schizoid boys and their controls, identified in the course of 20 years of clinical practice) and for 33 matched pairs of girls (comprising the total cohort of schizoid girls and their controls, of whom 17 were followed up). The case notes were those of a busy, all-purpose, child psychiatry department during the years 1962–1982; case note data had not been systematically collected; and the main rater was not "blind." But a second rater, "blind" to the childhood data, rated a subset of case notes for schizoid children and their matched controls. With the exception of "unusual fantasy" which was rare, especially in girls, interrater reliabilities (weighted kappa) ranged from 0.43 to 1.0 with a mean of 0.73 (Wolff, 1991; Wolff & McGuire, 1995).

The mean age at referral of the schizoid children was 9.8 years for boys and 10.0 years for girls and their mean maximum tested IQ (Wechsler Intelligence Scale for Children or Binet form "L") was 109 and 103, respectively (Wolff, 1991; Wolff & McGuire, 1995).

Among 32 schizoid boys, 16 presented with symptoms of common child psychiatric disorders, including conduct disorder, mixed conduct and emotional disorder, school refusal, soiling, and hyperkinetic syndrome. Six presented with educational failure. In only 10 did the core features of schizoid personality itself form part of the presenting symptoms. These were (1) lives in a fantasy world, eccentric, has a single interest (electronics); solitary, and introspective; (2) had a delusional episode, cannot mix socially, lives in a persecutory dream world, does not want to go to school, restless, odd movements; (3) elective mutism, socially withdrawn, picks at himself, fights at school, associates with a wild boy, stammers, is enuretic; (4) elective mutism, poor mixer; (5) obstinate, obsessional questioning, insensitive to feelings of others, noisy and objectionable, always interrupts at home, friendless, too quiet at school, cannot get off to sleep at night, lacks initiative; (6) callous about father's disability, falsely told speech therapist (treating his stammer) that his parents were dead, excessively unguarded, good at creative writing, gave talk on astronomy at school, joined railway society, refuses to play team games, temper tantrums at school (threatens to throw things), withdrawn and a poor mixer (only one friend), obsessional habits, makes little eye contact when talking to others; (7) elective mutism, a loner, shy, avoids school sports, afraid to sleep alone, hyperkinetic, explosive if crossed, aggressive and threatening under stress, once threatened mother with a poker; (8) solitary, others gang up on him, mimics other boys, sullen and aggressive, loses control and screams, restless, attention seeking, very objective about himself, has enjoyed modern classical music since age 3; (9) repetitive, even perseverative, obstinate, sometimes sits alone in the dark, talks nonsense to himself, is too unguarded, under stress, threatens to burn the school down, keen on music in an adult way, knows about "the olden days," does not want to be "a Scottish boy," wets himself daily; (10) restless, flares up for no reason, concentrates only when interested, difficult to shift from his own goals, has fixed ideas since infancy, likes solitary play with lego, cannot hold a rational conversation, only talks about *his* concerns, destroys other children's belongings, has difficulty expressing his thoughts, cannot cope in school playground, hits and pushes, but without malice, is extroverted and too unguarded, does not pick up social cues, but is not withdrawn or solitary and popular with other children, in the classroom puts his hands over his ears, seems to lack normal anxiety, gets frustrated and often cries.

Among schizoid girls comorbidity was even more common, 24 out of 33 presenting with other child psychiatric disorders and 5 with educational failure. Conduct disorder as a presenting complaint was equally common in schizoid and control boys (in 5 out of 32 in each group), but it was more common in schizoid girls (11 out of 33) than in their matched controls (3 out of 33). Pure emotional disorder occurred in only 1 schizoid boy and 4 schizoid girls, compared with 10 and 10, respectively, among their controls. Asperger (1944), too, had drawn attention to the frequent occurrence of conduct disorders, even "maliciousness," in the children he described.

Of the core features we had identified, being a "loner" (rated as "yes" or "no" on the basis of case note and school descriptions of the child as being "solitary," "a poor mixer," "can't make friends," "a loner") and having "unusual fantasies" (rated on a 3-point scale, on the basis of comments such as "romances," "can't tell truth from fiction," "tells fantastic stories") significantly differentiated schizoid girls and boys from their matched controls. Having special interest patterns (rated on a 3-point scale on the basis of comments on the child's special interests and/or the forming of collections) differentiated highly between schizoid and control boys but was rare among the girls and did not significantly distinguish schizoid girls from their matched controls in childhood. In adult life, too, proportionally fewer women than men were found to have such interests. Impaired empathy, excessive sensitivity, and odd styles of communication, all, as predicted, characteristic features of schizoid children in later life (see later), could not be rated from the case notes because they had rarely been recorded, especially in the control groups.

An important finding was that significantly more schizoid than control children had specific developmental delays of language, educational, or motor functioning, serious or multiple in 15/32 schizoid boys compared with 4/32 of controls and in 13/33 schizoid girls compared with 1/33 of controls. Asperger (1944) too found both clumsiness and educational delays to be common in his children. In our groups, three schizoid boys but no schizoid girls and no controls had had earlier symptoms suggestive of autism, but never the full syndrome beginning under the age of 3 years. Three schizoid boys and three schizoid girls had been electively mute. One schizoid boy and one schizoid girl but no controls had had serious developmental language delays, including receptive language in the case of the boy. These children, both of normal intellectual ability, did not differ symptomatically from other schizoid children, and by the time of the follow-up, their language had greatly improved.

Overall, schizoid girls had more comorbidity, especially conduct disorder, than did boys and were significantly more conduct disordered than their matched controls. Both in childhood and later life, schizoid girls were characterized by exceptionally high rates of antisocial behavior (see later).

These differences between boys and girls in childhood may in part have been due to referral bias. If, like high-functioning autism (McLennan, Lord, & Schopler, 1993), schizoid personality shows itself less obviously in girls, one might expect the onset of social malfunctioning in girls to be later, as Asperger (1944) thought, and schizoid girls disturbed enough to merit a psychiatric referral, to have more adverse circumstances and constitutional difficulties, as well as more comorbidity. In fact, there was no difference in the age of referral of boys and girls: usually within the school years. And there was no evidence from the case notes for an excess of obstetric difficulties or organic cerebral impairment in either schizoid girls or boys compared with their matched controls. But the schizoid girls did have more comorbidity and came from a less privileged social background, with possibly more environmental adversities in comparison with their controls, than did the boys. They were also of marginally lower tested intelligence than schizoid boys, significantly so at follow-up, boys with schizoid personality having been of higher intelligence and socioeconomic background than the general population of clinic attenders (Wolff & McGuire, 1995).

PROGNOSTIC VALIDATION STUDIES

For the purpose of our follow-up studies, we devised a detailed, structured, focused psychiatric interview lasting about 2 hours (with a detailed glossary) designed to capture our postulated core features of schizoid personality disorder, as well as an overall rating of schizoid personality disorder, and ratings of psychiatric morbidity, work adjustment, friendships, intimate relationships, and social integration. In particular, we devised questions with probes to assess solitariness, empathy, emotional detachment, sensitivity, rigidity of mental set, and unusual styles of communication, as well as mystical, religious, and unusual perceptual experiences. Some ratings were self-ratings on the part of the subject, and others were made by the interviewer according to the glossary.[1]

It must be remembered that this interview was devised in the late 1970s, before the newer psychiatric diagnostic classifications existed, and before relevant instruments for measuring personality disorders were available.

The interviews with proband and control subjects in our first follow-up study was conducted by a psychiatrist "blind" to the childhood diagnosis and childhood data; interrater reliabilities were adequate (Wolff & Chick, 1980). In this study of 22 schizoid boys and 22 controls at a mean age of 22 years and after a mean interval of 12 years, 18 former schizoid patients were correctly identified as "definitely" and two as "doubtfully" schizoid. Only one control boy was misdiagnosed as schizoid and two schizoid boys as not so affected. Moreover, the five core features identified in childhood also differentiated very significantly between the two groups in adult life as did one other symptom: an unusual fantasy life. The childhood syndrome therefore had the feature of chronicity associated with personality disorder. This first follow-up also established that schizoid children in later life were not "introverted." Their scores on Eysenck's extra/introversion scale were the same as those of their controls and of the normal population. But a test for "psychological construing," that is, for the attribution of emotions and motivations to people in photographs, differentiated schizoid young men significantly from their matched controls and was related to their interview ratings of having impaired empathy (Chick, Waterhouse, & Wolff, 1979).

---

[1]For example, empathy "refers to the subject's ability to be aware of the feelings, thoughts and wishes of other people and to adapt his own responses accordingly. The subject may know he cannot easily understand how others feel and get on to their wavelength. He may feel clumsy about his social interactions not knowing what is appropriate, or he may merely act inappropriately and even hurtfully. Rate this paying special attention to the subject's intimate relationships with parents, siblings, spouse and closest friend, as well as to his more casual relationships with acquaintances and to the contact he was able to achieve with yourself." This feature was rated on a 4-point scale ranging from "average empathy" to "extreme impairment of empathy or callousness." The interviewer had to provide examples of communications on which this rating was based.

A second follow-up at a mean age of 27 years, by a social worker, again "blind" to the childhood data and diagnosis, also distinguished significantly between schizoid and control groups on overall diagnosis and core features (Wolff, Townshend, McGuire, & Weeks, 1991). On this occasion, the schedule for schizotypal personalities (SSP) (Baron, Asnis, & Gruen, 1981; Baron, Gruen, Asnis, & Kane, 1983) was incorporated into the semistructured interview and showed that 75% of schizoid men and women fulfilled DSM-III (American Psychiatric Association, 1980) criteria for this disorder (Wolff et al., 1991; Wolff & McGuire, 1995). This instrument has, more recently, been found to be of good reliability and with moderate sensitivity and specificity compared with a clinical consensus diagnosis (Benishay & Lencz, 1995). In addition, auditory P-300 and eye-tracking responses were recorded.

A clinical assessment of handedness showed a nonsignificant excess of left handedness or ambidexterity among schizoid boys (13/30 compared with 5/25 controls) (Wolff, 1998).

Although schizotypal personality disorder was found in the majority of our schizoid children grown up, their auditory evoked potentials and smooth pursuit eye tracking were no different from those of the controls and from a population control group (Blackwood et al., 1994). An explanation for this unexpected result comes from a study by Keefe et al. (1997) who found that eye-tracking deficits in relatives of patients with schizophrenia are not related to either schizotypal symptoms or attentional deficits as measured by the continuous performance test. The authors suggest that eye tracking and attentional deficits should be regarded as separate genetically based components of a schizophrenia-related phenotype.

An important finding from a clinical point of view was that our schizoid children were in adult life far less impaired in psychosocial functioning than people currently given a diagnosis of AS (Tantam, 1986, 1988a, 1991), appearing to resemble very closely Asperger's (1944) original case descriptions. Schizoid children grown up did have increased rates of treatment for psychiatric disorders in adult life compared with their control group of other referred children grown up, and their rate of working harmoniously at their expected level of occupation and, in boys, the rate of having had an intimate sexual relationship, was significantly reduced. But their rates of living independently, of marriage, and of stability of employment were not statistically different from those of the controls. Only one of 49 schizoid children personally followed up was in residential care, compared with over half the 60 patients diagnosed as having AS, studied by Tantam (1988b).

Two conclusions follow for the clinician: (1) there is a group of children, not as clearly impaired as children with autism or AS as currently defined (World Health Organization, 1992, 1993; American Psychiatric Association, 1994), who need to be diagnosed because their more subtle, underlying difficulties are long lasting, and schools and families need to accommodate to the children's special personality make-up; and (2) their overall outcome is reasonably good.

CHANGING DIAGNOSTIC CONCEPTS

The term "schizoid" was coined by Eugene Bleuler (see Nannarello, 1953) to describe shut-in, suspicious, sensitive people within the normal range of personality variation. Such characteristics Bleuler found in the premorbid histories of half his patients with schizophrenia who, even as children, stood out because they could not play with others, followed their own ways instead, and were regarded as strange, even "crazy," by other children because of their odd, intellectual characteristics. Kretschmer (1925) too used this term to describe a personality type found to excess premorbidly in schizophrenic patients and in their biological relatives (see Wolff, 1995). In 1926 Ssucharewa (for a translation see Wolff, 1996) wrote the first clinical account of six boys, who exactly resembled Asperger's (1944) cases, as well as our own, and whom she labeled as having a schizoid personality disorder.

In the more recent diagnostic classifications, beginning with DSM-III (American Psychiatric Association, 1980), the term "schizoid" has become more restricted, and the new category of schizotypal personality disorder was devised for personality characteristics found to excess in the biological relatives of schizophrenic patients and previously subsumed under the more general category of schizoid personality disorder. In fact, Szatmari (Nagy & Szatmari, 1986) described 20 children as schizotypal and recognized their similarity to our own cases, as well as to Asperger's (1944) and Wing's (1981). Their features were social isolation, social anxiety, magical thinking, bizarre preoccupations, poor rapport, and odd speech. The authors suggested the disorder may be a mild form of Kanner's autism or a variant of adult schizophrenia, or neither. Two of the 20 children developed schizophrenic illnesses in later life. Subsequently Szatmari dropped the term "schizotypal" in favor of AS.

Our work began before these developments took place and we have, rightly or wrongly, continued to use the term "schizoid" in its older, broader sense. From the start we realized that our children resembled Asperger's own cases in all respects, except that he found the full syndrome only in boys. Asperger himself stressed the children's giftedness, the frequent association with maliciousness, the unusual fantasy engaged in by some of the children, and the fact that the social disability tends to decrease in adult life when, despite continuing difficulties in intimate relationships, work adjustment may be excellent. This is in marked contrast to more recent accounts of people with AS (e.g., by Tantam, 1986, 1991; Wing, 1992) who were rarely able to lead independent lives, were very rarely in continuous employment, and hardly ever married. Tantam (1986) shared Wing's preference for classifying AS among the pervasive developmental disorders, and the majority of his subjects had the triad of impairments typical of autism in early childhood, although not necessarily beginning under the age of 3 years. Most of his cases also scored highly on a measure for schizoid/schizotypal personality. Tantam considered these personality features to be secondary to the underlying developmental disorder.

SCHIZOID PERSONALITY AND CURRENT DIAGNOSTIC CRITERIA FOR THE PERVASIVE DEVELOPMENTAL DISORDERS OF CHILDHOOD, INCLUDING ASPERGER SYNDROME

The first question here is whether the children we described and followed up are best considered as having a personality disorder beginning in childhood, or as suffering from a pervasive developmental disorder. Lorna Wing (1981) considered the latter classificatory term to be more useful for the children she described as having AS and this has been widely accepted. In part this preference stems from the aversion child psychiatrists rightly have to diagnostic labels that appear to carry an ominous prognosis (e.g., for schizophrenia). There are, however, two reasons for preferring the schizoid/schizotypal label for the children we have studied, unless the category of AS is specifically modified to include these children and the personality disorders they display.

First, although the children appear to be like those in Asperger's (1944) own account, they do not, as a group, fit the diagnostic categories of AS as defined in ICD-10 and DSM-IV. They do not have the abnormalities of reciprocal social interaction, nor the restrictive, repetitive, stereotyped patterns of behavior *"as for autism."* Our children's features *resemble* those of autism qualitatively but are by no means the same, and it is unclear as yet whether the difference is purely quantitative. Asperger (1979) himself thought that the syndrome of autistic psychopathy he described was different from Kanner's autism.

ICD-10 criteria include the absence of clinically significant general delay in spoken or receptive language or cognitive development; and they include circumscribed interests or restricted, repetitive, and stereotyped behavior patterns. An exclusion criterion is schizotypal disorder, but the definition includes schizoid disorder of childhood and autistic psychopathy (World Health Organization, 1992, 1993). DSM-IV criteria (American Psychiatric Association, 1994) also exclude significant general delay of language and cognitive development; indicate that the disturbance causes clinically significant impairment in social, occupational, or other areas of functioning; and differentiates the disorder from schizoid personality.

Some of our children did have early language delays and/or abnormalities, occasionally severe. One boy and one girl among the 65 children whose childhood case notes were analyzed had had serious developmental dysphasia which improved over time. And a few among those not personally followed up had had a below-normal IQ. Ehlers and Gillberg (1993) too found that the criterion of "no general delay in language and cognitive development" would have excluded a few of the cases of AS they found in a population survey. The association of severe early language delay with social impairments has been established in a follow-up study of 20 boys who, in early childhood, had had severe developmental language disorders. In adult life, many were socially "odd," with few intimate relationships, and two had developed a paranoid psychosis (Mawhood, 1995; Rutter & Mawhood, 1991). The case vignettes suggest that these children were similar to our schizoid children, but more seriously impaired in later life, perhaps because as a group they were of lower intelligence.

Children without early language delays and at the lower end of the IQ range within our schizoid group would have met ICD-10 and DSM-IV criteria for AS, except that they also fulfilled the criteria for schizoid and/or schizotypal personality disorders. Attempts to identify distinct subgroups among our schizoid young people, either by factor analysis or by inspection of the data, were not successful (Wolff, 1995). The exclusion criteria of schizotypal or schizoid personality disorders in the diagnosis of AS would thus exclude our group of schizoid children from this category (and even some of Tantam's cases), although our children resembled Asperger's own cases very closely.

In ICD-10, the criterion of circumscribed interest patterns or restricted and stereotyped behavior does not really capture the often very sophisticated special interests of our schizoid young people. In the most highly intelligent of the schizoid men, such interests formed the basis for a successful career choice: in astrophysics and graphic design. Only in a few of the less intellectually gifted could their special interests be described as restricted and repetitive.

Finally, an unusual fantasy life, occasionally amounting to pathological lying and the adoption of aliases, was prominent in some of our cases, as indeed it was in Asperger's original cases too (Asperger, 1944), and should be mentioned as a diagnostic feature of AS, if the schizoid group here described is to be included within this diagnostic category. As Klin and Volkmar (1997) make clear, the diagnosis of AS has, by different workers, been defined in varying ways, and according to current diagnostic criteria, it cannot unequivocably be differentiated from high-functioning autism.

Although the residual category PDD-NOS (DSM-IV) might be appropriate for our children, it is intended for subthreshold autistic syndromes whose symptoms appear in the first year of life (Mesibov, 1997; Towbin, 1997). This did not apply to our cases. We had only 3 children out of 65 whose case records were scrutinized who had symptoms of autism, but always short of the full triad and not beginning before the age of 3 years. PDD-NOS is a somewhat vague concept, to be used as a "temporary location" (Towbin, 1997) for disorders not fully characterized and not readily located on the spectrum from autism to normality. It appears to me to be altogether too broad a category to capture the quite well-defined symptom picture described in this chapter.

The children we have studied might be thought to fit the clinical pictures described under two other diagnostic labels: multiplex developmental disorder and semantic–pragmatic syndrome. The former term has been applied to a subgroup of children with pervasive developmental disorders who are impaired in their social relationships, including that with the primary caregiver; who are subject to episodes of intense anxiety or anger; and to recurrent episodes of disorganized thinking. They lack empathy, have poor frustration tolerance, and score highly for "bizarre" behavior (Cohen, Paul, & Volkmar, 1986; Towbin, 1997). In a recent validation study (van der Gaag, 1993), a group of children given this diagnosis were followed up. They differed from high-functioning autistic children by having a later onset of their disturbance, a higher verbal IQ, more "psychotic" thinking, more suspiciousness, and more aggressive behavior. They were less impaired than autistic children on measures of empathy and aloof and rigid behavior, and they had experienced more environmental stress. Both in childhood and in later life they appeared to be more seriously disturbed than our children: all had required inpatient child psychiatric care, and their later psychosocial functioning was poor. Two of 12 cases developed schizophrenia in late adolescence and a further 6 fulfilled the criteria for schizoid or schizotypal personality disorder at that time.

The validity of the semantic–pragmatic syndrome has recently been questioned. Both Towbin (1997) and Gagnon, Mottron, and Joanette (1997) indicate that this diagnostic term has been developed by speech and language pathologists and that they and the clinicians working in child psychiatric clinics may have failed to recognize the similarities of the children selectively referred to them. Gagnon et al. (1997) suggest that the diagnosis of semantic–pragmatic syndrome is equivalent to high-functioning autism. Some of our children might have fulfilled the rather varied symptomatic criteria described for this syndrome, but little would be gained from using this term.

A *second reason* for not choosing to classify our children within the pervasive developmental disorder category was because it seemed illogical to apply a different diagnostic label to the same condition according to whether it is seen in childhood or in adult life. Although our children often had specific developmental disorders from an early age, they did not come to psychiatric attention until middle childhood. Most of them in later life fulfilled the criteria for schizotypal personality disorder. The majority, as we shall see, remained free of serious mental illness, and the risk for later schizophrenia was small. But it is relevant to explore whether the premorbid childhood picture of people who develop schizophrenia in later life bears any resemblance to that of our schizoid children.

The evidence here is still sketchy. Schizoid and schizotypal personality characteristics have been found to excess at adolescence in patients, especially men, with schizophrenia (Foerster, Lewis, Owen, & Murray, 1991); and psychiatrically referred children who later develop schizophrenia were recorded as having "incongruous" behavior as well as specific developmental delays (Zeitlin, 1991). Sadly, the high-risk studies of children of schizophrenic parents have not generally focused on the clinical picture of the children, but, rather on their neuropsychological functioning and disorders of attention. Moreover, children who developed schizophrenia spectrum disorders were sometimes specifically excluded. In the New York High-Risk study, for example (Cornblatt, Dworkin, Wolf, & Erlenmeyer-Kimling, 1996), premorbid social isolation often preceded schizophrenia but was not the main focus of the study, and in the Copenhagen High-Risk study (Olin et al., 1998), 35.5% of later schizophrenic illnesses in the high-risk group were predicted by abnormal scores on a somewhat nonspecific teacher questionnaire enquiring about social isolation at school. Hollis (1996) too considered high-risk studies to have been disappointing in pinpointing the childhood antecedents of schizophrenia. In his own case-control study of the antecedents of juvenile onset schizophrenia, he found an excess of children with specific developmental language delays affecting expressive and receptive language, specific developmental motor impairments, and abnormalities of social development, in particular poor peer relationships, shyness, and social withdrawal (Hollis, 1995). A recent review of childhood-onset schizophrenia (Jacobsen & Rapoport, 1998) also documents conspicuous premorbid developmental disorders: 60% of the National Institute of Mental Health childhood-onset schizophrenia sample had developmental disorders of speech or language, and 34%, in contrast to adult onset schizophrenia, had transient symptoms of pervasive developmental disorder such as hand flapping and echolalia. And the British National birth cohort studies revealed that children who in later life developed schizophrenia were later in walking, had more speech problems, lower educational test scores, more solitary play preferences in early childhood, and, at 7 years, more socially inappropriate behavior and difficulty picking up social conventions than did nonschizophrenic controls (Jones, Rodgers, Murray, & Marmot, 1994; Done, Crow, Johnstone, & Sacker, 1994). It appears then that the precursors of schizophrenic illness consist both of solitariness and impaired social skills as well as specific developmental delays, including language delays.

In summary, the children we have described could be classified either as having a schizoid/schizotypal personality disorder or as having Asperger's autistic psychopathy according to the original description of this syndrome (Asperger, 1944). The current diagnostic category of AS, however, would be appropriate only if the criteria both in DSM-IV and ICD-10 were modified. The modifications necessary to include schizoid children would be (1) to omit the exclusion criterion of clinically significant delays in speech and language, (2) to omit the exclusion criteria of schizoid and schizotypal disorders, (3) to specify the less severe social impairments and the more sophisticated all-absorbing interests in comparison with autism, and (4) to include a criterion for unusual fantasy. The wider category of PDD-NOS is too vague to do justice to the clinical picture of our children.

It must be said also that the concepts of pervasive developmental disorder and personality disorders of the schizoid/schizotypal kind may not be as discrepant as current classifications suggest. Schizophrenia is now regarded as a neurodevelopmental disorder with a major genetic contribution to its etiology (Jones & Murray, 1991; Weinberger, 1995).

SCHIZOID PERSONALITY IN CHILDHOOD AND LATER PSYCHIATRIC MORBIDITY: THE LINK WITH SCHIZOPHRENIA

To determine whether there is a link between the syndrome we described and the later development of schizophrenia, a records survey was undertaken of all psychiatric hospital admissions in Scotland of the total cohorts of 109 schizoid men and 32 schizoid women and of their matched controls of other psychiatrically referred children who were then over 16 years of age (Wolff, 1992, 1995). In addition, we made a search in the local psychiatric hospitals for any in- and outpatient records of these people. The psychiatric records found were abstracted and DSM-III-R diagnoses (American Psychiatric Association, 1987) were applied by a single rater who was, unfortunately, not "blind." Because of small numbers, diagnostic categories were combined into schizophrenia, major affective illness, minor psychiatric illness, any personality disorder, alcohol and drug misuse, mental subnormality, conduct disorder, and admission for suicide attempt only.

Four schizoid boys had developed schizophrenia, compared with one control (who had had no premorbid schizoid features). Three schizoid girls but no controls had also developed this illness. Overall, 5.0% of schizoid young people and 0.7% of the controls had developed schizophrenia at a mean age of 26.5 years, compared with an estimated population prevalence rate in the United Kingdom by 27 years of 0.31–0.49% (Done, Johnstone, Frith, Golding, & Shepherd, 1991). One former girl patient, diagnosed as both schizoid and depressed in childhood, developed a serious bipolar illness and died after throwing herself off a train.

The numbers are small but suggest that the later risk for schizophrenia in our schizoid children, while sufficiently low for the clinician to give a good prognosis in childhood, is about 10 times greater than that of other referred children and of the general population. This, together with their clinical features in childhood and later life, especially their excess of schizotypal personality disorder at follow-up, support the idea that these children may have a schizophrenia spectrum disorder.

The mean maximum tested IQ in childhood of the seven schizoid people who later developed schizophrenia (84) was lower than that of the 134 who did not (103), and this agrees with the finding of significantly impaired intelligence (in fact 84.2) in children who develop schizophrenia in adult life (Russell, Munro, Jones, Hemsley, & Murray, 1995). Among our seven schizoid children who later developed schizophrenia, definite childhood evidence for organic brain dysfunction had been recorded in three and possible evidence in one further case. This too agrees with current views of schizophrenia as a neurodevelopmental disorder (Jones & Murray, 1991; Weinberger, 1995).

Mention must here be made of the fact that 2 of the 32 schizoid boys personally followed up had a transient delusional and hallucinatory state in childhood (consonant with the features of schizotypy) in response to what were for them particularly stressful experiences. These symptoms responded well to psychotropic medication. Although one of the boys suffered from two subsequent minor affective illnesses, neither developed a psychosis in later life.

The psychiatric records survey confirmed the findings of our first follow-up study that schizoid children in later life make significantly more use of psychiatric services than do other child psychiatric clinic attenders and have increased rates both of suicide and suicidal actions. The first follow-up had, in addition, shown an excess of depressive symptoms in schizoid children grown up (Wolff & Chick, 1980), often thought to be a reaction to their awareness of their social difficulties. The rate of suicide in our total cohorts of schizoid men and women was 4.0% compared with none among the controls, and a population prevalence rate by the same age of 0.0026%.

SCHIZOID PERSONALITY AND DELINQUENCY IN LATER LIFE

Our two follow-up studies of schizoid boys in adult life (Wolff & Chick, 1980; Wolff et al., 1991; Wolff, 1995) revealed no statistically significant differences between them and their controls in self-reports of either delinquent behavior or excessive drinking. If anything, at a mean age of 27 years, nonsignificantly more young men in the control than in the schizoid group had had (verified) contact with law-enforcing agencies.

Only 17 schizoid girls and no controls had been personally interviewed at 27 years of age (Wolff & McGuire, 1995; Wolff, 1995). Their self-reports of delinquent behavior and of excessive drinking were similar to those of schizoid men. This suggests that they were in fact an excessively delinquent group, because women usually have lower rates than men both of delinquent conduct and of excessive drinking.

The Scottish Criminal Records Office undertook a computer search for recorded offenses in our total cohorts of 109 schizoid boys and 32 schizoid girls then over the age of 16 years, and of their matched controls (Wolff,

1992, 1995). Not surprisingly, in all groups of these psychiatrically referred children grown up, the percentage of people with any convictions was greater than that expected for the general population of the same mean age: 32% of schizoid men and 34.5% of schizoid women had recorded convictions, compared with 34.5% and 15.5% of the controls. Comparable population norms were 22% for men and 5% for women. Schizoid women thus had exceptionally high rates of criminality. The mean number of offenses for schizoid and control men were 10.8 and 12.2, respectively, but for women they were 4.9 and 1.6. Moreover, about a third of male schizoid and control offenders had been in prison, as had a third of female schizoid offenders, whereas none of the female control offenders had had a custodial sentence.

There was no difference in the nature of offenses between the schizoid and control groups, and, in particular, by a mean age of 26.5 years, none had committed a particularly violent crime. But some 3 years after the survey, one of the young men in the schizoid group had entered the home of a housewife by posing as a priest, attacked her with a poker, and sexually assaulted her (Wolff, 1992, 1995). This highly intelligent young man had been a charming but totally solitary child with a serious specific developmental learning difficulty. He had always been unpredictably aggressive and his childhood was punctuated by repeated exclusions from school. He came from an affectionate and united family, his mother subject to depressive illnesses, his father socially withdrawn and reacting aggressively to the boy's misdemeanors.

We next looked for childhood predictors of conviction after the age of 16 (Wolff, 1995) within the smaller groups whose childhood case records had been analyzed. In the control group of boys and girls this was associated with childhood contacts with the juvenile justice system, with manual working-class status of the family, with delinquency in other family members, and with conduct disorder in the child him- or herself. In the schizoid group, later conviction was also associated with childhood contact with the juvenile justice system, and with conduct disorder of the child. It was not related to the family's occupational status or to delinquency in other family members. In contrast to the controls, later convictions in the schizoid group were particularly strongly associated with aggressive behavior in childhood. The one feature that appeared to protect against later delinquency, both in the schizoid and in the control groups, was a clinical presentation in childhood with a pure emotional disorder. This was found in 20 of the 65 children in the control group but in only 5 of the 65 schizoid children.

HELPFUL TREATMENT INTERVENTIONS

In the absence of controlled treatment outcome studies, this section is based on clinical experience alone.

The first helpful intervention is to recognize the condition. Then it is important to convey to child, parents, and teachers that the difficulties stem from the child's personality makeup. The identification of similar traits in other members of the family can be reassuring because affected parents have usually managed their lives quite well and hope for improvement of the child's future life adjustment can have a more realistic basis. It is also important to make it clear from the outset that neither the parents nor ill will on the part of the child are to blame for the problem. It needs to be stressed that the child's basic personality features are not likely to change and that the family and the school will have to accommodate to his or her special needs.

On the other hand, treatment of associated symptoms—of specific educational delays, of aggressive outbursts, stealing, depression, or, much more rarely, hyperkinesis and attention-deficit disorders, or delusional experiences—should be actively pursued and can be very effective. The treatment and interventions so clearly outlined by Klin and Volkmar (1997) for AS apply also to the children we have described.

Special educational measures are often needed. Affected children may find the hurly-burly of playtime in a crowded playground intolerable and need to be allowed to seek refuge in a quiet place instead. Often, too, they are helped by being excused from taking part in team games. Remedial teaching is indicated for the frequently associated specific educational impairments, and small group teaching is recommended when a noisy classroom is more than the child can cope with. If it is difficult to motivate a child for prescribed classwork, the curriculum may need to be built around the child's special interests. If there is severe educational retardation in relation to age and intelligence, or if the child's school behavior is intolerable because of aggressive outbursts, eccentricities provoking to other children, or other symptoms such as oppositional behavior, depression, stealing, or school refusal (often a reaction to the child's inability to tolerate even mild pressures for social conformity to ordinary school life), special schooling will have to be arranged.

Behavioral treatment approaches for aggressive outbursts can be very effective, especially if carried out in the school setting, and *social skills training* can help to improve peer relationships. *Medication* for associated hyperkinesis is as helpful as for other hyperkinetic children and short-term medication with psychotropic drugs is indicated during transient delusional and/or hallucinatory phases which occasionally occur. Long-term medication has, in my view, no place in the treatment of these children.

But the primary tasks of psychiatrist or psychologist are twofold: to provide very *long-term, even if infrequent, support* for the family as they negotiate the child's path through the school years and into further education and a working life and to *act as the child's advocate* in relation to his or her school and the school psychological services. Here a diagnostic label of "AS," now a well-known diagnosis, may be more helpful in facilitating access to services than the rather vague label of "constitutional personality disorder," even though strict diagnostic criteria for AS may not be fulfilled.

It is also important to maintain an optimistic stance: both Asperger and we ourselves found that the children's adjustment improves with age, once the pressures for conformity, always greatest during the school years, are at an end and the young people can find their own niche in life. The outlook is particularly good for schizoid children of high ability and when there is no comorbid aggressive conduct disorder.

One mother whose son is now grown up looked back on her years of clinic attendances and of her son's school difficulties as follows:

> "He could never understand why there was a problem. He didn't really enjoy being at school and trying to learn what other people wanted him to learn nor the way they tried to do it. He always wanted to go his own way. He hasn't basically changed. It's just easier when you're not at school. He has a detached appreciation of things. [He's] . . . a nonconformist and if you press [him] too far, you'll disturb him. He now knows that . . . [coming to the clinic] helped me to be confident that my analysis of him was reasonably correct . . . The school always said, 'You're encouraging him. We can't go on making exceptions of him.' "

This mother was keen to see me at the time of the follow-up

> "because [there are] a lot of individuals with basically nothing wrong with them but at the extreme of personality . . . and I wanted to be sure that people knew about such children and could support them and their parents in the face of school advice to insist on conformity, which really makes matters worse."

SCHIZOID PERSONALITY IN RELATION TO THE CRIMINAL JUSTICE SYSTEM

People who have committed apparently inexplicable crimes, and who may come from a stable family background are sometimes described in the media as "loners." Rarely is the account sufficient for a diagnosis to be made, even if psychiatric assessments are quoted.

But there have been several descriptions in the literature of violent patients in secure hospitals who were later diagnosed as having AS (Baron-Cohen, 1988; Mawson, Grounds, & Tantam, 1985); and an account of monozygotic twin girls with elective mutism ("the Silent Twins"), who developed schizophrenic illnesses in early adult life and were admitted to a secure hospital because of serious fire raising (Wallace, 1986), suggests that they would almost certainly have been diagnosed as having a schizoid/schizotypal personality disorder.

Schizotypal traits and developmental disorders have been found to excess among institutionalized, seriously delinquent youngsters (Hollander & Turner, 1985). And a study of personality disorders in a population of adult serious offenders confined to either prison or a secure hospital (Coid, 1989) found many with multiple DSM-III personality disorders. Borderline and antisocial personality disorders, usually associated with early family adversity, were the commonest, often with accompanying paranoid personality disorder. Schizoid and schizotypal personality disorders were much rarer and tended to be associated with evidence of neuropsychological abnormalities and, in a few cases, with clear features of AS and bizarre preoccupations which led to the subsequent criminal behavior.

Thus, a number of seriously delinquent people in the criminal justice system fall into the diagnostic categories of schizoid, schizotypal disorders, or AS, but, as we have seen, prospectively, children diagnosed as having schizoid personality disorder rarely commit serious crimes.

Much more common, both in childhood and in later life, is less serious delinquent behavior, which, as noted, occurs no more often among schizoid boys and young men than among other referred boys. But schizoid girls are excessively antisocial both in childhood and in later life and more often find their way into prison. This suggests that among women offenders, especially among those in prison, there may be some who, whatever the associated psychopathology, have a schizoid personality disorder which may well go unrecognized.

Although the numbers were small, one feature of the delinquency of our schizoid people in childhood and in later life, and in men as well as women, was skilled pathological lying and the adoption of aliases or even a false identity (Wolff, 1995). This should alert clinicians to the possibility of a schizoid diagnosis in people who present in this way.

Clinical experience indicated that in schizoid children, conduct disorder is often a response to what they experience as excessive pressure for conformity at school. In a less demanding school setting, such behavior often ceases. But a small minority of these children are aggressively delinquent whatever their environment and may then be exposed to the juvenile justice system.

Psychiatrists and psychologists have considerable influence on judicial decisions about young people. In my experience, schizoid children fare better when custody is demanded by the court, if they can be admitted to a small residential school or psychiatric unit, where not all the residents are delinquent so that the level of aggression is low, where the staff is well trained in the care of disturbed children; and the staff/child ratio is high. Schizoid children often do badly in large, noisy institutions for delinquent youngsters, where levels of bullying and violence are likely to be high and there is little opportunity for privacy. One former schizoid patient, an aggressive boy from a dysfunctional family, spent his most stable years as a well-liked member of a small residential school for children with emotional and behavioral difficulties. He deteriorated when he had to leave because he had outgrown the school's age range. His violent outbursts increased, he had numerous convictions, and he killed himself while in prison when he was 25.

An even greater problem is posed when, rarely, a schizoid person has committed a serious, violent or sexual assault or arson. Three issues then have to be considered:

1. Should the offender, like offenders with a psychotic illness at the time of the crime, be regarded as not fully responsible for his actions?
2. What is the risk of future dangerous behavior?
3. If custody is required for the protection of society, should prison or a secure hospital be the preferred option?

It is my view that because the impairments of the capacity for empathy and judgment and the idiosyncratic, obsessional preoccupations of some schizoid offenders with weaponry or poisons are constitutionally determined, such offenders should not be held fully responsible for their actions. On the other hand, they are less likely than other offenders with experientially engendered antisocial personality disorders to undergo radical transformations with time and treatment of their thought processes and of their capacity for moral behavior. They may thus remain a danger to others longer than other antisocial people.

The issue of confinement in hospital or prison is likely to be dealt with differently in different cultures. In the United Kingdom, in part in response to the human rights lobby, but also as a consequence of a rather narrow interpretation of the "treatability" clause in our mental health legislation, there has been a move away from admitting sociopathic offenders to hospital, yet those with schizoid/schizotypal personality disorder in addition to their sociopathy may adjust better to life in a secure hospital than to life in prison (for a discussion of these issues, see Wolff, 1995).

WHAT ARE THE LINKS BETWEEN SCHIZOID PERSONALITY IN CHILDHOOD, AUTISM, AND SCHIZOPHRENIA?

The Links with Autism

The individual features of schizoid personality in childhood certainly resemble the symptoms of autism. Both conditions present with qualitative abnormalities of reciprocal social interactions, unusually intense circumscribed interests and repetitive activities, and abnormalities in verbal and nonverbal communication. In a few cases of high-functioning autism and of severe schizoid disorder associated with a low-normal or below-normal IQ, it may be difficult to decide which diagnosis is the more appropriate. Many of Wing's and Tantam's cases of AS had the features of autism in the past. Yet in our group of less impaired schizoid children, only a minority had had autistic symptoms in early childhood and never the complete syndrome. What is more, whereas the features of our children resembled those of autism, they were not the same. Deficits in social interaction did not markedly affect our children's attachments to their parents; peer relationships were the most impaired. Our children's special interest patterns were often sophisticated, quite unlike the repetitive, stereotyped behaviors and utterances of autistic children. And the unusual modes of communication of our former patients were, in most cases, unlike those of autistic children, not immediately apparent to everyone but had to be carefully looked for. In addition, our schizoid children were not, like autistic children, deficient in imaginative play capacities. On the contrary, many engaged in unusual imagination and fantasy.

Yet, clear genetic links have been established between childhood autism and both AS and schizoid personality. Autism and AS have been found in members of the same families (van Krevelen, 1963; Gillberg, 1991; de Long & Dwyer, 1988), and Piven et al. (1990) reported social and cognitive deficits, similar to but milder than those of autistic people, among grown-up siblings of autistic patients.

In a controlled, "blind" study of parents of autistic children and parents of children with other handicaps, we found significantly more parents of autistic children to have mild schizoid personality traits and also to be more "intellectual" (Wolff, Narayan, & Moyes, 1988; Narayan, Moyes, & Wolff, 1990). Subsequently, Landa et al. (1992) found parents of autistic children more often than parents of controls to have atypical social patterns of behavior, in particular, disinhibited social communication, awkward or inadequate expression of ideas, and odd verbal interaction, all features resembling the language abnormalities we found in our schizoid young people. And Piven et al. (1994) found parents of autistic children to be more aloof, tactless, and unresponsive than parents of children with Down syndrome.

Twin studies of autistic children have shown that nonaffected identical twins more often than expected have cognitive and social deficits, milder but similar to those of autism itself (Folstein & Rutter, 1988; Bailey, Phillips, & Rutter, 1996). The labels "lesser variant" or "broader phenotype" of autism have been applied to these disorders. Bolton et al. (1994) found an excess of biological relatives of autistic people with the "lesser variant of autism," in addition to the expected very small excess of childhood autism itself. This lesser variant consisted of subtle impairments of social interaction (including lack of friendships and reciprocity and impaired conversation and social disinhibition) and communication (including language delay, articulation disorder, reading retardation, and spelling difficulties), together with repetitive stereotyped behavior (circumscribed interests). The language problems were usually outgrown, but the social difficulties often became more apparent in later life. The authors found only one sibling to have AS, perhaps because most subjects with the lesser variant did not meet the criteria for AS because of their associated language delays. The features of the broader phenotype have clear similarities with those of the schizoid children described here, although the case descriptions provided by Le Couteur et al. (1996) for affected twin partners of autistic people suggest that these were of lower intelligence, psychosocially more impaired, and with greater language disabilities than our schizoid children.

The current view is that autism and its broader phenotype may have a multifactorial genetic basis (Rutter, 1998), and are distinct from the other forms of social abnormality, especially schizotypal personality and other schizophrenia spectrum disorders (Bailey et al., 1996; Rutter, 1996). Yet such a distinction can be made only on the basis of improved studies of the clinical picture of children later diagnosed as schizotypal and/or schizophrenic and on advances in molecular genetics. The neurodevelopmental nature of autism and other pervasive developmental disorders is stressed. Yet schizophrenia itself and its antecedents are now recognized as falling within this group of disorders.

The Links with Schizophrenia

There have as yet been no systematic family genetic studies of either AS or schizoid personality disorder of childhood. Asperger (1944), Gillberg (1989), and we ourselves (Wolff, 1995) documented the apparent excess of Asperger/schizoid personality traits among the parents of affected children, and a genetic etiology is generally assumed.

We have proposed earlier that the symptoms of our young people with schizoid personality disorder fulfill the criteria of the DSM-IV Type A personality disorders and are equivalent to schizophrenia spectrum disorders. We also found that among our schizoid children, more than expected developed schizophrenic illnesses in later life.

Implications of the Suggested Links with both Autism and Schizophrenia

A genetic association of schizoid/AS and allied disorders with both autism and schizophrenia seems at first sight to go against the evidence that there is no excess of schizophrenia among the biological relatives of autistic people and that autism is not among the psychiatric disorders of relatives of schizophrenic patients. Moreover, despite a number of reports of such a development, autistic children are found to be no more likely than other children to develop later schizophrenic illnesses (Volkmar & Cohen, 1991).

It is now thought that both autism and schizophrenia are determined by several genes acting together, and that the obstetric impairments often associated with both conditions may be the result of genetic vulnerabilities to antenatal hazards (Bolton et al., 1994; McGrath & Murray, 1995).

To reconcile the possibility of a common genetic factor or factors for autism and schizophrenia (manifesting with variable expressivity as features of schizoid/schizotypal/AS disorders) with the observation that autism and schizophrenia do not co-aggregate in families, we would need to postulate that for autism as well as for schizophrenia another gene (or genes), different for each condition, is also among the necessary causes.

Folstein et al. (1999) have recently suggested that several genes interact to cause autism, that these may segregate independently, and have different manifestations. It may well be that the same holds for schizophrenia, and that there is a common genetic basis for some of the social impairments and developmental delays found in people affected by either condition and in their biological relatives. These impairments and developmental delays are of course also seen in other people, as in the children described in this chapter.

CONCLUSIONS

It is important, from a clinical and research point of view to recognize that current diagnostic criteria for AS are likely to identify only the more seriously impaired patients within the groups described by Asperger (1944), Ssucharewa (1926), and ourselves. More mildly affected children and adults, some of whom are gifted, need to have the nature of their basic difficulties recognized as constitutionally determined, so that their symptoms are not erroneously attributed to faulty upbringing. The diagnosis may be obscured by comorbidity. Associated specific developmental disorders will need special educational provisions, and associated conduct and other disorders require realistic treatment approaches. Care is needed to preserve and foster the children's special interests and gifts, and they and their families often need psychiatric or psychological support for many years. Although the children are not as impaired as children currently given an AS diagnosis, the problems they pose to their families and schools can be formidable.

From a research point of view, family studies of AS, as currently defined, are now needed to discover whether among the biological relatives of such individuals there is an excess with less severe disorders of the schizoid type here described, and whether there is an excess also of schizophrenia and schizophrenia spectrum disorders. The use of currently available questionnaire and interview measures of personality disorders, especially schizotypal, schizoid, and paranoid disorders, in these families will be revealing. The relationship between schizoid personality in childhood and delinquency needs to be further explored, as does the relationship between schizoid personality associated with high intelligence and special gifts and achievements.

From a classificatory viewpoint, it may be difficult to reconcile the fact that schizoid personality disorder in childhood appears to lie at one end of the autistic spectrum, where it merges with normal personality variation, although there is also evidence for its relatedness to the schizophrenia spectrum. Etiologically the problem is less serious. Both schizophrenia and autism are now thought of as neurodevelopmental disorders with a genetic basis, probably involving several genes. And people with both schizophrenia and autism are thought to have some psychological and language deficits in common (Frith & Frith, 1991; Baltaxe & Simmons, 1992). Family history studies of the less seriously affected, schizoid children would establish whether there is genetic overlap between schizoid personality, AS and autism on the one hand and schizophrenia on the other.

REFERENCES

American Psychiatric Association. (1980). *Diagnostic and statistical manual of mental disorders* (3rd ed.). Washington, DC: Author.

American Psychiatric Association. (1987). *Diagnostic and statistical manual of mental disorders* (3rd ed., rev.). Washington, DC: Author.

American Psychiatric Association. (1994). *Diagnostic and statistical manual of mental disorders* (4th ed.). Washington, DC: Author.

Asperger, H. (1944). Die "Autistischen Psychopathen" im Kindesalter. *Archiv für Psychiatrie und Nervenkrankheiten, 117,* 76–136.

Asperger, H. (1979). Problems of infantile autism. *Communication, 13,* 45–52.

Bailey, A., Phillips, W., & Rutter, M. (1996). Autism: Towards an integration of clinical, genetic, neuropsychological and neurobiological perspectives. *Journal of Child Psychology and Psychiatry, 37,* 89–126.

Baltaxe, C., & Simmons, J. Q. (1992). A comparison of language issues in high functioning autism and related disorders with onset in childhood and adolescence. In E. Schopler & G. B. Mesibov (Eds.), *High-functioning individuals with autism* (pp. 201–225). New York: Plenum.

Baron, M., Asnis, L., & Gruen, R. (1981). The schedule for schizotypal personalities (SSP): A diagnostic interview for schizotypal features. *Psychiatry Research, 4,* 213–228.

Baron, M., Gruen, R., Asnis, L., & Kane, J. (1983). Familial relatedness of schizophrenia and schizotypal states. *American Journal of Psychiatry, 140,* 1437–1442.

Baron-Cohen, S. (1988). An assessment of violence in a young man with Asperger's syndrome. *Journal of Child Psychology and Psychiatry, 29,* 351–360.

Benishay, D. S., & Lencz, T. (1995). Semistructured interviews for the measurement of schizotypal personality. In A. Raine, T. Lencz, & S. A. Mednick (Eds.), *Schizotypal personality* (pp. 463–479). Cambridge: Cambridge University Press.

Blackwood, D. H. R., Muir, W. J., Roxborough, H. M., Walker, M. T., Townshend, R., Globus, N., & Wolff, S. (1994) "Schizoid" personality in childhood: Auditory P-300 and eye tracking responses at follow-up in adult life. *Journal of Autism and Developmental Disorders, 24,* 487–500.

Bleuler, E. (1950). *Dementia praecox or the group of schizophrenias* (J. Zinkin, Trans.). New York: International University Press. (Original work published 1911)

Bleuler, M. (1954). [Letter]. *American Journal of Psychiatry, 111,* 382–383.

Bolton, P., Macdonald, H., Pickles, A., Rios, P., Goode, S., Crowson, M., Bailey, A., & Rutter, M. (1994). A case-control family history study of autism. *Journal of Child Psychology and Psychiatry, 35,* 877–900.

Chick, J. (1978). *Schizoid personality in childhood: A follow-up study.* Master's thesis, University of Edinburgh.

Chick, J., Waterhouse, L., & Wolff, S. (1979). Psychological construing in schizoid children grown-up. *British Journal of Psychiatry, 135,* 425–430.

Cohen, D. J., Paul, R., & Volkmar, F. R. (1986). Issues in the classification of pervasive developmental disorders: Towards DSM-IV. *Journal of the American Academy of Child Psychiatry, 25,* 213–220.

Coid, J. (1989). Psychopathic disorders. *Current Opinion in Psychiatry, 2,* 750–756.

Cornblatt, B. A., Dworkin, R. H., Wolf, L. E., & Erlenmeyer-Kimling, L. (1996). Markers, developmental processes and schizophrenia. In M. F. Lenzenweger & J. J. Hangaard (Eds.), *Frontiers of developmental psychopathology* (pp. 125–147). Oxford: Oxford University Press.

de Long, G. R., & Dwyer, J. T. (1988). Correlation of family history with specific autistic subgroups: Asperger's syndrome and bipolar affective disease. *Journal of Autism and Developmental Disorders, 18,* 593–600.

Done, D. J., Johnstone, E. C., Frith, C. D., Golding, J., & Shepherd, P. M. (1991). Complications of pregnancy and delivery in relation to psychosis in adult life: Data from the British perinatal mortality survey sample. *British Medical Journal, 302,* 1576–1580.

Done, J. D., Crow, T. J., Johnstone, E. C., & Sacker, A. (1994). Childhood antecedents of schizophrenia and affective illness: Social adjustment at ages 7 and 11. *British Medical Journal, 309,* 699–703.

Ehlers, S., & Gillberg, C. (1993). The epidemiology of Asperger syndrome: A total population study. *Journal of Child Psychology and Psychiatry, 34,* 1327–1350.

Foerster, A., Lewis, S. W., Owen, M. J., & Murray, R. M. (1991). Premorbid adjustment and personality in psychosis: Effects of sex and diagnosis. *British Journal of Psychiatry, 158,* 171–176.

Folstein, S. E., Gilman, S. E., Landa, R., Hein, J., Santangelo, S. L., Piven, J., Lainhart, J., & Wzorek, M. (1999). Predictors of cognitive test patterns in Autism families. *Journal of Child Psychology and Psychiatry, 40,* 1117–1128.

Folstein, S., & Rutter, M. (1988). Autism: Familial aggregation and genetic implications. *Journal of Autism and Developmental Disorders, 18,* 297–331.

Frith, U. (1991). "Autistic psychopathy" in childhood. (U. Frith, Trans., and Annot.). In U. Frith (Ed.), *Autism and Asperger syndrome* (pp. 37–92). Cambridge: Cambridge University Press.

Frith, C. D., & Frith, U. (1991). Elective affinities in schizophrenia and childhood autism. In P. E. Bebbington (Ed.), *Social psychiatry: Theory, methodology and practice* (pp. 65–88). London: Transaction.

Gagnon, L., Mottron, L., & Joanette, Y. (1997). Questioning the validity of the semantic–pragmatic syndrome diagnosis. *Autism, 1,* 37–55.

Gillberg, C. (1989). Asperger syndrome in 23 Swedish children. *Developmental Medicine and Child Neurology, 31,* 520–531.

Gillberg, C. (1991). Clinical and neurobiological aspects of Asperger syndrome in six family studies. In U. Frith (Ed.), *Autism and Asperger syndrome* (pp 122–146). Cambridge: Cambridge University Press.

Hollander, H. E., & Turner, F. D. (1985). Characteristics of incarcerated delinquents: Relationship between developmental disorders, environmental and family factors, and patterns of offence and recidivism. *Journal of the American Academy of Child and Adolescent Psychiatry, 24,* 221–226.

Hollis, C. (1995). Child and adolescent (juvenile) schizophrenia: A case control study of premorbid developmental impairments. *British Journal of Psychiatry, 166,* 489–495.

Hollis, C. (1996). Childhood antecedents of schizophrenia. *Schizophrenia Monitor, 6,* 1–5.

Jacobsen, L. K., & Rapoport, J. L. (1998). Research update: Childhood onset schizophrenia: Implications of clinical and neurobiological research. *Journal of Child Psychology and Psychiatry, 39,* 101–113.

Jones, P., & Murray, R. (1991). Aberrant neurodevelopment as the expression of the schizophrenia genotype. In P. McGuffin & R. Marray (Eds.), *The new genetics of mental illness* (pp. 112–129). Oxford: Butterworth-Heinemann.

Jones, P., Rodgers, B., Murray, R., & Marmot, M. (1994). Child developmental risk factors for adult schizophrenia in the 1946 birth cohort. *Lancet, 344,* 1398–1402.

Keefe, R. S. E., Silverman, J. M., Mohs, R. C., Siever, L. J., Harvey, P. D., Friedman, L., Roitman, S. E., Du Pre, R. L., Smith, C., Schneider, J., & Davis, K. L. (1997). Eye-tracking, attention, and schizotypal symptoms in nonpsychotic relatives of patients with schizophrenia. *Archives of General Psychiatry, 54,* 169–176.

Klin, A., & Volkmar, F. R. (1997). Asperger's syndrome. In D. J. Cohen & F. R. Volkmar (Eds.), *Handbook of autism and pervasive developmental disorders* (pp. 94–122). New York: Wiley.

Kraepelin, E. (1919). *Dementia praecox and paraphrenia* (R. M. Barclay, Trans.). Edinburgh: Livingstone.

Kretschmer, E. (1925). *Physique and character: An investigation of the nature of constitution and of the theory of temperament* (W. J. H. Sprott, Trans.). London: Kegan Paul, Trench & Trubner.

Landa, R., Piven, J., Wzorek, M. M., Gayle, J. O., Chase, G. A., & Folstein, S. E. (1992). Social language use in parents of autistic individuals. *Psychological Medicine, 22,* 245–254.

Le Couteur, A., Bailey, A., Goode, S., Pickles, A., Loeber, R., & Eaves, L. (1996). A broader phenotype of autism: The clinical spectrum in twins. *Journal of Child Psychology and Psychiatry, 37,* 785–801.

Mawhood, L. (1995). *Autism and developmental language disorder: Implications from a follow-up in early adult life.* Unpublished doctoral dissertation, University of London.

Mawson, D., Grounds, A., & Tantam, D. (1985). Violence and Asperger's syndrome: A case study. *British Journal of Psychiatry, 147,* 566–569.

McGrath, J., & Murray, R. (1995). Risk factors for schizophrenia: From conception to birth. In S. R. Hirsch & D. R. Weinberger (Ed.), *Schizophrenia* (pp. 187–205). Oxford: Blackwell Science.

McLennan, J. D., Lord, C., & Schopler, E. (1993). Sex differences in higher functioning people with autism. *Journal of Autism and Developmental Disorders, 23,* 217–227.

Mesibov, G. (1997). What is PDD-NOS and how is it diagnosed? *Journal of Autism and Developmental Disorders, 27,* 497–498.

Nagy, J., & Szatmari, P. (1986). A chart review of schizotypal personality disorders in children. *Journal of Autism and Developmental Disorders, 16*(3), 351–367.

Nannarello, J. J. (1953). Schizoid. *Journal of Nervous and Mental Diseases, 118,* 237–249.

Narayan, S., Moyes, B., & Wolff, S. (1990). Family characteristics of autistic children: A further report. *Journal of Autism and Developmental Disorders, 20,* 523–535.

Olin, S-C. S., Mednick, S. A., Cannon, T., Jacobsen, B., Parnas, J., Schulsinger, F., & Schulsinger, H. (1998). School teacher ratings predictive of psychiatric outcome 25 years later. *British Journal of Psychiatry, 172*(Suppl. 33), 7–13.

Piven, J., Gayle, J., Chase, G., Fink, B., Landa, R. Wzorek, M., & Folstein, S. (1990). A family history study of neuropsychiatric disorders in the adult siblings of autistic individuals. *Journal of the American Academy of Child and Adolescent Psychiatry, 29,* 177–184.

Piven, J., Wzorek, M., Landa, R., Lainhart, J., Bolyon, P., Chase, G. A., & Folstein, S. (1994). Personality characteristics of parents of autistic individuals. *Psychological Medicine, 24,* 783–795.

Russell, A. J., Munro, J., Jones, P. B., Hemsley, D. H., & Murray, R. M. (1995). A longitudinal follow-up of IQ in a sample of adult schizophrenics who presented to psychiatric services during childhood and adolescence. *Schizophrenia Research, 15,* 132–133.

Rutter, M. (1996). Autism research: Prospects and priorities. *Journal of Autism and Developmental Disorders, 26,* 257–275.

Rutter, M. (1999). Autism: Two-way interplay between research and clinical work. *Journal of Child Psychology and Psychiatry, 40,* 169–188.

Rutter, M., & Mawhood, L. (1991). The long-term psychosocial sequelae of specific developmental disorders of speech and language. In M. Rutter & P. Casaer (Eds.), *Biological risk factors for psychosocial disorders* (pp. 233–259). Cambridge, UK: Cambridge University Press.

Ssucharewa, G. E. (1926). Die Schizoiden Psychopathien im kindesalter. *Monatschrift fuer Psychiatrie und Neurologie, 60,* 235–261.

Tantam, D. (1986). *Eccentricity and autism.* Unpublished doctoral dissertation, University of London.

Tantam, D. (1988a). Lifelong eccentricity and social isolation I: Psychiatric, social and forensic aspects. *British Journal of Psychiatry, 153,* 777–782.

Tantam, D. (1988b). Lifelong eccentricity and social isolation II: Asperger's syndrome or schizoid personality disorder? *British Journal of Psychiatry, 153,* 783–791.

Tantam, D. (1991). Asperger's syndrome in adulthood. In U. Frith (Ed.), *Autism and Asperger syndrome* (pp. 147–183). Cambridge, UK: Cambridge University Press.

Towbin, K. E. (1997). Pervasive developmental disorder not otherwise specified. In D. J. Cohen & F. R. Volkmar (Eds.), *Handbook of autism and pervasive developmental disorders* (pp. 123–147). New York: Wiley.

Van der Gaag, J. R. (1993). *Multiplex developmental disorder: An exploration of borderlines on the autistic spectrum.* Master's thesis, University of Utrecht.

van Krevelen, D. Arn. (1963). On the relationship between early infantile autism and autistic psychopathy. *Acta Paedopsychiatrica, 30,* 303–323.

Volkmar, F. R., & Cohen, D. J. (1991). Comorbid association of autism and schizophrenia. *American Journal of Psychiatry, 12,* 1705–1708.

Wallace, M. (1986). *The silent twins.* Harmondsworth, Middlesex, UK: Penguin.

Weinberger, D. R. (1995). Schizophrenia as a neurodevelopmental disorder. In S. R. Hirsch & D. R. Weinberger (Eds.), *Schizophrenia* (pp. 293–323). Oxford: Blackwell Science.

Wing, L. (1981). Asperger's syndrome: A clinical account. *Psychological Medicine, 11,* 115–129.

Wing, L. (1992). Manifestations of social problems in high-functioning autistic people. In E. Schopler & G. B. Mesibov (Eds.), *High-functioning people with autism* (pp 129–142). New York: Plenum.

Wolff, S. (1991). "Schizoid" personality in childhood and adult life. III: The childhood picture. *British Journal of Psychiatry, 159,* 629–635.

Wolff, S. (1992). Psychiatric morbidity and criminality in "schizoid" children grown-up: A records survey. *European Child and Adolescent Psychiatry, 1,* 214–221.

Wolff, S. (1995). *Loners: The life path of unusual children.* London: Routledge.

Wolff, S. (1996). The first account of the syndrome Asperger described? *European Child and Adolescent Psychiatry, 5,* 119–132.

Wolff, S. (1998). Unpublished data. Edinburgh, Scotland: University of Edinburgh Department of Psychiatry

Wolff, S., & Chick, J. (1980). Schizoid personality in childhood: A controlled follow-up study. *Psychological Medicine, 10,* 85–100.

Wolff, S., & McGuire, R. J. (1995). Schizoid personality in girls: A follow-up study—What are the links with Asperger's syndrome? *Journal for Child Psychology and Psychiatry, 36,* 793–817.

Wolff, S., Narayan, S., & Moyes, B. (1988). Personality characteristics of parents of autistic children: A controlled study. *Journal of Child Psychology and Psychiatry, 29,* 143–153.

Wolff, S., Townshend, R., McGuire, R. J., & Weeks, D. J. (1991). "Schizoid" personality in childhood and adult life II: Adult adjustment and the continuity with schizotypal personality disorder. *British Journal of Psychiatry, 159,* 620–629.

World Health Organization. (1978). *Mental disorders: Glossary and guide to their classification in accordance with the ninth revision of the international classification of diseases.* Geneva: Author.

World Health Organization. (1992). *I.C.D.: The ICD-10 classification of mental and behavioural disorders—Clinical descriptions and diagnostic guidelines.* Geneva: Author.

World Health Organization. (1993). *International classification of diseases: Tenth revision.* Chapter V. Mental and behavioral disorders (including disorders of psychological development). Diagnostic criteria for research. Geneva: Author.

Zeitlin, H. (1991). Childhood development and schizophrenia. In C. Eggers (Ed.), *Schizophrenia and youth: Etiology and therapeutic consequences* (pp. 66–77). Berlin: Springer.

IV

Assessment, Treatment and Intervention, and Adulthood

11

Assessment Issues in Children and Adolescents with Asperger Syndrome

AMI KLIN
SARA S. SPARROW
WENDY D. MARANS
ALICE CARTER
FRED R. VOLKMAR

Children and adolescents with Asperger syndrome (AS) exhibit problems in multiple areas of development. Very much like individuals with autism, unusual developmental profiles are common, and the potential for confusion and misinterpretation of findings is great. Although the major principles of assessment are the same in both autism and AS (Klin et al., 1997), in AS one encounters a narrower range of IQ distribution and formal language skills on the one hand and a superficial competence thanks to a typically fluent and even verbose communication style on the other hand. The evaluator is presented with unique opportunities and challenges: whereas the assessment of basic intellectual and language skills is considerably more easy to perform in AS than in "classical" autism, the important areas of weakness might involve exactly those components of functioning that are the most difficult to assess. For example, there are no optimal standardized assessments to measure prosody in speech and pragmatics. There is a need, therefore, for considerable clinical skill and experience in the use of more informal procedures. The goal is not to stop at a simple list of standardized test results but to attempt to capture the disability as it affects the individual in his or her day-to-day life. Therefore, it is critical to obtain information from parents and professionals who, as a result of their daily contact with the child, observe the child in situations that are much more challenging than the one-on-one supportive testing environment of the clinic.

Clinicians and parents alike often ask for "the testing protocol for Asperger syndrome." The expectation is that there is a protocol which, if properly completed, is going to answer the question of whether a child or adolescent has or does not have AS. Such a protocol, however, does not yet exist. The best diagnostic instruments in the field were not developed with the intent of defining an algorithm for AS; rather, the parameters of diagnosis are defined for autism. It is likely that these instruments, or variations thereof, will be improved to encompass the clinical phenomena more typically associated with AS. However, such a protocol will have to await the emergence of a more solid body of research on the validation of the syndrome (see Chapter 1, this volume). It is important to note that differential diagnosis is only one component of the evaluation conducted for the purpose of defining the priorities of the intervention program, and probably not the most important area.

The absence of well-established and validated "ringing bells" for the diagnosis of AS has prompted some clinicians to adopt simplistic findings (e.g., of IQ profiles) to be the differential signposts for the condition, particularly vis-à-vis autism. Although it is important to be aware that certain profiles in neuropsychological testing are more likely to be associated with AS (e.g., Klin, Volkmar, Sparrow, Cicchetti, & Rourke, 1995), just as some typical profiles have become associated with autism (e.g., Dawson, 1983; Siegel, Minshew, & Goldstein, 1996), it is important that these different areas of assessment (e.g., differential diagnosis and neuropsychological testing) remain independent. Otherwise, we are likely to reify our own expectations using a circular style of reasoning without advancing our understanding of the different manifestations of high-functioning social disabilities. And for a given child, such simplistic generalization may prompt clinicians to adopt rushed and premature diagnostic conclusions, blurring the uniqueness of the child's distinct profile.

In this context, clinicians should also be aware that by simply associating a name to a complex clinical presentation, the understanding of a child's individualized profile of challenges is not necessarily advanced. This in fact can render the assessment irrelevant, as directives for the educational professionals who will be working with the child cannot be derived simply from a diagnostic assignment. Even though progress in the various diagnostic, neuropsychological, and neurobiological issues discussed elsewhere in this volume is likely to contribute considerably to assessment procedures, such developments will not replace the evaluation process from the more practical viewpoint of assembling data about individualized needs and strengths that will guide the compilation of specific recommendations for treatment and intervention. These practical considerations in the assessment of children and adolescents with AS are the subject matter of this chapter.

Our discussion focuses on the school-age child because children with AS typically present for assessment relatively late in development, often because their unique disabilities tend to go unnoticed beforehand (Volkmar, Klin, Schultz, Pauls, & Cohen, 1996). Also, diagnostic issues are even more complicated in younger children with high-functioning social disabilities. This does not mean that symptoms are undetectable in preschool years; in fact, a comprehensive review of the child's development often reveals some warning signals that antedated the parents' or educators' stated serious concerns and the time they first sought a referral. However, in the absence of major cognitive delays or difficulties in language acquisition, preschool referrals tend to focus on unspecified behavioral problems such as attention deficits or difficulties in social integration. Enhanced awareness of the condition, combined with better diagnostic techniques for the younger child, will likely increase detection of AS in younger children, which in turn is likely to help researchers to gain more detailed knowledge of the unique aspects of preschool development in AS. Until then, however, more general guidelines for children with autism and pervasive developmental disorders should be followed in preschool evaluations (e.g., Klin et al., 1997; Marcus & Stone, 1993).

GENERAL PRINCIPLES FOR ASSESSMENT

AS, like other pervasive developmental disorders, involves delays and deviant patterns of behavior in multiple areas of functioning. To thoroughly evaluate all relevant domains, different areas of expertise, including overall developmental functioning, neuropsychological features, and behavioral status, are required. Hence, the clinical assessment of individuals with this disorder is most effectively conducted by an experienced interdisciplinary team adopting a transdisciplinary approach. Both the unique contributions of each discipline (e.g., child psychologist, speech and language pathologist, and child psychiatrist) and the redundancy resultant from the behavioral observations obtained by different clinicians can result in a more comprehensive and accurate view of the child's needs and assets.

A few principles should be made explicit prior to a discussion of the various areas of assessment. First, given the complexity of the condition, importance of developmental history, and common difficulties in securing adequate services for children and adolescents with AS, it is important that parents are encouraged to observe and participate in the evaluation (Morgan, 1984). This guideline helps to demystify assessment procedures, avails the parents of shared observations that can then be clarified by the clinician, and fosters parental understanding of the child's condition. All these can then help the parents evaluate the programs of intervention offered in their community. Second, evaluation findings should be translated into a single coherent view of the child: Easily understood, detailed, concrete, and realistic recommendations should be provided. When writing their reports, clinicians should strive to express the implications of their findings to the child's day-to-day adaptation, learning, longer-term well-being, and vocational training. Third, the lack of awareness of many mental health and educational professionals of the disorder, its features, and associated disabilities often necessitates direct and continuous contact on the part of the evaluators with the various agencies to secure and implement recommended interventions. This is particularly important in the case of AS, as most of these individuals have average IQ levels and are often not thought of as in need for special programming. Conversely, as AS becomes a more well-known and perhaps fashionable label, it may be applied in an often unwarranted fashion by practitioners who intend to convey only that their client is currently experiencing difficulties in social interaction and in peer relationships. As the disorder is meant as a serious and debilitating developmental syndrome impairing the person's capacity for socialization and not as a transient or mild condition appearing late in a child's life, parents should be briefed about the present unsatisfactory state of knowledge about AS and the common confusions of use and abuse of the diagnostic concept currently prevailing in the mental health community. This should help them in their postevaluation reading of materials related to AS, which, otherwise, can be extremely confusing. Ample opportunity should be given to clarify misconceptions and to establish a consensus about the child's abilities and disabilities, which should not be simply assumed under the use of the diagnostic label (Shea, 1993).

In the majority of cases, a comprehensive interdisciplinary assessment involves the following components: a thorough developmental and health history, psychological and communication assessments, and a diagnostic examination including differential diagnosis. Further consultation regarding behavioral management, motor disabilities, other neurological concerns, psychopharmacology, and assessment related to advanced studies or vocational training may also be needed.

HISTORY

A careful developmental and health history should include information related to pregnancy and the neonatal period, early development and characteristics of development, and medical and family history. A review of available records including previous evaluations should be performed and the results compared to obtain a sense of course of development. In addition, information on several other specific areas should be directly obtained because of their importance in the diagnosis of AS. These areas include a careful history of onset/recognition of the problems, development of motor skills, language and communication patterns, and special interests (e.g., favorite occupations, unusual skills, and collections). Particular emphasis should be placed on social development, including past and present problems in social interaction, patterns of attachment to family members, development of friendships, play behaviors, self-concept, and mood presentation.

Questions about development can be framed for parents around a specific time or well-remembered event, such as the child's first or subsequent birthdays, the movement to a new house, or any other important family event that is likely to improve the reliability of the parent's account. The most useful questions tend to address specific everyday situations that parents can describe in detail. This type of response allows the clinician to make a judgment about the quality of the child's behavior (Le Couteur et al., 1989) and has the advantage of not requiring the parents to make general statements regarding the normalcy or abnormality of the child's behavior. Instead, the focus is on real examples of behavior, about which parents have been shown to provide accurate descriptions (Schopler & Reichler, 1972). The process of taking the history should convey to parents a sense that the information they provide is both helpful and welcome; the history-taking process can help the clinician establish a collaborative relationship with parents.

Whereas the child's history is best obtained during a direct interview with the parents, developmental and behavioral inventories may be forwarded to the parents prior to their first visit to elicit and frame observations which can then be further elaborated with the help of the examiner. When parents are willing to share videotapes of representative situations at home or at school, the videotapes may provide essential historical and behavioral information for the purpose of differential diagnosis. They also complement the observations obtained in the more structured environment of the clinic. Parents should be included in the actual evaluation process in at least two complementary ways: (1) as informants for semistructured diagnostic interviews (e.g., the Autism Diagnostic Interview—Revised; Lord, Rutter, & Le Couteur, 1994) (see later) and (2) as observers who can contextualize the behaviors exhibited by the child during the evaluation.

PSYCHOLOGICAL ASSESSMENT

This component aims at establishing the overall level of intellectual functioning, profiles of psychomotor functioning, verbal and nonverbal cognitive strengths and weaknesses, style of learning, and independent living skills. At a minimum, the psychological assessment should include assessments of intelligence and adaptive functioning, although the assessment of more detailed neuropsychological skills can be of great help to further delineate the child's profiles of strengths and deficits. Academic achievement is often assessed as part of school-based evaluations, and, therefore, is not reviewed here. At any rate, the procedures involved in the academic testing of children with AS do not usually require modifications from those utilized with typical children. As for personality assessment, although more traditional techniques using projective testing may be of help in further understanding the child's personality, functioning style, and integrity of thought processes, priority is probably better placed on the unique and more directly relevant issues such as circumscribed preoccupations (their interference with general learning and social adjustment), compensatory strategies of adaptation, social cognition (processing of social information), understanding one's role in social interaction and establishment of relationships, and mood presentation.

A description of results should include not only quantified information but also a judgment as to how representative the child's performance was during the assessment procedure, and a description of the conditions that are likely to foster optimal and diminished performance. For example, the child's responses to the amount of structure imposed by the adult, the optimal pace for presentation of tasks, successful strategies to facilitate learning from modeling and demonstrations, effective ways of containing off-task and maladaptive behaviors such as cognitive and behavioral rigidity (e.g., perseverations, perfectionism, and ritualized behavior), distractibility and impulsivity (e.g., difficulty inhibiting irrelevant responses, tangentiality), and anxiety, are all important observations that can be extremely useful for designing an appropriate intervention program.

The following discussion on the various measures used to assess relevant domains of psychological functioning in children with AS highlights those instruments and procedures that have proven to be of particular usefulness in the assessment of children with high-functioning social disabilities.

Intelligence

Although definitions of intelligence are almost as numerous as there are theorists who strive to define the concept (Kaufman, 1994), there is a high degree of consensus among psychologists as to what specific, operationalized capacities should be measured to obtain a useful indicator of a child's intellectual level (Snyderman & Rothman, 1987). These include verbal and nonverbal reasoning or abstract/conceptual thinking, problem solving, fund of knowledge, mathematical competence, memory, mental speed, and perceptual discrimination. Most intelligence batteries currently in use include these areas in varying degrees. The various instruments differ, however, in terms of emphasis placed on linguistic skills, speed of performance (i.e., timed tasks), reliance on visual or auditory presentation, and number of constructs tested.

Among the various intelligence batteries currently in use, the age-proven Wechsler scales, including the Wechsler Preschool and Primary Scale of Intelligence—Revised (WPPSI-R; Wechsler, 1989), the Wechsler Intelligence Scale for Children, third edition (WISC-III; Wechsler, 1992), and the Wechsler Adult Intelligence Scale, third edition (WAIS-III; Wechsler, 1997), provide the standards for the testing of intelligence in terms of psychometric properties, standardization procedures, and extent of research. Most children presenting for assessment with a differential diagnosis of AS are capable of completing the age-appropriate version of these scales.

Due to the preponderance of scatter (i.e., marked variability in subtest scores) in the intelligence profiles of children with autism-related conditions (McDonald, Mundy, Kasari, & Sigman, 1989), global indices of verbal and performance functioning may misrepresent these children's cognitive abilities. Depending on the degree and nature of the scatter, factor scores (as discussed by Kaufman, 1994) may provide a more accurate description of the child's functioning. However, even factor scores may be biased by the presence of isolated strengths or weaknesses. It is, therefore, important to avoid a misrepresentation of the child's intellectual profile as a result of averaging highly discrepant scores, which could mask the child's unique strengths and deficits.

That notwithstanding, the Wechsler scales' division of the various tasks into Verbal and Performance (visual–perceptual) scales offers a useful conceptualization of the child's profile. The profiles of higher-functioning children and adolescents with autism and AS appear to differ from the profiles obtained for lower-functioning children with autism, whose verbal scores are usually lower than the performance scores (e.g., Prior, 1979). How exactly they differ has been the subject of some controversy, as different studies have yielded different results (e.g., Ehlers et al., 1997; Klin et al., 1995; Ozonoff, Pennington, & Rogers, 1991; Siegel et al., 1996). It is likely that the inconsistency in research results might be attributed, at least partially, to varying diagnostic procedures and definitions used by the different researchers (see Chapters 1 and 2, this volume). However, it does appear that whereas Verbal and Performance IQs of nonretarded individuals with autism are fairly comparable (e.g., Ozonoff et al., 1991; Siegel et al., 1996), Verbal and Performance IQs of those with AS may differ favoring the former (e.g., Ehlers et al., 1997; Klin et al., 1995). More detailed subtest score analyses appear to show that while in autism there are peaks on visual–constructive skills (e.g., particularly on the Block Design subtest), in AS peaks are obtained in verbally mediated tasks (e.g., Information). Tasks requiring visual–perceptual speed with motor output appear to be a weakness in both populations. It should be noted, however, that research studies in this area are usually cross-sectional rather than longitudinal; the little information available does appear to suggest that in AS overall score profiles may change over time, for example, as a result of the child's acquisition of compensatory strategies in areas of weakness (Volkmar, Klin, Schultz, Bronen, Marans, Sparrow, & Cohen, 1996). In this context, it is important to emphasize that IQ testing should be used sparingly, not only to avoid subjecting the child to unnecessary testing but also to avoid carryover or learning effects, in which the child becomes familiar with some tasks and stimulus materials as a result of repeated testing.

Regardless of the controversy over general population profiles, the individualized results of intellectual testing can be of help in revealing a particular learning style. For example, many children with AS appear to use verbal mediation when performing nonverbal tasks; this natural compensatory strategy can be expanded and nurtured so that the child learns to use this skill more broadly (e.g., in creating scripts for decoding nonverbal social information). In the same vein, the inclusion of a verbal task examining the child's understanding of social conventions (Comprehension) and a nonverbal task exploring the child's ability to sequence social situations (Picture Arrangement) helps determine the level of discrepancy between the child's comprehension of social situations presented verbally and pictorially (Dean, 1977). Differences in scores on Block Design and Object Assembly favoring the former may indicate that the child is more competent on nonverbal problem-solving tasks that involve parts/whole analysis and has all the information necessary for the problem's solution available, in contrast to tasks that require the mental representation of the goal (i.e., the complete puzzle figure) and the completion of a self-generated hypothesis-testing procedure. The former may be seen as a more rote form of learning, contrasting with the latter which appears to include "executive" aspects (see discussion on executive functions, later). Similarly, a more detailed analysis of Digit Span scores may reveal a highly discrepant result for digits forward and backward, again, probably indicating that the child is more comfortable with rote recall than with mental manipulation of digits (a "working memory" task). However, interpretations based on single tasks, or even a direct comparison between two tasks, should not take place in isolation; there is a need to obtain as much information about a given hypothesis as possible and viable. In sum, it is important that the evaluator make an effort to understand the child's performance in more detail, beyond overall scores, and with a view toward translating test findings into insights into the child's learning style and possible internal resources that can be used in the child's educational program.

Adaptive Functioning

Adaptive functioning refers to capacities for personal and social self-sufficiency in real-life situations. The importance of this component of the clinical assessment cannot be overemphasized. Its aim is to obtain a measure of the child's typical patterns of functioning in familiar and representative environments such as the home and the school, which may contrast markedly with the demonstrated level of performance and presentation in the clinic. It provides the clinician with an essential indicator of the extent to which the child is able to use his or her potential, as measured in the assessment, in the process of adaptation to environmental demands. A large discrepancy between intellectual level and adaptive level signifies that a priority should be made of instruction within the context of naturally occurring situations in order to foster and facilitate the use of skills to enhance quality of life.

The most widespread measurement of adaptive behavior is provided by the Vineland Adaptive Behavior Scales (Sparrow, Balla, & Cicchetti, 1984a). The Vineland assesses capacities for self-sufficiency in various domains of functioning including Communication (receptive, expressive, and written language), Daily Living Skills (personal, domestic, and community skills), Socialization (interpersonal relationships, play and leisure time, and coping skills), and Motor Skills (gross and fine). These capacities are assessed on the basis of the individual's current daily functioning using a semistructured interview administered to a parent or other primary caregiver. The Vineland is available in three editions: a survey form to be used primarily as a diagnostic and classification tool (Sparrow et al., 1984a), an expanded form for use in the development of individual education or rehabilitative planning (Sparrow et al., 1984b), and a classroom edition to be used by teachers (Sparrow, Balla, & Cicchetti, 1985). Whereas the norms of the survey and the expanded editions range from infancy to adulthood, the norms of the classroom edition range from young childhood to the age of 12 only. Among the various editions, the expanded form is the most useful in the case of children with autism-related conditions, whose level of adaptive functioning is usually much lower than their demonstrated intellectual level (Volkmar, Carter, Sparrow, & Cicchetti, 1993). Using the child's developmental level as a point of reference, this form makes possible for the clinician to plan intervention on the basis of those skills the child should have acquired given his or her intellectual level. Because the items of the Vineland were selected on the basis of their immediate relevance to real-life adaptation and are modifiable, the skills described therein can be readily incorporated into the child's intervention plan.

Although several research studies (e.g., Volkmar, Sparrow, Goudreau, Cicchetti, & Cohen, 1987; Volkmar et al., 1993) have helped delineate the usual profile obtained for children with autism, Vineland data for individuals with AS are still scant, although the results do not appear to differ significantly from the those obtained for individuals with high-functioning autism, with the exception of the Communication domain (which appears higher) and the Motor domain (which appears lower) in AS (Klin, 1997). Scores on the Socialization domain are almost invariably the lowest among the various domain scores. The discrepancy between Vineland composite scores and IQ scores can be extremely large, with gaps of three standard deviations favoring the latter being fairly commonplace, forcefully suggesting that these individuals are unable to translate their cognitive strengths into real-life adaptation skills. The gap between scores on the Socialization domain and IQ scores can be even larger, again highlighting the magnitude of these individuals' social disability, particularly in light of their cognitive resources. Recently, Vineland norms for individuals with autism have become available (Carter et al., 1998), highlighting the importance of employing special population norms when evaluating children with autism. There is a possibility that a similar effort restricted to the more able group of individuals with autism and related conditions might be equally beneficial, although this is still in the future.

Neuropsychological Assessment

Along with intelligence batteries, neuropsychological assessment may be used to complement a psychological assessment when there are concerns about specific patterns of behavioral deficits (e.g., attention and impulsivity), when there are indications of possible identifiable neurological involvement affecting specific brain systems, or in order to explore the nature of a child's learning disability in detail. The specific choice of neuropsychological tests usually reflects the neuropsychologist's own training and experience; several comprehensive batteries are available, but because they were usually developed initially for use with adults, their usefulness with children can at times be limited (Pennington, 1991). Similarly, the psychometric properties of these tests, including the availability of solid norms for children, can be quite poor. More recently, however, several partial batteries or single tests have become available, which are easy to administer and interpret, some of which are now becoming computer based, facilitating the work further by providing detailed results of the child's performance. Regardless of the specific tests used, the following constructs are usually included in neuropsychological assessments, although the given areas should, of course, follow a rationale based on available data and referral questions. Specific tests are provided for the sake of illustration of a possible battery.

Laterality

As laterality is usually required for the interpretation of psychomotor tasks, and as it can reveal minor signs of neurological vulnerability, the assessment of lateralization of functions including handedness, footedness, and eyedness is usually performed. The Edinburgh Handedness Test (Oldfield, 1971), which provides a quick quantified assessment of lateralization, has been shown to have adequate validity and reliability coefficients (Williams, 1986).

Motor Skills

Although there is some controversy over whether individuals with AS differ in terms of motor functioning from individuals with high-functioning autism (e.g., Ghaziuddin, Butler, Tsai, & Ghaziuddin, 1994). There is little controversy over the fact that motor skills are often deficient relative to their overall IQ. For younger children, the Bruininks–Oseretsky Test of Motor Proficiency (Bruininks, 1978) can provide useful measures of gross and fine motor skills, particularly if one of the referral concerns has to do with motor incoordination (e.g., the child is thought to be "clumsy" or tends to "bump into other children"). It is important to note, however, that measures of motor skills might not necessarily reflect the magnitude of the motor-related problems displayed by individuals with AS, as many motoric behaviors are heavily dependent on cognitive functions (e.g., imitation), social understanding (e.g., adjustment to other people's posture), and social gracefulness (e.g., adjustment of gait patterns to the conversational partner's movements) (see Chapter 3, this volume), all of which are deficient in this population.

The Beery–Buktenica Developmental Test of Visual–Motor Integration (VMI; Beery, 1989) and the Bender Visual Motor Gestalt Test (Bender, 1938) provide a quick assessment of the child's graphomotor skills, perceptual accuracy, and hand–eye coordination. Perseverative behaviors, laterality problems, and distortions indicative of neurological involvement may also be revealed (Stellern, Vasa, & Little, 1976). The Purdue Pegboard (Tiffen, 1968) provides a timed measure of visual–motor coordination that can reveal further information about lateralization functions.

Even though standard measures of motor functioning may be helpful in further understanding the motoric deficits presented by a child, the focus of the evaluation should be on how these deficits hinder the child's learning of adaptive skills (e.g., fastening buttons, tying shoelaces, writing, and using assistive technology such as computer-based devices or electronic organizers). Similarly, an evaluation of motor skills should not focus only on the traditional areas outlined previously. Issues of body awareness and motor planning, for example, can be very disabling to a child. Whenever problems in areas such as these arise, the consultation with an occupational therapist can be very helpful (see later).

Attention

Although individuals with AS are often initially referred for assessment due to attentional concerns, it is often the case that the problems involve more selective attention, internal distractions, and inhibition of irrelevant or otherwise prepotent responses rather than more generalized distractibility and impulsivity as in attention-deficit/hyperactivity disorder (ADHD) (Klin &

Volkmar, 1997). In other words, the problem is often *not* that the child has difficulties focusing on most things (in fact, the child may become overly focused on specific activities); rather, it is difficult to get the child to pay attention to what the adult wants him or her to pay attention to. Therefore, results on attention tasks should not be interpreted in isolation. That notwithstanding, standard measures of attention may help the clinician further elucidate the nature of attentional problems. One of the current attentional tasks available is the Vigil Continuous Performance Test (CPT; Cegalis, 1993), which is a computer-administered measure of sustained visual attention and motor response inhibition; there is an analogous version in the auditory modality. The visual CPT is normed for children and adults, and there are currently no norms for the auditory CPT.

Visual–Spatial Perception

The standard intelligence batteries typically include visual–spatial problem-solving tasks, which are tasks that combine visual–spatial perception, problem-solving strategy generation, speed of mental processing, and motor coordination. At times, particularly if there is suspicion of right-hemisphere dysfunction, it is worth administering motor-free visual perceptual tasks. A useful test in this area is, for example, the Benton Judgment of Line Orientation (Benton, Hannay, & Varnay, 1975), which has been shown to have good validity (Riccio & Hynd, 1992) and reliability (Benton, Hamsher, Varnay, & Spreen, 1983). Also, there is now a good neurofunctional model of this task based on blood flow studies (Hannay, Falgout, & Leli, 1987).

Verbal and Visual Memory

Besides providing important information in respect to learning capacities, measures of verbal and nonverbal memory can also be of help in differentiating lateralized brain dysfunction. One excellent instrument in this area is the California Verbal Learning Test (CVLT; Delis et al., 1987), a computer-assisted, normed test of learning and remembering of verbal material. Its reliability coefficients are excellent (Delis, Kramer, Kaplan, & Ober, 1987), and it has been shown to differentiate individuals with right versus left brain dysfunction. A large number of visual memory tests are available, as part of intelligence batteries (e.g., the Bead Memory subtest of the Stanford–Binet Intelligence Scale, 4th edition; Thorndike, Hagen, & Sattler, 1986), memory batteries, or more specialized experimental procedures. The availability of both verbal and visual memory measures can be of help in further delineating the child's learning style and in choosing the optimal forms of teaching and assistive materials (e.g., when making a decision as to whether or not to employ visual aides) (e.g., Hodgdon, 1995).

Executive Functions

Among the most established neuropsychological findings in studies of individuals with AS is the observation that they present with significant executive function (EF) deficits (Pennington & Ozonoff, 1996). Executive functions denote a range of specific neuropsychological abilities, including, among others, cognitive flexibility, inhibition of prepotent but irrelevant responses, adjustment of behavior using environmental feedback, extracting rules from experience, selection of essential from nonessential information, and upholding in one's mind both a desired goal and the various steps required to accomplish it (i.e., working memory). One of the most direct implications of deficits in EF concerns the well-known real-life difficulties that these individuals encounter in organizing their activities, completing tasks in an efficient manner, avoiding getting stuck in counterproductive routines, and learning from their ongoing experiences.

Even though the Wisconsin Card Sorting Test (WCST; Grant & Berg, 1948) has been traditionally the EF test battery of choice, a number of newer batteries named with colorful geographic names such as the Tower of Hanoi, the Tower of London, and the Stockings of Cambridge are now available. These newer tasks are based on similar principles, but there is an additional emphasis on forward planning skills. Ozonoff (1998) has recently provided a detailed account of measures to assess EF with a focus on more able individuals with autism and related disorders.

Several other neuropsychological tests can be of help in providing further details or evidence for specific learning disabilities or neurological dysfunction, such as mental rotation tasks, face perception tasks, and others. The length and content of any neuropsychological protocol, however, should be based on specific questions that can be answered by specific tests and can be justified in cost–benefit terms.

Social–Emotional Functioning

Traditional projective methods of personality assessment are typically not useful in the evaluation of children with severe social disabilities because of these children's typical overconcreteness. Nevertheless, at least a few studies (e.g., Dykens, Volkmar, & Glick, 1991) have demonstrated the usefulness of projective instruments such as the Rorschach Inkblot Test (Exner, 1991) in helping to clarify the nature of thought problems in higher-functioning autistic individuals. More commonly, though, the use of simpler projective techniques such as drawings as well as play sessions may be more revealing with regard to social–cognitive skills, emotional presentation, and intrapsychic preoccupations that are typically not explored during other sections of the evaluation involving a conversational format. It should be noted, however, that these data can only be appropriately interpreted within the context of the child's developmental skills.

Drawings may provide a wealth of information about cognitive level, interests, primary attachments, and understanding of social life. Several guidelines should be kept in mind in both requesting the child to draw and interpreting the work produced. The child should have an opportunity to draw spontaneously before a specific request is made. The resultant work may be a perseverative interest which may range from, for example, an oval stroke drawn repeatedly, to meaningful figures representing inanimate objects such as a clock or a piece of machinery. This work should be analyzed in terms of its perseveration quality, salience of social vis-à-vis inanimate elements, visual–perceptual coherence, and presence of unusual qualities given the child's age and developmental level. The child should then be requested to draw a person, him- or herself, and his or her family. This work can be analyzed in terms of traditional cognitive scoring systems (Harris, 1963), but also, and more importantly, in terms of the difference in quality between the inanimate and the social drawings. Particular attention should be paid to the sense of coherence of the human body, differentiation of physical properties (e.g., younger and older, smaller and bigger, and male and female), affective representation, and any other emotional quality represented in the drawing. It is also important to question the child about the drawing, as often what appears as indistinguishable strokes may actually represent the child's effort to comply with the request to draw a person. At times, the child's work may represent a specific circumscribed interested (e.g., on plate tectonics or on the solar system), which are not well depicted in the drawings but about which the child may talk at length with great richness of detail. It is also important to question the parents about the child's drawing patterns, as sometimes the child's work may reflect either a well-rehearsed and practiced item or a constant preoccupation.

Play activities offer innumerable opportunities to explore aspects of the child's development and behavior. These include cognitive quality (e.g., functional/manipulative vs. representative and imaginative) and the presence of role play (Fein, 1981), which may characterize the child's ability to take the perspective of others. This is an essential social–cognitive skill necessary for adequate interaction with others and for the development of self-understanding (Selman, Lavin, & Brion-Meisels, 1982). If opportunities to observe these phenomena are not available in the child's spontaneous play, the examiner may initiate play situations in order to directly explore the child's understanding of social–emotional phenomena. For example, a puppet setting can be used to elicit the child's responses to situations of joy and distress, as well as to explore the child's ability to impute mental states (e.g. beliefs and intentions) to others and predict their behavior accordingly (i.e., to have a "theory of mind") (Baron-Cohen, 1995).

COMMUNICATION ASSESSMENT

Although significant abnormalities of speech and language are not typical of AS, at least three conspicuous phenomena in such individuals' communication patterns are of clinical interest (Klin & Volkmar, 1997). First, speech may be marked by poor prosody, although inflection and intonation may not be as rigid and monotonic as in autism (Fine, Bartolucci, Ginsberg, & Szatmari, 1991). Individuals with AS often exhibit a constricted range of intonation patterns that is used with little regard to the communicative functioning of the utterance (assertions of fact, humorous remarks, etc.). Rate of speech may be unusual (e.g., too fast) or may lack fluency (e.g., jerky speech), and such individuals often show poor modulation of volume (e.g., voice is too loud despite physical proximity to the conversational partner). The latter feature may be particularly noticeable in the context of a lack of adjustment to the given social setting (e.g., in a library or in a noisy crowd). Second, speech may often be tangential and circumstantial, conveying a sense of looseness of associations and incoherence. Even though in some cases this symptom may be an indicator of a possible thought disorder (Caplan, 1994; Dykens et al., 1991), more typically, the lack of contingency in speech is a result of the one-sided, egocentric conversational style (e.g., unrelenting monologues about the names, codes, and attributes of innumerable TV stations in the country), failure to provide the background for comments and to clearly demarcate changes in topic, and failure to suppress the vocal output accompanying internal thoughts. Third, the communication style of individuals with AS is often characterized by marked verbosity. The child or adult may talk incessantly, usually about a favorite subject, often in complete disregard to whether the listener might be interested, engaged, or attempting to interject a comment, or change the subject of conversation. Despite such long-winded monologues, the individual may never come to a point or conclusion. Attempts by the interlocutor to elaborate on issues of content or logic, or to shift the interchange to related topics, are often unsuccessful. These symptoms may be accounted for in terms of significant deficits in pragmatic skills and/or lack of insight into and awareness of other people's expectations. Yet, the challenge for the evaluator is to understand these communication problems developmentally, as strategies of social adaptation, and to measure the degree to which these problems interfere with the individual's social competency.

These more conspicuous clinical phenomena usually represent the resulting manifestations of a range of deficits in communication and social deficits (see Chapter 4, this volume), all of which require attention by the speech and language pathologist performing the communication assessment. The cluster of conversational skills to be examined include topic management (e.g., initiation, responsivity, maintenance, and elaboration and extension), turn-taking skills, clarification requests, quantity and quality of speech appropriate to situation, functional understanding of presupposition and perspective taking (e.g., knowledge of the intent of the speaker, accurate interpretation of perlocutionary and illocutionary intent, and offering of needed background information only), nonliteral language (e.g., inferencing, double meanings, idioms, metaphors, irony and sarcasm, and humor), and nonverbal communication (e.g., modulation of gaze, facial and bodily gestures, and posture). Individuals with AS are often pedantic and formal; they can also be inappropriately blunt, ignoring social conventions and making inaccurate judgments as to social cues. They can also provide misleading cues to conversational partners or consistently offer inordinate amounts of irrelevant information, unclear referents, or vague or tangential comments.

It is clear, therefore, that the communication assessment of individuals with AS should involve much more than the testing of speech and formal language (e.g., articulation, vocabulary, sentence construction, and comprehension). At a minimum, the assessment should examine nonverbal forms of communication (e.g., gaze and gestures), nonliteral language (e.g., metaphor, irony, absurdities, and humor), suprasegmental aspects of speech (e.g., patterns of inflection, stress, and pitch), pragmatics (e.g., turn taking and sensitivity to cues provided by the interlocutor), and content, coherence, and contingency of conversation. Particular attention should be given to perseveration on circumscribed topics, metalinguistic skills (Tager-Flusberg, 1989), reciprocity, and rules of conversation (Grice, 1975).

The assessment of communication patterns in individuals with AS is critical for an understanding of the person's strategies of adaptation in both the social realm and in terms of thought processes and learning. As individuals with AS may have age appropriate skills on many tests of formal language properties—articulation, fluency, grammatical form, vocabulary knowledge, reading decoding (e.g. Minshew, Goldstein, & Siegel, 1995)—a limited focus on more traditional aspects of speech and language may misrepresent the extent and importance of the communication deficits. In fact, findings are likely to be inconclusive at best and misleading at worst. More than in the case of other populations, therefore, the assessment approaches based on transactional, functional, and ecological models play an important role in the adequate assessment of communication skills in AS, with their emphasis on the understanding of communicative behaviors within the contexts in which they occur or the people to whom they are directed (Prizant, Schuler, Wetherby, & Rydell, 1997; Wetherby, Schuler, & Prizant, 1997).

Assumptions regarding language and communication deficits should not be made without adequate sampling across different contexts. In controlled conditions with explicit instructions, children may demonstrate abilities that are not always available to them in spontaneously occurring situations (e.g., Paul & Cohen, 1985). It is the inability to do so spontaneously when incoming stimuli (linguistic, social, and contextual) require rapid, online integration of information and flexible response that leads to breakdowns in communication. Discrepancies in communicative functioning between home, school, and the clinic are common; these may be due to level of comfort, familiarity (with examiner or setting), or the support of context or routine. Understanding the source of variability, when it is present, is the first step in determining how to advance the child's generalization and consistency of available or newly learned skills. Discrepancies in levels of function in one setting or another should lead to an objective to generalize optimal skill levels across settings.

Assessment Instruments

An assessment of the communication difficulties in an individual with AS should be performed within the context of the child's cognitive level and formal language capacities. The assessment of formal language skills should not require major adjustments in the evaluation procedures. Traditional batteries such as the Clinical Evaluation of Language Fundamentals—Third Edition (Semel, Wiig, & Secord, 1995) and the Test of Auditory Comprehension of Language—Revised (Carrow-Woolfolk, 1985) may supply the necessary background information for a better interpretation of higher level language skills. The selection of test batteries that focus on nonliteral language skills, flexible use of language for problem solving, and pragmatic skills, however, deserve closer scrutiny and more thoughtful consideration. Most of these constructs are probably better observed in real-life situations; nevertheless, some instruments can help the examination of available potential without which the interpretation of real-life observations might not be possible.

Among the tests of higher-level language and communication skills, the Test of Language Competence—Expanded Edition, may be of particular help (Wiig & Secord, 1989). This battery includes two levels covering the age range from 5 to 18 years. It focuses on skills such as interpreting and recognizing ambiguity, inferencing, conversational sentence production, and interpretation of figurative expressions. Both the Test of Problem Solving—Elementary (Zachman, Barrett, & Huisingh, 1984) and the Test of Problem Solving—Adolescents (Zachman, Barrett, Huisingh, Orman, & Blagden, 1991) provide helpful measures of the child's use of language for problem solving and reasoning, including the following functions: predicting outcomes, determining solutions, using content cues, making inferences, understanding why questions, analyzing, thinking independently, clarifying, empathizing, fair-mindedness, and understanding affect. These two batteries cover the age range from 6 to 17 years.

Although a formal assessment of pragmatic skills can be performed for children ages 5 to 13 using the Test of Pragmatic Language (Phelps-Terasaki & Phelps-Gunn, 1992), it is often the case that the performance of the child with AS in such structured testing might be at a higher level than one would observe in a more spontaneous situation. Therefore, even if this battery is used, it is important that an assessment of language in social interaction is conducted in less structured situations. The combination of formal and informal procedures can establish a solid basis from which to build social and communicative goals that can considerably enhance real-life skills in the social realm.

Observational Goals

Both when interacting with the individual with AS in the clinical setting and when observing him or her at school or maybe in the workplace, investigators should keep in mind a number of observational goals. These goals summarize the various vulnerabilities such individuals typically show in communicative exchange:

- The ability to manage conversational interchanges—topic management, initiation versus response ratios, shifting, maintenance, and extension.
- The ability to recognize and respond to clarification requests or to request clarification.
- The ability to demonstrate appropriate interactions that illustrate Grice's (1975) maxims of relevance (contingency), quantity, quality, and manner.
- The individual's ability to interpret nonliteral language accurately—humor, sarcasm, irony, indirect requests and polite forms; ambiguity, inferencing, implicature.
- The individual's ability to recognize indirect/polite forms.
- The awareness of the need for shifts in register that are person and context dependent—that is, style and manner (boss vs. peers, individual vs. group, familiar vs. unfamiliar partner; home vs. school/work; formal vs. informal, etc.).
- The individual's capacity to modulate tone and volume and other prosodic features according to place, topic or emotional valence.
- The individual's flexibility in dealing with a range of different situations and his or her capacity to use language to modulate the responses given (e.g., joining a group, disagreeing, and responding to frustration or hostility).
- The individual's ability to use language for purposes of learning or managing work routines, problem solving, predicting, reframing, and similar tasks.

In summary, a comprehensive communication assessment of individuals with AS should be based on knowledge of the unique, typical language and communication issues exhibited by individuals with this condition. Procedures should go much beyond the assessment of traditional, formal language skills (phonology, syntax, standardized measures of language comprehension and expression), although both the latter and cognitive status should inform the clinician's interpretation of deficits in higher-level language (e.g., metalinguistic skills) and in communication skills (e.g., social language use). Sampling of communication patterns should ideally take place in different environments, given the typical variability of communication competencies across settings. If this is not possible, there should be at least multiples sources of information providing data on the child's communication patterns in different environments and with different people who vary in familiarity to the child. Both formal assessment instruments and informal observations are necessary to obtain a thorough sampling of the child's communication skills. Although assessment batteries may provide useful data in the areas of nonliteral language and the use of linguistic *means* for problem solving, the assessment of both prosodic and pragmatic skills require more detailed informal observations obtained in more spontaneous, conversation-like situations.

DIAGNOSTIC ASSESSMENT

The diagnostic assessment involves the integration of information obtained in all components of the comprehensive evaluation, as well as a specific focus on issues of importance for differential diagnosis. The integration process should include primarily a synthesis of the behavioral observations obtained by the various clinicians involved in the evaluation, noticing the regularities and reconciling any points of inconsistency. Although a single coherent view of the child should emerge from this process, variability across settings and across people can be a characteristic element of the child's presentation, representing an important element to be considered when planning the educational program and other forms of treatment and intervention. The integration process should also consider the unique contributions of each component of the evaluation. The psychological assessment should provide overall as well as detailed levels of cognitive abilities, play patterns, and social cognitive capacities; this information should establish the parameters for expectations in the other areas of functioning, particularly social and communicative skills. The communication assessment should contribute measures of formal language skills as well as a detailed profile of social communication patterns, including prosodic and conversational skills; this information should not only inform the diagnostic process of the child's available language resources but also contribute directly to a formulation of the child's social disability. A detailed history, including patterns of language acquisition and social development, should not only inform the process of differential diagnosis—as onset patterns are an important element of the diagnostic criteria for AS—but also provide a sense of the child's unique developmental trajectory, successful and less successful educational experiences, as well as specific maladaptive behavioral patterns that have impeded the child's learning and social adjustment.

The diagnostic examination should also include observations of the child during more and less structured periods. This effort should take advantage of observations in all settings, including the clinic's reception area (e.g., contacts with other children or with family members) and the halls (e.g., how the child interacts initially with the examiners), as well as in the testing room during breaks, during periods of silence, or in otherwise unstructured situations. Quite often, the child's disability is much more apparent during such periods in which the child is not given any instruction and has no adult-imposed expectation as to how to behave. Specific areas for observation and inquiry include the patient's patterns of special interest and leisure time, social and affective presentation, quality of attachment to family members, development of peer relationships and friendships, capacities for self-awareness, perspective taking and level of insight into social and behavioral problems, typical reactions in novel situations, and ability to intuit other person's feelings and infer other person's intentions and beliefs. Problem behaviors that are likely to interfere with remedial programming should be noted (e.g., anxiety and temper tantrums). The child's ability to understand ambiguous nonliteral communications (particularly teasing and sarcasm) should be further examined, particularly in regard to the child's patterns of response (e.g., misunderstandings of such communications may elicit aggressive behaviors). Other areas of observation involve the presence of obsessions or compulsions, ritualized behaviors, depression and panic attacks, integrity of thought, and reality testing.

Unstructured observations may be obtained through conversational interviews or play, depending on the age and the developmental level of the person with AS. These settings allow for observations of important self-regulatory behaviors. For example, while engaged in play, one may observe the child's capacity for self-control and self-monitoring and the habitual patterns of behavior observed when the child is left to his or her own devices, as well as the need, or absence thereof, to include the examiner in play activities. Interviews should strive to re-create a naturalistic setting in which the person's spontaneous communication patterns become evident and a level of comfort is achieved so that child is capable of sharing thoughts about social experiences and relationships, insights into his or her role in other people's reactions to him or her, and topics of interest or favored activities that can reveal what the child's self-initiated leisure time consists of.

Diagnostic Instruments

A range of diagnostic instruments is available to aid in the diagnosis of autism-related conditions. These instrument vary in terms of comprehensiveness and nature of data collection (ranging from completion by teachers of yes–no ratings of diagnostic symptoms to semistructured interviews by a trained clinician that may last for several hours), psychometric properties (reliability and validity coefficients), and examiner requirements (e.g., from little or no expertise or training in autism to high levels of expertise and the need for formal training and demonstrated reliability performance relative to a gold standard) (see Lord, 1997, for a thorough review). However, none of the available instruments was developed with the intention of differentiating AS from other relevant developmental disabilities. In fact, all these instruments were developed to aid in the diagnosis of autism. Information derived from them can be of great help to the diagnostician interested in AS, but these instruments do not provide an algorithm for differential diagnosis. It is likely that with the increase in research knowledge about the validity of AS, including unique developmental trajectories and social and communication symptomatology, such algorithms will evolve from existing instruments or from modifications to existing instruments.

The absence of AS-specific diagnostic instruments, however, does not diminish the usefulness of some of the more comprehensive procedures for several reasons. First, the diagnosis of AS currently requires that the child does not meet criteria for autism (see Chapter 1, this volume). If results on the diagnostic instrument are positive for autism, this would theoretically preclude a diagnosis of AS (we emphasize the term theoretically in the absence of well-validated, AS-specific instruments, which itself is probably not surprising given the various controversies regarding the diagnosis). Second, diagnostic instruments may provide the structure necessary for the examiner to follow in order to cover the central symptomatology of autism-related conditions. This is important not simply to rate the child on the various defining criteria but to obtain a comprehensive profile of social, communication, and behavioral abnormalities in the child's presentation and to devise and prioritize the child's treatment plan. It is important to note that the great majority of autism-related diagnostic instruments were developed to be used with a specific range of the autistic population, and they can be very unhelpful if used with a different segment of this population. For example, there is little evidence that widespread instruments such as the Childhood Autism Rating Scale (CARS; Schopler, Reichler, & Renner, 1988) or the Autism Behavior Checklist (ABC; Krug, Arick, & Almond, 1980) can be of help in the diagnosis of higher-functioning individuals with autism or AS, as these instruments focus on a level of symptom severity that is not commonly found in this population.

Two diagnostic instruments can be of help in the diagnostic process involving individuals with high-functioning autism and AS: the Autism Diagnostic Interview—Revised (ADI-R; Lord et al., 1994) and the Autism Diagnostic Observation Schedule—Generic (ADOS-G; Lord, Rutter, & DiLavore, 1996). The ADI-R is a comprehensive, semistructured interview covering most developmental and behavioral aspects of autism and related conditions. The child's parent or caregiver serves as the informant. There is an algorithm keyed in to criteria for autism according to the fourth edition of the *Diagnostic and Statistical Manual of Mental Disorders* (DSM-IV; American Psychiatric Association, 1994). The ADI-R also provides a dimensional measure of severity of autistic symptomatology. Although interviews using the ADI-R may last on average between 2 or 3 hours, the effort is worthwhile given the resultant wealth of both historical and current data on the child's social, communication, and behavioral patterns. A positive element making the ADI-R more relevant to the diagnosis of individuals with high-functioning social disabilities is the fact that symptomatology is graded in terms of severity, making the instrument more sensitive to milder or more unique forms of social communicative dysfunction. The ADOS-G is a standard protocol for observation of social and communicative behaviors associated with autism. The instrument consists of a series of structured and semistructured presses for interaction, accompanied by coding of specific target behaviors associated with particular tasks and by general ratings of the quality of behaviors. The ADOS-G includes four modules, defined in terms of the child's expressive language capacities. Modules 3 and 4 are appropriate for children/young adolescents and young adults, respectively, with fluent speech. Therefore, in most cases, modules 3 and 4 would be applicable in the case of individuals with AS. The ADOS-G complements information obtained with the ADI-R, which is informant based. Like the ADI-R, the ADOS provides a measure of severity of autistic symptomatology. Diagnostic algorithms for autism have been recently developed, but these instruments cannot yet be used to diagnose AS.

Both the ADI-R and the ADOS-G were developed as investigator-based interviews to be used in research studies of autism. Researchers are required to participate in training workshops and to establish reliability with investigators from other centers. Both instruments require general experience in interviewing and working with individuals with autism. Although these various requirements signify that these two instruments will probably not be available to the general population of clinicians working with individuals with autism-related conditions, a large number of clinical researchers are already using them on a routine basis in both North America and elsewhere, including Europe, Latin America, and Asia. The major benefit of this development is that the diagnostic process in the pervasive developmental disorders is quickly becoming more uniform, thus making possible better communication among diagnosticians and enhancing comparability of research findings.

Differential Diagnosis

The differential diagnosis of AS involves primarily autism without associated retardation—that is, higher-functioning autism—(HFA) and pervasive developmental disorder not otherwise specified (PDD-NOS) in DSM-IV or atypical autism in the tenth edition of *International Classification of Disease* (ICD-10; World Health Organization, 1992; see Chapter 1, this volume, for a more extensive discussion). Although some authors might include personality disorders characterized by significant deficits in social–emotional functioning (e.g., schizoid personality disorder), such diagnoses do not take into account the developmental factors of AS that may prove to be of great importance for an understanding of its pathogenesis and course.

AS differs from HFA in that the onset is usually later and the outcome more positive. In addition, social and communication deficits are less severe, motor mannerisms are usually absent whereas circumscribed interests and verbosity are more conspicuous, motor "clumsiness" is apparently more frequently seen in AS, and there are some indications that family history of similar problems is more frequently reported in AS than in HFA.

The distinction between AS and PDD-NOS is problematic because, essentially, the latter is a residual category with no defining criteria. PDD-NOS is used to describe a rather large and heterogeneous group of children who do not meet strict criteria for autism but who exhibit a pattern of developmental and behavioral dysfunction similar to that observed in autism. Such children typically exhibit unusual sensitivities and affective responses in the presence of more differentiated social relatedness and better cognitive and communicative skills than do most autistic children (Volkmar & Klin, 1998). The ICD-10 definition of atypical autism, despite its attempt to operationally define the areas of "atypicality" (e.g., in age of onset and symptomatology) is also, essentially, a negative or subthreshold definition (i.e., not, or not quite, autism). From the information revealed in the few attempts to study this population (see Towbin, 1997, for a review), it is acceptable to conclude that if AS is strictly defined, it differs from the much more common PDD-NOS in that social, emotional, and communicative deficits are more severe and outcome is poorer in AS; circumscribed interests, verbosity, and motor "clumsiness" are more pronounced in AS; and the IQ range is probably more variable in PDD-NOS. Empirical evidence substantiating some of these observations was obtained in the autism/PDD DSM-IV field trials (Volkmar et al., 1994).

Comorbidity

Although discussions of co-occurrence of two or more separate child psychiatric conditions are complex and depend on a series of factors (see Chapter 7, this volume), discussions of comorbidity are particularly problematic in the context of AS, where the use of the diagnostic label has probably been less strict than in most other developmental disorders. In addition, given that the literature is still very much based on case studies or small case series, some anomalies may occur. For example, there have been at least four studies reporting the association between AS and Tourette syndrome (TS) (Berthier, Bayes, & Tolosa, 1993; Kerbeshian &

Burd, 1986; Littlejohns, Clarke, & Corbett, 1990; Marriage, Miles, Stokes, & Davey, 1993), conveying the impression that AS and TS may occur together frequently. Preliminary data on 99 subjects with AS (Volkmar, Klin, Schultz, Pauls, & Cohen, 1996), however, suggest that this co-occurrence is much less frequent than implied by these publications (only 2 of 99 patients with AS also had TS). Still, this rate is much higher than the prevalence rate of TS in the general population. Other disorders or symptoms appear to be much more prominent. The same set of preliminary data documented the co-presence of obsessive–compulsive disorder, depression, ADHD, and anxiety disorder in larger proportions. The co-occurrence of some disorders appear to be developmentally dependent. For example, ADHD is more often observed in younger children whereas depression is more often observed in older children, adolescents, and adults. The importance of identifying comorbid conditions or symptoms lies in the fact that some of these may be treated behaviorally, educationally, or psychopharmacologically (see Chapter 7, this volume).

FURTHER ASSESSMENTS AND CONSULTATIONS

Depending on the individual's age, level of functioning, stage in life, and profile and context of challenges, several additional forms of assessment and consultation may be appropriate.

Behavioral Assessment

Problematic patterns of maladaptive behaviors impeding the child's ability to learn, to relate adequately to others, and to adjust to the requirements of different settings may necessitate a study of the antecedents to these behaviors, circumstances in which these behaviors emerge, the contributory aspects of a given setting, and the effectiveness of approaches used to address them. In most situations, a functional analysis of the behavior or cluster of behaviors in question needs to be performed, typically under the supervision of a behavioral consultant with experience in working with individuals with autism-related conditions. Although this process is similar to the one employed in the case of individuals with autism of varying levels of function (Powers, 1997), children and adolescents with AS often possess resources, particularly verbal and cognitive abilities, that need to be capitalized on in order to maximize the effectiveness of the behavioral intervention plan. Therefore, behavioral assessments should not occur in isolation; rather, they should be an integral part of a more comprehensive process in which the individual's communication and behavioral abilities and disabilities are considered, so that both the behavioral treatment and the social and communication skills intervention can profit from and benefit the other.

Occupational Therapy and Assistive Technology

As many individuals with AS exhibit problems in fine motor skills, particularly in graphomotor abilities and speed of execution, as well as in motor planning, a more thorough occupational therapy assessment may be indicated to examine in more detail the person's needs in this area and to prescribe a set of practical intervention steps. The focus of this assessment should be on those skills that impinge more directly upon the person's acquisition of adaptive skills (e.g., dressing, grooming, and playing) and on academic performance (e.g., writing and drawing). For some individuals whose deficits also include organizational and other learning skills, an assistive technology assessment might be recommended (Raskind & Higgins, 1998). The goals of this assessment are to collect data pertinent to a prescriptive plan aimed at availing the student of an array of assistive devices, ranging from modified utensils to electronic organizers and computers, to advance his or her ability to accomplish academic goals and augment self-reliance and independence.

Family Assessment

The clinical focus on a child's disabilities may often lead to neglect of the fact that the child spends much of his or her time in the family setting, and that the presence of a child with disabilities in the family can place enormous burdens on family functioning in general (Marcus, Kunce, & Schopler, 1997) and on the various family members in particular, including siblings (Harris, 1994). Clinicians should always be available, in a supportive and resourceful manner, to address family's concerns not directly related to the child's being evaluated. In addition, a number of treatment issues directly impinging upon the child's functioning and program might need to be addressed in the context of the family, including parent training (Koegel, Bimbela, & Schreibman, 1996), behavioral interventions (Harris & Powers, 1984), burnout (Marcus, 1984), and advocacy (Surratt, 1984).

Vocational Assessment

The most important transitions for individuals with AS at the end of their school involve preparation for advanced studies or vocational training. Unfortunately, the school system is often lacking in preparing students for this transition, and parents often find themselves searching in a void for guidance in this process. Although professionals in the area of vocational assessment and job coaching are available in the community, the number of such professionals with expertise in the field of social disabilities is, unfortunately, extremely limited. Clinicians should be available to provide the guidance necessary to the students and their families by orienting vocational evaluators as to the important principles to be considered. For this purpose, the clinicians themselves need to become knowledgeable about principles of vocational assessment in the field of autism-related conditions (Hayes, 1987) and to learn about resources in the community and the options available to their clients (Gerhardt & Holmes, 1997) and aspects of their client's condition that may enhance or impede his or her success in advanced studies or in securing a job (see Chapter 12, this volume).

SUMMARY

The assessment of children and adolescents with AS is best conducted by an interdisciplinary team capable of covering the central developmental and symptomatological aspects of the condition. This team should be able to provide a comprehensive and coherent view of the child in terms of individualized strengths and needs that can be directly translated into a programmatic plan of treatment and educational intervention. The involvement of parents and educational professionals who can provide information on the child's functioning in more representative settings is crucial in this process. The assessment should include psychological, communication, and diagnostic components. The psychological component should include at a minimum detailed measures of cognitive functioning and of adaptive skills. The communication component should detail aspects of communication competence, including observations of prosodic patterns and conversational skills. The diagnostic component should integrate aspects of developmental history and current presentation with a view to define the major challenges impinging on the child's learning potential and social adjustment, as well as the behavioral strengths that can be capitalized upon in intervention. Clinicians should be aware of the major intervention resources available to individuals with AS, including social skills training programs, behavioral management approaches, family support techniques, and assistive technology, using the appropriate assessment procedure in their evaluation whenever the need for such resources becomes apparent. Throughout the assessment process, the focus should be on the child's individualized profile in terms of behavioral patterns and cognitive/communication resources. Adherence to this major focus should prevent the overemphasis on diagnostic assignment, which, in itself, is of limited value for the interventionist's effort to translate the assessment findings into a concrete program of treatment.

REFERENCES

Baron-Cohen, S. (1995). *Mindblindness: An essay on autism and theory of mind.* Cambridge, MA: MIT Press.

Beery, K. E. (1989). *Revised administration, scoring, and teaching manual for the Developmental Test of Visual–Motor Integration.* Cleveland, OH: Modern Curriculum Press.

Bender, L. (1938). *A Visual Motor Gestalt Test and its clinical use.* American Orthopsychiatric Association Research Monograph No. 3.

Benton, A. L., Hamsher, K. DeS., Varnay, N. R., & Spreen, O. (1983). *Contributions to neuropsychological assessment.* New York: Oxford University Press.

Benton, A. L., Hannay, H. J., & Varnay, N. R. (1975). Visual perception of line direction in patients with unilateral brain disease. *Neurology, 25,* 907–910.

Berthier, M. L., Bayes, A., & Tolosa, E. S. (1993). Magnetic resonance imaging in patients with concurrent Tourette's disorder and Asperger's syndrome. *Journal of the American Academy of Child and Adolescent Psychiatry, 32*(3), 633–639.

Bruininks, R. H. (1978). *Bruininks–Oseretsky Test of Motor Proficiency.* Circle Pines, MN: American Guidance Service.

Caplan, R. (1994). Thought disorder in childhood. *Journal of the American Academy of Child and Adolescent Psychiatry, 33*(5), 605–615.

Carrow-Woolfolk, E. (1985). *Test of Auditory Comprehension of Language—Revised.* Austin, Texas: Pro-Ed.

Carter, A. S., Volkmar, F. R., Sparrow, S. S., Wang, J. J., Lord, C., Dawson, G., Fombonne, E., Loveland, K., Mesibov, G., & Schopler, E. (1998). The Vineland Adaptive Behavior Scales: Supplementary norms for individuals with autism. *Journal of Autism and Developmental Disorders, 28*(4), 287–302.

Cegalis, J. (1993). *The Vigil Continuous Performance Test.* Nashua, NH: ForThought Ltd.

Dawson, G. (1983). Lateralized brain dysfunction in autism: Evidence from the Halstead–Reitan neuropsychological battery. *Journal of Autism and Developmental Disorders, 13*(3), 269–286.

Dean, R. S. (1977). Patterns of emotional disturbance on the WISC-R. *Journal of Clinical Psychology, 33,* 486–490.

Delis, D. C., Kramer, J. H., Kaplan, E., & Ober, B. A. (1987). *CVLT—California Verbal Learning Test.* San Antonio, TX: Psychological Corporation.

Dykens, E., Volkmar, F. R., & Glick, M. (1991). Thought disorder in high-functioning autistic adults. *Journal of Autism and Developmental Disorders, 21,* 291–231.

Ehlers, S., Nyden, A., Gillberg, C., Sandberg, A. D., Dahlgren, S. O., Hjelmquist, E., & Oden, A. (1997). Asperger syndrome, autism and attention disorders: A comparative study of the cognitive profiles of 120 children. *Journal of Child Psychology and Psychiatry, 38*(2), 207–217.

Exner, J. E., Jr. (1991). *The Rorschach: A comprehensive system, Vol. 2: Interpretation* (2nd ed.). New York: Wiley.

Fein, G. G. (1981). Pretend play in childhood: An integrative review. *Child Development, 52,* 1095–1102.

Fine, J., Bartolucci, G., Ginsberg, G., & Szatmari, P. (1991). The use of intonation to communicate in pervasive developmental disorders. *Journal of Child Psychology and Psychiatry, 32*(5), 771–782.

Gerhardt, P. F., & Holmes, D. L. (1997). Employment: Options and issues for adolescent and adults with autism. In D. J. Cohen & F. R. Volkmar (Eds.), *Handbook of autism and pervasive developmental disorders* (pp. 650–664). New York: Wiley.

Ghaziuddin, M., Butler, E., Tsai, L. Y., & Ghaziuddin, N. (1994). Is clumsiness a marker for Asperger Syndrome? *Journal of Intellectual Disabilities Research, 38*(5), 519–527.

Grant, D. A., & Berg, E. A. (1948). A behavioral analysis of degree of reinforcement and ease of shifting to new responses in a Weigle-type card sorting problem. *Journal of Experimental Psychology, 32,* 404–411.

Grice, P. (1975). Logic and conversation. In J. Cole & P. Morgan (Eds.), *Syntax and semantics: Speech acts* (pp. 41–59). New York: Academic Press.

Hannay, H. J., Falgout, J. C., & Leli, D. A., (1987). Focal right temporo-occipital blood flow changes associated with Judgment of Line Orientation. *Neuropsychologia, 25,* 755–763.

Harris, D. B. (1963). Children's drawings as measures of intellectual maturity: A revision and extension of the Goodenough Draw-a-Man Test. New York: Harcourt, Brace & World.

Harris, S. L. (1994). *Siblings of children with autism: A guide for families.* Bethesda, MD: Woodbine House.

Harris, S. L., & Powers, M. D. (1984). Behavior therapists look at the impact of an autistic child on the family system. In E. Schopler & G. B. Mesibov (Eds.), *The effects of autism on the family* (pp. 207–224). New York: Plenum.

Hayes, R. (1987). Training for work. In D. J. Cohen & A. M. Donnellan (Eds.), *Handbook of autism and pervasive developmental disorders* (pp. 360–370). New York: Wiley.

Hodgdon, L. (1995). Solving social-behavioral problems through the use of visually supported communication. In K. A. Quill (Ed.), *Teaching children with autism: Strategies to enhance communication and socialization* (pp. 265–286). New York: Delmar.

Kaufman, A. S. (1994). *Intelligent testing with the WISC-III.* New York: Wiley.

Kerbeshian, J., & Burd, L. (1986). Asperger's syndrome and Tourette syndrome: The case of the pinball wizard. *British Journal of Psychiatry, 148,* 731–736.

Klin, A. (1997, October 16). *Asperger's syndrome: Diagnosis and phenomenology.* Paper presented at the 44th annual meeting of the American Academy of Child and Adolescent Psychiatry, Toronto, Ontario, Canada.

Klin, A., Carter, A., Volkmar, F. R., Cohen, D. J., Marans, W. D., & Sparrow, S. S. (1997). Assessment issues in children with autism. In D. J. Cohen & F. R. Volkmar (Eds.), *Handbook of autism and pervasive developmental disorders* (pp. 411–447). New York: Wiley.

Klin, A., & Volkmar, F. R. (1997). Asperger's syndrome. In D. J. Cohen & F. R. Volkmar (Eds.), *Handbook of autism and pervasive developmental disorders* (pp. 94–122). New York: Wiley.

Klin, A., Volkmar, F. R., Sparrow, S. S., Cicchetti, D. V., & Rourke, B. P. (1995). Validity and neuropsychological characterization of Asperger syndrome. *Journal of Child Psychology and Psychiatry, 36*(7), 1127–1140.

Koegel, R. L., Bimbela, A., & Schreibman, L. (1996). Collateral effects of parent training on family interactions. *Journal of Autism and Developmental Disorders, 26*(3), 347–359.

Krug, D. A., Arick, J. R., & Almond, P. J. (1980). Behavior checklist for identifying severely handicapped individuals with high levels of autistic behavior. *Journal of Child Psychology and Psychiatry, 21,* 221–229.

Le Couteur, A., Rutter, M., Lord, C., Rios, P., Robertson, S., Holdgrafer, M., & McLennan, J. D. (1989). Autism Diagnostic Interview: A standardized investigator-based instrument. *Journal of Autism and Developmental Disorders, 19,* 363–387.

Littlejohns, C. S., Clarke, D. J., & Corbett, J. A. (1990). Tourette-like disorder in Asperger's syndrome. *British Journal of Psychiatry, 156,* 430–443.

Lord, C. (1997). Diagnostic instruments in autism spectrum disorders. In D. J. Cohen & F. R. Volkmar (Eds.), *Handbook of autism and pervasive developmental disorders* (pp. 460–483). New York: Wiley.

Lord, C., Rutter, M., & DiLavore, P. (1996). *Autism Diagnostic Observation Schedule—Generic (ADOS-G).* Unpublished manuscript, University of Chicago.

Lord, C., Rutter, M., & Le Couteur, A. (1994). Autism Diagnostic Interview—Revised: A revised version of a diagnostic interview for caregivers of individuals with possible pervasive developmental disorders. *Journal of Autism and Developmental Disorders, 24*(5), 659–685.

Marcus, L. M. (1984). Coping with burnout. In E. Schopler & G. B. Mesibov (Eds.), *The effects of autism on the family* (pp. 313–326). New York: Plenum.

Marcus, L. M., Kunce, L. J., & Schopler, E. (1997). Working with families. In D. J. Cohen & F. R. Volkmar (Eds.), *Handbook of autism and pervasive developmental disorders* (pp. 631–649). New York: Wiley.

Marcus, L. M., & Stone, W. L. (1993). Assessment of the young autistic child. In E. Schopler, M. E. Van Bourgondien, & M. M. Bristol (Eds.), *Preschool issues in autism* (pp. 149–174). New York: Plenum.

Marriage, K., Miles, T., Stokes, D., & Davey, M. (1993). Clinical and research implications of the co-occurrence of Asperger's and Tourette syndrome. *Australian and New Zealander Journal of Psychiatry, 27*(4), 666–672.

McDonald, M. A., Mundy, P., Kasari, C., & Sigman, M. (1989). Psychometric scatter in retarded, autistic preschoolers as measured by the Cattell. *Journal of Child Psychology and Psychiatry, 30*(4), 599–604.

Minshew, N. J., Goldstein, G., & Siegel, D. J. (1995). Speech and language in high-functioning autistic individuals. *Neuropsychology, 9*(2), 255–261.

Morgan, S. (1984). Helping parents understand the diagnosis of autism. *Journal of Developmental and Behavioral Pediatrics, 5*(2), 78–85.

Oldfield, R. C. (1971). The assessment and analysis of handedness: The Edinburgh Inventory. *Neuropsychologia, 9*, 97–113.

Ozonoff, S. (1998). Assessment and remediation of executive dysfunction in autism and Asperger syndrome. In E. Schopler, G. B. Mesibov, & L. J. Kunce (Eds.), *Asperger syndrome or high-functioning autism?* (pp. 263–289). New York: Plenum.

Ozonoff, S., Pennington, B. F., & Rogers, S. J. (1991). Executive function deficits in high-functioning autistic individuals: Relationship to theory of mind. *Journal of Child Psychology and Psychiatry, 32*(7), 1081–1105.

Paul, R., & Cohen, D. (1985). Comprehension of indirect requests in adults with mental retardation and pervasive developmental disorders. *Journal of Speech and Hearing Research, 28*, 475–479.

Pennington, B. F. (1991). *Diagnosing learning disorders: A neuropsychological framework*. New York: Guilford Press.

Pennington, B. F., & Ozonoff, S. (1996). Executive functions and developmental psychopathology. *Journal of Child Psychology and Psychiatry, 37*(1), 51–87.

Phelps-Terasaki, D., & Phelps-Gunn, T. (1992). *Test of Pragmatic Language*. Austin, TX: Pro-Ed.

Powers, M. D. (1997). Behavioral assessment of individuals with autism. In D. J. Cohen & F. R. Volkmar (Eds.), *Handbook of autism and pervasive developmental disorders* (pp. 448–459). New York: Wiley.

Prior, M. (1979). Cognitive abilities and disabilities in infantile autism: A review. *Journal of Abnormal Child Psychology, 7*, 357–380.

Prizant, B. M., Schuler, A. L., Wetherby, A., & Rydell, P. (1997). Enhancing language and communication development: Language approaches. In D. J. Cohen & F. R. Volkmar (Eds.), *Handbook of autism and pervasive developmental disorders* (pp. 572–605). New York: Wiley.

Raskind, M. H., & Higgins, E. L. (1998). Assistive technology for postsecondary students with learning disabilities: an overview. *Journal of Learning Disabilities, 31*(1), 27–40.

Riccio, C. A., & Hynd, G. W. (1992). Validity of Benton's Judgment of Line Orientation Test. *Journal of Psychoeducational Assessment, 10*, 210–218.

Schopler, E., & Reichler, R. J. (1972). How well do parents understand their own psychotic child? *Journal of Autism and Childhood Schizophrenia, 2*, 387–400.

Schopler, E., Reichler, R. J., & Renner, B. R. (1988). *The Childhood Autism Rating Scale (CARS)*. Los Angeles: Western Psychological Services.

Selman, R. L., Lavin, D. R., & Brion-Meisels, S. (1982). Troubled children's use of self-reflection. In F. C. Serafica (Ed.), *Social–cognitive development in context* (pp. 62–99). New York: Guilford Press.

Semel, E., Wiig, E., & Secord, W. (1995). *Clinical Evaluation of Language Fundamentals—Third Edition*. San Antonio, TX: Psychological Corporation.

Shea, V. (1993). Interpreting results to parents of preschool children. In E. Schopler, M. E. Van Bourgondien, & M. M. Bristol (Eds.), *Preschool issues in autism* (pp. 185–198). New York: Plenum.

Siegel, D. J., Minshew, N. J., & Goldstein, G. (1996). Wechsler IQ profiles in diagnosis of high functioning autism. *Journal of Autism and Developmental Disorders, 26*(4), 389–406.

Snyderman, M., & Rothman, S. (1987). Survey of expert opinion on intelligence and aptitude testing. *American Psychologists, 42*, 137–144.

Sparrow, S. S., Balla, D., & Cicchetti, D. (1984a). *Vineland Adaptive Behavior Scales, Expanded edition*. Circle Pines, MN: American Guidance Service.

Sparrow, S. S., Balla, D., & Cicchetti, D. (1984b). *Vineland Adaptive Behavior Scales, Survey edition*. Circle Pines, MN: American Guidance Service.

Sparrow, S. S., Balla, D., & Cicchetti, D. (1985). *Vineland Adaptive Behavior Scales, Classroom edition*. Circle Pines, MN: American Guidance Service.

Stellern, J., Vasa, S. F., & Little, J. (1976). *Introduction to diagnostic–prescriptive teaching and programming*. Glen Ridge, NJ: Exceptional Press.

Surratt, J. E. (1984). Advocacy: Effectively changing the system. In E. Schopler & G. B. Mesibov (Eds.), *The effects of autism on the family* (pp. 129–143). New York: Plenum.

Tager-Flusberg, H. (1989). A psycholinguistic perspective on language development in the autistic child. In G. Dawson (Ed.), *Nature diagnosis and treatment* (pp. 92–118). New York: Guilford Press.

Thorndike, R. L., Hagen, E. P., & Sattler, J. M. (1986). *Guide for administering and scoring the Stanford–Binet Intelligence Scale: Fourth edition*. Chicago: Riverside.

Tiffen, J. (1968). *The Purdue Pegboard Test*. Chicago, IL: Science Research.

Towbin, K. E. (1997). Pervasive developmental disorder not otherwise specified. In D. J. Cohen & F. R. Volkmar (Eds.), *Handbook of autism and pervasive developmental disorders* (pp. 123–147). New York: Wiley.

Volkmar, F. R., Carter, A., Sparrow, S. S., & Cicchetti, D. V. (1993). Quantifying social development in autism. *Journal of the American Academy of Child and Adolescent Psychiatry, 32*, 627–632.

Volkmar, F. R., & Klin, A. (in press). The pervasive developmental disorders. In H. Kaplan & B. Sadock (Eds.), *Comprehensive textbook of psychiatry* (7th ed.). Baltimore, MD: Williams & Wilkins.

Volkmar, F. R., Klin, A., Schultz, R. B., Bronen, R., Marans, W. D., Sparrow, S. S., & Cohen, D. J. (1996). Grand Rounds in Child Psychiatry: Asperger's syndrome. *Journal of the American Academy of Child and Adolescent Psychiatry, 35*(1), 118–123.

Volkmar, F. R., Klin, A., Schultz, R., Pauls, D., & Cohen, D. J. (1996, October 22–27). *Symposium on Asperger's syndrome: Diagnosis, neuropsychology, neuroimaging, and genetic aspects.* Presented at the 43rd annual meeting of the American Academy of Child and Adolescent Psychiatry, Philadelphia.

Volkmar, F. R., Klin, A., Siegel, B., Szatmari, P., Lord, C., Campbell, M., Freeman, B. J., Cicchetti, D. V., Rutter, M., Kline, W., Buitelaar, J., Hattab, Y., Fombonne, E., Fuentes, J., Werry, J., Stone, W., Kerbeshian, J., Hoshino, Y., Bregman, J., Loveland, K., Szymanski, L., & Towbin, K. (1994). DSM-IV autism/pervasive developmental disorder field trial. *American Journal of Psychiatry, 151,* 1361–1367.

Volkmar, F. R., Sparrow, S. S., Goudreau, D., Cicchetti, D., & Cohen, D. J. (1987). Social deficits in autism: An operational approach using the Vineland Adaptive Behavior Scales. *Journal of the American Academy of Child and Adolescent Psychiatry, 26*(2), 156–161.

Wechsler, D. (1989). *Manual for the Wechsler Preschool and Primary Scale of Intelligence—Revised.* San Antonio, TX: Psychological Corporation.

Wechsler, D. (1992). *Manual for the Wechsler Intelligence Scale for Children, 3rd edition.* San Antonio, TX: Psychological Corporation.

Wechsler, D. (1997). *Manual for the Wechsler Adult Intelligence Scale, 3rd edition.* San Antonio, TX: Psychological Corporation.

Wetherby, A., Schuler, A. L., & Prizant, B. M. (1997). Enhancing language and communication development: Theoretical Foundations. In D. J. Cohen & F. R. Volkmar (Eds.), *Handbook of autism and pervasive developmental disorders* (pp. 513–538). New York: Wiley.

Wiig, E., & Secord, W. (1989). *Test of Language Competence—Expanded edition.* San Antonio, TX: Psychological Corporation.

Williams, S. M. (1986). Factor analysis of the Edinburgh Handedness Inventory. *Cortex, 22,* 325–326.

World Health Organization. (1993). *International classification of diseases: Tenth revision.* Chapter V. Mental and behavioral disorders (including disorders of psychological development). Diagnostic criteria for research. Geneva: Author.

Zachman, L., Barrett, M., & Huisingh, R. (1984). *Test of Problem Solving—Elementary.* East Moline, IL: Lingui-Systems.

Zachman, L., Barrett, M., Huisingh, R., Orman, J., & Blagden, C. (1991). *Test of Problem Solving—Adolescent.* San Antonio, TX: Psychological Corporation.

12

Treatment and Intervention Guidelines for Individuals with Asperger Syndrome

AMI KLIN
FRED R. VOLKMAR

Most of this volume is concerned with diagnostic, neuropsychological, and neurobiological issues related to Asperger syndrome (AS). The uncertainty regarding the validity of the condition, the limitations of current research, and the confusion prevalent in clinical practice can all be very disconcerting to parents and educational professionals alike, whose primary focus is on how to provide services to one specific child. Although this chapter builds on current knowledge and clinical experience, it does not presuppose a consensus on any of the other issues discussed in the other sections of this book. In other words, regardless of the specific nosological status of AS, and even regardless of whether this diagnosis applies flawlessly to a given individual, there are certain guidelines for intervention that are thought to be helpful in devising treatment programs for individuals with severe social disabilities with relative strengths in cognitive and language functioning. Intervention programs should never be based solely on a given diagnosis; rather programs should be highly individualized to address a specific child's needs while capitalizing on the child's assets. Therefore, even though treatment programs for individuals with AS do not require the resolution of the vexing questions of diagnosis and etiology, they do require a thorough understanding of the specific individual's profile of skills and deficits in areas important for learning, for communicating and relating with others, and for acquiring independent living skills.

The aim of this chapter is not to provide a scholarly review of the work available on educational and behavioral interventions for individuals with severe social disabilities. Instead, this chapter provides a series of suggestions to be considered when planning and implementing the intervention program for a given person. Readers interested in more details about the various topics addressed are referred to the original cited materials. Although the research literature on interventions for individuals with AS is still scant, several helpful texts are available that portray different approaches and provide a wealth of concrete ideas and teaching strategies for individuals with this or similar conditions (e.g., Attwood, 1998; Myles & Simpson, 1998; Quill, 1995; Schopler & Mesibov, 1992; Schopler, Mesibov, & Kunce, 1998). Equally helpful materials can be accessed in the literature of interventions for children with learning disabilities (e.g., Minskoff, 1994; Minskoff & DeMoss, 1994), whose profile often includes a social disability component of varying degrees (Gresham, 1992). In this context, the treatment guidelines outlined by Rourke (1989, 1995) for children with Nonverbal Learning Disabilities (NLD) is of particular importance given that there appears to be some areas of convergence in both learning and social style between what is referred to as NLD and AS (Klin, Sparrow, Volkmar, Cicchetti, & Rourke, 1995). Other chapters in this volume provide additional relevant information (e.g., Chapter 7 discusses drug treatments).

Understandably, the needs of children with autism and the support services available to address these needs—from special education schools, to model programs and research data on intervention approaches—have become associated with a profile of severe social disability usually accompanied by equally severe cognitive and language limitations and behavioral challenges. As a result, parents of individuals with AS often find themselves unable to profit from the considerable resources associated with the term "autism," because their children's needs and challenges as well as their strengths are quite different. This historical development has resulted in a void of support services for more able children with social disabilities and their families, who, to some extent, have become orphans in a system primarily categorized in terms of autism on the one hand and the more academically based learning disabilities or mainstream education on the other hand. There is little doubt that this situation has been the main motivator for the proliferation of regional and national parent support organizations coalescing around the terms "Asperger syndrome," "higher-functioning autism," or "higher-functioning pervasive developmental disorders." The following set of treatment and intervention guidelines accompanies this trend by extracting the principles and strategies that are thought to be uniquely suited to address the needs of individuals with AS and their families.

SECURING AND IMPLEMENTING SERVICES

The authorities who decide on entitlement to services are sometimes unaware of the extent and significance of the disabilities involved in AS. Proficient verbal skills, overall IQ usually within the normal or above normal range, and a solitary lifestyle often mask outstanding deficiencies observed primarily in novel or otherwise socially demanding situations, thus decreasing other people's perception of these children's salient needs for supportive intervention. Thus, active participation on the part of the clinician, together with parents and possibly an advocate, to forcefully pursue the patient's eligibility for services is often needed. It is the case, however, that educational professionals are becoming increasingly more aware of the condition, not in small part because of the extremely effective dissemination of information being carried out by parent support organizations armed with Internet Web sites and the latest clinical and research literature. Also, the apparent increased use of the term "Asperger syndrome" by clinicians has led to an increase in referrals for special education services and has forced educators to pursue further training of their personnel and restructuring of services to better cater to children with this unique profile of severe social and communication disabilities in the presence of cognitive and language strengths. Unfortunately, this development is uneven in different parts of North America, and it is still common for parents to confront denial of services because the child is seen as "too bright," "too verbal," or "doing very well academically."

Individuals with AS have been identified in the past with different diagnostic concepts, which at times considerably frustrate their parents' effort to secure adequate services. For example, through our partnership with the Learning Disabilities Association of America we were able to learn that many individuals with AS or related conditions were diagnosed as learning disabled (with the occasional accompanying notes highlighting the presence of some "eccentric features"); this nonpsychiatric diagnostic label is often much less effective in securing services. Parents of children with AS who carry a diagnosis of autism or pervasive developmental disorders not otherwise specified (PDD-NOS) often had to contend with educational programs designed for much lower-functioning children, thus failing to have their children's relative strengths and unique disabilities properly addressed. Yet another large number of individuals with AS were sometimes characterized as exhibiting "social–emotional maladjustment" (SEM), or "social–emotional disturbance" (SED), an educational label often associated with conduct problems and willful maladaptive behaviors. These individuals were often placed in educational settings for individuals with conduct disorders, thus allowing for possibly the worst mismatch, namely, the bringing together of individuals with a naïve understanding of social situations and individuals who can and do manipulate social situations to their advantage without the benefit of self-restraint. In other words, the perfect victims placed with the perfect victimizers.

Not that individuals with AS may not present with significant maladaptive and disruptive behaviors in social settings; however, these behaviors are often a result of their narrow and overly concrete understanding of social phenomena and the resultant overwhelming puzzlement they experience when required to meet the demands of interpersonal or group social life. As a result, the social maladaptive behaviors exhibited by individuals with AS should be looked at in the context of a thoughtful and comprehensive intervention needed to address their social disability—as a curriculum need—and not as punishable, willful behaviors deserving suspensions or other disciplinary measures that in fact mean very little to them, punish them for their disability, and only exacerbate their already poor self-esteem.

It is often helpful for the child's advocates to bring to the school authorities' attention the fact that the child can look better or worse depending on the setting in which he or she is observed. Situations in which the child may be observed in optimal adjustment to the school setting tend to be highly structured and routinized or otherwise academically driven situations. Situations that maximize the visibility of the condition include unstructured social situations (particularly with same-age peers) and novel situations requiring intuitive or quick-adjusting social problem-solving skills. The same observation applies to the clinicians conducting the evaluation intended to ascertain the need for special services: Such an evaluation should include detailed interviews with parents and professionals knowledgeable of the child in naturalistic settings (e.g., home and school) and, if possible, direct observations of the child in unstructured periods such as recess time or otherwise unsupervised settings (see Chapter 11, this volume).

Finally, it is not uncommon for the focus of educational professionals' concern to center around a child's increasingly challenging behavioral problems, including noncompliance, anxiety, disruptive behaviors such as "talking back," interrupting classroom activities, "bothering" other children, or even verbal aggression or otherwise "acting out." Resources are often allocated to address the disruptive behaviors, including the assignment of an aide, disciplinary measures, behavioral management aimed at extinguishing the problematic behaviors, and, at times, despair, which then includes contacting outside specialists and considering removal of the child from school to a self-contained placement or even home-bound schooling. What is often lacking in this effort is the consideration of the behaviors in question as, at least partially, a result of the child's social disability. If this paradigm shift is effected, the solution for the disruptive behaviors is often found in a more comprehensive program of action, which gives center stage to the social disability and its impact on the child's capacity for adjusting to the demands of everyday life at school. No doubt, some of these steps might still have to be taken, but by implementing them as if the social disability was not there, such a strategy is more likely to result in escalation of behavioral difficulties and in increase of general frustration to all those involved, including the child.

GENERAL EDUCATIONAL INTERVENTION SETTING

Although one of the main social policy debates in special education has focused on whether children with special needs such as autism and related conditions should be in a self-contained or a mainstream environment (Burack, Root, & Zigler, 1997), most professionals would agree that these children are best provided with a continuum of services built around the child's individual needs (Harris & Handleman, 1997). The reality of available services in a given region, however, often determine what might be the specific mix of specialized and inclusive experience that is adequate, if not optimal, for a given child. Whereas self-contained settings may be best equipped to provide the specialized services a socially disabled child needs, these settings often fail to provide enough experiences with typical peers from whom a child may model appropriate behaviors and learn to function in a "real-life" environment. Regular school environments may provide the latter but may not have the resources to address the former. There are no inherent flaws in either model as successful intervention program can be provided in either setting provided there is an effort to optimize individualized services, expanding, creating, training, monitoring, and empirically evaluating the program over time.

Parents of individuals with AS often ask the question, "Where are the best schools for children with this condition?" Although some special education schools have been developing some special expertise in this area, in most situations the answer to this question is more complex, as there are virtually no schools that identify themselves as "AS schools," nor would it be probably a good thing that only segregated settings could provide the specialized educational intervention. Both private and public school settings can provide a good program. This section deals with the elements of an adequate program, not necessarily where this program should be provided, as the possibilities are wide open. The absence of readily identified schools serving bright children with severe social disabilities makes the process of securing an appropriate program quite difficult for both parents and clinicians seeking the right placement. Detailed state registers are often lacking, and the parents and/or clinicians are left to deal with this issue on their own. Quite often, an effective partnership is established between the child's caregivers and the school district authorities, although at times there is mistrust and even litigation. To avoid adversarial relationships, all people involved should make an effort to acquaint themselves with the following factors involved in securing or providing appropriate placement and programming for children with social disabilities:

1. *The range of services available in the region.* Educational managers should have a detailed knowledge of all resources available within their immediate jurisdiction as well as in a wider contiguous region and make this information available to all those involved in the process, but parents should make an attempt to visit the various suggested educational placements and service providers available to obtain firsthand knowledge and feelings about them, including the physical setting, staffing, adult/student ratio, range of special/support services, children mix, and so forth.

2. *Knowledge of model programs.* Parents and professionals should make an effort to locate programs (public or private) that are thought to provide high-quality services according to local experts, parent support organizations, or other parents. Regardless of whether the program is an option for the given child, knowledge of such programs may provide all those concerned with a model and criteria with which to judge the appropriateness of the program in discussion for the specific child.

3. *Knowledge of the rights and duties of all those involved in the process leading to educational placement.* It is crucial that parents become acquainted with their legal rights in order to become effective advocates for their children (Berkman, 1997), and it is equally important that the school authorities establish their own knowledge base of appropriate services so that fringe or otherwise questionable educational practices unsupported by any data are not forcefully introduced into a program because of legal pressure. Discussions likely to produce consensual agreement tend to be based on detailed and individualized knowledge of a child's needs, which refrain from ideological statements (e.g., treatment X is good for all children, regardless of the child's profile), and seek to evaluate existing services while not precluding the creation of new ones. An evolving partnership between parents, educational professionals, and specialists in the various components of the educational program is needed, which includes mechanisms of self-evaluation and empirical monitoring, and which leads to a periodic adjustment of goals, discarding ineffective approaches and testing new ones.

When reviewing the appropriateness of a given program for a bright child with social disabilities, the infrastructure of educational resources should be the focus of discussion, including the available resources that will serve the given child. The following specifications are usually thought to be positive and necessary resources, which, however, may vary in content from place to place:

1. Although a relatively small setting is usually preferable, regardless of the size of the program, the setting should provide ample opportunity for individual attention, individualized approach, and small work groups. At times, a compromise is reached by placing a socially disabled child in a large setting accompanied by a paraprofessional aide. This alternative is only helpful if there is an infrastructure of expertise and support for

the child beyond the immediate presence of the aide; the absence thereof places undue responsibility on a less trained person, however gifted he or she might be. As a result, the aide rather than supporting the child inclusion in the program might end up serving as a virtual partition between the child and peers, constantly redirecting, mediating, or otherwise containing the child.

2. An essential aspect of the available educational infrastructure concerns the availability of a communication specialist with a special interest in pragmatics and social skills training, who can be available for individual and small-group work, and who also can make communication and social skills training intervention an integral part of all school activities, implemented at all times, consistently, and across staff members, settings, and situations. This professional should also act as a resource to the other staff members and an advocate of the social and communication skills training aspect of the curriculum.

3. There should be opportunities for social interaction and promotion of social relationships in fairly structured and supervised activities. By building social contact around a common interest or activity, the pressure of unstructured social exchange is lessened, making the experience more likely to be successful. Of course, there should be naturalistic interaction as well, although the availability of different configurations of social settings—from individual work to small groups to structured larger group activities to unstructured large natural gatherings such as recess time or lunch—makes it possible to practice social skills in one setting and then to apply them in others. It also allows for frequently troublesome situations to be identified in larger settings and then brought into the small therapeutic setting for correction, skill building, practice, and rehearsal.

4. There should be a concerted effort to promote the acquisition of real-life skills in addition to the academic goals. The norm in individuals with AS (Klin, 1997) is to exhibit a significant discrepancy between cognitive potential (i.e., IQ) and their ability to translate this into adaptive functioning (i.e., constructive real-life behaviors consistently performed to meet the demands of everyday life). Although it is always encouraging to document a child's potential, longer-term goals including the child's prospects for vocational accomplishment and independent living require higher-level adaptive skills than are usually found in this population. Therefore, adaptive skills should be one of the central points of any program for a child with AS.

5. There should be a willingness to adapt the curriculum content and requirements to provide flexible opportunities for success, to foster the acquisition of a more positive self-concept, and to foster an internalized investment in performance and progress. Assignments, projects, and so on, should be evaluated in terms of their contribution to the child's longer-term educational goals rather than being enchained to inflexible (e.g., credit) requirements. This may mean that the individual with AS is provided with in-

dividual challenges in his or her areas of strengths, and with individualized programs in his or her areas of weakness. For example, given the fact that individuals with AS often excel in certain activities, social situations may be constructed to allow the child the opportunity to take the leadership in the activity, explaining, demonstrating, or teaching others about it. Such situations are ideal to help the individual with AS to (a) take the perspective of others, (b) follow conversation and social interaction rules, and (c) follow coherent and less one-sided goal-directed behaviors and approaches. In addition, by taking the leadership in an activity, the individual's self-esteem is likely to be enhanced, and the child's (usually disadvantageous) position vis-à-vis peers is for once reversed. When this initiative is entertained, however, appropriate preparation should take place, so that the result obtained is not the reverse of the envisioned goal because of undue pressure placed on the child.

6. Children with AS are often overwhelmed by the day-to-day pressures of life at school. One proactive way of addressing this issue is to make available to the child a sensitive in-school counselor who can focus on the individual's emotional well-being and serve as the "safe address" to the child, and who can coordinate services, monitor progress, serve as a resource to other staff members, and be an effective and supportive liaison with the family.

GENERAL INTERVENTION STRATEGIES

Strategies of intervention—including teaching practices and approaches, behavioral management techniques, strategies for emotional support, and activities intended to foster social and communication competence—should be conceived and implemented in a thoughtful, consistent (across settings, staff members, and situations), and individualized manner. Equally important, the benefit (or lack thereof) of specific recommendations should be assessed in an empirical fashion (i.e., based on an evaluation of events observed, documented, or charted), with useful strategies being maintained and unhelpful ones discarded in order to promote an ongoing adjustment of the program to the specific conditions of the individual child with AS. The following suggestions may be helpful when considering the optimal approaches to be adopted. It should be noted, however, that there are different degrees of concreteness and rigidity, paucity of insight, social awkwardness, communicative one-sidedness, and so forth, characterizing individuals with AS and that the particular circumstances and patterns of strength and weakness all require consideration. Care providers should embrace the wide range of expression and complexity of the disorder, avoiding dogmatism in favor of practical, individualized, and commonsense clinical judgment. The following general recommendations are ones which require thoughtful individualized adjustment:

1. Problem-solving skills in general but also concepts and helpful behavioral routines should be taught in an explicit and sometimes rote fashion using a parts-to-whole teaching approach, often couched in verbal instruction, and presented and rehearsed in such a way that the verbal steps are in the correct sequence for the behavior to be effective.

2. Specific problem-solving strategies should be taught for handling the requirements of frequently occurring troublesome situations. Training should also be necessary for recognizing situations as troublesome and for applying learned strategies in discrepant situations.

3. The individual with AS should be instructed on how to identify a novel situation and to resort to a preplanned, well-rehearsed list of steps to be taken. This list should involve a description of the situation, retrieval of pertinent knowledge, and step-by-step decision making. When the situation permits (another item to be explicitly defined), one of these steps might be reliance on the counselor's, a friend's, or an adult's advice, including a telephone consultation;

4. Social awareness should be cultivated at every opportunity, focusing on the relevant and essential aspects of given situations and pointing out the marginal or irrelevant aspects contained therein. Discrepancies between the individual's perceptions regarding the situation in question and the perceptions of others should be made explicit.

5. An important priority in the program is to foster generalization of learned strategies and social skills. This is also one of the main challenges (e.g., Gaylord-Ross, Haring, Breen, & Pitts-Conway, 1984; Ihrig & Wolchik, 1988). Although a great deal of attention and research has been invested in generalization technology in the field of behavioral therapies (Powers, 1997), less knowledge is available in the crucial areas of social and communication skills training. But this situation is changing, and new research studies are now becoming available in this area as well (e.g., Gena, Krantz, McClannahan, & Poulson, 1996; Taylor & Harris, 1995). From a programming perspective what is important is to define generalization explicitly as a goal to be achieved, including the various specific strategies to be implemented and the goals in the light of which the success of the program will be measured.

6. Self-evaluation should be encouraged, but it is important that this process is done in a concrete and explicit fashion concerning day-to-day behaviors, and not on the basis of insight-oriented, more fundamental reappraisal of oneself, which might frustrate the child and/or further exacerbate negative self-feelings. Awareness should be gained into which situations are easily managed and which are potentially troublesome. This is especially important with respect to perceiving the need to use prelearned strategies in appropriate situations. Self-evaluation should also be used to strengthen self-esteem, but this should be done by way of choosing or restructuring the situations to promote success. The goal here is to teach the children about

the situations in which they are more likely to present themselves in a position of strength rather than a position of vulnerability or weakness;

7. The link between specific frustrating or anxiety-provoking experiences and negative feelings should be taught to the individuals with AS in a concrete, cause–effect fashion, so that they are able to gradually increase insight into their feelings and have more control over the situations that usually result in negative feelings or otherwise emotional pressure. In this context, it is also important to promote awareness of the impact of their actions on other people's reactions and feelings, to gain increased control over the result of their social experiences.

8. Adaptive skills intended to increase self-sufficiency should be taught explicitly with no assumption that general explanations might suffice or, as noted, that the children will be able to generalize from one concrete situation to similar ones. Rule sequences for shopping and using transportation, for example, should be taught verbally and repeatedly rehearsed. There should be constant coordination and communication between all those involved in order to maximize consistency. A list of specific adaptive behaviors to be taught may be derived from results obtained with the Vineland Adaptive Behavior Scales, Expanded Edition (Sparrow, Balla, & Cicchetti, 1984), which assess adaptive behavior skills in the areas of Communication, Daily Living (self-help) Skills, Socialization, and Motor Skills. As the behaviors listed in the Vineland are normed, it is possible to extract from this instrument all skills that the individual should be exhibiting given his or her cognitive level and then to incorporate these skills in the child's program. The Vineland may also be used to gauge progress in adaptive skill development using a test–retest model after a meaningful period (e.g., at the end of two consecutive school years).

9. Additional teaching guidelines should be derived from the individual's profile of neuropsychological assets and deficits. The major areas of neuropsychological focus should be motor, fine motor, and visual–motor coordination, including graphomotor skills, visual–spatial attention, perception, problem-solving and memory skills; auditory/verbal attention, learning, reasoning, and memory; cross-modal integration of information, and executive functions (see later). Specific intervention techniques should aimed at remediating or circumventing the identified difficulties by means of compensatory strategies, usually of a verbal nature. However, the goals established for intervention based on neuropsychological findings should be broad based, with a view to address central aspects of the social disability. For example, if significant motor, sensory-integration, or visual–motor deficits are corroborated during an evaluation, the individual with AS should receive physical and occupational therapies, but not only should these therapies focus on traditional techniques designed to remediate these deficits but also they should promote the learning of visual–spatial concepts (e.g., order, causation, sequencing, and left–right orientation), real-life navigation

issues (e.g., how to get somewhere), and time concepts, pairing narratives and verbal self-guidance to the actual physical activity taking place. Another adequate goal to be advanced in occupational therapy intervention is to teach self-help skills (e.g., dressing and grooming) and to promote the optimal utilization of assistive technology (e.g., computer-based skills; see later discussion). Other neuropsychological deficits such as difficulties in processing visual sequences or in interpreting visual information simultaneously with auditory information, particularly in social situations, should be addressed by promoting increased reliance on verbal mediation (e.g., having a script) and on explicit routines for seeking relevant information (e.g., having a stepwise routine to be followed including looking at the other person's eyes or listening to the person's voice for explicit cues). Cross-modal integration is of particular importance as, for example, it is important not only to be able to interpret other people's nonverbal behavior correctly but also to interpret what is being said in conjunction with these nonverbal cues (Minskoff, 1980a, 1980b; Rourke, 1989; 1995).

SOCIAL AND COMMUNICATION SKILLS TRAINING

Almost universally, the most important component of the intervention program for individuals with AS involves the need to enhance communication and social competence. This emphasis does not reflect a societal pressure for conformity or an attempt to stifle individuality and uniqueness. Rather, this emphasis reflects the clinical fact that most individuals with AS are not loners by choice, and that there is a tendency, as children develop toward adolescence, for despondency, negativism, and sometimes, clinical depression, as a result of the individual's increasing awareness of personal inadequacy in social situations, and of repeated experiences of failure to make and/or maintain relationships (Klin & Volkmar, 1997). The typical limitations of insight and self-reflection vis-à-vis others often preclude spontaneous self-adjustment to social and interpersonal demands. Therefore, there is a need to teach social and communication skills, explicitly, at all times, as an integral part of the program and as its major priority. Training in communication and social skills usually does not imply that the child will eventually acquire communicative or social spontaneity, naturalness, and gracefulness. It does, however, better prepare the individual with AS to cope with social and interpersonal expectations, thus enhancing their effectiveness as conversational partners, as potential friends or companions, and as employable professionals. Many adults with this condition are not given an opportunity to exhibit their considerable talents and skills because of failure during the interview stage of job applications; earlier in life they might be lost in a vicious cycle of misguided attempts to pursue goals that are incompatible with their profile of strengths and weaknesses, leading to repeated experiences of failure and a resultant poor view of themselves. Limited insight might also signify that the person may pursue an irrelevant course of action. For example, after being turned down in several job interviews, talented college graduates might attempt to pursue a manual job that requires considerable eye–hand coordination skills, manual dexterity, improvisation in novel situations, and speed of execution, all skills usually found to be weaknesses in these individuals' profiles. Feeling the burden of failure in what they might see as a "menial" job not commensurate with their educational training, they might pursue an additional degree, only to repeat this cycle next time they approach the job market. Unless issues of social presentation and competence are adequately addressed, including what to do in specific situations such as lunch or free-time periods, the chances for vocational satisfaction are lessened.

The observation that social and communication skills building is the core intervention component for individuals with AS and related social disabilities is certainly not new (Mesibov, 1984, 1986). However, this emphasis in the literature has not necessarily translated into more readily available educational programs and resources. And even though school systems are increasingly more aware of this issue, and parents are repeatedly told of the importance of social and communication skills training, the situation in the field is still quite frustrating for all those concerned, service providers and consumers alike. Until recently, the immediate reason for this state of affairs had to do with the lack of a readily available program of intervention in this area; more recently, however, there has been a small, but important, upsurge of ideas and strategies for social skills building (e.g., Baron-Cohen & Howlin, 1998; Gray, 1995; Hodgdon, 1995; Koegel & Koegel, 1995), including some initial treatment studies (e.g., Ozonoff & Miller, 1995). The reality, however, is that the number of professionals trained to implement such a curriculum, or even to train educational professionals on the fundamentals of this approach, is still quite minimal, leaving both educational managers and parents in a dire quandary, namely, how to include what is being promoted as the most important component of any program for individuals with social disabilities without access to the knowledge base in this area, and even less access to professionals who feel comfortable carrying out the social-skills-building program. Clearly, without a concerted effort to develop this area as a discipline in which a much larger number of professionals are trained, curricula are developed, and research data are produced, this situation will not be easily changed, and is likely to worsen before it starts to get better, hopefully as a result of clinicians', educational managers', and parents' pressure. At present, the professionals who would appear to be at the greatest advantage to play the central role in this area are speech and language therapists with a special interest in pragmatics or conversational skills, although other mental health or educational professionals could certainly be equally proficient. The issue, of course, is that all these professionals require training not only in social and communication skills training but also in the unique challenges posed by bright individuals with severe social disabilities.

Although there are a few prepackaged social skills programs available commercially, they are of limited effectiveness because they are not based on the specific experiences of a given socially disabled child. Also these packages tend to promote prosocial skills in children whose difficulties do not require the much more intensive and explicit intervention needed in AS. However, it is important for the special educator to become acquainted with these materials as some resources can be of great help in specific areas (e.g., in expanding the vocabulary of emotions, in playing cooperative games, in social problem solving).

Although there are several established approaches to social and communication skills training, there are still few research data available on their effectiveness. This situation is improving, albeit slowly, with a trickle of research studies that have been published in the past few years (e.g., Ozonoff & Miller, 1995; Pierce & Schreibman, 1997; Thorp, Stahmer, & Schreibman, 1995). Excellent reviews of social and communication skills training are available (e.g., Prizant, Schuler, Wetherby, & Rydell, 1997; Quill, 1995; Twachtman, 1995), including the use of behavioral approaches in promoting social development (Matson, Benavidez, Compton, Paclawskyj, & Baglio, 1996). However, these reviews often focus on principles and general techniques rather than providing a readily applicable and accessible practical approach. As a result, professionals working in the front line often request the translation of these principles into a "package," "instruction manual," or an otherwise concrete plan to follow in their effort to serve their clients.

Such concrete, adjustable "packages" are now also becoming available. Following are some examples that focus on more able individuals with social disabilities. It should be noted, however, that excellent programs have been described for the promotion of social and communication skills in individuals with autism who exhibit significant cognitive and language deficits (e.g., Carr et al., 1994; Koegel & Koegel, 1995). Several aspects of these programs may be applicable to more able socially disabled individuals as well.

1. *Social Stories.* One of the most interesting, recent approaches for social skills training in autism and related conditions is the work of Gray and colleagues (Gray, 1995; Gray et al., 1993; Gray & Garand, 1993), who use visual and written materials and techniques based on situations from a child's actual experience to teach social skills. The individualization of the instructional process, combined with the use of written and videotape resources, and the fact that this approach grew from direct school-based work with individuals with social disabilities, makes it an attractive option for special educators.

2. *Visual strategies for improving communication.* This approach, which was developed by Hodgdon (1995, 1996), is in fact a compilation of effective visual tools and resources to aid the child in both communicating more effectively and better understanding the communication demands imposed by the surrounding social environment. It capitalizes on autistic children's typical visual–spatial strengths to compensate for their social and communication deficits. The major resource book (Hodgdon, 1996) provides concrete ideas and examples that can be readily adopted in the classroom. It is important to note, however, that these techniques may not be optimal for students whose visual–spatial processing skills are a weakness rather than a strength.

3. *Social perception skills training.* Minskoff and colleagues (Minskoff, 1987, 1994; Minskoff & DeMoss, 1994) developed two programs focused on social perception skills training for adolescents and adults. One of the very attractive elements of this program is that it focuses on social skills judged by employers as critical for job success.

4. *Teaching theory of mind (ToM).* Capitalizing on the ToM research in autism (Baron-Cohen, Tager-Flusberg, & Cohen, 1993), several attempts have been made to teach children underlying social cognitive principles necessary to infer the mental states of others (e.g., beliefs, intentions, and feelings)—that is, to acquire ToM skills. Although studies to date have shown that despite improvement on children's performance on experimental tasks there is apparently little improvement on general social competence (Ozonoff & Miller, 1995) or in communication competence (Hadwin, Baron-Cohen, Howlin, & Hill, 1997), the potential of this approach has not yet been properly evaluated. A practical guide is now available on this approach (Baron-Cohen & Howlin, 1998).

There are several core elements in these various approaches and in specialized clinical practices serving children and adolescents with social disabilities. The following strategies are often included in social and communication skills training:

1. *Awareness of conventional pragmatic or conversation rules* are central to every program, including topic selection, ways of marking topic shifts, and the ability to consistently provide the necessary amount of background information for an unfamiliar listener. This goal can be advanced by helping the child appreciate who is likely to be more interested or familiar with various topics. For example, relatives are more interested in and acquainted with topics related to the family than strangers; same-age peers are likely to be more interested in and familiar with topics related to movies, games, TV shows, and so on, than are adults. On the other hand, same-age peers are not likely to be interested in discussing more circumscribed topics

such as deep-sea marine biology or politics, or any special interest the child with AS may have that is likely to be unusual or eccentric to same-age peers. These unusual topics are more likely to be of interest to adults and teachers. It is helpful to foster the child's awareness of the varying interests of his or her friends by developing a list of preferred topics and less preferred topics for each individual friend. This goal is sometimes advanced by means of letter composition, where the child writes a letter to a friend, to a same-age acquaintance, to a relative, to an unfamiliar adult, to a celebrity, and so on.

2. *Appropriate "reading" of social cues* is a necessary precursor for generating appropriate comments, for adjusting to social demands, for determining the listener's perspective, reactions, and so on, and for maintaining a level of reciprocity without which there is communication breakdown (e.g., the listener may leave, become upset, or have unfavorable impressions of the speaker). For example, the child needs to be able to monitor the relative interest of his or her listener so he or she can make a decision as to whether the listener may be appreciating the exchange on a given topic or whether a new topic should be introduced. In this context, verbal instructions on how to interpret other people's social behavior are often helpful, following explicit guidelines accompanied by repeated rehearsal and practice, initially in a rote fashion and gradually moving toward variations of the initial practice situations. The meaning of eye contact, gaze, and various inflections, as well as tone of voice and facial and hand gestures, at times, needs to be taught in a fashion not unlike the teaching of a foreign language; that is, all elements should be made verbally explicit and appropriately and repeatedly drilled. The same principles should guide the training of the individual's expressive skills. Concrete situations should be exercised in the therapeutic setting (individually, or, preferably, in small groups) and gradually tried out in naturally occurring situations. All those in close contact with the individuals with AS should be made aware of the program so that consistency, monitoring, and contingent reinforcement are maximized. Of particular importance, encounters with unfamiliar people (e.g., making acquaintances) should be rehearsed until the individual is made aware of the impact of his or her behavior on other people's reactions to him or her. Techniques such as practicing in front of a mirror, listening to the recorded speech, watching a videorecorded behavior, and so forth, should all be incorporated in this program. Videotaped feedback, in particularly, has been found to be a useful medium for advancing this goal given the potential for pausing the picture and highlighting specific visual cues in a more explicit manner. Social situations contrived in the therapeutic setting that usually require reliance on visual–receptive and other nonverbal skills for interpretation should be used and strategies for deciphering the most salient nonverbal dimensions inherent in these situations should be offered and practiced. The following nonverbal social cues should be included in the program: (a) setting: the child needs to be made aware of where the interaction is taking

place, what expectations (e.g., volume of voice, style of speech) are associated with that setting (e.g., school playyard, church service); (b) body proximity: how to position oneself when engaged in conversation, the meaning of different postures, and what information can be gained from such cues; (c) facial, bodily, and voice emotional expressions: individuals with AS often require explicit instruction on the need to pay attention to affective expressions in all modalities, and on how to decode these separately, and, even more important, on how to integrate this set of cues into a meaningful context; and (d) special instruction is often needed with nonverbal cues providing the context of nonliteral forms of communication, including teasing, irony, and sarcasm, as well as figures of speech and humor. Other emotional tones of speech (e.g., excitement and anger) may also require instruction.

3. *Self-monitoring in conversation* often needs to be taught, with a view toward helping the child to adjust speech style in terms of setting (e.g., more or less formal) and volume (e.g., when a loud voice, say in a sports game, is appropriate and when a whisper, say in a funeral, is expected), as well as rate and rhythm, inflection modulation, stress for emphasis, and so on. The child may also need to be taught on how to adjust speech depending on proximity to the speaker and number of people and background noise.

These goals are often advanced in the context of individual, small-group (up to three students), or slightly larger (up to six students) social skills training groups using a range of specific techniques. In Gray's (1995) approach, for example, "Comic Strip Conversations" visually highlight the feelings and intentions of each speaker using color (e.g., red for teasing statements and green for friendly statements). By representing the emotional expression of the characters' statements, thoughts, and feelings, the perspective of those individuals becomes more readily apparent. "Topic Boxes" is another useful strategy: In this activity, a topic is drawn out of a box for both the socially disabled student and a peer or therapist to comment on while drawing attention to different opinions about these topics. Such specific techniques are organized under the more general "social review strategies," which include the following steps: (1) identification of a target social situation known to be problematic for the student; (2) gathering information about what the student already knows about that situation (including both helpful knowledge about setting, perceptions, interpretations, expectation, as well as unhelpful knowledge or absence thereof); (3) sharing observations of nonverbal cues, interpretations of a given situation, and so on, with other people in the group including peers and therapist; (4) practice of newly acquired knowledge and behaviors in the context of one-to-one exchanges, group interaction, watching videotapes, and casual conversation; and (5) generalization of skills to a variety of contexts under some supervision, so that the student's progress can be determined and outstanding or new problematic areas can be identified as situations to be revisited in the small, therapeutic environment.

In summary, the effort to develop the individual's skills with peers in terms of managing social situations should be a priority in any social and communication skills training program. This development should include *topic management* (to expand and elaborate on a range of different topics initiated by others, shifting topics, ending topics appropriately, and feeling comfortable with a range of topics that are typically discussed by same-age peers), *flexibility in social interaction* (to recognize and use a range of different means to interact, mediate, negotiate, persuade, discuss, and disagree through verbal and nonverbal means), *perception of nonverbal social cues* (to attend to and correctly understand the meaning of gaze, gestures, voice, and posture), *appreciation of social expectations associated with a given setting* (to be aware of the implications of where and with whom the social situation is taking place and to correctly derive the appropriate set of behaviors to that setting), and *operational knowledge of the language of mental states and related phenomena* (to make inferences, to predict, to explain motivation, and to anticipate multiple outcomes so as to increase the flexibility with which the person both thinks about and uses language with other people).

ORGANIZATIONAL SKILLS

Among the most established neuropsychological findings in studies of individuals with AS is the observation that they present with significant executive function (EF) deficits (Pennington & Ozonoff, 1996; Ozonoff, 1998). EFs denote a range of specific neuropsychological abilities, including, among others, inhibition of prepotent but irrelevant responses, adjustment of behavior using environmental feedback, extracting rules from experience, selection of essential from nonessential information, and upholding in one's mind both a desired goal and the various steps required to accomplish it. One of the most direct implications of deficits in EF concerns the well-known real-life difficulties that these individuals encounter in organizing their activities, in completing tasks in an efficient manner, in avoiding getting stuck in counterproductive routines, and in learning from their ongoing experiences. Some parents sometimes described their children as being devoid of a "pilot" or "navigator," requiring help with trivial matters such as shopping and completing homework assignments, despite being otherwise quite bright.

Such difficulties can be impairing, resulting in school failure or an inability to achieve a minimal level of community-related independent living skills. A lack of appreciation of these difficulties often results in giving students with AS long-term open-ended assignments and other forms of unstructured homework which they are unable to perform, not because they have difficulty with the subject but because they have problems producing a realistic stepwise plan on how to achieve their goal and then following the various steps to implement the plan. The combination of social and EF difficulties also result in problems with grooming, scheduling, and a long list of fundamental adaptive behavioral skills.

There are at least two forms of treatment and intervention to be considered in regard to these difficulties. The first approach uses computer-based cognitive rehabilitation packages that take the student along a series of exercises promoting each of the EF areas as well as other neuropsychological capacities underlying EF. Although this form of intervention has been shown to have positive impact on real-life skills in individuals with neurologically based disorders (e.g., Chen, Thomas, Glueckauf, & Bracy, 1997), the data on individuals with autism-related conditions are still scant. The second approach switches the focus from underlying neuropsychological capacities to the real-life situations in which the organizational skills deficits are most problematic for a given individual. This approach involves the identification of a person's frequently troublesome situations in which organizational skills are required and then the use of an assistive tool or approach to remediate the given problem. Specific remediation strategies range from creating lists or scripts detailing a stepwise approach to achieve a given goal and rehearsing with the individual the implementation of that list to the creation of pictorial schedules and reminders to the use of assistive technology (see next section). The latter usually provides the student with a readily available tool such as an electronic organizer or laptop computer, which gives the student immediate access to, for example, short-term and long-term schedules, homework assignments containing details of steps to be accomplished, in the order that they need to be completed for achieving the goal, and writing programs that organize narrative structure, elicit topics to be covered, and so on.

ASSISTIVE TECHNOLOGY

Assistive technology (AT) refers to the use of computer-based resources developed for individuals with disabilities. Although traditionally the focus has been on students with sensory and physical impairment, this focus has expanded considerably in the past few years, including also individuals with learning disabilities (Bryant & Bryant, 1998; Raskind & Higgins, 1998). AT was recognized by Congress as a viable need for people with disabilities when it passed the Technology-Related Assistance to Individuals with Disabilities Act in 1988, and reauthorized the legislation in 1994 (Bryant & Seay, 1998). This development has resulted in numerous services benefitting a wide range of individuals with disabilities (Lewis, 1998); the legislation mandating accessibility of this technology to students with disabilities has also led to increasing dissemination of these resources in school programs (Smith, 1998).

Unfortunately, there is still very little documentation on the use of AT in the field of autism and related conditions, particularly in regard to more able students who do not require basic enabling devices to operate a computer, to learn basic language skills, and so on. Nevertheless, individuals with AS and related conditions do exhibit many disabilities which can be effectively addressed by means of computer-based resources. Given the natural affinity with computers that these children often exhibit, this medium can be used to promote learning and adaption in a range of important areas. First, graphomotor difficulties are often found in AS; sometimes, students cannot complete their assignments, or they cannot properly expand their thoughts and learning because they are required to write their work by hand, resulting in a laborious, untidy, and frustrating process. Although handwriting should be addressed in occupational therapy, from a longer-term perspective, it does not make sense to enchain the student's learning to whatever he or she will be able to handwrite. The various commonplace tools available for grammatically correct writing and the more specialized software capable of eliciting and structuring the student's work, combined with enabling devices such as special keyboards or mouse, offer a long-term empowering strategy to deal with writing deficits. Second, as previously noted, individuals with AS often exhibit significant organizational and self-management deficits. Software designed to provide the student with clear schedules, task organizers, ready-made routines (or algorithms) for completion of frequent tasks, and so on, can be of great help to these students. Third, communication between home and school as well as between settings of the school, components of behavioral management programs such a reinforcement or reward menus, and other elements of the educational intervention can be written or programmed directly onto the student's computer or organizer; as the device travels with the child, the tool can become a readily available support to the child, empowering him or her in these various settings and promoting transfer of information among the various professionals and family members. Fourth, proficiency in computer-related skills allows the student to independently access sources of information for general purpose as well as for school use (e.g., using the Internet), to initiate some social contact in a less stressful fashion by communicating with others by means of electronic mail, to promote self-initiative and self-reliance in the context of the child's own interests, and so forth. Although there is always a concern that computer-related activities can further exacerbate social isolation, it does not need to be this way. For example, classroom-based activities can and should involve several students acting in collaboration, where group results require the coordination among each member of the group. For older individuals, computer-based skills may allow them vocational possibilities not hitherto available. For example, some of our adult clients have established their own Internet businesses, whereas others work in this field for a wide range of agencies, from mental health centers to libraries or schools.

Despite the potential of AT for individuals with social disabilities, and the fact that the use of enabling technology is mandated whenever a case can be made of its benefits to a given child with disabilities, there is no compilation of resources currently available from the perspective of autism, AS, and related conditions. The number of AT professionals and consultation services is still limited. Therefore, parents, clinicians, and educational professionals are often left to learn on their own about what might be applicable in the case of a given child, which is a daunting task for the noninitiated. The most well-known clearing house agency for dissemination of AT information is probably *Closing the Gap,* which can be accessed through the Internet. A review of the efficacy of AT, its applications, and easily accessible resources are badly needed in the field of AS and related conditions.

ACADEMIC CURRICULUM

The curriculum content should be decided based on long-term goals, so that the usefulness of each item is evaluated in terms of its long-term benefits for the individual's socialization skills, vocational potential, and quality of life. Emphasis should be placed on skills that correspond to relative strengths for the individual as well as skills that may be viewed as central for the person's future vocational life (e.g., writing skills, computer skills, and science). If the individual has an area of special interest that is not so circumscribed and unusual as to prevent its use in prospective employment, such an interest or talent should be cultivated in a systematic fashion, helping the individual to acquire strategies of learning (library, computerized data bases, Internet, etc.). Specific projects can be set as part of the person's credit gathering, and specific mentorships (topic related) can be established with staff members or individuals in the community.

This approach is necessary to avoid the common situation in which an inflexible school credit system is applied, enforcing the teaching of academic subjects that are only marginally related to the future life of a student with a social disability. Quite often, this inflexible approach leads to a great deal of frustration and, eventually, to the student's failure and loss of motivation, sacrificing the whole school experience for the sake of complying with irrelevant requirements. Given that motivation, self-initiative, and a positive self-concept are the main goals to be maximized, special modifications of assignments can enable a student to complete the requirements of a given a class successfully. For example, if the goal of an English class is to teach composition, the actual topic for research should tailor the student's intrinsic interests. A student failing an English course because the topic of research is, for example, standard novels, may succeed if the topic is shifted to, for example, a science-related topic.

BEHAVIORAL MANAGEMENT

Individuals with AS often exhibit different forms of challenging behavior. It is crucial that these behaviors are not seen as willful or malicious; rather, they should be viewed as connected to the individual's disability and treated as such by means of thoughtful, therapeutic, and educational strategies rather than by simplistic and inconsistent punishment or other disciplinary measures that imply the assumption of deliberate misconduct. Specific problem-solving strategies, usually following a verbal rule or algorithm, may be taught for handling the requirements of frequently occurring, troublesome situations (e.g., involving novelty, intense social demands, or frustration). As noted, training is usually necessary for recognizing situations as troublesome and for selecting the best available learned strategy to use in such situations. Anxiety management is, at times, an important component of intervention and may include both behavioral procedures such as desensitization and rehearsal and psychopharmacological treatment.

The general guidelines for behavioral management, including data collection procedures necessary for a functional analysis of problematic behaviors, intervention approaches including the use of reward systems, and evaluation protocols to gauge the success of specific approaches, should follow the established guidelines of behavioral assessment and therapy (e.g., Powers, 1997). In this process, it is helpful to compile a list of frequent problematic behaviors such as perseverations, obsessions, interrupting behaviors, or any other disruptive behaviors and then to devise specific guidelines to deal with them whenever the behaviors arise. These guidelines should be discussed with the individual with AS in an explicit, rule-governed fashion and all professionals involved should be aware of the program so that clear expectations are set and consistency across adults, settings, and situations is maintained. Ad hoc approaches are likely to result in improvised reactions to the student's behaviors, reinforcement of maladaptive patterns of behavior and consequent escalation, and insecurity as to how to act on the part of the adults. A proactive approach that makes the management of problematic behaviors an integral component of the general program of intervention is clearly preferable, increasing predictability and consistency, two important factors in any behavioral management approach.

VOCATIONAL TRAINING

Often, adults with AS may fail to meet entry requirements for advanced education or for jobs in their area of training because of their poor interview skills, social disabilities, eccentricities, or anxiety-related vulnerabilities. Therefore, an important aspect of vocational training concerns the acquisition of social skills in all areas involved in applying for an advanced educational degree or a job. The skills to be targeted include grooming and presentation and application letter writing, as well as every aspect of the interview process. Equally important, individuals with AS should be trained for and placed in jobs for which they are not neuropsychologically impaired, and in which they will enjoy a certain degree of support and shelter. College experience is facilitated by individual tutorial systems, where a faculty member and perhaps a peer, can act as immediate resources to the student, both being available and seeking frequent, periodic contact in order to monitor the student's progress and well-being. A similar situation should be available in job placement, where individual supervision and support should be provided by a supervisor or coworker who is aware that, at least initially, the guidance required will extend to areas other than the specific work apprenticeship. It is usually preferable that the job does not involve intensive social demands.

As originally emphasized by Asperger (1944), it is necessary to foster the development of existent talents and special interests in a way as to transform them into marketable skills. However, this is only part of the task to secure (and maintain) a work placement. Equal attention should be paid to the social demands defined by the nature of the job, including what to do during meal breaks, contact with the public or coworkers, or any other unstructured activity requiring social adjustment or improvisation. Excellent reviews on vocational possibilities and strategies for vocational training are available in the literature (e.g., Gerhardt & Holmes, 1997; Van Bourgondien & Woods, 1992). However, the number of knowledgeable professionals available as job coaches, as well as the public resources available in this area, is still quite limited; equally frustrating is the absence of good compilations of appropriate college, vocational training, and independent living programs, all of which are of crucial importance to adults with AS and their families, who are left to find their own way by means of independent research. It is hoped that one of the major priorities of parent support organizations and clinicians alike will be to pool resources and knowledge in an easily accessible medium.

PSYCHOTHERAPY

Although insight-oriented psychotherapy is not usually helpful, it does appear that fairly focused and structured counseling can be useful for individuals with AS and related conditions, particularly in the context of alleviating overwhelming experiences of sadness, negativism, or anxiety; problem-solving specific frustrations in regard to vocational goals and placement; and promoting family functioning and ongoing social adjustment (Pope, 1993). The psychotherapeutic relationship can be used to address concrete issues related to the patient's well-being, from practical, independent living problems to self-management and more intimate interpersonal problems, including sexuality and fantasy life.

SELF-SUPPORT GROUPS

As individuals with AS are usually self-described loners despite an often intense wish to make friends and have a more active social life, there is a need to facilitate social contact within the context of an activity-oriented group (e.g., church communities, hobby clubs, and self-support groups) (Mesibov, 1992). Although there is little published documentation on the effects of self-support groups, the available information suggests that individuals with AS enjoy the opportunity to meet others with similar problems, finding reassurance and a sense of identify in the group. However, this experience is not universal, and some individuals prefer to avoid association with others with similar problems. Others still fail to relate to any commonalities among group members and, consequently leave the group. It is also important to acknowledge that relationships established during group activities may not carry over to other settings, in which the group members themselves, rather than the therapist or group leader, would have to initiate the contact.

CONCLUSION

Individuals with AS and their families have to contend with the fact that public awareness of this condition, including its unique disabilities and strengths and the resources available for educational and other services, is still limited. The recent proliferation of parent support groups coalescing around the terms "Asperger syndrome," "high-functioning autism," or "high-functioning pervasive developmental disorders" reflect the fact that individuals with AS have in the past been offered a choice between insufficient services for students with academically based learning disabilities, services for children with autism who are at a much lower level of general functioning, or, still, services for children with conduct problems, whose needs are totally different and incompatible with AS. These gaps in awareness and in services are slowly being corrected, although there is still much to be done in terms of producing a more research-based body of knowledge on effective interventions and in terms of considerably augmenting the resources available, including training of professionals, restructuring of current educational curricula, and better preparation of students for the demands of independent living. This chapter highlights some core components of any educational and treatment program for individuals with AS. As part of the approach presented here, social and communication skills training and the acquisition of adaptive skills take center stage. It advances the principle that our educational and treatment goals should focus on the longer-term goals of promoting increased social opportunities, of better capitalizing on the individuals' natural talents and on vocational satisfaction and independent-living skills, as well as on their general emotional well-being.

REFERENCES

Asperger, H. (1944). Die "Autistischen Psychopathen" im Kindesalter. *Archiv für Psychiatrie und Nervenkrankheiten, 117*, 76–136.

Attwood, A. (1998). *Asperger's syndrome: A guide for parents and professionals.* Philadelphia: Kingsley.

Baron-Cohen, S., & Howlin, P. (1998). *Teaching children with autism to mind-read: A practical guide for teachers and parents.* New York: Wiley.

Baron-Cohen, S., Tager-Flusberg, H., & Cohen, D. J. (Eds.). (1993). *Understanding other minds: Perspectives from autism.* Oxford: Oxford University Press.

Berkman, M. (1997). The legal rights of children with disabilities to education and developmental services. In D. J. Cohen & F. R. Volkmar (Eds.), *Handbook of autism and pervasive developmental disorders* (pp. 808–827). New York: Wiley.

Bryant, D. P., & Bryant, B. R. (1998). Using assistive technology adaptations to include students with learning disabilities in cooperative learning activities. *Journal of Learning Disabilities, 31*(1), 41–54.

Bryant, B. R., & Seay, P. C. (1998). The Technology-Related Assistance to Individuals with Disabilities Act: Relevance to individuals with learning disabilities and their advocates. *Journal of Learning Disabilities, 31*(1), 4–15.

Burack, J. A., Root, R., & Zigler, E. (1997). Inclusive education for students with autism: Reviewing ideological, empirical, and community considerations. In D. J. Cohen & F. R. Volkmar (Eds.), *Handbook of autism and pervasive developmental disorders* (pp. 796–807). New York: Wiley.

Carr, E. G., Levin, L., McConnachie, G., Carlson, J. I., Kemp, D. C., & Smith, C. E. (1994). *Communication-based intervention for problem behaviors: A user's guide for producing positive change.* Baltimore: Brookes.

Chen, S. A., Thomas, J. D., Glueckauf, R. L., & Bracy, O. L. (1997). The effectiveness of computer-assisted cognitive rehabilitation for persons with traumatic brain injury. *Brain Injury, 11*(3), 197–209.

Gaylord-Ross, R. J., Haring, T. G., Breen, C., & Pitts-Conway, V. (1984). The training and generalization of social interaction skills with autistic youth. *Journal of Applied Behavior Analysis, 17*(2), 229–47.

Gena, A., Krantz, P. J., McClannahan, L. D., & Poulson, C. L. (1996). Training and generalization of affective behavior displayed by youth with autism. *Journal of Applied Behavior Analysis, 29*(3), 291–304.

Gerhardt, P. F., & Holmes, D. L. (1997). Employment: Options and issues for adolescents and adults with autism. In D. J. Cohen & F. R. Volkmar (Eds.), *Handbook of autism and pervasive developmental disorders* (pp. 650–664). New York: Wiley.

Gray, C. A. (1995). Teaching children with autism to "read" social situations. In K. A. Quill (Ed.), *Teaching children with autism: Strategies to enhance communication and socialization* (pp. 219–242). New York: Delmar Publishers Inc.

Gray, C., Dutkiexicz, M., Fleck, C., Moore, L., Cain, S. L., Lindrup, A., Broek, E., Gray, J., & Gray, B. (Eds.). (1993). *The social story book.* Jenison, MI: Jenison Public Schools.

Gray, C., & Garand, J. (1993). Social stories: Improving responses of students with autism with accurate social information. *Focus on Autistic Behavior, 8,* 1–10.

Gresham, F. M. (1992). Social skills and learning disabilities: Causal, concomitant, or correlational? *School Psychology Review, 21*(3), 348–360.

Hadwin, J., Baron-Cohen, S., Howlin, P., & Hill, K. (1997). Does teaching theory of mind have an effect on the ability to develop conversation in children with autism? *Journal of Autism and Developmental Disorders, 27*(5), 519–37.

Harris, S. L., & Handleman, J. S. (1997). Helping children with autism enter the mainstream. In D. J. Cohen & F. R. Volkmar (Eds.), *Handbook of autism and pervasive developmental disorders* (pp. 665–675). New York: Wiley.

Hodgdon, L. (1995). Solving social-behavioral problems through the use of visually supported communication. In K. A. Quill (Ed.), *Teaching children with autism: Strategies to enhance communication and socialization* (pp. 265–286). New York: Delmar.

Hodgdon, L. (1996). *Visual strategies for improving communication. Volume 1: Practical supports for school and home.* Troy, MI: QuirkRoberts.

Ihrig, K., & Wolchik, S. A. (1988). Peer versus adult models and autistic children's learning: Acquisition, generalization, and maintenance. *Journal of Autism and Developmental Disorders, 18*(1), 67–79.

Klin, A. (1997, October 16). *Asperger's syndrome: Diagnosis and phenomenology.* Paper presented at the 44th Annual Meeting of the American Academy of Child and Adolescent Psychiatry, Toronto, Ontario, Canada.

Klin, A., Sparrow, S. S., Volkmar, F. R., Cicchetti, D. V., & Rourke, B. P. (1995). Asperger syndrome. In B. P. Rourke (Ed.), *Syndrome of nonverbal learning disabilities: Neurodevelopmental manifestations* (pp. 93–118). New York: Guilford Press.

Klin, A., & Volkmar, F. R. (1997). Asperger's syndrome. In D. J. Cohen & F. R. Volkmar (Eds.), *Handbook of autism and pervasive developmental disorders* (pp. 94–122). New York: Wiley.

Koegel, R. L., & Koegel, L. K. (Eds.). (1995). *Teaching children with autism: Strategies for initiating positive interactions and improving learning opportunities.* Baltimore: Brookes.

Lewis, R. B. (1998). Assistive technology and learning disabilities: Today's realities and tomorrow's promises. *Journal of Learning Disabilities, 31*(1), 16–26.

Matson, J. L., Benavidez, D. A., Compton, L. S., Paclawskyj, T., & Baglio, C. (1996). Behavioral treatment of autistic persons: A review of research from 1980 to the present. *Research in Developmental Disabilities, 17*(6), 433–65.

Mesibov, G. B. (1984). Social skills training with verbal autistic adolescents and adults: A program model. *Journal of Autism and Developmental Disorders, 14,* 395–404.

Mesibov, G. B. (1986). A cognitive program for teaching social behaviors to verbal autistic adolescents and adults. In E. Schopler & G. B. Mesibov (Eds.), *High-functioning individuals with autism* (pp. 143–156). New York: Plenum.

Mesibov, G. B. (1992). Treatment issues with high-functioning adolescents and adults with autism. In E. Schopler & G. B. Mesibov (Eds.), *Social behavior in autism* (pp. 265–303). New York: Plenum.

Minskoff, E. H. (1980a). A teaching approach for developing nonverbal communication skills in students with social perception deficits. Part I. *Journal of Learning Disabilities, 13,* 118–124.

Minskoff, E. H. (1980b). A teaching approach for developing nonverbal communication skills in students with social perception deficits. Part II. *Journal of Learning Disabilities, 13,* 203–208.

Minskoff, E. H. (1987). *Pass Program: Programming appropriate social skills.* Fishersville, VA: Woodrow Wilson Rehabilitation Center.

Minskoff, E. H. (1994). *TRACC Workplace Social Skills Program.* Fishersville, VA: Woodrow Wilson Rehabilitation Center.

Minskoff, E. H., & DeMoss, S. (1994). Workplace social skills and individuals with learning disabilities. *Journal of Vocational Rehabilitation, 4*(2), 113–121.

Myles, B. S., & Simpson, R. L. (1998). *Asperger syndrome: A guide for educators and parents.* Austin, TX: Pro-Ed.

Ozonoff, S. (1998). Assessment and remediation of executive dysfunction in autism and Asperger syndrome. In E. Schopler, G. B. Mesibov, & L. J. Kunce (Eds.), *Asperger syndrome or high-functioning autism?* (pp. 263–289). New York: Plenum.

Ozonoff, S., & Miller, J. N. (1995). Teaching theory of mind: a new approach to social skills training for individuals with autism. *Journal of Autism and Developmental Disorders, 25*(4), 415–33.

Pennington, B. F., & Ozonoff, S. (1996). Executive functions and developmental psychopathology. *Journal of Child Psychology and Psychiatry, 37*(1), 51–87.

Pierce, K., & Schreibman, L. (1997). Multiple peer use of pivotal response training to increase social behaviors of classmates with autism: Results from trained and untrained peers. *Journal of Applied Behavior Analysis, 30*(1), 157–160.

Pope, K. K. (1993). The pervasive developmental disorder spectrum: A case illustration. *Bulletin of the Menninger Clinic, 57,* 100–117.

Powers, M. D. (1997). Behavioral assessment of individuals with autism. In D. J. Cohen & F. R. Volkmar (Eds.), *Handbook of autism and pervasive developmental disorders* (pp. 448–459). New York: Wiley.

Prizant, B. M., Schuler, A. L., Wetherby, A., & Rydell, P. (1997). Enhancing language and communication development: Language approaches. In D. J. Cohen & F. R. Volkmar (Eds.), *Handbook of autism and pervasive developmental disorders* (pp. 572–605). New York: Wiley.

Quill, K. A. (Ed.). (1995). *Teaching children with autism: Strategies to enhance communication and socialization.* New York: Delmar.

Raskind, M. H., & Higgins, E. L. (1998). Assistive technology for postsecondary students with learning disabilities: An overview. *Journal of Learning Disabilities, 31*(1), 27–40.

Rourke, B. P. (1989). *Nonverbal learning disabilities: The syndrome and the model.* New York: Guilford Press.

Rourke, B. P. (1995). Treatment program for the child with NLD. In B. P. Rourke (Ed.), *Syndrome of nonverbal learning disabilities: Neurodevelopmental manifestations* (pp. 497–508). New York: Guilford Press.

Schopler, E., & Mesibov, G. B. (Eds.). (1992). *High functioning individuals with autism.* New York: Plenum.

Schopler, E., Mesibov, G. B., & Kunce, L. J. (Eds.). (1998). *Asperger syndrome or high-functioning autism?* New York: Plenum.

Smith, D. C. (1998). Assistive technology: Funding options and strategies. *Mental and Physical Disabilities Law Report, 22*(1), 115–23.

Sparrow, S. S., Balla, D., & Cicchetti, D. (1984). *Vineland Adaptive Behavior Scales, Expanded edition.* Circle Pines, MN: American Guidance Service.

Taylor, B. A., & Harris, S. L. (1995). Teaching children with autism to seek information:

Acquisition of novel information and generalization of responding. *Journal of Applied Behavior Analysis, 28*(1), 3–14.

Thorp, D. M., Stahmer, A. C., & Schreibman, L. (1995). Effects of sociodramatic play training on children with autism. *Journal of Autism and Developmental Disorders, 25*(3), 265–82.

Twachtman, D. D. (1995). Methods to enhance communication in verbal children. In K. A. Quill (Ed.), *Teaching children with autism: Strategies to enhance communication and socialization* (pp. 133–162). New York: Delmar.

Van Bourgondien, M. E., & Woods, A. V. (1992). Vocational possibilities for high-functioning adults with autism. In E. Schopler & G. B. Mesibov (Eds.), *High-functioning individuals with autism* (pp. 227–239). New York: Plenum.

13

Adolescence and Adulthood of Individuals with Asperger Syndrome

DIGBY TANTAM

When treating adolescents and young adults with Asperger syndrome (AS) the clinician faces the variability of the disorder which is caused by the variability of the core symptoms and the adjustments that sufferers make to them. Adolescence and young adulthood are periods of considerable social change and new social demands, such as the transition from school to work, starting and consolidating sexual relationships, and leaving home. These transitions are problematic for people with AS because of their handicap as well as their awareness that others thrive from the social opportunities they find so difficult. It has been said that the "mildness" of the handicap in AS is what makes its emotional and social impact so severe. Mothers of young children with AS sometimes say, "The worst part is that he doesn't look handicapped, so people think he's naughty." At a later age, there is usually no doubt that something is wrong with the person with AS—peers are far more searching in their social demands than are people who are either of the next or of an earlier generation—but the AS is still attributed to a moral defect, not just by others but also by the person with AS.

There is little clinical experience and research information about adults with AS. I have therefore relied on my own experience with young adolescents or young adults with suspected AS whom I have seen over the last 16 years, in most cases to confirm or refute the diagnosis. Detailed records have been kept of more than 100 of these patients. Because this chapter is a distillation of such clinical experience, it is written in the first person to a greater extent than is usual.

I followed up a number of these patients over a 10-year period. In the course of this follow-up, I realized that AS is truly a developmental disorder. The problems associated with it, and its severity, change at different stages in development. I also realized that the emotional consequences of the disorder have a much greater affect on outcome than is commonly recognized.

In this chapter, I try to do the following:

1. Describe the difficulties that adolescents and adults with AS have in terms that are linked to diagnosis by the practitioner but that will also throw light on the experience of AS for the individual with AS and his or her caregivers.
2. Recommend management strategies whenever I think that there is sufficient evidence for them.
3. Consider some of the developmental factors that impinge upon AS.
4. Emphasize how clinicians can assist individuals with AS, parents, and other caregivers to come to terms with AS to develop successful compensatory strategies.

Because of lack of knowledge about AS, particularly in adults, most of this chapter is devoted to the description, which I divide into three parts. The first part considers the impairments most likely to be at the core of AS. The second part considers how some individuals with AS cope with this core syndrome. The third part considers other people's reactions and how these can increase or diminish the disability of a person with AS.

WHAT IS ASPERGER SYNDROME?

Mr. Black threw himself into the river Trent when his campaign for the abolition of British summertime failed. When asked why he did it, he explained that putting clocks forward an hour in summer and back an hour in winter caused wear and tear to their mechanisms, which shortened their life. John Green collects books about steam and thinks about it constantly. However, he cannot bear people mentioning steam or even, sometimes, the 19th century. John thinks that the fate of steam power was tragic: It had so much promise, yet it was swept aside by the internal combustion engine. William Brown has been living in a high-security hospital most of his life, since strangling and drowning a 14-year-old school fellow. His main activity is to recollect his life in songs—singing a series of songs in chronological order, each one contemporary to a month or a year of his past. When I saw him he had just finished a successful series, which had lasted for 3 days. Mr. Gold memorized weather records and knew that certain days—May 11, for example—had had, over the previous 20 years, low rates of sunshine. He dreaded these days, always hoping that the statistical trend would be bucked, but, as it rarely was, he usually spent the day in a "suicidal" state.

Each of these men suffered a lifelong developmental disorder, likely to be diagnosed in Europe as AS named after the Viennese psychiatrist who described "autistic psychopathy" in 1944 (Asperger, 1944). Each of them had also developed an ordering principle for their lives. Steam power, songs, weather, and time are different "special interests"—as these preoccupations are called—but they have some features in common. In the past, it has been assumed that the principal common factor is that they are pursued as purely private interests, and that they indicate that people with AS are emotionally detached from others. Some people think that AS is synonymous with schizoid personality disorder (Wolff, 1991). Epidemiological studies suggest that emotional and social detachment—usually called aloofness in this literature—is often associated with "core" autism, or "Kanner syndrome" than with AS, however (Waterhouse et al., 1996).

When analyzing the special interests of people with AS, other common features emerge. Their complexity and originality vary according to intelligence. Special interests often involve the mastery of a classification or a method of enumeration and its application to large-scale or unpredictable phenomena (e.g., names and populations of capital cities, heights of mountains, records of sporting achievements, laws of astrophysics or meteorology, and train timetables). The interest may assist the person with AS to find his or her way in the world. A man working at a garden center memorized the names of over 50 varieties of carrot. Mr. Gold believed that sunshine determined mood, and because his mother suffered from anxiety and, as a result was moody, he set himself to be able to predict how much sunshine to expect.

The repetitiveness of the list making and other systematic activities that are required for the pursuit of special interests is soothing to many people with AS. But this is not the only emotional investment that people with AS have. John Green's interest in the vanishment of steam is of a piece with the fascination of other people with AS with the underdog, or the neglected. Interests in murderers, old recordings, or the restoration of old machines are common. The interest may also be commemorative, linked to a memory of a happier time. Many people with AS like to memorize hit parades of bestselling pop records, but they are rarely interested in the current hit parade as in the period when their mothers were young and less careworn.

I have highlighted special interests because they are vivid and often the features that first engage clinicians' attention. They are not, however, always salient in a person with AS, which indicates an immediate clinical challenge when assessing people with AS. Each one is an individual, more so than people without AS. There is therefore considerable heterogeneity in the presentation and many of the problems of a person with AS.

This raises questions about the nosological status of the syndrome. There is no consensus as yet about (1) whether there is a single impairment that underlies all cases of AS, (2) whether it is related to that of autism, and (3) what the single impairment is. My experience and reading of the current research suggest that there is an autistic spectrum and that the common feature of everyone on this spectrum is an abnormality in nonverbal communication (Tantam, 1992). I have argued that the early indications of this abnormality are the failure of the child to attend to others' nonverbal communication (Tantam, 1992) and subsequently to allow their gaze to be redirected by others' gestures and the failure of imitation.

Whether or not these are primary impairments, the child with AS does not "latch on" to social interactions around him or her. In the previously cited article, I argued that this failure to latch on might have adverse developmental consequences. These could be as diverse as a lack of social attention, a misunderstanding of social status, a failure to process faces efficiently, and the acquisition of common sense at the expense of "original thought."

Some of these adverse developmental consequences are so often present in AS that they constitute a "core syndrome." The core syndrome includes impairments that may stand in the way of making relationships with others and may sometimes cause offense to other people. However, a failure to make relationships or offending are not core symptoms of AS. They are secondary problems (considered in the second part of this chapter) which may or may not occur, depending on the resources of the person with AS and of his or her family or caregivers. These secondary problems may also be caused by other disorders, including emotional and familial disorders. The extent to which these secondary problems become serious or incapacitating is also influenced by people's reactions to them (considered in the third part of this chapter).

DIAGNOSTIC ASSESSMENT

Ethical Considerations

Parents often initiate even when the person with AS is an adult. Thus, examiners must take special care to safeguard the patient's right to a confidential assessment, and it is often useful to negotiate with the patient how much involvement parents should have before the assessment takes place or an appointment is set. Fortunately, it is rare for people with AS to keep a parent, or a caregiver, from being involved. With the patient's permission, I obtain further information, particularly about early development, from a person other than the patient, and I often take the opportunity of counseling parents or caregivers about AS. Parents may ask about the diagnosis, prognosis, and treatment of an adolescent or an adult with AS and may sometimes suggest that this information should be given to them alone and not to the individual with AS.

When that happens, first I ask permission of the person with AS to see his or her parents and discuss these matters with them. Then, I ask the patient whether or not he or she wishes to have the same information that I give the parents about his or her condition. I also offer to send the individual with AS a copy of my letter to the referring doctor. However, I assume that it may sometimes be harmful for a person with AS to perceive him- or herself as having a medical condition which is likely to be lifelong and for which there is no specific treatment. My approach is influenced by the values prevailing in the practice of medicine in the United Kingdom and may not be appropriate in other countries. However, clinicians need to know how to solve the conflicting ethical demands of beneficence and autonomy.

Other Considerations during Assessment

Children with autism are often regarded as unreliable as informants because of their lack of self-reflectiveness, and child psychiatrists rely heavily on parents. General psychiatrists, on the other hand, rarely interview parents, let alone take a detailed developmental history from them. My approach is to first see the patient on his or her own, even if I am assessing a less able person with autism, who has no usable language. This enables me to make an assessment of communicative behavior, affect, and physical status. People with AS have usable language, although they may be too anxious, uncertain about why they are seeing me, or preoccupied with conversational rituals to be able to give a good history. It is rarely necessary to take a full psychiatric history from the patient, and, indeed, reliance on the patient's own perception of his or her disability may be misleading—a possible reason for the underdiagnosis of AS in general psychiatry clinics. I routinely ask about friends, and routinely I am told that the person has them even when I know that he or she does not. Such is the social stigma attached to emotional isolation. Careful inquiry about what constitutes friendship ("Does John ever come round to your house?") can be revealing. Asking for the first names of friends is also useful (sometimes a person will say, "You are my friend"). I also ask about how a person has spent his or her most recent period of leisure in an attempt to uncover special interests. Such a question is not always successful if a person feels stigmatized because of his or her special interests. Often, the best clue to a special interest is how the interview opens. A person might say, "Do you know the time?" or "Is it the 13th today?," which may indicate a particular interest in clocks or the calendar, for example.

It is important to see at least one parent after seeing the person with AS. There is a temptation to underestimate the concern of the person with AS about this interview, and I always give the person the opportunity to be present. I base my developmental history on a questionnaire derived from the Handicaps and Behaviour Schedule (Lund, 1989), which was originally developed by Lorna Wing and her colleagues. With their permission, I recast selected items as questions and then conduct a reliability study by asking parents to complete the questionnaire sent to them in the mail and interviewing them at an interval of several months using the same items. Only items in which scores were significantly concordant were retained (Tantam, 1991).

Nowadays I usually ask parents to complete the questionnaire before they attend, and then I review it with them. This allows me to check items which are unclear and also puts parents in touch with their concerns. Often, parents have some knowledge of AS before they seek an interview. A developmental history stretching back, sometimes 30 years, is clearly open to inaccuracy. Knowledge of AS might also influence parents' memories. Bias and inaccuracy can be counteracted in two ways: (1) by arriving at a tentative diagnosis before reviewing the developmental history and (2) by comparing parents' assessments of current communicative behavior with one's own observations.

There is substantial disagreement about different diagnostic criteria for AS when applied to adolescents and when applied to adults (Ghaziuddin, 1992). However, an adolescent meeting these diagnostic criteria might have been quite different in early childhood. A child may, for example, progress out of a classical Kanner-type autism in early childhood to reach an AS adjustment in adolescence, or he might always have had the symptoms of AS. Researchers often exclude children with a significant history of language delay from a diagnosis of AS, but clinicians may be more interested in the current profile of difficulties, irrespective of their origins, and may want to diagnose AS even if there is a history of language delay. Diagnostic criteria oriented toward researchers may therefore differ from those oriented to clinicians.

Clinical experience is consistent with Wing and Gould's (1979) classic epidemiological study indicating the co-occurrence of a triad of social impairments, and that sufferers from this triad may be diagnosable as having Kanner's syndrome, AS, or a continuum of disorders in between. More able people with the triad ("high-functioning" in the U.S. literature) have social adjustment problems different from those of their less able fellow sufferers and are less likely to have associated handicaps, but the cutoff point between the more and the less able is fuzzy. Cluster analyses often throw up a high-functioning cluster (Klin, Volkmar, Sparrow, Cicchetti, & Rourke, 1995), but the discriminating variables tend to be nonspecifically associated with social relatedness and, therefore, severity but do not indicate a core syndrome distinct to AS. Without better information about natural history and without any markers of specific etiology linked to syndromal descriptions, it is meaningless to be prescriptive about what part of the autistic spectrum constitutes AS. Even the cases that Asperger himself described, although recognizably more able people with autism (Marsden, Kalter, & Ericson, 1974), seem quite heterogeneous in the extent of their impairments.

A more valuable approach to clinical assessment, and possibly to research, is to consider dimensions of impairment within the population of more able people with autism. The dimensions that I consider are those of the core syndrome (see Table 13.1).

THE CORE SYNDROME

The triad of social impairments (Wing & Gould, 1979) is increasingly recognized (see Chapter 15, this volume) as the best approximation to the clinical features common to everyone on the autism spectrum, and therefore I have based the constituents of the core syndrome on the triad with some modifications. These include separating language from nonverbal communication, and relabeling "social impairment" as "impaired intersubjectivity." Because of the robust association of AS and motor incoordination, I have also added the latter to the list.

Nonverbal Communication

Abnormalities of nonverbal communication are readily detectable in almost everyone with an autistic spectrum disorder and in my view constitute a necessary criterion for the disorder. Communication is, clearly, two-way and impairments may occur in both expression and interpretation. However, one deficit may be particularly marked, giving rather different clinical presentations.

Deficits in nonverbal communication may affect one "channel" specifically, such as facial expression or tone of voice, or all channels. In autism, although one channel may be egregiously affected, it is usual to find that there is impairment of all channels of expression, including face expression, posture, gesture, voice prosody, and gaze behavior. It is harder to assess interpretation deficits, but studies of people with autism suggest that the interpretation of tones of voice is as affected as the more commonly tested interpretation of facial expression. This suggests that the impairment is due to a defect in expressive competency rather than a failure of performance in a particular channel—the nonverbal equivalent of a dysphasia rather than a dysarthria.

TABLE 13.1. The Core Syndrome of AS

- Impaired nonverbal communication
- Impaired speech and language
- Impaired intersubjectivity
- Idiosyncratic, stereotyped, asocial interests and activities
- Incoordination

Impaired Nonverbal Expression

Many people with AS have impaired expression in all the channels mentioned in the previous section. Voluntary emotional expression of people with AS may be less impaired than involuntary expression so that people with AS may be able to read with expression even though their tone of voice in conversation is conspicuously monotonous. Similarly, in conversation, people with AS may smile or produce other voluntary facial expressions in conversation, but they will not show the involuntary play of expression that constantly accompanies speech in the conversation of nonautistic people. It seems to be the lower two-thirds of the face that is particularly affected. It is even characteristic of the impairment of nonverbal expression in autism that it is anomalous and not just deficient. Abnormal voice prosody includes the characteristic sing-song intonation of autism in which the pitch of the voice either does not drop at the end of phrases, as normal in English speech, or may even rise, giving a questioning quality. The rhythm of speech and the accent may also be abnormal: Native English speakers with AS may sometimes speak with a "foreign" accent. Other abnormal expressions involving other channels include facial grimacing, idiosyncratic gestures which may have a jerky quality and are not integrated into speech or the exchange of gaze, postural shifts with a choreiform quality, and taking up position in relation to other people at an inappropriate interpersonal distance.

> Richard was a tall, rather thin man with unusual athetoid gestures, manneristic jerks of his neck, and grimaces of his face. His voice was indefinably accented and often had a querulous character as the pitch of his voice rose at the end of every statement. He began the interview by talking about himself in the most personal way, and without hesitation, often referring to his interests in astrophysics and classical history. He showed no guile and no barrier to converse with me, a stranger. He had worked for a number of years in a job he had obtained through his father's contacts and was also a member of a Christian group for which he proselytized in his local neighborhood. He described himself as having "hundreds" of friends, but on closer questioning he considered everyone that he had met and talked to a friend. Family members were very fond of him, although they could find him wearing particularly when in times of stress, he became much more rigid in his pursuit of daily routine and also repeatedly questioned them about future events.

Impaired Nonverbal Interpretation

Impaired nonverbal expression produces a conspicuously odd appearance which other people quickly pick up, even if they cannot identify its cause. Impaired nonverbal interpretation—a defect in the ability to decode other people's nonverbal expressions—only affects behavior indirectly and is therefore much more difficult to spot. There is strong evidence of impairment in the interpretation of facial expression in less able people with autism although some uncertainty about the degree to which this is a specific impairment or whether it is a part of a more general cognitive deficit. Preliminary experiments indicate impaired face interpretation (Scott, 1985) and impaired ability to link tone of voice and facial expression in AS.

If the social impact of impaired expression is oddity, the impact of impaired interpretation is a lack of empathy, which may be attributed by other people to malice (i.e., to a moral defect) rather than to a disorder. Elsewhere (Tantam, 1995) I have argued that there are two stages in the normal development of empathy. In the first stage, an emotional expression in another triggers a corresponding emotion in the infant and the infant empathizes with others unselectively. In the second stage, cultural and social factors lead to some of these responses being suppressed so that the child learns only to feel empathetic toward certain groups, or in certain situations. I argued that the lack of empathy associated with personality disorder is a result of overinhibition of spontaneous empathic responses, but that the lack of empathy in autism is due to a failure of development of empathy at the first stage and an impairment in the ability to interpret emotional expressions.

> Tom was described as a "little angel." He had blond hair and a serene and unlined face. His voice, posture, and face were unremarkable, but, as the interview progressed, it became apparent that they were also inexpressive. I had read considerable background detail about Tom and knew that he had been expelled from one school for having pushed a child who could not swim into a pond and was suspended from another, special, school because he had been constantly disruptive in the classroom. Tom described several of his classmates as his friends, but according to his teachers, he was shunned by other children. His parents said that he never had a friend, nor had Tom ever been close to his younger brother. In fact, Tom had once tried to push his toddler brother downstairs. I asked whether Tom was attached to his parents. Would he, for example, be distressed if his mother were upset by something not connected with him? They were sure that he would not and remembered an occasion when his mother was acutely ill and had been carried out of the house on a stretcher and Tom asked who would cook dinner now that mother was no longer going to be at home. Direct testing, using posed photographs of facial expression, showed that Tom could differentiate a happy expression from others, but he confused "surprised" with "no expression," "angry" with "surprised," and "disgusted," and "frightened" with sad.

The Fifth Child

Doris Lessing (1989) wrote this novel with the intensity that would normally be expected of a real-life account. A well-off, liberal couple with four children decide to have a fifth. At first, he seems not to belong to them or to recognize any attachment to them or to their values. Professionals are at a loss. He is prone to temper outbursts and tyrannizes the household. He seems to be an able child but does not use his intelligence and delights to hang out with the rough boys who are failing academically. An anomalous feature of the book is that he dominates this group. If this were real life, it would be expected that he would be exploited by them. "Fifth children" are not uncommon, at least not in my practice; they are the adolescents who become uncontrollable, who are malicious, sometimes cruel, and always inexplicable.

Previously, many of them would have been diagnosed as having antisocial personality disorder. The reason that they are referred to me is that many have a developmental history typical of a pervasive developmental disorder, and some have been diagnosed as having AS. I find that many of them have an impaired ability to interpret nonverbal cues, particularly the cues of social distress. Sometimes there is a history of family disruption during early childhood, and it is possible that this had an effect on the acquisition of empathy. However, direct testing often indicates the kinds of errors found in Tom's case, described earlier.

The disabilities of this group of hard-to-place people are only now becoming recognized. They pose serious problems in education, health, and other settings because they often relate to others by "outrage." I address this matter later in the chapter.

Etiology of Impaired Nonverbal Communication

There has been regular speculation, since Damasio, Maurer, Damasio, and Chui (1980) suggested that AS is the consequence of childhood onset aprosodia, occurring as a result of nondominant hemisphere lesions. A recent, complementary hypothesis has been that the low-empathy form of AS is a consequence of prospagnosia from infancy, presumably of cerebral origin (Kracke, 1994). There are important differences, however, between the pattern of symptoms of cerebral lesions and those of AS. For example, when a person with AS mimics someone else's speech (i.e., the individual repeats exactly what the other person said), he or she usually reproduces the prosody as well as the words, even though his or her own spontaneous prosody may be abnormal. Consistent nondominant cerebral lesions are not found on neuroimaging in AS, and when there is a cerebral lesion it may lead to a clinical picture that is significantly different from AS.

Cerebral lesions may be associated with speech meeting the criteria of Rapin (1996) for "verbal dyspraxia," except that Rapin confines this description to cases in which there are no focal brain lesions. It is of interest to note that according to Rapin, verbal dyspraxia is never associated with autism. The impairment of nonverbal expression may also differ in detail from that of a person with AS in that the amount of expression may be reduced but not its timing. Tantam, Holmes, and Cordess (1993) analyzed the nonverbal expressions of adults with AS and found that the opposite was true of them: The amount of expression was not significantly reduced, but its timing was. In particular, people with AS tended not to respond by looking at someone to whom they were talking when the other person was doing something so-cially "interesting," such as beginning to talk or looking at them. Others have since made consistent findings (Leekam, Hunnisett & Moore, 1998; Willemsen-Swinkels, Buitelaar, Weijnen, & Engeland, 1998). This social gaze response (Tantam, 1992; see also Baron-Cohen et al., 1995) may be sub-cortically mediated. The impairment of nonverbal interpretation in AS may also be due to a failure to link social significance and perception, as a result of the failure of subcortical processes. Amygdalectomized subjects have a comparable impairment which Adolphs, Tranel, Damasio, and Damasio (1995) suggest is due to a failure to link representations of facial expressions with representations of fear.

Management of Impaired Nonverbal Communication

Some reports suggest that shaping social responses in young children has been effective in attenuating autistic impairment in a number of cases (Lovaas & Smith, 1989), but the procedures used are not suitable for adoles-cents and adults with AS, even though they have similar impairments. It is common for adolescents with AS to make an unexpected, rapid improve-ment in their social functioning. My clinical experience shows that parents' judgments of increased social understanding is associated with an improve-ment in nonverbal expression and in peer relationships. Interaction with peers has the potential to be more rewarding after the onset of adolescence than it was in childhood, but it is also more socially demanding. People with AS who make long-term intimate relationships are exceptional, but when this happens it appears to accelerate social development. In schizophrenia, a disorder in which nonverbal expression is also impaired, although for other reasons, social interaction also appears to be effective in reducing the accu-mulation of negative symptoms. These strands of evidence, albeit tenuous, do, therefore, point to the importance of peer relationships in providing suf-ficient reward for a person with AS to overcome obstacles in social relation-ship and in providing a framework for shaping nonverbal communication.

Impaired Speech and Language

Although unimpaired language is one of the defining characteristics of AS, speech is not normal. Forty-six socially impaired people who met the criteria for autistic spectrum disorders were rated for errors in conversational speech. Syntactic errors were defined to be the use of phrases or clauses that were not "well-formed," and semantic errors were defined to be the use of well-formed but nonsensical phrases or clauses. Most of the latter were nonsensical because of the inclusion of a neologism, for example, "I saw a Norish yesterday," "Norish" being a particular type of electricity pylon. Syntactic abnormalities were correlated with a developmental history of delayed speech comprehension, and both were correlated with the presence in infancy of other characteristics suggestive of Kanner syndrome, or more severe autism. Semantic and pragmatic abnormalities occurred in the whole series. A similar differentiation has been proposed by Rapin (1996), one of the originators of the term "semantic–pragmatic disorder," who divided developmental language disorders into three categories and indicated that the most frequent form—phonological/syntactic deficit disorder—also occurred in autism, and that semantic–pragmatic disorder occurred in isolation and in association with various developmental disorders including AS. In practice, it is not easy to distinguish syntactic from other types of abnormality. Pronominal reversal is often taken to be a syntactic disorder, but Asperger (1979) particularly cited pronominal reversal as an example of speech abnormality and attributed it to a failure of role taking.

Speech production is often impaired in AS. There may be an attempt to speak on inspiration as well as expiration, suggesting that the cause may be the problems in integrating motor elements into a complex performance. Dysfluencies are also common, often being covered up by fillers such as "ums" and "ahs."

Assessment of Speech and Language Abnormalities

Experienced teachers and practitioners often underestimate semantic difficulties in AS, and may neglect them during assessment. Neologisms are most often the names of things or categories which are important to the person with AS (e.g., radio aerials or pylons of a particular kind) and are usually easy to spot. The absence of names, typically those of superordinate categories, is harder to identify but may underlie the difficulty that people with AS have in learning. Generalizing from knowledge acquired in one situation to another and using metaphor are examples of semantic difficulty that people with AS may have. They both represent a problem of intention, which is: not apprehending the rule or principle that ties together the meanings of a word.

Etiology of Speech and Language Abnormalities

Wittgenstein proposed that meaning is in the use of words, implying that the competent language user has a representation of the situations, including the social situations, in which certain words are used. If this view is correct, semantic competence relies on social competence. For example, knowing when to wear formal clothes is a social competence that underlies the semantic category "interview." Language impairment in autism may therefore follow from social impairment.

The alternative viewpoint is that speech and nonverbal communication are mediated by different centers or "modules." The Wittgensteinian unitary model implies a single spectrum of autistic severity, from the least able, whose capacity for social interaction would be sufficiently impaired for their acquisition of language to be jeopardized, to the most able, Asperger group, who would have sufficient social competence to be able to acquire language but not to manage the more subtle aspects of social interaction, such as speech pragmatics. The modular approach would suggest that there is a contingent relationship between language impairment and autism. If only the language module malfunctions, pure developmental language disorder is produced, and if only the (putative) social competence module or modules malfunction, pure "autism" is produced. In life, where malfunction is assumed most often to occur as a result of intrauterine or, perhaps perinatal, damage, larger areas of brain are more likely to be involved, and so several modules will end up malfunctioning, leading to a contingent association between cognitive functioning, impaired language, and impaired social competence.

Epidemiological studies may provide data that could distinguish these two models. Until then, the second model—that language and social competence are developmentally distinct—seems the most useful clinically. It provides an explanation for adults who had severe speech impairments with features of autism until the age of 4 or 5 years but who then acquired speech and became indistinguishable from adults whose development was always typical of AS. The modular approach also emphasizes the fact that there are two social signaling systems—language and nonverbal communication—and that one can be used to supplement and, to a degree, substitute for, the other.

Management of Speech and Language Difficulties

Pragmatic abnormalities may be conspicuous. They contribute to the apparent disinhibition of some people with AS who may ask personal questions of the interviewer or may volunteer indiscreet information about themselves or their parents. Pragmatic abnormalities may also increase the impression of immaturity, combined with pedantry, that many people with AS have. Cognitive difficulties that parallel pragmatic speech problems include a fussiness and search for precision about concepts, which is doomed to failure because no definition exists for them, only competence in their use. People with AS may have study or examination problems as a result and may need help in apportioning time and in developing strategies for getting to the gist of a topic or a question.

On the other hand, words may provide people with AS with social understanding that they do not have intuitively. Clear, nonmetaphorical descriptions of why people react as they do, or how to behave in particular situations, can be useful guides for a person with AS who is at a loss and may help to prevent emotional upset or social breakdown.

Concrete or literal interpretations may also be the basis for the originality and humor of people with AS. Some years ago, a eulogy was broadcast on the radio in the United Kingdom about an eccentric man who moved into a small caravan and located himself at the end of the broadcaster's garden. The eccentric man was later interviewed by social services and referred to a psychiatrist. The broadcaster asked his neighbor how the examination had gone, but he was laughing too much to be able to answer the question. Eventually, the source of the humor was revealed: The psychiatrist was called "Maddox" (or Mad Docs) and his prospective patient, on hearing the name, had been so overcome with laughter that the nurse in charge of the outpatient clinic had asked him to leave.

Impaired Intersubjectivity

Research criteria for AS according to the tenth edition of *International Classification of Disease* (ICD-10; World Health Organization, 1992) include "impaired nonverbal expression" with "a relative lack of peer relationships, lack of social or emotional reciprocity, and a lack of shared enjoyment or attention" under the subheading of "qualitative impairments in social interaction," which is said to be present if any two of the listed impairments are present. This suggests that the impairments are linked.

Friendship—a close relationship with a peer—demands the most social understanding of any relationship because mutuality is one of the requirements for friendship (Argyle, 1986), and it is in its absence that a lack of social understanding is mostly detected. A lack of peer relationships may result from such a wide range of conditions that it cannot be considered to have a specific relation to AS.

Although the other deficiencies mentioned are more specific, they are not so easy to interpret. From the clinical assessor's point of view there are at least two separate elements: an impairment of what Trevarthen (1979) termed intersubjectivity, and a lack of attention. Attentional deficits do not seem to be as much of a problem in adulthood as they are in childhood, when they may result in selective auditory responding and the adoption of idiosyncratic learning strategies. Failure of intersubjectivity is a much more obtrusive impairment after childhood.

Seventy-seven percent of the AS subjects for whom I have detailed developmental records were described by their parents as being "unaware of other people" at some time in their childhood, and 75% were still unaware at the time of the interview, in late adolescence, or early adulthood. Awareness may develop as the social adjustment of a person with AS improves and may be painful when it does so.

A 22-year-old man diagnosed with AS had a particular interest in aerodynamics and made and rode go-karts with carefully sculpted farings to reduce drag as much as possible. During late adolescence, he became self-conscious about these designs and, as his parents described, at about the same time, he became more sociable and aware of their feelings. The parents thought that this represented a significant improvement, but the patient himself became anxious that he could no longer withdraw into his private world of special interests to cope with stress, and that, in consequence, he was more vulnerable than he had been before.

People with AS may develop discursive rules to learn to regulate their social behavior. These rules may be quite rigid and stereotyped when AS is associated with mild learning difficulty but are more flexible and, therefore, powerful in the most able. They work best when the person with AS is interacting with older people, with caregivers who are prepared to do the work of understanding themselves, or with children who are less socially demanding. The successful application of rules requires a person to get some feedback about how other people are feeling. If this is not possible because of a lack of empathy, other strategies to minimize the impact of social understanding may be used. One of these strategies is to create large and predictable social effects by acting to "outrage" other people, which I discuss in a later section on aggression.

Etiology of Impaired Intersubjectivity

Karmiloff-Smith, Klima, Bellugi, Grant, and Baron-Cohen (1995) argue that there is a dissociation between impairments in communication and in social understanding, citing Williams syndrome, in which good social understanding coexists with communicative deficits, as an example. This would be consistent with the idea that there is a specific "module" concerned with intersubjectivity—Baron-Cohen (1994) terms it the "theory of mind module"—which may be impaired independently of damage to impairment of nonverbal communication. It is, however, possible that particular timing or a specific type of impairment in nonverbal communication is required to impair the development of intersubjectivity. Impairments occurring later in infancy or those that spare some aspect of social interaction may not prevent the development of intersubjectivity and may therefore conceal the association between earlier impaired nonverbal communication and impaired intersubjectivity. Hobson (1990) has argued that there is an association between impaired intersubjectivity and communicative abnormalities, although he proposes that it is the impaired intersubjectivity that leads to the other problems, and not vice versa as argued here.

What certainly seems true in adults is that there is considerable variation in the association between the impairment of nonverbal communication and the impairment of empathy, intuition about appropriate social behavior, and other measures of the quality of social interaction. This suggests that other developmental factors influence intersubjectivity. Clinical experience suggests that people with AS are susceptible to the same developmental influences as others in this development, and that family factors, social practice, and socialization experiences all play a part. These factors are considered in more detail in the section on social factors.

Theory of Mind

Researchers have found that people with severe autism have deficits in their ability to construct a theory of mind and therefore are unable to put themselves into the minds of another. Defects in the theory of mind have been repeatedly demonstrated in less able people with autism but less consistently in a higher-functioning group (Bowler, 1992). The samples used in the confirmatory studies have been matched for verbal intelligence, but it still remains a possibility that language is even more impaired in the less able group than the testing suggests. Language, and not a distinct theory-of-mind module, may be the reason for failure on theory-of-mind tasks. This would be consistent with the success of people with AS on the same tasks and on more demanding tasks designed to make allowance for the higher intelligence of the AS group.

This is not to say that people with AS do not have unusual "theories of mind," or at least theories about people. The theories usually seem "stripped down," as if developed by a psychologist or anthropologist naïve to the culture. For example, a person with AS recently told me about her proxemic theory. She had observed that when people lined up, they left a gap between themselves and the person in front, and that this gap was substantially larger in the case of men standing behind women. She used this information to jump lines, by looking for this combination and pushing in behind the woman nearest the front who was followed by a man.

Theory of the World

People with AS who pass theory-of-mind tasks should not be assumed to have the same theories about the world as others. Bowler (1992), for example, showed that the people with AS whom he tested were less likely to use mental state terms. As in everything else that they do, it seems that people with AS have to develop their own models of the world. This may be because they cannot identify with others so they imbibe from them their ways of looking at the world. People with AS, like people with other autistic spectrum disorders, may be good mimics, but they are not good imitators. They may reproduce exactly what others have said and others' tones of voice, even when they cannot modulate their own tone of voice when they are speaking for themselves. But they do not make themselves temporarily into another person, as imitation requires.

As Hobson (1990) pointed out in relation to autism, people with AS do not make the sharp distinction between people and things that is normally expected. Objects may have animistic power, and people may be measured like objects.

> Mr. White had been ill-treated in a community where he had been placed, and this had rocked his life to its foundations. He felt that he could not recover from it and was confronted by his own powerlessness. In the subsequent years, he developed a passion for steamships and for steam power generally. He explained it to me one day in this way: Steam had been a good source of power, but it had been discarded, for no good reason. He felt that it had been badly treated, and he wanted to reinstate it. The books on steam that he owned had a special importance. They were power. When they had to be moved, he became almost overwhelmingly anxious because their power was waning.

> Mr. Scarlet had gone to visit relatives in Sierra Leone. When he came back I asked him about them. He had not seen them since he was very little. When I asked him what he thought of them, he answered that his grandfather was 42 inches, and his uncle was 46 inches. Mr. Scarlet, who had a fascination for boxing records, had assessed his male relatives on a metric system that was, arguably, for him, one of the most easily grasped measures of male status, girth.

From these and other examples, I have concluded that people with AS are not lacking in intersubjectivity, but their subjectivity is suffused through the world in which they live and is not restricted to close, personal others.

Management of Impaired Intersubjectivity

Possible approaches that have been used in other fields to increase interpersonal sensitivity are cognitive approaches, social skills training, and counseling or psychotherapy. Training in the theory of mind increases theory-of-mind skills but not other social skills. Social skills training does not generalize to other settings (see Chapter 12, this volume) although some generalizable effects have been achieved from role play and sociodrama.

Psychotherapeutic approaches have been extensively applied in autism by psychoanalysts with the belief that autism was a psychogenic disorder. The aim has been to cure autism, but there is no widely accepted evidence that this can be achieved by psychological means; however, it may be that the psychotherapeutic approach contains a valuable element of education about interpersonal skill. The conflict between the psychodynamic and the biological explanations of autism may have prevented workers with a biological orientation from seeing the value of this educational element. Clinical experience suggests that a problem-solving counseling approach, which incorporates education about interpersonal skills, may be helpful, although more formal evaluation should be done.

Empathy training has been used in other fields, for example, in the treatment of pedophiles. It may have a place in the management of the person with AS who has reduced empathy, but this has yet to be evaluated.

Other types of psychotherapy or counseling do have a place in the treatment of emotional disorder in AS and I consider them later.

Idiosyncratic, Stereotyped, Asocial Interests and Activities: Mastery through Predictability

Repetition seems to be intrinsically attractive to anyone with autism. It has been speculated that this is a consequence of frontal lobe abnormality, but it does not have the character of perseveration. Most people find some satisfaction in regular movement or regular sensory stimulation, for example, that provided by music or dance. The social nature of these activities makes them unappetizing to people with AS, but it may be that they obtain a similar satisfaction from spinning tops and watching the drum of a washing machine, or in other highly predictable pursuits. The more intellectually able a person with AS is, the more likely he or she is to find satisfaction in conceptual repetition (e.g., making lists).

I have already considered the psychological importance of special interests to people with AS. They are not a universal feature of the disorder, being more often associated with impaired nonverbal expression than with impaired nonverbal interpretation. Their complexity is often in proportion to intelligence. Many of the special interests that typify AS involve repeating the same facts or rehearsing the same memories, and it can trigger fury if something has changed (e.g., the time of a television program). Repetitive questioning is a related activity and, like special interests, it becomes worse when a person is anxious. This suggests that one of the benefits of repetition is anxiety reduction.

However, special interests are not just about anxiety. They are play equivalents, and, like play, they have a mastery element to them. I believe that people with AS value them because they provide a map of the human world which is otherwise such a closed book. Size of cities, records, birthdays, top-20 lists, waist measurements—all numbers that my patients with AS have memorized—may all be attempts to find a powerful quantitative clue to society. For a person with AS, knowing the largest city or the tallest building puts a bound on human endeavor and may represent some sense of mastery over the unpredictability of other people.

Motor Incoordination

Recent studies indicate that people with AS are as clumsy as other people with autism, despite being less impaired than them in other respects. It is difficult to be precise about the origins of the clumsiness. Clinical tests of coordination may be normal. Gestural copying is often impaired, as is the ability to catch a thrown ball or to throw a ball back accurately (see also Chapter 5, this volume). Movements involving the whole body seem to be more impaired than those involving a body part, suggesting that the problem may be in integrating the elements of a complex movement. Riding a bicycle is a developmental task that many people with AS find difficult. Many people with AS also have a degree of apraxia and find it difficult to copy other people's actions. Some of their apparent incoordination may actually be movement idiosyncracy, because they do not model their actions or gait on those of other people. Although many people with AS have good visuospatial skills and may indeed think visually, eye–hand (visuomotor) skills seem to be impaired. Learning motor skills is also often delayed but performance of over-learnt skills once acquired may be excellent.

Managing Motor Incoordination

It is not known whether teaching people with AS to be more coordinated would help other impairments. I know of one case in which there seemed to be a definite reduction of AS behavior following regular attendance at a gym class. Its effects on adults have not been tested.

Differential Diagnosis of the Core Syndrome

Of the adolescents and adults referred to me for assessment of AS on whom I have kept detailed records, 9% had received a previous diagnosis of schizophrenia, 14% a diagnosis of obsessive–compulsive disorder (OCD), and a substantial number a diagnosis of Nonspecific Learning Disabilities. Many were on medication despite their being no known treatment for the core impairments. Few had been diagnosed as having a schizoid personality disorder, although it is one of the alternative diagnostic formulations cited in the literature (Wolff & Chick, 1980).

The diagnosis of schizophrenia is most often made on the basis of negative symptoms and in the absence of a developmental history. In each case, the developmental history demonstrated that expressive abnormalities were apparent well before schizophrenia, even childhood-onset schizophrenia (McKenna et al., 1994), could be expected to develop. Diagnostic difficulty may arise when there is no reliable developmental history, and when a person with apparent AS reports abnormal ideas and experiences.

The difficulty of distinguishing idiosyncratic reports of nonpsychotic experiences from the reports of psychotic symptoms is considered in a later section.

OCD and AS overlap in their symptoms. OCD may be comorbid with AS, and this is apparent when an episode of disorder is superimposed on lifelong rigidity and stereotyped behavior. When this happens there may be some contingent factor which triggers the OCD.

> William has AS but is less ritualistic than many people with the disorder. When he was 11, his father developed dysentery while abroad, and the family became preoccupied about hygiene and hand washing. Shortly afterward, he went away to boarding school and began to compulsively wash his hands.

AS may also be mistaken for OCD if the infant onset is not recognized and the communicative abnormalities are overlooked. OCD arising in someone with an anankastic personality presents the most diagnostic difficulty. Resistance to rituals may be a distinguishing feature: It is usually much less in AS than in OCD. Rituals in AS are usually comforting and there may be a mounting pleasurable excitement that precedes them. Compulsive rituals are preceded by anxiety.

There are some forms of eccentricity which are not due to communicative impairments arising from a developmental disorder. Some seem to be reactions to life events, as Eliot's fictional portrait of the miser Silas Marner indicates; others may be associated with psychiatric disorders other than AS.

Schizoid personality disorder is a diagnosis often associated with eccentricity. However, it is a source of considerable diagnostic confusion. The disorder described in ICD-10 (World Health Organization, 1992) is very different from the descriptions of schizoid personality disorder in use by psychotherapists, which are derived from Fairbairn (1952). The ICD-10 definition stresses coldness, indifference to other's opinions, and insensitivity. Fairbairn's description stresses oversensitivity to others and lack of persistence. These features appear in ICD-10 anxious (avoidant) personality disorder and have been more frequent in people whom I have seen whose social isolation has been attributed to long-standing personality traits rather than a primary autistic impairment.

Anxious (avoidant) personality disorder leads to marked proneness to social anxiety, which can result in isolation at school, victimization, and, in adolescence and adulthood, an eccentric social adjustment which may be mistakenly attributed to AS. However, avoidant personality disorder is associated with impaired social performance or impaired social competence. Nonverbal communication and the intuitive application of social understanding are unaffected.

When oversensitivity is the major feature, a diagnosis of narcissistic personality disorder may be more appropriate. Narcissistic personality disorder may also lead to social isolation if a person's oversensitivity to slight or humiliation leads to social avoidance and a hostile unwelcoming manner with an apparent lack of empathy. However, nonverbal communication and social intuition are unaffected.

Paranoid personality disorder may be associated with eccentricity and a lack of empathy for others and may sometimes be mistaken for AS. I find that the "fifth child syndrome" (as mentioned earlier) may be misdiagnosed as antisocial personality disorder but rarely vice versa. Mild learning disability may be apparent as an impairment in social relationships and may lead to a misdiagnosis of AS. The pattern of developmental delay in learning difficulty may be patchy, but there is no selective impairment of communication and motor development as there is in AS. Nonverbal communication is impaired in learning disabilities because there may be some poverty of expression and a lack of interpretative skill. However, the level of these abilities will be in keeping with the person's overall level of ability.

AS has been associated with chromosomal abnormalities, metabolic disorders, and neurological disorders. The symptoms of fragile-X syndrome are similar to those of autism, and if a person is only mildly affected and therefore, has only a mild learning disability, he or she may be referred for assessment for AS. A family history of learning disability in men suggests the possibility of fragile-X, and the person's affected DNA segment should be tested (Willemsen et al., 1995). Genetic counseling should be undertaken before a chromosome analysis is carried out.

All of the above conditions may occur in association with autistic spectrum disorders, which makes the differential diagnosis of AS complicated. This is particularly true of personality disorders. The emotional difficulties that a person with schizoid personality disorder has may be identical to those that a person with AS acquires, often because of adverse social consequences that result from having AS. These emotional difficulties are considered in more detail in the later section on emotional disorders.

Investigation of Core Syndrome

It is rare for congenital neurological conditions to present for the first time in adult life. It is also rare for people with AS to arrive at adulthood without having had some investigation of their condition, even though a diagnosis may not have been made. If a lifelong medical record is available, investigations may not need to be repeated. In the absence of such a record when there is doubt about the diagnosis, for example, because of a history of epilepsy, physical and psychological screenings are necessary (see Table 13.2). If abnormalities are found, further investigation is necessary.

TABLE 13.2. First-Line Investigation of Primary Impairments in AS

Investigation	Justification
Full physical examination	May detect focal neurological signs, skin lesions, joint elasticity. Useful for estimating poor coordination.
Psychometry	Gives objective evidence about learning ability. Pattern of scores often less helpful than expected, but verbal superiority to performance subtests typical of AS. Can incorporate standardized tests of empathy.
CT scan	May detect focal lesions. Not good for visualizing posterior fossa. May be more acceptable than MRI.
EEG	Particularly useful if there is a history of epilepsy. May give nonspecific evidence of focal lesions.
Chromosome screen	Many, if rare, chromosome abnormalities associated with AS. May need to precede with genetic counselling if screening for heritable condition such as fragile X.

Reactions to the Core Syndrome

The primary impairments of AS obstruct normal social interactions and may, therefore, prevent the formation of social relationships which are believed to be especially important in laying the foundations of personality. It is not clear whether early social experience has an effect on the person in later life, but if childhood attachment does affect adult social relationships, it is likely that some of the difficulties of adults with AS are due to this early disruption. Disrupted social interaction certainly leads to contemporaneous failure to make relationships in later life, with consequent social stigmatization, and a lack of support or even rejection. These can lead to other consequential disabilities which can contribute to the handicap, albeit secondarily. Table 13.3 shows some of these secondary disabilities.

TABLE 13.3. Personal Reactions to AS

Personal reaction	Problem behavior
Antisocial behavior	Aggression and "malice"; outrage
Impaired social relationships	Loneliness; adopting a marginal lifestyle
Substance misuse	
Sexual dysfunction	Fetishism
Emotional disorder	Anxiety; depression; panic disorder

Antisocial Behavior

The proportion of people with AS who present conduct problems or become offenders is unknown. In my experience, some offenses are rarely associated with AS, as with theft, for example. Sexually motivated crimes are also unusual and, when they occur, may be a consequence of a lack of understanding on the part of the person with AS. People with AS may be aggressive and commit offenses against other people, but it is unclear how frequently and what proportion of people with AS are at risk of doing so. Many people with AS have a hypertrophied sense of right and wrong and are unusually conscientious and unwilling to break the law, although this does not preclude isolated instances of lawbreaking which the person with AS feels are justified. People with AS are also more likely to be the victims than the perpetrators of aggression.

There have been numerous case reports of people with AS who have been violent, including some in this chapter. These case reports have been criticized as giving a selective, and therefore inaccurate, picture of the risk (Ghaziuddin, Tsai, & Ghaziuddin, 1991). One possible explanation for these different perspectives is that although violent behavior is not more common in people with AS than it is in the general population, persistent violence by a person with AS is a particularly difficult problem, which is more likely to lead to a long-term institutional placement, and that people with AS may therefore be overrepresented in psychiatric settings. For example, men with AS were overrepresented in a survey of one U.K. secure hospital (Scragg & Shah, 1994) and their needs were largely unrecognized.

Violence by a person with AS often has some special features. It may be triggered by idiosyncratic stimuli nourished by rumination over past slights; displaced from provoking the person onto a safer target at a later date; and uninhibited by empathic response to the intended victim's fear. Sometimes the explanation for violence may be similar to that given by Raskolnikov in Dosteyevsky's *Crime and Punishment*: that it is of an "experimental" nature.

> A girl of 19 had struggled at a series of private schools without being recognized as an individual with AS. Her parents split up and her father remarried during this period. When a half sister was born, the girl became very attentive to the baby but also began to wonder what would happen if the baby became ill. The patient mixed ground glass in the baby's food on two occasions to test this out.

> A boy of 13 became fascinated by the possibility of killing a schoolmate. He selected a boy and made one undetected attempt to harm him. Subsequently, he drowned the same boy in a pond.

Both of these people were hard put to give explanations for their actions, but they were able to describe something of what they wanted. In both cases, they wanted to experience a sense of mastery over another person and also to test whether their predictions about how others would behave in such extreme circumstances would be borne out in practice.

Reactions to extremes are easier to predict than are reactions to milder stimuli, because there is less room for individual variation. This may be the basis of the outrage that attracts some people with AS. Outrageous actions include transparent lies, provocative aggression, classroom disruption, and any simple action likely to produce an extreme, and therefore predictable, response.

> A boy called his grandmother to tell her, in an unsuccessfully disguised voice, that her husband had been killed in a car accident. Her husband had been at work and had not been involved in any accident, which became apparent as soon as he arrived home a few hours later.

Sexual Dysfunction

People with AS may be overtly sexually active, although they rarely succeed in having relationships with others and, if they do, they are almost always the seduced rather than the seducer, unless their relationship is with another person with AS or autism. However, the assumption that most people with AS are asexual may represent an unwillingness on the part of the professional and of the individual with AS to talk about this aspect of life. It may also be a result of the fetishistic orientation of the sexual activity. One patient described becoming excited when imagining dress shirts being torn, another became excited when he wore tight, wrinkle-free trousers, and another was stimulated by the word "enchantment" and wrote prose incorporating this word into different phrases which he would read.

Substance Abuse

The misuse of alcohol or drugs may be one way in which an adult with AS deals with his or her anxiety, although it is not known how often this problem occurs.

Emotional Disorders

Emotional disorders are overrepresented in AS. They may make all aspects of the core syndrome seem more severe. Many people with AS may grieve for loss of their home, their relatives, or their caregivers and yet not have this grief recognized.

Ms. Blue constantly tore her clothes until the workers in the hostel where she lived took away her own things, and bought her new clothes. She had been living in the hostel for about a year and this problem had begun shortly after she arrived. She could not explain her behavior but cried during much of the interview and asked repeatedly if she could go back home to live with her parents. It seemed that Ms. Blue was rending her clothes in grief.

Depression may be common. Deliberate self-harm is rare, although suicide may occur. Most people with AS are anxious much of the time, and their behavior may be motivated by the desire to avoid anxiety. Panic is a variant of anxiety that may be difficult to recognize because the attacks of anxiety may not be accompanied by physical causes or effects and may be disconnected to events.

A man in his 30s, whose AS was diagnosed in adulthood, complained of odd, indescribable sensations in his legs. He sometimes accused his mother of touching him, even when she was at some distance from him. He had no other symptoms suggestive of psychosis. The onset of the paresthesiae in his legs was associated with great agitation and the gradual spread of abnormal sensation centripetally. It was only when his mother described the onset of an "attack" as coming when the patient was about to leave the house to go to the shops that its association with anxiety became apparent. Neuroleptic medication did not reduce the frequency of the symptoms, but fluoxetine did, and comorbid panic disorder was diagnosed.

Anxiety may sometimes be severe and lead to a schizophreniform psychosis. The differential diagnosis may be difficult, as unusual thoughts may be translated as delusions and unusual sensory experiences as hallucinations. First-rank symptoms may occur, even in remitting disorders which do not appear, in the long run, to be schizophrenia.

Schizophrenia should only be diagnosed after careful assessment, as negative symptoms may not easily differentiate the two. Passivity symptoms may also occur when people with AS are highly aroused, but they do not indicate the onset of a psychosis and should not lead, in themselves, to a diagnosis of schizophrenia.

A young man suspected of AS, but not previously diagnosed, enrolled in a university away from his hometown, living in a student residence hall. New students had no classes during the first week and traditionally, drank in excess, were noisy, and made friends. Within 24 hours, the young man was convinced that his mind could be read, that the people on the television were enacting his thoughts, and that there was some hidden conspiracy behind everything that was happening, which his parents, but not he, knew about. His symptoms continued until he returned home, at which time they remitted completely. He took a year off and then reenrolled at his home university. He was anxious and lost some sleep before the start of the term and on the third day visited another friend in residence hall. He developed delusional mood and was treated with a low dose of chlorpromazine. The mood persisted, as did a high level of arousal, behavioral disorganization, and insomnia. He was admitted to a psychiatric unit and settled down after a week still on the chlorpromazine. Family and individual counseling began, and apart from a slight increase in anxiety during his first examination, he has remained well for 18 months. Neuroleptics were discontinued, and he remained well at follow-up 1 year later.

The treatment of psychosis is not changed by being associated with AS. Lithium appears to be as effective at preventing relapse of bipolar illness as it is in nonautistic people, although there may be greater risk in using this medication if patients cannot be relied on to report side effects. Neuroleptics may worsen lack of emotional expressiveness because of the Parkinsonian akinesia that they produce and should be avoided except in the short-term management of overarousal or acute psychotic symptoms. The atypical neuroleptics, which have fewer extrapyramidal effects, may be more advantageous for this reason, but there has been insufficient assessment of their use in AS to be able to recommend them.

Helping People with their Personal Reactions

Anxiety is often prominent in people with AS, and they want to know how to manage it. Making the environment, including the social environment, more predictable is particularly important. For many people with AS, managing anxiety is difficult, and medication may be necessary despite its limitations. The selective serotonin reuptake inhibitors (SSRIs) have been widely used, and have been found to be effective in reducing anxiety and, therefore, increasing adaptiveness. The SSRIs have the theoretical advantage of their reputed activity in OCD which has some overlap with AS ritualizing. Propranolol has fewer central effects, although it may cause insomnia, but it also seems to be less effective in AS. Neuroleptics are often used as anxiolytic agents. Neuroleptics have Parkinsonian side effects which may make the expressive abnormalities of people with AS worse and may cause tardive dyskinesia. The newer, atypical neuroleptics, such as sulpiride and risperidone, are thought to have less of these side effects and are increasingly used. However, their long-term effects in AS are unknown, and they are not free of the demotivating effect common to all the neuroleptics. It is therefore advisable in the majority of cases, to use them only for short-term urgent treatment.

Counseling can be helpful because it is designed to help someone with AS understand why other people do what they do, and how he or she can put this information to use in responding to difficult situations.

SOCIAL REACTIONS

The primary impairments of AS, and the psychological disabilities that ensue from them, have a powerful impact on others. Caregivers may feel helpless and, consequently, feel a need to push the person with AS away, or to react by becoming overinvolved. Peers and siblings may feel pushed aside due to the attention given to the person with AS or outraged by his or her behavior. Each of these reactions impinges upon the person with AS, for whom they may create further problems, or "tertiary handicaps." Some of the most important are the behavioral and emotional problems that result from victimization.

Victimization

Of the people with AS on whom I have detailed records, 64% were reported by their parents as being bullied or teased at school. Bullying involved being aggressive, tearing clothes, opening a boy's fly in the street (something that girls do rather than boys), or spitting on someone. Teasing involved names suggestive of social isolation, such as "monster" or "machine." Teasing was sometimes extended to other family members. People with AS might deal with bullying by being aggressive themselves, often inflaming the situation further.

It is difficult to know why AS creates such hostility in others. The worst period is, in my experience, the early years at secondary school (i.e., 11–15 years old). One factor may be the attribution of the actions of the person with AS to malice rather than to disability. I know of two cases in which classes were prepared for the entry of a boy with AS, who was moving because of being bullied at another school, by being told that the new boy had a medical condition which affected his ability to relate to others. In both cases, there was little subsequent bullying.

Enslavement by Routine

Handicaps may also arise because the person with AS has not had enough social structure around him or her to contain their anxiety about change. This is particularly apparent when a person becomes dominated by his or her need to avoid change. Adherence to routine is frequent in AS, although its causes remain uncertain. I have discussed it as a psychological disability in a previous section, linking it to the lack of predictability about the world of a person with AS. Others have speculated that there is a primary impairment in autistic people, resulting in a failure to inhibit perseveration. However, the considerable variation in the severity of routine, and the different reactions of caregivers to it, suggest that social responses to the tendency to routinize also have a powerful impact. This section is headed "enslavement by routine" because that can be an accurate description of the extent to which the life of the person with AS and his or her family can be completely dominated by the avoidance of any change, such as might be created by a visitor at the home, a visit to a professional, home improvements or repairs, or holidays. Sometimes parents find themselves going along with their child's demands out of compassion or a willingness to put their own interests second to those of their child. Often, changes in routine trigger aggression, and parents avoid them in order to avoid aggressive confrontations.

PHYSICAL DISORDERS ASSOCIATED WITH AS

AS has been associated with aminoaciduria, with connective tissue disorder, and with Sotos syndrome. There are reports of autism associated with Duchenne muscular dystrophy (Komoto, Usui, & Otsuki, 1984; Portwood, Wicks, Slakey, Lieberman, & Fowler, 1981), and I have seen one case of AS associated with myotonic dystrophy. Congenital space-occupying lesions (e.g., those associated with neurofibromatosis and with tuberous sclerosis) may be associated with AS, as may Tourette syndrome.

I have seen more cases of thyroid disease in persons with AS and in their families than I would have expected. There is also an unusually high incidence of surgery to the genitals of children with AS, most often correction of a phimosis or orchidopexy for maldescended testicle.

There appears to be an association of AS with visual impairment. For example, I have seen two cases associated with congenital nystagmus. This might be explained by the social gaze hypothesis of AS considered in an earlier section. Reduced visual acuity will impair the child's ability to recognize social stimuli. AS also seems to be associated with motor disturbances caused by unrelated physical disorders. The associations of AS with ligamentous laxity and with muscular dystrophy are examples. Motor difficulties may contribute to impaired nonverbal expression and may be a reason for the association.

PSYCHIATRIC DISORDERS ASSOCIATED WITH AS
BUT NOT APPARENTLY CAUSED BY IT (COMORBIDITY)

There has been no epidemiologically based study of the prevalence of psychiatric disorder in patients with AS. Clinical experience is made unreliable by selection bias, although this may not affect the ratio of different disorders. Experience in my own clinic is that emotional and conduct disorders are common, but that may be a selection bias. These disorders are considered in more detail in a previous section.

When psychosis occurs in a person with AS, the possibility of schizophrenia is often raised. There is no evidence in the literature that schizophrenia is more common in people with AS than in the general population, and it may, indeed, be rarer. However bipolar affective disorder is more common, and the most likely explanation is that it is not a disability due to the AS but a comorbid disorder, perhaps resulting from genetic linkage. A familial association with bipolar disorder has also been reported (DeLong & Nohria, 1994). It is interesting to note that bipolar disorder also seems to be more common in the families of people with OCD and with Tourette syndrome.

Bipolar disorder occurring in a person with AS will respond to conventional treatment once it is recognized.

GUIDELINES FOR PARENTS

Parents often initiate the referral of a person with AS, even if that person is a young adult. Often, parents act as the patient's advocate for many years and wish to have a diagnosis to enable them to continue to do so. Parents rarely want further information about specific aspects of management. There is often a lack of information, and I try to address this issue at the first interview.

The way I present information to parents depends on their previous knowledge of AS and on their psychological approaches. However, the message usually contains the following information:

- AS is thought by many people to be a subtype of autism.
- The basic problem is in nonverbal communication and in understanding how to react to other people.
- People with AS often make improvements in their social adjustment well into adult life.
- AS is not caused by poor upbringing.
- Other people's responses can affect the behavior and emotions of someone with AS.
- Depression and anxiety can occur.
- People with AS often compare themselves unfavorably to their peers.
- Many people with AS feel marginalized.
- Many people with AS are victimized, particularly at school.
- Further information about AS may be obtained from local or national autistic societies, in those countries in which they exist, or, increasingly, from the Internet. (See the Appendix at the end of the book.)
- Associated problems may need special, additional help.

It is difficult to come to a realistic appraisal of the abilities of one's own child, but it is important that parents of people with AS try to do so because expectations that are too high lead to disappointment and possibly criticism on the part of parents and loss of self-esteem for the person with AS. Expectations that are too low may also be harmful, leading to a failure to make use of a person's full potential. The low expressed emotions approach that works in schizophrenia also appears to work in AS. Clear expectations, low critical comments, low emotional demand, and the avoidance of overinvolvement are all good principles. The latter is particularly difficult. It is easy for parents to become enmeshed with their child's problems because the adult with AS seems so indifferent to his or her own best interests. It is realistic that parents of people with AS assume that their affected children are less responsible and more in need of protection than are their peers with the same chronological or mental age. However, it is essential that parents draw back from total involvement. Enmeshment is the quickest way to burn out.

DEVELOPMENTAL PERSPECTIVE

The greatest fluctuations in AS are due to changes in personal reactions to problems and, to a lesser degree, to social reactions, which are consequent to the core syndrome. This is most apparent in the developmental crises that people with AS may experience, often at times of psychosocial transition, as between infancy and primary school; at about 7 years old in the United Kingdom; at the start of secondary school at 11 or 12 years old; at the time of examinations before leaving school at 16, 17, or 18 years old; or immediately after school, adjusting to work, further education, or the loss of the school day.

Rapid developmental improvements may occur in late infancy, perhaps associated with the acquisition of language, and in late adolescence, but social development occurs throughout the 20s and 30s.

As AS knowledge becomes more widespread, middle-aged men whose marriages or careers are failing are increasingly becoming aware of AS tendencies that have been present but did not cause major social difficulties earlier in life. This type of late disclosure of AS may become a greater problem in the future.

The occurrence of such late disclosures indicates how substantial an effect emotional factors can have on the disability associated with AS. Counseling is helpful in dealing with these emotional problems and should be used.

PROGNOSIS

Little is known about the prognosis in AS, and there have been no long-term follow-up studies published in which current criteria of AS have been used to select the sample. The available information comes from follow-up studies of autism, comparisons of current state with retrospective information about early childhood, and case reports. This rather motley information does, however, seem to support Asperger's own assertion that AS has a good prognosis, although the meaning of this statement needs to be qualified.

The primary impairment in AS does not seem to worsen and may improve. This may be true of all aspects of the impairment. Parents may, for example, report greater expressiveness over the years, a reduction of extreme preservation of sameness, growing intersubjectivity and empathy, and less incoordination. A crude comparison of those who have most improved with those who have least improved, compared with their reported childhood status, among the people with AS that I have seen demonstrated that social contact with peers was associated with good prognosis. It is possible that improvement allowed greater social contact rather than the social contact shaping social behavior and producing improvement, but anecdotal evidence also indicates that a peer relationship, for example, in a long-standing sexual relationship does reduce impairment. The key element may be the social demand that is associated with peer interaction: Peers do not make explicit demands, but they also make few allowances.

ACKNOWLEDGMENT

I am grateful to my patients and their families for teaching me not only about autism but also about coping with suffering and isolation. Case descriptions cited in this chapter are amalgamated from different people, and none therefore correspond to a particular individual. All names and other identifying details have been changed. I am also grateful to Emmy van Deurzen for long and insightful discussions about the Dasein of Asperger syndrome.

REFERENCES

Adolphs, R., Tranel, D., Damasio, H., & Damasio, A. R. (1995). Fear and the human amygdala. *Journal of Neuroscience, 15,* 5879–5891.

Argyle, M. (1986). The skill, rules, and goals of relationships. In G. Gilmour & S. Duck (Eds.), *The emerging field of personal relationships* (pp. 23–29). London: Academic Press.

Asperger, H. (1944). Die "Autistischen Psychopathen" im Kindesalter. *Archiv für Psychiatrie und Nervenkrankheiten, 117,* 76–136.

Asperger, H. (1979). Problems of infantile autism. *Communication, 13,* 45–52.

Baron-Cohen, S., Campbell, R., Karmiloff-Smith, A., Grant, J., & Walker, J. (1995). Are children with autism blind to the significance of the eyes? *British Journal of Developmental Psychology, 13,* 379–398.

Bowler, D. M. (1992). "Theory of mind" in Asperger's syndrome. *Journal of Child Psychology and Psychiatry, 33,* 877–893.

Damasio, H., Maurer, R. G., Damasio, A., & Chui, H. (1980). Computerized tomographic scan findings in patients with autistic behaviour. *Archives of Neurology, 37,* 504–510.

DeLong, R., & Nohria, C. (1994). Psychiatric family history and neurological disease in autistic spectrum disorders. *Developmental Medicine and Child Neurology, 36*, 441–448.

Fairbairn, W. (1952). *Psychoanalytic studies of the personality.* London: Tavistock.

Ghaziuddin, M. (1992). Brief report: A comparison of the diagnostic criteria for Asperger Syndrome. *Journal of Autism and Developmental Disorders, 22*, 651–656.

Ghaziuddin, M., Tsai, L. Y., & Ghaziuddin, N. (1991). Brief report: Violence in Asperger syndrome, a critique. *Journal of Autism and Developmental Disorders, 21*, 349–354.

Hobson, R. P. (1990). On acquiring knowledge about people and the capacity to pretend: Response to Leslie. *Psychological Review, 97*, 114–121.

Karmiloff-Smith, A., Klima, E., Bellugi, U., Grant, J., & Baron-Cohen, S. (1995). Is there a social module? Language, face processing, and theory of mind in individuals with Williams syndrome. *Journal of Cognitive Neuroscience, 7*, 196–208.

Klin, A., Volkmar, F. R., Sparrow, S., Cicchetti, D., & Rourke, B. P. (1995). Validity and neuropsychological characterization of Asperger syndrome: Convergence with nonverbal learning disabilities syndrome. *Journal of Autism and Developmental Disorders, 36*, 1127–1140.

Komoto, J., Usui, S., & Otsuki, S. (1984). Infantile autism and Duchenne muscular dystrophy. *Journal of Autism and Developmental Disorders, 14*, 191–195.

Kracke, I. (1994). Developmental prosopagnosia in Asperger syndrome: Presentation and discussion of an individual case. *Developmental Medicine and Child Neurology, 36*, 873–886.

Leekam, S. R., Hunnisett, E., & Moore, C. (1998). Targets and cues: Gaze-following in children with autism. *Journal of Child Psychology and Psychiatry and Allied Disciplines, 39*(7), 951–962

Lessing, D. (1989). *The fifth child.* London: Paladin.

Lovaas, O. I., & Smith, T. (1989). A comprehensive behavioural theory of autistic children: Paradigm for research and treatment. *Journal of Behavior Treatment and Experimental Psychiatry, 20*, 17–29.

Lund, J. (1989). Measuring behaviour disorder in mental handicap. *British Journal of Psychiatry, 155*, 379–383.

Marsden, G., Kalter, N., & Ericson, W. A. (1974). Response productivity: A methodological problem in content analysis studies in psychotherapy. *Journal of Consulting and Clinical Psychology, 42*, 224–230.

McKenna, K., Gordon, C. T., Lenane, M., Kaysen, D., Fahey, K., & Rapoport, J. L. (1994). Looking for childhood-onset schizophrenia: The first 71 cases screened. *Journal of the American Academy of Child and Adolescent Psychiatry, 33*, 636–644.

Portwood, M. M., Wicks, J., Slakey, S., Lieberman, J., & Fowler, W. (1981). Psychometric evaluations in muscular dystrophy. *Archives of Physical Medicine and Rehabilitation, 62*, 531.

Rapin, I. (1996). Practitioner review: Developmental language disorders: A clinical update. *Journal of Child Psychology and Psychiatry and Allied Disciplines, 37*, 643–655.

Scott, D. W. (1985). Asperger's syndrome and nonverbal communication: A pilot study. *Psychological Medicine, 15*, 683–687.

Scragg, P., & Shah, A. (1994). Prevalence of Asperger's syndrome in a secure hospital [see comments]. *British Journal of Psychiatry, 165*, 679–682.

Tantam, D. (1991). Asperger's syndrome in adulthood. In U. Frith (Ed.), *Autism and Asperger's syndrome* (pp. 147–183). Cambridge: Cambridge University Press.

Tantam, D. (1992). Characterizing the fundamental social handicap in autism. *Acta Paedopsychiatrica, 55*, 83–91.

Tantam, D. (1995). Empathy, persistent aggression, and antisocial personality disorder. *Journal of Forensic Psychiatry, 6*, 10–18.

Tantam, D., Holmes, D., & Cordess, C. (1993). Nonverbal expression in autism of Asperger type. *Journal of Autism and Developmental Disorders, 23*, 111–133.

Trevarthen, C. (1979). Communication and cooperation in early infancy: A description of primary intersubjectivity. In M. Bullowa (Ed.), *Before speech: The beginning of interpersonal communication* (pp. 321–347). Cambridge: Cambridge University Press.

Waterhouse, L., Morris, R., Allen, D., Dunn, M., Fein, D., Feinstein, C., Rapin, I., & Wing, L. (1996). Diagnosis and classification in autism. *Journal of Autism and Developmental Disorders, 26*, 58–86.

Willemsen, R., Mohkamsing, S., de Vries, B., van den Oweland, A., Mandel, J., Galjaard, H., & Oostra, B. (1995). Rapid antibody test for fragile X syndrome. *Lancet, 345*.

Willemsen-Swinkels, S. H., Buitelaar, J. K., Weijnen, F. G., & Engeland, H. (1998). Timing of social gaze behavior in children with a pervasive developmental disorder. *Journal of Autism and Developmental Disorders, 28*(3), 199–210.

Wing, L., & Gould, J. (1979). Severe impairments of social interaction and associated abnormalities in children: Epidemiology and classification. *Journal of Autism and Developmental Disorders, 9*, 11–29.

Wolff, S. (1991). "Schizoid" personality in childhood and adult life. I: The vagaries of diagnostic labelling. *British Journal of Psychiatry, 159*, 615–620, 634–635.

Wolff, S., & Chick, J. (1980). Schizoid personality disorder in childhood: A controlled follow-up study. *Psychological Medicine, 10*, 85–100.

World Health Organization. (1992). *The ICD-10 classification of mental and behavioral disorders* (10th ed.). Geneva: Author.

V

Perspectives on Research and Clinical Practice, and Parent Essays

14

Perspectives on the Classification of Asperger Syndrome

PETER SZATMARI

Johnny was first seen at 4 years of age. His parents' main concerns were speech delay, eating habits, and behavioral problems. In terms of speech, Johnny was virtually mute. He said his first words at 18 months but since that time has not shown any progression in language development. Johnny did not shake his head in answer to "yes" or "no" and he did not point or use gestures. He also showed marked impairments in social responsiveness; for example, he did not look at people directly, was not very affectionate with them, and has never really developed an emotional bond with adults other than his mother. He did not enjoy the attention of other people and would not direct his parent's attention to toys or to other objects of interest. Johnny did not show distress or anxiety on separation and was described by his mother as an extremely passive, unresponsive, placid baby. He did not play with other children but preferred to play by himself. He also showed a preference for solitary, repetitive activities that have a high sensory component, such as splashing water on his hands and spinning wheels. Johnny liked to smell the hair and face of his parents and to squeeze their heads. He did not develop any pretend or symbolic play but liked to clap his hands, jump up and down, and flick his fingers in front of his eyes. He liked to line up cars and became quite upset if this line was disturbed in any way. He also had a fascination with sounds, lights, and shiny objects. Johnny would become quite upset with small changes in his daily routine, such as taking a different route to school or having to put on long pants rather than shorts.

"Solitariness, temper tantrums and a fanatical interest in religious ritual were the principal marks of a boy age 12 and a half—Peter. . . . He went to bed at 9 pm but did not fall asleep until midnight and insisted on one of his parents remaining by his bedside all the while. At mealtimes he frequently refused to stay at table, alleging as his reason for this that his mother 'did not eat right' or 'was not dressed right.' He had 'church on the brain.' His main topics of conversation were ecclesiastical and his principle recreation out of school hours was rehearsing church services. His knowledge of these matters was said by his mother to be astonishingly detailed, and when he went to church, he would find fault with the minutiae of the service. He had no friends of his own and said that he did not want any. If his parents invited another boy to the home, he 'sat and talked quite nice to him,' but he would not accept invitations in return. . . . He had the habit of harping on one theme to the intense and frequently expressed annoyance of his parents—for example, he would talk for hours to his cat saying 'nice boy' over and over again ad nauseam. His school report said; 'the boy is obedient, quiet and inoffensive; in fact, the one thing that strikes us is that he is apathetic, dreamy and slow on the uptake. In some subjects—English and drawing, he is in advance of his years; in others, arithmetic, he is slow and backward. When he first came here, he kept somewhat aloof but he is now mixing gradually with the other boys.'

"In appearance, he was a well groomed but thin and sallow complexioned boy, who carried himself in a slovenly fashion with bent shoulders and looked older than his years. He had a glum expression and he did not talk spontaneously at the interviewer but only in answer to questions and then rather briefly. He did not look his interlocutor in the eye but usually looked at the ground instead. In reply to questions, he admitted his interest in religious ritual. His reading beside the Bible, consisted almost exclusively of Shakespeare and Mark Twain. He was not interested, he said, in such papers as 'Chums' or 'Boy's Own' paper or tales of adventure."

*   *   *

Do these two children have the *same* disorder or do they have a *different* disorder? At one level, these two children are very different, and it does not take years of training to discern this. One child is mute; the other talks fluently. One child is completely withdrawn from social interaction; the other is able to interact with others but does so in an unusual fashion. One child is fascinated with concrete objects, such as cars, lights, and hair; the other is fascinated with more esoteric subjects, such as church services, Shakespeare, and the writings of Mark Twain. The first child might be classified as having autistic disorder and was recently seen in the clinic. The second child, who might just as reasonably be classified as having Asperger syndrome (AS), was seen in 1924 at Guy's Hospital in London and was described in the 1947 edition of the psychiatric textbook of Henderson and Gillespie as having "schizoid" personality disorder (pp. 616–621).

In spite of these differences, these two children share impairments in social reciprocity, in communicating with others, and in having a preference for doing the same thing over and over again. What they share at a more fundamental level is a primary disinterest in intersubjectivity—the world of other people and their place in it. Instead, they are fascinated with concrete or conceptual objects for their own sake, not as a means of establishing relationships with other people. Much of this book is taken up with whether Johnny and Peter have the "same" or a "different" disorder. This question, which sounds so simple on the surface, is in fact quite complicated. In many ways, our inability to answer this question conclusively confronts us with the extraordinary limitations of our vocabulary, our conceptualization of the developmental disabilities, and the criteria we use to validate current classification systems.

What does it mean when we say "two disorders are different"? Different at the level of simple symptoms and behaviors or different at a more fundamental level of mechanism and process? What evidence would we need to decide whether two disorders are the same or different, and is it even possible to marshal such evidence given our current state of knowledge? It is generally accepted that for two disorders to be different, they should vary on characteristics independent of the diagnostic criteria (Rutter, 1978). These characteristics include causation, outcome, and response to treatment, though etiology often takes precedence as the most important distinguishing feature. The problem is that our knowledge of etiology is so limited and our study designs for causation so narrow in scope that it is difficult to provide conclusive answers. Indeed, will it *ever* be possible to decide whether two disorders are the same or different in the absence of perfectly conclusive evidence? As a result of these and other considerations, I argue that for some distinctions it is more important to evaluate the *usefulness* of diagnostic distinctions rather than their validity.

HISTORICAL BACKGROUND

Children with social-communication impairments and eccentric behavior have been recognized for many years. Such children are often diagnosed as having a psychiatric illness or a "personality disorder." There is indeed a superficial similarity with schizophrenia in that the children are socially withdrawn and have odd communication and thought patterns. Asperger (1944) preferred to conceptualize the children that he described as having a "personality disorder" characterized by the same type of autistic withdrawal that is seen in schizophrenia. But he did not consider the disorder a form of psychosis. Although Asperger's work became well-known in Europe, it was cited in only a few English-speaking journals (Van Krevelen, 1971) until Lorna Wing (1981) published her case series of AS patients.

Table 14.1 illustrates the differing impact that work on AS and autism has had since that publication. The table illustrates that the number of pa-

TABLE 14.1. Number of Articles Published in Medline[a] since 1981

	AS	Autism
1981–1985	8	581
1986–1990	33	893
1991–1995	61	1019
1996–1997	35	443

[a]using key words "Autism" and "Asperger syndrome"

pers appearing in MEDLINE on autism has doubled over a 10-year period. In contrast, the number of papers appearing under the heading of Asperger syndrome has only increased to 15–20 papers a year. By far the vast majority of these papers have either been single case reports (Burgoine & Wing, 1983; Mawson, Grounds, & Tantam, 1985) or, more recently, case–control studies comparing AS children with those with autism on various neuropsychological indices and measures (Ozonoff, Rogers, & Pennington, 1991; Gillberg, 1989; Szatmari, Bartolucci, & Bremner, 1989; Szatmari, Archer, Fisman, Streiner, & Wilson, 1995; Eisenmajer et al., 1996). There are no outcome or treatment studies. Reading the introduction of these papers shows a singular focus on deciding whether AS and autism are "separate disorders" or "on a continuum" of severity (Schopler, 1996).

As the case vignette of Peter illustrates, clinical descriptions of odd and eccentric children have appeared in the literature well before Asperger published his paper. Indeed, Sula Wolff has provided a translation of "the first account of the syndrome Asperger described" in a paper that appeared in 1926 (Ssucharewa & Wolff, 1996). This paper describes six boys with schizoid disorder and draws heavily on Kretschmer's (1925) early work. Although it is always difficult to make diagnoses from case reports, it certainly does appear as if this is the same group of children described by Asperger some 20 years later. Sula Wolff herself has published a number of papers, and more recently a book, on schizoid children in which she makes the convincing argument that in spite of some differences in severity, children with schizoid disorder and AS represent the same group of children (Wolff, 1995).

Kanner's work on infantile autism, on the other hand, became extremely well-known soon after his paper was published in 1943. He originally thought of infantile autism as an early form of schizophrenia, also borrowing the term "autism" from Bleuler. His descriptions were precise enough to be useful in classifying a large number of children who had previously been difficult to understand. Children with autism were also described well before Kanner's 1943 paper but usually appeared in books on mental handicap and the "idiot savant." The famous case of the "genius" at Earlswood who produced meticulous drawings of naval ships and was obsessed with being a naval captain is one famous example (Tredgold, 1937).

Thus, AS and autism as diagnostic categories arise from two rather separate traditions within the history of child psychiatry and have different historical routes.

Many of the individuals described by Wing (1981) in her classic paper originally met criteria for autism, suggesting that the new term was merely a description of some children with autism at a later stage of development. Thus, she did not use it as a diagnostic term in the sense of a mutually exclusive category. However, others soon recognized that the descriptions also fit children who would not meet the official criteria for autism. The first case-control studies comparing children with autism and AS on clinical features appeared in 1989 and demonstrated that the most important distinguishing feature between the disorders was language development (Gillberg, 1989; Szatmari et al., 1989). The problem with these studies was that the criteria for diagnosing AS were not specified, so the extent to which the differences were a function of the way the groups were originally defined could not be established. The next step was to specify explicit criteria for AS and then to compare the groups on variables independent of the defining criteria. However, as pointed out by Ghaziuddin, Tsai, and Ghaziuddin (1992) the diagnostic criteria used by various authors differed from each other so it was difficult to reach a consensus.

The third revised edition of the *Diagnostic and Statistical Manual of Mental Disorders* (DSM-III-R; American Psychiatric Association, 1987) did not mention AS as a diagnostic category; instead the disorder was conceptualized as a type of pervasive developmental disorders not otherwise specified (PDD-NOS). The draft version of the tenth edition of *International Classification of Disease* (ICD-10, World Health Organization, 1992) did, however, contain criteria for AS that were very similar to those used for autism except that children with AS could not have clinically significant language or cognitive delay. The PDD committee for DSM-IV reviewed the literature on AS and concluded that the evidence that it was a "valid" disorder was both inconsistent and equivocal, although it was recognized that there was very little evidence of good quality either way (Szatmari, 1992, 1997). In the DSM-IV field trial, 48 individuals with AS were identified and differed from those with autism on the basis of IQ and certain symptoms and behaviors. As a result of these data and the literature review, a decision was made to include AS as a category in DSM-IV (American Psychiatric Association, 1994) with the specific comment that the diagnostic validity of the disorder was unknown. The intent was to stimulate further research and to recognize that the term was being used by parents and clinicians, whether or not scientists could agree on its validity.

More recent studies have now used these DSM-IV criteria to evaluate AS. One important finding is that these criteria are virtually unworkable. Indeed, Miller and Ozonoff (1997) have shown that the children described by Asperger himself would not meet DSM-IV criteria. The difficulty is that according to the manual, a child who meets criteria for both autism and AS is given preferentially a diagnosis of autism. Miller and Ozonoff (1997) found that the children described by Asperger also met criteria for autism, a finding similar to one reported by us (Szatmari et al., 1995) using a contemporary sample of children. In other words, DSM-IV conceptualizes the disorders as mutually exclusive, a view different from that originally held by Wing. The sensible decision to have autism take precedence over a diagnosis of AS in DSM-IV was taken to ensure that AS children were as different from autism as possible, but it was not based on any empirical evidence. In fact, the criteria for autism were designed to differentiate children with autism from those with *non-PDD disorders*, not from children within the PDD spectrum. As a result, the criteria are perhaps overinclusive and make no mention of specific types of social and communication impairments that could be used to differentiate PDD subtypes. We have shown that by modifying the criteria slightly and by reversing the hierarchy rule (i.e., by saying that children who meet criteria for both autism and AS are given a diagnosis of AS), children with AS can be identified and are different from children with autism on measures of autistic symptoms, social competence, and language abilities (Szatmari et al., 1995). A new series of studies is now needed to refine the diagnostic differentiation and to see whether differences between AS and autism also exist on other measures of etiology, outcome, and response to treatment.

EVALUATING THE CLASSIFICATION OF THE PERVASIVE DEVELOPMENTAL DISORDERS

How is one to classify children who present with behaviors falling within the autistic triad and how does one decide that the classification is valid (Cohen, Paul, & Volkmar, 1986)? Building a classification system is in many ways like building a house, although too often the house is built on shifting sands. One starts with a foundation of disorders that have been historically accepted as valid and as providing clinically useful information. These fundamental disorders represent broad concepts and include the developmental, emotional, and behavior disorders. The criteria for establishing the validity of these have been well described by Robins and Guze (1970) and later by Rutter (1978), Blashfield and Draguns (1976), Skinner (1981), and Cantwell (1982) and are now universally accepted. To be valid, a "new disorder" must differ from an "older," more established, disorder on variables that are *independent* of the defining characteristics. Furthermore, these independent variables must not be trivial but must relate to clinically important distinctions with respect to etiology, natural history, associated features, and response to treatment. To be valid, two disorders must differ on all these domains as well as meeting the tests of independence and nontriviality. These rules of evidence have worked well in establishing that autism is a valid disorder, distinct from the other emotional and behavioral disorders of childhood and from childhood schizophrenia. These rules have also worked very well in distinguishing emotional disorders from conduct disorders. Why? Presumably, because these are broad categories in which differences in etiology are so great that they translate into large effect sizes with respect to differences in natural history and response to treatment. It is important, however, to realize that none of our research designs is unequivocally able to establish etiology or causation. This would require either true experiments or the identification of specific genetic mutations. At best, we must resort to cross-sectional and longitudinal designs that suggest certain correlates or risk factors are associated with one category of disorder rather than another. There are no absolute differences in child psychiatry, only differences of degree. Once these quantitative differences are of a sufficient effect size, they *appear* like categorical differences, but it is very important to recall that there is always some observed overlap between disorders on clinical symptoms, risk factors, outcome, and response to treatment. This overlap is the result not only of measurement error but also of the enormous variation seen in child development.

However, these rules of evidence have proved relatively unsuccessful in establishing clear differences *within* the major subcategories of disorder. For example, conduct, oppositional, and attention-deficit disorder are now subsumed under the disruptive behavior disorders (American Psychiatric Association, 1994). In reality, children with these disorders share many symptoms, risk factors, outcome (Hinshaw, 1992) and treatment response (Klein et al., 1997). In fact, some children with oppositional disorder go on to have conduct disorder (Biederman et al., 1996). There are differences to be sure, but again these are quantitative rather than qualitative differences. Nevertheless, the distinction between the types of disruptive behavior disorders has proven to be clinically *useful* as long as it is also recognized that overlap can and does exist. The problem is even more acute with respect to the anxiety disorders of childhood, for which DSM-IV now lists several types. However, these disorders share a common family history (Bernstein, Borchardt, & Perwien, 1996), a similar outcome (Bernstein et al., 1996), and a good response to some treatment methods (Kendall et al., 1997). Their distinctiveness relies primarily on different symptom patterns, but these differences have not yet translated into major differences with respect to etiology, natural history, or response to treatment. Nevertheless, clinicians feel that, by and large, these clinical distinctions are *useful* without necessarily being valid. There is enough variation in outcome and response to treatment that thinking about these disorders differently is helpful, though this may not always be so as knowledge accumulates.

The difficulty is that the evidence for diagnostic validity relies too heavily on finding differences in etiology between two disorders. The language trap is to think of disorders as "things" rather than descriptions of a developmental process. Children do not have "autism" in the same way they have a strep throat. Our classification system is built on the medical model. We tend to think of symptoms and behaviors as external representations of some hidden reality or etiology that lies elusive and beyond our grasp. Nevertheless, the signs and symptoms we describe are supposed to be reliable and accurate indicators of that underlying disease mechanism. That is probably an overly simplistic view as etiological mechanisms are likely much more complicated and involve the interaction of multiple risk and protective factors through complex causal chains leading to one, or perhaps several, final common pathways. Once we get behind the broad categories of disorder and begin to think of distinctions within the disruptive behavior disorders, within the anxiety and affective disorders, and within the pervasive developmental disorders, this notion of "distinct" etiological mechanisms translating into variation in clinical features, outcome, and response to treatment is overly simplistic and leads to unhelpful debates as to whether one subtype of disorder is the "same" or "different" from another.

At some level, autism and AS *must* share etiological risk mechanisms. There now seems reasonably good evidence that autism is a genetic disorder caused by multiple interacting genes (Szatmari, Jones, Zwaigenbaum, & MacLean, 1998). It would not at all be surprising if the genes for autism did not overlap (to some extent) with the genes for AS. Even if the genes were totally distinct, it is highly likely that the phenotypical effects of those genes would overlap and disrupt the same brain systems. There are likely to be some differences, but these would be quantitative, not qualitative, and not of the same magnitude as the difference between, for example, autism and anxiety disorder. Let us suppose the genes for autism and AS are different but the brain systems are the same, or alternatively, the genes are the same but (because of other modifying factors) these genes affect the brain at different points in development. What would we then conclude; is AS the same or, different than autism? In this context, the criteria for *same* and *different* are somewhat arbitrary. Thinking of the problem in terms of "same and different" is a conceptual and linguistic trap that will not provide a way ahead for further research and clinical practice. It may be more accurate to think of several (many or a few?) causal chains that overlap and diverge at different points but ultimately coalesce into a final common pathway with enormous phenotypical variation.

Neither is it terribly useful to think of these disorders as on a "continuum." PDD is a disorder of multiple impairments in socialization, communication, and play with added impairments in cognitive abilities. On which of these domains are the disorders on a continuum? Moreover, two disorders may be on a continuum yet so quantitatively different that it is still clinically useful to make the distinction between them. Mild transient dysphoria is on a continuum with endogenous depression, yet the distinction between them is still useful with respect to using antidepressant medication or supportive counseling. Similarly, AS and autism may be on a continuum with respect to severity of symptoms and etiological mechanisms, yet there may be enough variation in their outcome that it is still clinically useful to parents and clinicians to distinguish the disorders. Indeed, in some ways, children with AS are *more* severe than those with autism as the discrepancy between their intellectual potential and their actual adaptation in terms of socialization and communication is so very marked; they look so "normal" but their behavior is so "odd." There is also some evidence that adolescents with AS have more symptoms of anxiety and depression than do children with autism (Szatmari et al., 1989), although the mechanism for this finding may be only that they have the ability to communicate their distress more readily. In this context, they have the more *severe* disorder because they have better communication skills. It all depends on what dimension of severity one is talking about.

Given the scanty empirical evidence, it is probably premature to lump or split AS and autism. An alternative to conceptualizing these as separate disorders or on a continuum is to think of different developmental pathways or trajectories. Although children with autism and AS may share an etiological process, there may be a difference in either their rate of development or the appearance and disappearance of certain PDD-like behaviors and symptoms. By definition, children with AS develop some functionally useful speech by 3 years of age. This may put them on a different developmental pathway or trajectory than other children with PDD, in particular, those with autism or atypical autism who develop speech after 3 years. Once children with AS are on this particular developmental pathway, they then develop at a certain rate associated with the bizarre preoccupations, fluent but pragmatically impaired speech, and certain types of social impairments that are characteristic of children with AS and differentiate them from the pathway of children with autism (Szatmari, Bryson, et al., 1998). Once a subgroup of children with autism develop language, albeit at a later age, they may then join the developmental pathway of the children with AS except that they would lag behind in terms of their development. Some children with autism who develop fluent language may eventually catch up to those with AS and might resemble them more and more with increasing age. This would account for the cross-sectional differences seen early on which might attenuate with increasing age (Eisenmajer et al., 1996). Autistic children who do not develop fluent language would then fall farther and farther behind. The diagnostic category (AS) becomes a marker of the onset of fluent language, which is in reality an important prognostic marker. Seen in this context, then, the difference between children with autism and AS may lie primarily in the domain of outcome and natural history. The size of the differences on outcome may vary with age so that, in turn, the clinical usefulness of the distinction may vary with age as well. In contrast to criteria for diagnostic validity, the *usefulness* of the clinical distinction is not an absolute characteristic of the classification system.

The issue here is that the distinctions we make between disorders must be, above all, clinically useful. If they are also valid (in the sense described by Rutter and others) it is an added bonus, but without clinical utility, clinical distinctions are meaningless. Clinical distinctions *may* not be valid yet are still useful. Two "disorders" may share a common etiology, may overlap with respect to symptomatology, and may overlap with respect to outcome, but it may still be clinically useful to planning treatment to make that clinical distinction, even if one cannot emphatically say that one disorder is the "same" or "different" than the other.

Essentially, AS is a type of pervasive developmental disorder and, with autism, shares impairments in social reciprocity, in communication, and in having a preference for repetitive, solitary activities. The main distinguishing characteristics have to do with the formal aspects of language development (i.e., when speech develops) and the level of expressive and receptive language abilities. If that distinguishing characteristic is associated with clinically significant differences in outcome and with differences in treatment needs, then the clinical distinction is useful. But this does not say that children with AS have normal language development. They patently do not. Their expressive and receptive language skills are often just below average, but, more important, they have significant and profound disturbances in prosody and the pragmatics of communication (Fine, Bartolucci, Szatmari, & Ginsberg, 1994) that is, in the use of intonation, in initiating and sustaining a conversation, and in the use of cohesive devices and other linguistic structures.

In fact, given our current level of understanding it may be more useful to differentiate AS from autism on the basis of clinical features that are associated with large differences on outcome. This would involve defining diagnostic criteria by model building not by hypothesis testing; first identify factors that account for the greatest variation in outcome and then translate these factors into diagnostic criteria. These factors will most certainly include some aspect of language development but may also involve other measures of age of onset or certain types of social impairment. Diagnostic criteria are not usually arrived at in this way, but for subtypes of disorder this may be the approach that maximizes the clinical utility of diagnostic differentiation. Ultimately, diagnostic criteria should be based on response to treatment, but this may not yet be possible for disorders such as PDD.

ASPERGER SYNDROME AND OTHER DISORDERS OF ATYPICAL DEVELOPMENT

One of the other controversies is the relationship between AS and disorders other than autism. Descriptions of unusual, socially impaired, and eccentric children have appeared in the literature for many years. Reading the clinical descriptions of children with atypical personality development (Rank, 1949), schizoid and schizotypal disorders (Wolff, 1995), semantic pragmatic disorders (Bishop, 1989), right-hemisphere syndromes (Weintraub & Mesulam, 1983), Nonverbal Learning Disabilities (Klin, Volkmar, Sparrow, Cicchetti, & Rourke, 1995), and, more recently, multiple complex developmental disorders and multiple developmental impairments (van der Gaag et al., 1995) makes one wonder whether the same children are being described under very different diagnostic labels.

Wing's concept of the autistic triad consisting of impairments in socialization, social communication, and social play has had an extraordinary impact on calling attention to this group of children (Wing & Gould, 1979). Autism as described originally by Kanner, and later more precisely by Rutter, can be easily identified in its extreme forms. We now know that these early definitions of autism were somewhat restrictive and more representative of younger and lower-functioning autistic children. As they develop, more able children with autism show a diminution in social isolation, an increasing competence in communication, and an intense interest in more abstract concepts rather than concrete objects. But there were also children who *never* showed the early "classic" manifestations of autism and who presented initially with those symptoms seen in older persons with autism. These milder manifestations of autism are just now being recognized.

It is also true that it is relatively easy to identify children with extreme forms of language disorder, schizophrenia, dyslexia, and so on. However, as these children were identified, clinicians have become aware that not all children fit the "classic" picture of these disorders either, just as not all children fit the description of classic autism. These children are in the borderland between the various developmental disorders and, to be sure, share many clinical features. Identified by language pathologists, they became children with semantic–pragmatic disorder; identified by neuropsychologists, they became children with Nonverbal Learning Disabilities; identified by psychiatrists, they were labeled as having schizoid or schizotypal personality disorder; identified by psychoanalysts, they were those with atypical development. On the one hand, this plethora of terms represents a diagnostician's nightmare, but on the other hand, it is true that the psychopathology of these children is being recognized and their disability made a legitimate object of scientific study. However, before these terms are adopted as clinically useful, it must be shown that the children differ from those with AS in meaningful ways, even if it is difficult to identify differences on etiology. When comparing two disorders, both of which are ill defined, it is difficult to interpret the findings, particularly if there are few differences between the groups. In comparing diagnostic categories, at least *one* should be well defined. The first priority in the field is to establish the boundaries (if any) between autism and AS and then decide whether useful distinctions exist between AS and these other disorders outside the PDD spectrum.

CONCLUSION

I have tried to make three points in this chapter:

1. Descriptions of odd and eccentric children have appeared in the literature well before Asperger published his paper.
2. It may be more helpful to assess the clinical usefulness of the diagnostic category instead of its validity.
3. An alternative to seeing autism and AS as the same or different is to think of different but potentially overlapping developmental trajectories.

What I have not discussed are the criteria for clinical usefulness; how does one decide whether the clinical distinctions between diagnoses are useful or not?

It is clear that in contrast to discussions of diagnostic validity, etiology is not as relevant to clinical utility as are assessments of natural history and response to treatment. To be useful, a diagnostic distinction should be associated with clinically important differences on outcome and treatment response. Even here criteria are needed in assessing whether a quantitative difference on outcome is of sufficient size to be useful. How big a difference in outcome in social competence between AS and autism should we accept as "big enough"? This is a determination that should include parents and individuals with autism and AS themselves, not only researchers. Measurement studies are needed to determine the "minimally significant difference" that is considered clinically important by parents and, in some circumstances, the patients themselves. This sort of analysis is frequently done in randomized control trials of medical treatments (Redelmeier, Guyatt, & Goldstein, 1996). Up to now, we have not included family members in the evaluation of our classification system. Yet they need to tell us whether the clinical distinctions we make are ultimately useful or not.

A classification system must do more good than harm to patients and families. How do parents of young children feel when their children receive a diagnosis of autism or AS? What are the barriers to service experienced by parents of both groups? Is it easier to get services with a diagnosis of autism or one of AS? How important is it to get the "right" diagnosis in terms of long-term outcome? All these questions are important and also need to be addressed in evaluating the recent classification of the PDDs and whether AS is a useful clinical diagnosis. These questions extend well beyond narrow notions of differences in etiology but are equally important and should not be ignored. Moreover, such questions may be easier to answer than those pertaining to etiology, which are the focus of current evaluations of diagnostic validity. A classification system cannot be useful unless it is valid, but it can be valid and quite useless. In discussions of AS, we need to move beyond narrow questions of "same" or "different." These mysterious children have been with us a long time and have puzzled both parents and clinicians. Sometimes the accumulation of knowledge is painfully slow, but it is gratifying that we know more today than we did even 5 years ago.

REFERENCES

American Psychiatric Association. (1987). *Diagnostic and statistical manual of mental disorders* (3rd ed., rev.). Washington: Author.

American Psychiatric Association. (1994). *Diagnostic and statistical manual of mental disorders* (4th ed.). Washington: Author.

Asperger H. (1944). Die "Autistischen Psychopathen" im Kindesalter. *Archiv für Psychiatrie und Nervenkrankheiten, 117,* 76–136.

Bernstein, G. A., Borchardt, C. M., & Perwien, A. R. (1996). Anxiety disorders in children and adolescents: A review of the past 10 years. *Journal of the American Academy of Child and Adolescent Psychiatry, 35,* 1110–1119.

Biederman, J., Faraone, S. V., Milberger, S., Jetton, J. G., Chen, L., Mick, E., Greene, R. W., & Russell, R. L. (1996). Is childhood oppositional defiant disorder a precursor to adolescent conduct disorder? Findings from a four-year follow-up study of children with ADHD. *Journal of the American Academy of Child and Adolescent Psychiatry, 35*(9), 1193–1204.

Bishop, D. (1989). Autism, Asperger's syndrome, and pragmatic semantic disorder: Where are the boundaries? *British Journal of Disorders of Communication, 24,* 107–121.

Blashfield, R. K., & Draguns, J. G. (1976). Evaluative criteria for psychiatric classification. *Journal of Abnormal Psychology, 85,* 140–150.

Burgoine, E., & Wing, L. (1983). Identical triplets with Asperger's syndrome. *British Journal of Psychiatry, 143,* 261.

Cantwell, D. P. (1982). Diagnostic validity of the hyperactive child (attention deficit disorder with hyperactivity) syndrome. *Psychiatric Developments, 1,* 277–300.

Cohen, D. J., Paul, R., & Volkmar, F. R. (1986). Issues in the classification of pervasive developmental disorders. Toward DSM-IV. *Journal of the American Academy of Child and Adolescent Psychiatry, 25,* 213.

Eisenmajer, R., Prior, M., Leekam, S., Wing, L., Gould, J., Welham, M., & Ong, B. (1996). Comparison of clinical symptoms in autism and Asperger's disorder. *Journal of the American Academy of Child and Adolescent Psychiatry, 35,* 1523–1531.

Fine, J., Bartolucci, G., Szatmari, P., & Ginsberg, G. (1994). Cohesive discourse in pervasive developmental disorders. *Journal of Autism and Developmental Disorders, 24*(3), 315–329.

Ghaziuddin, M., Tsai, L. Y., & Ghaziuddin, N. J. (1992). Brief report: A comparison of the diagnostic criteria for Asperger syndrome. *Journal of Autism and Developmental Disorders, 22,* 643–649.

Gillberg, C. (1989). Asperger syndrome in 23 Swedish children. *Developmental Medicine and Child Neurology, 81,* 520–531.

Henderson, D. K., & Gillespie, R. D. (1947). *A textbook of psychiatry for students and practitioners* (6th ed.). London: Oxford University Press.

Hinshaw, S. P. (1992). Externalizing behavior problems and academic underachievement in childhood and adolescence: Causal relationships and underlying mechanisms. *Psychological Bulletin, 111*(1), 127–155.

Kanner, L. (1943). Autistic disturbances of affective contact. *Nervous Child, 2*, 217–250.

Kendall, P. C., Flannery-Schroeder, E., Panichelli-Mindel, S. M., Sutham-Gerow, M., Hein, A., & Warman, M. (1997). Therapy for youths with anxiety disorder: A second randomized clinical trial. *Journal of Consulting and Clinical Psychology, 65*(3), 366–380.

Klein, R. G., Abikoff, H., Klass, E., Ganeles, D., Seese, L. M., & Pollack, S. (1997). Clinical efficacy of methylphenidate in conduct disorder with and without attention deficit hyperactivity disorder. *Archives of General Psychiatry, 54*(12), 1073–1080.

Klin, A., Volkmar, F. R., Sparrow, S. S., Cicchetti, D. V., & Rourke, B. P. (1995). Validity and neuropsychological characterization of Asperger syndrome. *Journal of Child Psychology and Psychiatry, 36*, 1127–1140.

Kretschmer, E. (1925). *Physique and character: An investigation of the nature of constitution and of the theory of temperament* (W. J. H. Sprott, Trans.). London: Kegan Paul, Trench & Trubner.

Mawson, D., Grounds, A., & Tantam, D. (1985). Violence and Asperger's syndrome: A case study. *British Journal of Psychiatry, 147*, 566–569.

Miller, J. N., & Ozonoff, S. (1997). Did Asperger's cases have Asperger disorder? A research note. *Journal of Child Psychology and Psychiatry, 38*(2), 247–251.

Ozonoff, S., Roger, S. J., & Pennington, B. F. (1991). Asperger's syndrome: Evidence of an empirical distinction from high-functioning autism. *Journal of Child Psychology and Psychiatry, 32*, 1107–1122.

Rank, B. (1949). Adaptation of the psychoanalytic technique for the treatment of young children with atypical development. *American Journal of Orthopsychiatry, 19*, 130–139.

Redelmeier, D. A., Guyatt, G. H., & Goldstein, R. S. (1996). Assessing the minimal important difference in symptoms: A comparison of two techniques. *Journal of Clinical Epidemiology, 49*, 1215–1219.

Robins, E., & Guze, S. B. (1970). Establishment of diagnostic validity in psychiatric illness: Its application to schizophrenia. *American Journal of Psychiatry, 126*, 983–987.

Rutter, M. (1978). Diagnostic validity in child psychiatry. *Advances in Biological Psychiatry, 2*, 2–22.

Schopler, E. (1996). Are autism or Asperger syndrome different labels or different disabilities? *Journal of Autism and Developmental Disorders, 26*, 109–110.

Skinner, H. A. (1981). Toward the integration of classification theory and methods. *Journal of Abnormal Psychology, 90*, 68–87.

Ssucharewa, G. E., & Wolff, S. (1996). The first account of the syndrome Asperger described? [Die schizoiden Psychopathien im Kindesalter]. *European Child and Adolescent Psychiatry, 5*(3), 119–132.

Szatmari, P. (1992). The validity of autistic spectrum disorders: A literature review. *Journal of Autism and Developmental Disorders, 22*, 583–600.

Szatmari, P. (1997). Pervasive developmental disorder not otherwise specified. In T. A. Widiger (Eds.), *DSM-IV source book* (Vol. 3, pp. 43–54). Washington, DC: American Psychiatric Press.

Szatmari, P., Archer, L., Fisman, S., Streiner, D. L., & Wilson, F. (1995). Asperger's syndrome and autism: Differences in behavior, cognition and adaptive functioning. *Journal of the American Academy of Child and Adolescent Psychiatry, 34*(12), 1662–1670.

Szatmari, P., Bartolucci, G., & Bremner, R. (1989). Asperger's syndrome and autism: Comparisons on early history and outcome. *Developmental Medicine and Child Neurology, 31,* 709–720.

Szatmari, P., Bryson, S. E., Streiner, D. L., Wilson, F. J., Archer, L., & Ryerse, C. (1998). *The two-year outcome of preschool children with autism and Asperger syndrome.* Submitted manuscript.

Szatmari, P., Jones, M. B., Zwaigenbaum, L., & MacLean, J. E. (1998). Genetics of autism: Overview and new directions [Special issue]. *Journal of Autism and Developmental Disorders, 28*(5), 363–380.

Tredgold, A. F. (1937). *Mental deficiency* (6th ed.). Baltimore, MD: Williams & Wilkins.

Van der Gaag, R. J., Buitelaar, J., Van den Ban, E., Bezemer, M., Njio, L., & Van Engeland, H. (1995). A controlled multivariate chart review of multiple complex developmental disorder. *Journal of the American Academy of Child and Adolescent Psychiatry, 34*(8), 1096–1106.

Van Krevelen, D. A. (1971). Early infantile autism and autistic psychopathy. *Journal of Autism and Child Schizophrenia, 1,* 82.

Weintraub, S., & Mesulam, M. M. (1983). Developmental learning disabilities of the right hemisphere: Emotional, interpersonal, and cognitive components. *Archives of Neurology, 40,* 463.

Wing, L., & Gould, J. (1979). Severe impairments of social interaction and associated abnormalities in children: Epidemiology and classification. *Journal of Autism and Developmental Disorders, 9,* 11–29.

Wing, L. (1981). Asperger's syndrome: A clinical account. *Psychological Medicine, 11*(1), 115–129.

Wolff, S. (1995). *Loners: The life path of unusual children.* London, Routledge.

World Health Organization. (1992). *The ICD-10 classification of mental and behavioural disorders—Clinical descriptions and diagnostic guidelines.* Geneva: World Health Organization.

15

Past and Future of Research on Asperger Syndrome

LORNA WING

Since the publication of my paper on Asperger's work (Wing, 1981) I have felt like Pandora after she opened the box. Fred Volkmar and Ami Klin note that more than 100 papers on Asperger syndrome, the term I used in my first paper and adopted in the tenth revision of *International Classification of Diseases* (ICD-10; World Health Organization, 1992), have now been published. In the United Kingdom, the use of the diagnosis in clinical practice seems to have increased at a remarkable rate. My original purpose, as someone just beginning to consider the nature of this condition, was to emphasize the strong possibility that the syndrome was part of the autistic spectrum and that there were no clear boundaries separating it from other autistic disorders. However, since then, various workers have tended to the belief that Asperger syndrome and autism are different conditions—quite the opposite of my intention. Two misunderstandings have contributed to this. First, Asperger did emphasize the special skills of the children he described, but he wrote, in his original long paper (Asperger, 1944/1991) that the "autistic personality . . . also occurs in the less able, even in children with severe mental retardation" (pp. 58–59). Later in the paper he notes a "smooth transition . . . to those mentally retarded people who show highly stereotyped automaton-like behaviour" (p. 75). He included, in this description, calendar calculators and those showing feats of rote memory, such as knowing all the tram-lines in Vienna. As Uta Frith (1991) remarked in a footnote to her translation, "this important insight . . . has often been overlooked, even by Asperger himself in his later papers" (p. 59). It was, I must confess, overlooked by myself in my 1981 paper but corrected in later publications (Wing, 1996, 1998). Second, Asperger wrote that parents did not recognize their child's problems until the child was 3 years old or older; sometimes not until the child started school. However he observed in his first paper that the characteristic features are found from the second year of life. Uta Frith, in her footnote, points out that "this statement is so well buried in the text that it has been overlooked. Instead, the belief has persisted that Asperger's cases show normal development, especially in language, up to three years or later" (p. 67).

Eric Schopler (1998), who was one of the workers who recognized the overlap of Asperger syndrome and autism, was critical of the publicity given to Asperger's work in my paper and of the choice of the term "syndrome." He wrote, "The premature use of the Asperger syndrome label serves as a seriously flawed model for how psychiatric diagnostic categories are formed. It should have been left in the investigative state until a valid sub-group had been established. It appears to me that premature use of the Asperger syndrome label has had far more negative consequences than positive, slowing down what progress in understanding and treatment of autism has been accomplished to date" (p. 397). It is perhaps a little difficult to know how Asperger's ideas could have been put into "the investigative state" until papers discussing its nature had been published. In any case, the model Schopler criticizes is more or less how all diagnostic concepts in psychiatry have evolved.

I agree with the points made by Schopler concerning the relationship of Asperger syndrome and high-functioning autism. On the other hand, in our clinical work, my colleagues and I see many children and adolescents such as the ones Asperger described. Their parents will not consider a diagnosis of autism, but what they have heard about Asperger syndrome strikes a chord with them. We also see a small but steady flow of adults who come to seek advice for themselves because something they have read or heard makes them think they have Asperger syndrome. When the diagnosis is confirmed and the implications, positive as well as negative, are discussed, in almost all cases the individual concerned is immensely relieved to have an explanation of why he (or occasionally she) has felt different from others all his life. They are mostly willing to accept the relationship to autism when this is put into context. Sometimes we have seen, together with their wives, husbands wanting a diagnosis for themselves, and both have felt happier and closer to each other once they know the reasons for their past problems. Occasionally, we are approached by individuals with university degrees, who have reached high levels in their chosen professions. They seek help because they have become alarmed when an upward move away from paperwork to tasks demanding social interaction has been suggested. This has brought them face-to-face with their pattern of skills and limitations, and in their search for self-understanding, they have come across the concept of Asperger syndrome. They benefit from a clear diagnosis and open discussion. Some ask for a letter to show their employers to explain why they have decided to refuse what looks like a highly desirable promotion, and they have been able to continue in the type of work that suits them best. This is one of the most satisfying aspects of our clinical work. Such individuals would never have asked for a referral if the only label available had been autism as it is usually described. Awareness of Asperger's perceptive ideas on management and education has led to increasing understanding of the needs of children and adults with average or high cognitive ability who have autistic disorders. This is the case whether they can be classified as Asperger syndrome or as high-functioning autism on any of the various criteria available. Whatever the academic pros and cons, it is the consequences for the clinical field that have justified bringing Asperger's work into focus. On this point, I strongly disagree with Schopler. It may be that experience in the United Kingdom is very different from that in the United States, but this seems rather unlikely. However, this does *not* imply that autism and Asperger syndrome can be neatly separated from each other.

HISTORY

The history of autistic spectrum disorders is, like most things in life, a muddled series of chance events. As noted by Peter Szatmari (Chapter 14, this volume), clinicians had known children with social and communication disorders and odd behavior for many years before Kanner's and Asperger's descriptions were published. In the 19th century, such children were described as "insane."

From the beginning of the 20th century, many investigators have tried to discern specific syndromes among the large pool of individuals who have in common impairments of social interaction and social communication skills. Szatmari also points out that each professional started from the background of his or her particular interest and type of clinical practice. Each tended to pick certain features from the complex clinical picture on which to base his or her idea of a syndrome.

Robinson and Vitale (1954) described children with "circumscribed interests." Margaret Mahler (1952), as a psychoanalyst, worked with children who showed what she called "empty clinging." Heller (see Hulse, 1954) was concerned with children who regressed after a period of apparently normal development. De Sanctis (1908) and Earl (1943) described individuals with catatonic behavior. Leo Kanner (1943, 1973), in his clinical practice as a child psychiatrist, saw young children who were aloof and indifferent to people and who had elaborate repetitive routines. Hans Asperger, as a pediatrician with a special interest in remedial education, described children whose odd social interaction and communication meant that they had problems with education and could not fit into the social groups of their peers. Elizabeth Newson (1983), an educational psychologist, has suggested that children with "pathological demand avoidance" should be grouped together as their pattern of behavior and their educational needs differ in many ways from those of children with more typical autistic spectrum disorders. Dorothy Bishop, from the perspective of her research in language development, describes in Chapter 9 (this volume) children with "semantic–pragmatic disorder." Sula Wolff (1995, Chapter 10, this volume) discusses children with "schizoid personality disorder of childhood" who have high levels of ability and whose clinical picture overlaps with that of the most able children described by Asperger. Bryon Rourke, Katherine Tsatsanis, and colleagues (Rourke, 1982, 1989; Chapter 8, this volume) have studied children with a pattern of nonverbal learning difficulties and social impairment that they believe indicates right-hemisphere dysfunction. Gillberg and his colleagues (Gillberg, 1992; Ehlers & Gillberg, 1993; Gillberg & Gillberg, 1989) described a somewhat similar group of children with deficits in attention, motor control, and perception (the "DAMP" syndrome) who had originally been given the label of "minimal brain dysfunction" (MBD). Both Rourke and Gillberg recognize the considerable overlap of their respective groups with Asperger syndrome. All of these workers were, so to speak, fishing in the same pool of social and communication disorders, but, because of their specific foci of interest, their catches were different in some ways though overlapping in others.

THE RELATIONSHIP OF ASPERGER SYNDROME AND AUTISM

It is, of course, possible that any one of these professionals might, by chance, have identified a specific syndrome unrelated to the others. It is equally, or perhaps more, likely that none of them did. Much attention has been given to the similarities and differences between Asperger syndrome and autism. Peter Szatmari asks the important question, What is meant by the statement that "disorders are different"? I (Wing, 1998) listed the various levels at which differences could in theory be defined, ranging from the most fundamental level of original aetiology, via neuropathology and neuropsychology, to overt behavior and response to treatment. The conclusion was that there were no consistent and reproducible differences between Asperger syndrome and autism at any of these levels, however each was defined, apart from those that were the direct consequences of the criteria used. For example, Sally Ozonoff and Elizabeth McMahon Griffith (Chapter 2, this volume) describe the inconsistent results of published research in neuropsychology. They discuss the difficulties of separating the effects of cognitive and language ability when comparing groups classified as having Asperger syndrome or autism.

Confusion in Diagnostic Criteria

The difficulty of defining criteria for diagnosis is a recurring theme throughout the volume. Various contributors note that the use of different diagnostic systems leads to lack of comparability among studies and is a major source of confusion in interpretation of the research that has been done. Some suggest that the solution is the adoption of a standard set of criteria. Asperger (1944) did not specify diagnostic criteria for his group of children, so, as discussed by Fred Volkmar and Ami Klin, different authors have made different proposals. Although various neurological and psychological abnormalities have been reported, the findings tend to be inconsistent and no definitive relationships with diagnostic subgroups have been established. In consequence, the criteria for autistic spectrum disorders have to be in terms of behavioral features, which are hard to operationalize. Furthermore, there are a large number of behavioral features making up the clinical pictures, and each of these can be manifested in a wide range of ways. Apart from the social and communication impairments that are accepted as the core of the spectrum, there is no way of knowing which of the other features should be included among the essential criteria. For example, should one of the criteria be motor coordination problems, and, if so, what kind? Should odd reactions to sensory input be included, and, if so, what modalities? How important are special skills, special interests, and repetitive routines? Should motor stereotypies be included, and, if so, which ones? In the end, the choice must be arbitrary but with the hope that independent measures will justify the selection. To date, none of the suggested definitions has been independently validated.

The criteria according to ICD-10 and *Diagnostic and Statistical Manual of Mental Disorders*, fourth edition (DSM-IV; American Psychiatric Association, 1994) for the subgrouping of the so-called pervasive developmental disorders are particularly unsatisfactory. Peter Szatmari (Chapter 14, this volume) gives cogent reasons why the criteria for Asperger syndrome in these systems are unworkable. Rebecca Landa (Chapter 4, this volume) points out the confusion resulting from the criteria referring to language in autism and Asperger syndrome, which are phrased in ways that are not mutually exclusive. For example, a child may have words by 2 years and phrase speech by 3 (Asperger syndrome) but still fit the criterion of abnormal functioning in social communication before 3 years (autism). Eisenmajer et al. (1996) found that 22 clinicians whose diagnostic practices were studied evidently based their diagnoses of Asperger syndrome on Asperger's descriptions of current behavior rather than the early history of speech development. The children they diagnosed fulfilled criteria for autism but were diagnosed as Asperger syndrome.

Among the children and adults referred to the Elliot House diagnostic and assessment center, we have seen many individuals who resembled Asperger's descriptions, some of whom had no delay in speech development. But hardly any meet the other ICD-10 and DSM-IV developmental criteria for this syndrome, namely, normal development of self-care, adaptive skills, and curiosity before 3 years of age (Leekam, Libby, Wing, Gould, & Gillberg, in press). Motivation to acquire and use self-care and adaptive skills is conspicuous by its absence in children with autistic spectrum disorders, however high their level of cognitive ability. This is compounded in some by motor clumsiness. These difficulties contribute to the failure to achieve independence in adult life even in some individuals who have university degrees.

The closely similar ICD-10 and DSM-IV criteria have moved a long way from Asperger's own descriptions. This would not matter if (1) these criteria were easy to apply in clinical practice, (2) they had some external validity, and (3) they were given some name other than Asperger syndrome. Unfortunately, they do not meet any of these requirements. Ami Klin, Fred Volkmar, and Sara Sparrow, in their Introduction to this volume, point out, rightly, that answers to current problems of classification cannot be found by returning to Kanner's and Asperger's original papers. However, if new diagnostic constructs are suggested and evaluated, they should be given new names. A great deal of the present confusion arises from the use of the original eponymous labels for constructs that differ in breadth and/or content. Thus, at least some of the rise in reported prevalence rates of "autism" can be attributed to the fact that the earliest studies used Kanner's original criteria whereas later studies used other criteria that are much wider, while still referring to "autism" as if all the criteria were the same (Wing, 1993).

Evidence from Clinical Case Studies

Over the last 10 years, my colleagues and I at the Elliot House diagnostic center have seen nearly 700 children and adults with autistic spectrum disorders. We have collected information on family background; perinatal history; developmental history from infancy covering self-care and other practical skills, schoolwork, impairments of social interaction, communication and imagination, and motor coordination; responses to sensory stimuli; and stereotypies and repetitive routines and, for adolescents and adults, psychiatric history and details of any forensic problems. To do this we have used current and previous versions of the Diagnostic Interview for Social and Communication Disorders (DISCO), which is a semistructured interview designed to collect information in a systematic form. The information can be coded for computer analysis. The current version of the DISCO is being used in a series of studies and has been found to have high interrater agreement (work to be published). From this clinical and research experience, a number of conclusions have been drawn, three of which are relevant to this discussion. First, any combination of clinical features can occur although some patterns are more common than others. There are certain constraints, such as the impossibility of detecting pronoun reversal in a child who has no speech, but otherwise no combination is impossible. Any of the features described by Kanner (1943, 1973) can occur in individuals who fit Asperger's description and vice versa. Second, the clinical picture changes with increasing age. The degree of change varies greatly among individuals but change does occur and affects the overall clinical picture. For example, a child can begin life with typical Kanner's syndrome and grow into the pattern described by Asperger. Eisenmajer et al. (1998) found that, in high-functioning children with autistic spectrum disorders, language delay was associated with more severe autistic symptoms in their early years. However, by the time they were approaching puberty, age of language onset no longer predicted the way autistic symptoms were manifested, apart from an association between language delay and lack of looking and smiling when socially approached. Third, different types of autistic spectrum disorders can be found within one extended family. If two or more siblings are affected, the details of their clinical pictures may be very different (Bowman, 1988). Such variation can be found even among monozygotic twins or triplets (Burgoine & Wing, 1983).

FUTURE DIRECTIONS FOR RESEARCH

The conclusion from the previous discussion must be that there is little point in continuing to pursue the question whether Asperger syndrome and autism are the same or different disorders.

Classification

The most reasonable approach to classification is to recognize that although there may be sub-groups that are specific and separate at some level of discourse, at present these have not been identified. Any psychological function can be disordered in its development, either alone or in combination with others. Social impairment is one among many such problems, but it has received particular attention and is the core feature of the autistic spectrum disorders whatever diagnostic criteria are used. Any of the other specific developmental disorders (e.g., reading problems, poor motor coordination, expressive speech problems, and visuospatial difficulties) could also be selected as the core feature of a wide group of disorders. Dorothy Bishop's selection of semantic–pragmatic disorder in Chapter 9 is an example. Whatever disability is chosen as the core, the groups thus formed would overlap to varying extents with all the others. Doubtless there are specific conditions to be found among the groups, but the available evidence suggests that the basic causes and neuropathologies do not map onto the clinical features in any clear way (Rapin, 1994).

Why select for special attention the group of those with social impairment? The reason is that this type of developmental disorder results in such severe, strange, and striking effects on behavior, separating individuals with the disorder from their social community. Such difficulties occur even in those with good cognitive ability, as graphically described by Digby Tantam (Chapter 13, this volume).

In our practice at Elliot House, we have found that the best way to record and convey basic information concerning individuals in the group of those with social impairment is to rate them on three separate dimensions. The first is the quality of social interaction. Wing and Gould (1979) suggested the following subtypes: "aloof and indifferent to others," "passive acceptance of social approaches," and "active but odd, inappropriate approaches to others." Wing (1988) added a fourth subgroup comprising high-functioning individuals who have acquired social rules through intellectual learning rather than through interaction and who apply the rules rigidly (p. 93). The second dimension is the level of ability in verbal skills, and the third is the level of nonverbal and practical skills. This basic descriptive classification has to be supplemented with other information concerning, for example, motor, sensory, emotional, and behavioral problems. Known causes, such as Retts syndrome or tuberose sclerosis, would be recorded separately, as would apparent age of onset. (The real age of onset tends to be difficult or impossible to ascertain.) This is far more helpful for practical purposes than any of the available systems of classification. The clinical picture changes with age, so the classification on the different dimensions may also have to change. This need to change can be avoided only if the classification is made to depend on behavior in, for example, the preschool years. This may be shown to have relevance for some kinds of research but is no use for planning programmes and services for older children and adults.

The problem with adopting this kind of practical, multidimensional approach to subgrouping is that it does not fit into the conventional pattern used for the classification of psychiatric disorders in the ICD and DSM systems. These classification systems are based on the "specific disease" type of medical model, which fits so well the conditions due to bacteria and viruses. However, there are other medical models that might fit developmental disorders better, such as that used for injuries and accidents, which can result in any combination of types and sites of lesions.

Causes and Pathology

From the point of view of research into causes and pathology, in-depth examination of specific aspects of autistic spectrum disorders is likely to be more productive than pursuing differences between autism and Asperger syndrome. For example, in Chapter 3 (this volume) on motor functioning, Isabel Smith argues for a more analytical approach in order to identify the mechanisms underlying observable performance. Experience at Elliot House has shown the wide variation in types and severity of motor problems, ranging from marked clumsiness in all motor tasks to poor coordination observable only when the individual tries to take part in team games. Detailed analysis of this feature would include development of tests and methods of observation, subtyping, correlation with other features found in autistic spectrum disorders, examination of the various physical and psychological functions involved in motor performance, and developmental history and course over time. Work of this kind would be helpful in identifying methods of remediation or compensation as well as increasing understanding of the underlying pathology.

The communication and language impairments found in the autistic spectrum disorders are of particular interest. Rebecca Landa (Chapter 4, this volume on social language) and Dorothy Bishop (Chapter 9, this volume, on semantic–pragmatic disorder) discuss an important aspect of the impairments found in autistic spectrum disorders and related conditions. Bishop explores the question whether all children with semantic–pragmatic disorder should be classified as having an autistic spectrum disorder. She argues that in some children with semantic–pragmatic problems, the clinical picture lies outside though close to the boundaries of autistic conditions. It would be helpful to extend the research on these children by examining their developmental history from infancy, covering all the areas that are relevant for the autistic spectrum and other communication disorders, and to follow them up into adolescence and adult life. The early developmental history would help to clarify the relationship with autistic spectrum disorders. However, the true depth of social impairment is often not revealed until an individual is exposed to the demands of adulthood. It is from the perspective of adult life that it is possible to see what types of education and support during childhood would have been helpful as preparation for the postschool years.

Interest in social impairment has led to the development of the theory-of-mind hypothesis (Baron-Cohen, 1988). In their chapter, Ami Klin, Robert Schultz and Donald Cohen (in press) highlighted a fundamental question concerning the nature of the theory-of-mind deficit. Does understanding that others have thoughts and feelings develop in the first few years of life on the basis of growing perceptual and cognitive skills, or is there a built-in preference for, and expectations associated with, people rather than things, present from birth or soon after? Elucidation of the mechanisms involved would have important theoretical and practical implications.

It would be of great interest and value to study the development, or lack thereof, of social responses in children with autistic disorders in the first days or weeks of life. The problem with work of this kind is that the diagnosis of such conditions cannot be made at birth, and the comparatively low prevalence would necessitate extremely large numbers of subjects. One method of increasing the chances of finding sufficient numbers of babies likely to develop an autistic spectrum disorder, used by Baron-Cohen, Allen, and Gillberg (1992), is to include infant siblings of children known to be affected. Even using this method, such a study would be a large and difficult undertaking, but if it yielded significant results, it could be of considerable value for early diagnosis and early intervention. The detection of abnormalities so early in life might also give clues to the underlying neuropathology.

Francesca Happé, Uta Frith, and their colleagues (Happé et al, 1996) are studying the areas of the medial prefrontal cortex of the brain that are active when an individual is trying to solve problems requiring the use of theory of mind. The adults taking part are those with autistic spectrum disorders who are high functioning, regardless of their ICD-10 or DSM-IV subgroups (Uta Frith, 1999, personal communication). Differences from normal volunteers have been found. The results can be linked with the theory of "weak central coherence" in autistic disorders (Frith, 1989; Frith & Happé, 1994). This is the hypothesis that individuals with autistic disorders fail to integrate information into context, leading to the inability to extract the higher-level meaning. The inability to plan and to predict the consequences of actions that is most easily observed in more able people with autistic spectrum disorders also supports the hypothesis that some regions of the prefrontal cortex are involved, as discussed by Robert Schultz, Lizabeth Romansky, and Katherine Tsatsanis (Chapter 6, this volume; Klin et al., in press).

These authors' research into the functions of the amygdala and its role in attaching emotion to environmental stimuli appears to be highly relevant to all autistic disorders, not just Asperger syndrome. People with these disorders experience intense, raw emotions of fear, rage, and, sometimes, ecstasy. The problem is that these responses tend not to be aroused by the social and personal stimuli that have emotional meaning for most human beings. Instead, individuals with autistic disorders respond with anxiety, anger, or pleasure to objects or events that are special to them but may seem irrelevant to others. They may be terrified of a pair of yellow curtains, infuriated if a visitor does not arrive at the exact second they were expected, or transported with delight while staring at electricity pylons. Finding the neural basis of these idiosyncratic responses would add much to our understanding of autistic disorders.

The abnormalities of responses to sensory stimuli, particularly sound and touch, are another aspect of autistic spectrum disorders that might yield interesting findings if examined in depth.

One theme developed by several contributors to this volume, with which I an in complete agreement, is the importance of recognizing that just as there are no clear borderlines between subgroups within the autistic spectrum, there are also no clear boundaries with the conditions around the fringes of the spectrum. Fred Volkmar and Ami Klin warn against simplistic concepts of Asperger syndrome versus autism. They emphasize the multidimensional nature of the relationships and they advocate the inclusion, in research on the autistic spectrum, of other disorders that share some of the features. Susan Folstein and Susan Santangelo recommend this wide approach in relation to genetic studies, as does Dorothy Bishop in relation to semantic pragmatic language disorder. Gillberg (1992) developed the hypothesis that autistic disorders were part of a much wider class of disorders of empathy.

It should be emphasized that, for research, it is essential to give detailed information concerning the subjects taking part, so that comparisons with the results of other studies are possible. This can be done without having to select subjects based on ICD-10 or DSM-IV criteria.

This list of possible topics for research is by no means exhaustive. It is intended as an illustration of what might be fruitful areas for investigation.

EDUCATION AND TREATMENT OF CHILDREN

An important part of our work at Eliot House is to advise on educational needs and placements. We have found that the ICD-10 and DSM-IV subgroups are of no use for planning education, behavior management, occupation, leisure activities, or designing services. A flexible approach, in which different ways of subgrouping are used depending on the purpose of the exercise, is much more appropriate. For example, for education and prognosis in adult life, grouping on the three dimensions of quality of social interaction and verbal and nonverbal ability, as described previously, is particularly relevant. In the United Kingdom, many teachers and caregivers have found this descriptive classification helpful in working with individuals with autistic spectrum disorders.

The aims of educational research include finding useful methods of assessment and defining the principles underlying specialized methods of education and how these can be adapted to individual needs. Ami Klin and Fred Volkmar raise the question of the best type of school for children with Asperger syndrome. I prefer to rephrase this question to ask about education for children with autistic spectrum disorders who have average or high levels of cognitive ability, as long experience has shown that their educational needs are not related to the subgroup diagnosis they are given. In the United Kingdom there is one school that specializes in educating children of this kind. A few other schools have a particular interest in and experience with such children. However, many of the children are placed in mainstream schools with or without special support. This sometimes works well but can be a disaster, especially if no diagnosis has been made, the staff have no experience with autistic spectrum disorders, and the child is teased and bullied by his or her peers. Detailed studies are needed to show the effects of different educational placements and different educational and environmental approaches, such as those outlined by Ami Klin and Fred Volkmar (Chapter 12, this volume) and Wing (1996). At present there is no shortage of firmly held beliefs but a serious dearth of established facts.

SERVICES FOR ADULTS

On leaving school, some high-functioning adults live at home with their parents doing nothing, some are found places in residential care homes that may or may not be specialized, and some obtain paid employment, with or without the help of a supported employment scheme. Research into the factors leading to different outcomes in adult life, including the effects of the methods of helping described by Digby Tantam (Chapter 13, this volume), would be of practical value. Variables that markedly affect the quality of life of the adults are the level of insight into their problems, the degree to which they want to make social relationships, and how far they feel they have succeeded in doing so. Wanting a partner of the opposite sex adds special poignancy to the situation of those who try to interact and fail. Ways of helping individuals to come to terms with loneliness and frustration pose particular problems for those undertaking counseling of high-functioning adults with autistic spectrum disorders.

PSYCHIATRIC CONDITIONS

As emphasized by Tantam, any kind of psychiatric condition can complicate autistic spectrum disorders. These are easier to diagnose in high-functioning adults with enough speech to describe their symptoms. Schizophrenia is very rare but can occur. Depression is particularly common and suicide rates are higher than would be expected for the general population. As pointed out by Andres Martin, David Patzer, and Fred Volkmar (Chapter 7, this volume), it is often not clear whether these psychiatric conditions are an expression of the disorder or represent comorbidity.

One particular complication of autistic spectrum disorders is not mentioned anywhere in this book. That is the appearance of severe catatonic and Parkinsonian features. Many of the features of autistic spectrum disorders overlap with those of catatonia and Parkinsonism. In a small minority of individuals, severe catatonic slowness and episodes of "freezing" develop in adolescence or early adult life. In a recent study of referrals to Elliot House who had autistic spectrum disorders, it was found that 17% of all those age 15 and over when seen had catatonic and Parkinsonian features of sufficient degree to severely limit their mobility, use of speech, and carrying out of daily activities. Because of referral bias, it is likely that this is an overestimate of the prevalence, but there is no doubt that catatonia does occur in some individuals with autistic spectrum disorders and is a serious problem for them and their caregivers. It appears that the development of catatonia is sometimes related to stresses arising from inappropriate methods of care and management. It was somewhat more common in those with mild or severe mental retardation but did occur in some who were high functioning. Those affected were significantly more likely to have been passive in social interaction than a comparison group, but otherwise no clues were found to explain why a minority reacted to adverse conditions in this particular way. No medical treatment was found to help those seen at Elliot House, though Realmuto and August (1991) reported that antidepressive medication was effective in two individuals with autism and catatonia. A structured, organized environment designed for people with autistic spectrum disorders and gentle prompting to take part in a program of appropriate activities has been found to reduce the severity of the condition, or at least to prevent further deterioration (Shah & Wing, 1999).

Research is needed on the epidemiology of psychiatric conditions occurring with autistic spectrum disorders, the factors that are associated with their onset and those affecting prognosis, and the effectiveness of different methods of treatment. The occurrence of severe catatonic and Parkinsonian features, even though they affect only a small minority, is of particular interest because of the implications for the neuropathology of both conditions (Wing & Shah, 1999).

CONTRIBUTIONS OF PARENTS AND INDIVIDUALS WITH AUTISTIC SPECTRUM DISORDERS

Books and articles by parents, including those in this volume, and by individuals with autistic spectrum disorders, are growing in number. They are an invaluable source of information and insight into the world of autism for research workers, educators, caregivers, and parents. Readers who have no personal experience of autism find the personal accounts fascinating and are more likely to be understanding and tolerant if they encounter odd autistic behavior. The writings are also evidence of the determination and courage with which the individuals concerned cope with loneliness and adversity.

FINAL THOUGHTS

To return to the subject of my introduction to this chapter, it is perhaps ironic that, having been responsible for using the term "Asperger syndrome" in my 1981 paper, I am now arguing strongly against its existence as a separate entity. The reason for its adoption in my first paper on the subject was to avoid the label of "autistic psychopathy" used by Asperger when writing in German. In his language, psychopathy refers to personality disorder, but in English it is often used as synonymous with antisocial psychopathy. I thought that "Asperger syndrome" was a neutral term that would suffice for the discussion but carried no particular implications for the nature of the pattern of behavior. Also, the eponym acknowledged Asperger's contribution to the understanding of the group of children he described. The trouble is that verbal labels have a strange tendency to take on an existence of their own, whatever the intentions of their coiner. If I were starting all over again, knowing what I now know, would I have used this label? Perhaps not. But it has served the purpose of widening prevailing concepts of autistic spectrum disorders. Would this have happened if I had referred to high-functioning autism, autism with average or high cognitive ability, or something similar? Probably not, but who knows? Should the term "Asperger syndrome" now be dropped completely? I do not know, because it still has its uses in clinical work. One thing is certain—when you open Pandora's box, there is no way of predicting the consequences.

REFERENCES

American Psychiatric Association. (1994). *Diagnostic and statistical manual of mental disorders* (4th ed.). Washington, DC: Author.

Asperger, H. (1991). "Autistic psychopathy" in childhood (U. Frith, Trans. and Annot.). In U. Frith (Ed.), *Autism and Asperger syndrome* (pp. 37–92). Cambridge: Cambridge University Press. (Original work published 1944)

Baron-Cohen, S. (1988). The autistic child's theory of mind. A case of specific developmental delay. *Journal of Child Psychology and Psychiatry, 30,* 285–297.

Baron Cohen, S., Allen, J., & Gillberg, C. (1992). Can autism be detected at 18 months? The needle, the haystack and the CHAT. *British Journal of Psychiatry, 161,* 839–843.

Bowman, E. P. (1988) Asperger syndrome and autism: The case for a connection. *British Journal of Psychiatry, 152,* 377–382.

Burgoine, E., & Wing, L. (1983). Identical triplets with Asperger syndrome. *British Journal of Psychiatry, 143,* 261–265.

De Sanctis, S. (1908). Dementia praecocissima catatonica oder katatonie des fruheren kindersalters? *Folia Neurobiologica, 2,* 9–12.

Earl, C. J. C. (1943). The primitive catatonic psychosis of idiocy. *British Journal of Medical Psychology, 14,* 230–253.

Ehlers, S., & Gillberg, C. (1993). The epidemiology of Asperger syndrome. A total population study. *Journal of Child Psychology and Psychiatry, 34,* 1327–1350.

Eisenmajer, R., Prior, M., Leekam, S., Wing, L., Gould, J., Welham, M., & Ong, B. (1996). Comparison of clinical symptoms in autism and Asperger's disorder. *Journal of the American Academy of Child and Adolescent Psychiatry, 35,* 1523–1531.

Eisenmajer, R., Prior, M., Leekam, S., Wing, L., Ong, B., Gould, J., & Welham, M. (1998). Delayed language onset as a predictor of clinical symptoms in pervasive developmental disorders. *Journal of Autism and Developmental Disorders, 28,* 27–534.

Frith, U. (1989). *Autism: Explaining the enigma.* Oxford: Blackwell.

Frith, U. (Ed.). (1991). *Autism and Asperger syndrome.* Cambridge: Cambridge University Press.

Frith, U., & Happé, F. (1994). Autism: Beyond "theory of mind." *Cognition, 50,* 115–132.

Gillberg, C. (1992). The Emmanuel Miller Memorial lecture 1991. Autism and autistic-like conditions: Subclasses among disorders of empathy. *Journal of Child Psychology and Psychiatry, 33,* 813–842.

Gillberg, I. C., & Gillberg, C. (1989). Asperger syndrome: Some epidemiological considerations. *Journal of Child Psychology and Psychiatry, 30,* 631–638.

Happé, F., Ehlers, S., Fletcher, P., Frith, U., Johansson, M., Gillberg, C., Dolan, R., Frackowiak, R., & Frith, C. (1996). "Theory of mind" in the brain. Evidence from a PET scan study of Asperger syndrome. *Clinical Neuroscience and Neuropathology, 8,* 197–201.

Hulse, W. C. (1954). Dementia infantilis. *Journal of Nervous and Mental Diseases, 119,* 471–477.

Kanner, L. (1943). Autistic disturbances of affective contact. *Nervous Child, 2,* 217–250.

Kanner, L. (1973). *Childhood psychosis: Initial studies and new insights.* Washington, DC: V. H. Winston & Sons.

Klin, A., Schultz, R., & Cohen, D. J. (in press). The need for a theory of theory of the mind in action: Developmental and neurofunctional perspectives on social cognition. In S. Baron-Cohen, H. Tager-Flusberg, & D. J. Cohen (Eds.), *Understanding other minds: Perspectives from autism and developmental cognitive neuroscience* (2nd ed.). Oxford: Oxford University Press.

Leekam, S. R., Libby, S., Wing, L., Gould, J., & Gillberg, C. (in press). Comparison of ICD-10 and Gilberg's criteria for Asperger syndrome. *Autism.*

Mahler, M. S. (1952). On child psychoses and schizophrenia: Autistic and symbiotic infantile psychoses. *Psychoanalytic Study of the Child, 7,* 286–305.

Newson, E. (1983). Pathological demand-avoidance syndrome. *Communication, 17,* 3–8.

Rapin, I. (1994). Introduction and overview. In M. L. Bauman & T. L. Kemper (Eds.), *The neurobiology of autism* (pp. 1–17). Baltimore: Johns Hopkins University Press.

Realmuto, G. M., & August, G. J. (1991). Catatonia in autistic disorder: A sign of comorbidity or variable expression? *Journal of Autism and Developmental Disorders, 21,* 517–528.

Robinson, J. F., & Vitale, L. J. (1954). Children with circumscribed interests. *American Journal of Orthopsychiatry, 24,* 755–764.

Rourke, B. P. (1982). Central processing deficiencies in children: Towards a developmental neuropsychological model. *Journal of Clinical Neuropsychology, 4,* 1–18.

Rourke, B. P. (1989). *Nonverbal Learning Disabilities: The syndrome and the model.* New York: Guilford Press.

Schopler, E. (1998). Premature popularization of Asperger syndrome. In E. Schopler & G. M. Mesibov (Eds.), *Asperger syndrome or high-functioning autism?* (pp. 385–399). New York: Plenum.

Shah, A., & Wing, L. (1999). *Understanding and managing catatonia in autism: A clinical perspective.* Manuscript submitted for publication.

Wing, L. (1981). Asperger's syndrome: A clinical account. *Psychological Medicine, 11,* 115–129.

Wing, L. (1988). The continuum of autistic characteristics. In E. Schopler & G. Mesibov (Eds.), *Diagnosis and assessment in autism* (pp. 91–110). New York: Plenum.

Wing, L. (1993). The definition and prevalence of autism: A review. *European Child and Adolescent Psychiatry, 2,* 61–74.

Wing, L. (1996). *The autistic spectrum: A guide for parents and professionals.* London: Constable.

Wing, L. (1998). The history of Asperger syndrome In S. Schopler, G. M. Mesibov, & L. J. Kunce (Eds.), *Asperger syndrome or high functioning autism?* (pp. 11–28). New York: Plenum.

Wing, L., & Gould, J. (1979). Severe impairments of social interaction and associated abnormalities in children: Epidemiology and classification. *Journal of Autism and Developmental Disorders, 9,* 11–29.

Wing, L., & Shah, A. (1999). *Catatonia in autistic spectrum disorders.* Manuscript submitted for publication

Wolff, S. (1995). *Loners: The life path of unusual children.* London: Routledge.

World Health Organization. (1992). *International classification of diseases: Tenth revision.* Chapter V. Mental and behavioral disorders (including disorders of psychological development). Diagnostic criteria for research. Geneva: Author.

16

Parent Essays
Introduction

Having a child with disabilities is associated with long-term challenges that are at times exasperating, at times devastating. We all know that, but parents know best. However, this is only part of the story. The four accounts provided by parents that follow expand on this theme but in colors that are at once a testimony to parents' endurance and resourcefulness and to their rejoicing in and celebration of their children's uniqueness and special victories. These accounts were beautifully composed, although the writing process itself was quick flowing, almost cathartic: a ready-made, unfolding story brewing in the minds of the parents for years and now gently told with the determination of the survivor and conqueror. The accounts bring the children alive, with their peculiarities and rigidities, but also with their endearing moments, their downright, striking successes, and most of all with boundless love. We find no better antidote to the fallacious tendency of some to equate children with their disabilities than to present the singularity of each of these children's life adventure.

Walter

JEANNE WALLACE

With all my efforts, I didn't think I would be experiencing yet another parent–teacher conference like this one, but here I was again, facing four puzzled, frustrated sixth-grade teachers. Walter had given me no indication of
any problems at school; in fact, according to him, he was doing quite well.
He should have been doing well. In fourth grade he had been identified as
gifted, and in fifth grade he had qualified for the Johns Hopkins sponsored
Center for Talented Youth Program. Yet the teachers were telling me that his
work was below grade level. It was hard to believe that just a few years ago,
these same teachers were gushing about Walter's older brother, Alex, a high
achiever and student body president. How could the pride and pleasure I
was feeling then give way to the resentment I was feeling now? Of course,
Walter was different, he himself admitted that he was a "nerd," but what
could he be doing at school to cause so much exasperation? Why couldn't
these teachers appreciate Walter for the great kid he is?

Just a few years earlier I had realized how much Walter was like his
grandfather, a brilliant, eccentric chemical engineer. Walter's grandfather,
raised in a wealthy European family, had managed to escape France with
many of his assets just days before it fell to the Nazis, because he had long
anticipated that it would happen that way. One of his most outstanding eccentricities had to do with his aversion to high-pitched sounds. He spent
much of his time working and relaxing in two large soundproof boxes, constructed for him at work and at home. In addition to the relief from noise,
the boxes provided the solitude he needed. At the dinner table we would
hear long dissertations on scholarly subjects delivered in a monotonous,

heavily accented voice. Walter was beginning to give similar speeches. But I didn't want Walter to grow up to be like his grandfather. In spite of his achievements, including a patent for dairy creamer, he was, in many ways, a prisoner of his rigidity and rituals, and I hoped that Walter would be not be such a loner. I knew one other man, a biostatistician, who seemed so much like Walter and his grandfather that I used to wonder if we were somehow related. He also isolated himself and was so unyielding in his habits that, despite his high abilities, working with him was difficult. I was determined to protect Walter from the difficulties these men faced on a daily basis.

And so as I sat in the conference, I heard the usual complaints: Walter's horrific handwriting, crude three-line classroom essays when other kids produced pages, zero credit for assignments never turned in, and the rudeness—"Walter tries to be funny, but he's so insensitive he gets obnoxious." And then the samples of his work . . .

Science Reports
[written illegibly]

Sharks—I don't see the point of dissecting sharks. They were smelly. I didn't like shark dissection.

Bridge Engineering—Bridges was boring. I don't see the point of watching some older person tell you what you already know. But then again, that's the problem with the rest of school.

Bread Mold Experiment—People already know moldy bread smells bad. We don't have to stink up the classroom to prove it. I didn't like the bread decomposition.

If only they were willing to take into consideration the unassigned pieces that I had coaxed him to write at home.

The Truth About the Bermuda Triangle
By Walter (age 9)

The truth about whatever flies over the Bermuda Triangle is this:

First of all, the Loch Ness Monster vacations in the Bermuda Triangle. The Monster is very nice and well mannered. It eats whatever it can find. It is very happy and wants to help people. It also has relatives.

It has a father, the Lake Michigan Monster. The father is very much like its son. The father has a brother, the Lake Erie Monster. They have a cousin, the Amazon River Monster. The cousin has an uncle, the Bermuda Triangle Monster. This monster causes all the trouble. This monster is well mannered like its cousins, but it has a burping problem. When a plane comes to pet the Loch Ness Monster, the Bermuda Triangle Monster burps. The burp is so annoying that it destroys the body of a man, enlarges his head, and turns him to stone. To keep the stone head safe, the Loch Ness Monster puts it on Easter Island. This is what happens in the Bermuda Triangle.

But as the conference was winding to completion, I began hearing something different. Walter's demeanor and his body language at school were very strange. He was stiff when he walked, and in class he sat in a "fetal position." Sometimes he rocked his body side to side or rubbed his hands together repetitively. One teacher who had some special education experience suggested that perhaps there was something the school psychologist hadn't thought of when she tested him last year. "I don't think he's autistic, but . . . . "

It was then that I realized I had to restart the search for expertise I had abandoned 2 years earlier. After 1½ years' worth of weekly sessions with a respected child psychiatrist who characterized his problem as "he's just too bright," I had given up working with professionals who didn't get it. Instead, I devoted extra time to working and playing with Walter. I thought his obsession with playing computer strategy games was a big part of the problem. I took it upon myself to strictly limit the hours he was allowed to play, even though the professionals thought I shouldn't. Instead of spending endless hours with the computer, I persuaded him to write essays at home, to learn to play the flute, to play board games with me, to get into our swimming pool, or just to converse with me. This constant coaxing was a great strain. It took tremendous determination and patience, but I thought he had improved. Yet clearly, what I was doing was not enough. I would need to find professional help with a new direction. As before I felt bewildered, where could I turn now?

The revelation came a week later. Walter's father and I had begun our probe, speaking to psychologists and psychiatrists we knew. Upon hearing about our concerns, a psychiatrist acquaintance mused, maybe Walter had a developmental disability that had not been identified because he is so bright. She had recently seen a patient who seemed to be similar. He had Asperger syndrome. . . .

I entered it into the Yahoo search—Asperger syndrome (I wasn't sure of the spelling). When the description came up, I was astounded. I couldn't believe that the *Diagnostic and Statistical Manual of Mental Disorders* contained a diagnosis that described Walter so well. What a relief to find out the problem, but sobering to understand that we were dealing with a severe disability considered to be a form of autism. I felt foolish, too, here Walter's father and I were, two physicians, and we had never heard of Asperger syndrome. I spent much of the following 2 months exhaustively searching the Internet. Three and a half months later we arrived at the Yale University Child Study Center for Walter's evaluation.

There was nothing unusual about Walter's first 2 years of life. He met all the developmental milestones on time, even initiating speech slightly early. Friends would comment about how much he was like his older brother, only Alex was dark and Walter was blond and blue-eyed. Just as

Walter was turning 2, we left him in a resort camp each day during a vacation. He was the youngest and happiest camper there, quite a well adjusted 2-year-old. We noticed his first unusual behavior several months later. Walter began to spend hours with the video cassette recorder, inserting Disney cartoon videos. Although there was no logo distinguishing the video-cassettes from each other, he managed to identify each one correctly by decoding the words on the label. At about the same time he developed an interest in astronomy, amassing impressive knowledge for a child his age. We realized that Walter might have some unusual talents.

When he was 2½, Walter began preschool. Because he had done well in Mommy-and-me class, we were surprised that he had a difficult time, always remaining outside the group. He adjusted better when we switched to another preschool with a more structured curriculum. At age 3, he became determined to read. I found Walter once, sitting with a children's book, crying with frustration. We bought him the Learning Company software program, *Reader Rabbit*, and within a month he was reading fluently. After that he began to focus unusual concentration for his age on educational computer games, doggedly completing any we could find. One day when I left for work at 8 A.M., he was already sitting at the computer. When I returned at 4 P.M., he was sitting in the same place with wet pants, his lunch on the kitchen table untouched. By age 4, Walter had few interests outside computer games, Nintendo, and board games. Yet, he developed friendships with several boys his age.

Walter began kindergarten at age 5. By this time, he had read each volume of C. S. Lewis's *Narnia Chronicles* many times. Although he liked his teacher, she complained about his behavior constantly. She made it clear that she thought his problems stemmed from what was going on at home, and that it was wrong that we "forced him to learn to read at such an early age." By age 6, Walter had acknowledged that he was different from other children, sometimes expressing frustration that they were unable to share his skills and interests.

As he advanced from first to sixth grade, Walter showed little interest in school in spite of his very high cognitive abilities. His classroom work was fast, sloppy, and incomplete. Often he would neglect to turn in any assignment. Comparing a second-grade essay to several done in class in sixth grade, we could see that his classroom performance had actually deteriorated over his elementary school years. The earlier essay was legible, fairly well developed, and cohesive, whereas the sixth-grade work consisted of a few disjointed sentences written in faint chicken scratch. During this period Walter replaced any interest in school with tremendous passion for (1) computer strategy games, (2) science fiction books, (3) fact books, and (4) Mensa puzzles and riddles. When not sitting in front of the computer, he increasingly stayed in his room with his guinea pig, either reading or lying on his back on the floor kicking a large ball in the air. Convincing him to leave his room for an outing or to play outside required a great deal of patience and fortitude, usually met with the comment, "stupid and pointless."

Walter has always been reluctant to speak to adults and has been able to maintain eye contact only with his closest family members and friends. He seems to lack empathy and often displays inappropriate responses to emotional concepts. However, if asked to interpret a facial expression or how another person would feel, he often gets it right. Walter suffers in settings in which there is excessive social stimulation going on around him. We were shocked to see a videotape taken in his classroom for the Yale University Social Learning Disability Study. Walter had his head on the desk with his eyes closed during the entire period. Later his teachers admitted that this had been a frequent posture in class for several years.

Walter's physical movements are awkward. His manner of walking varies from a stiff gait, nose pointed up and arms held back to a wild stride with arms flailing. He has not yet mastered the skill of cutting his meat, spreading jam on bread, buttoning a shirt, or washing his hair. He considers personal hygiene simply a waste of time. In day-to-day situations, Walter seems to be completely unaware of body language. Yet, again, if asked to express what he thinks another person's body language is saying, he is often correct. He sometimes exhibits stereotypical movements like rocking, hand wringing, or repetitive tossing.

Among the positive experiences during Walter's grade-school years have been the flute lessons he began when he was 9. We had long been concerned about his difficulty in taking instruction from others, something we had attributed to his precocity. He just seemed to know such things as math and science concepts without having to be taught. We encouraged the flute lessons, thinking that he would have to learn in a stepwise fashion to master that skill. We had the good fortune to find his flute teacher, a patient, explicit mentor who truly enjoys working with Walter. It has taken constant encouragement, but Walter has continued to progress well with his music. This has been an experience that has made a difference.

We realize how lucky we are that Walter has consistently had two or three close friends. His friends seem to sincerely enjoy his company and actively pursue him. He can be fun to be around, and has an excellent sense of humor. However, the relationships are primarily built around computer games and are reminiscent of the parallel play of much younger children. Walter readily admits that he has no interest in most kids because they are "stupid." He is frequently unaware of other children's names.

We, Walter's parents, have enjoyed a close affectionate relationship with him. We love to be with him. He's been so clever, so knowledgeable, so full of dry humor, so quiet and undemanding. But, we have been concerned that he holds back emotions and inner thoughts. Often, what really seems to be on his mind are issues such as computer game strategies, mathematical concepts, or academic discourses in subjects ranging from ancient history to modern business concerns. Despite our pride in his unusual abilities, we feel sorry that he is missing many of the childhood experiences experienced by his siblings and peers.

But Walter has his own ideas of who he is and where he's going. Here is an excerpt from an autobiographical piece written when he was 11:

My name is Walter. I am an intelligent, unsociable, and adaptable person. I would like to dispel any untrue rumors about me. I am not edible. I cannot fly. I cannot use telekinesis. My brain is not large enough to destroy the world when unfolded. I did not teach my guinea pig to eat everything in sight (that is the unfortunate nature of a long haired, short haired guinea pig like mine, Chrono). I would like to tell of an experience that shows some of my character.

I am a rather adaptable person. This experience shows a bit of my adaptability. My family and I were in Mammoth, California on vacation this summer. On our first day, we went hiking. After several hours I no longer wanted to hike ever again. On the way back, I saw a giant rock with little rocks jutting out of it. People attached to cords were climbing it. I thought that I might want to do that later.

I did get a chance to climb the rock later. When my brother was mountain biking, I had nothing to do. I decided to climb the rock. I got strapped in, and grabbed hold of the first handhold. I was scared that I would fall, but I pressed on. At one point, the handhold I needed was to the left, and though my father was shouting to move left, I could not hear him. I was paralyzed with fear. I could not go up or down. Just before I would have jumped off, I tried to wedge myself between a crack that was formed by the intersection of my climbing course with another course. I was scared to death, but I walked sideways to the top. I had done it, and was never going to do it again.

The next day I did do it again. When I was finished, I saw an advertisement for a ropes course. I decided to inquire about it. I found that it was a giant ropes course with trees holding cables leading to sixty feet in the air. I wasn't sure if I could do it, but I wanted to try.

The next day my father and I found the group that was going to do the ropes course. The first thing the leader did was to ask each of us why we were there. I said, "I'm here to suffer!" Then we went to the spot in the woods where the course was. It had bridges and lines going from tree to tree leading to a platform sixty feet up. I wondered how we were to get to the platform. I then learned that we were going to climb the trees. I didn't think I could do it. I was filled with fear and awe. The trees had widely spaced rungs and sawed off branches. Unfortunately, they were placed randomly. It seemed impossible. I was relieved that we were attached to a safety system.

On the first course, I saw that I would have to climb a tree and then cross a narrow bridge to the platform. I thought that the tree was the hard part. I stepped up to the first rung and began to climb. Several times I lost my footing and almost fell. Several times I looked, almost paralyzed with fear, for the next rung. I finally made it to the bridge. I couldn't walk across the bridge. I had to crawl, looking down the whole time. That wasn't very reassuring. However, I made it. I was sixty feet in the air, and I had completed the first course. Then I wondered, how do I get down? I saw the person in front of me grab on to a stick on a line and gripping the stick, zoom down until he was out of sight. It looked rather frightening to me. The only thing that made me follow was that it seemed like a more viable plan than a kamikaze leap.

I zoomed four hundred feet, from sixty feet in the air, gripping a stick. It was exhilarating. Then I saw a tree ahead of me. When I thought I would make a painful crash, I hit a brake and slowed down. I then stopped, and climbed down a ladder to return to *terra firma* once again.

I was now no longer content to just do the easiest course. I was going to challenge myself to harder ones. I did each of the courses several times until it was time to leave. At the end, when our leader asked each of us what we had learned, I said, "I did not suffer. I learned a lot about what I could accomplish, about how to climb, and about my newfound fear of wood." That experience shows my adaptability in a scary situation.

The Yale University Child Center Social Learning Disability evaluation was highly professional and provided invaluable detailed information about Walter's strengths and weaknesses. The 20-page document has offered interventional recommendations for Walter's social growth and instruction that we would have been unable to obtain anywhere else. Nevertheless, a veil of depression came over us when we received the report. Now we understood the problem and had some idea of how we should proceed. But where could we find professionals who had the skill and willingness to work with us? I began searching for and interviewing speech and language therapists, behavioral therapists, counselors, and others. Putting together a well-integrated program for Walter seemed to be impossible. And then there was the problem of school. Walter was about to enter junior high school. So far, his peers accepted him as a very smart, eccentric kid, but I didn't think that such tolerance would continue for the next several years. And what about the junior high school teachers? There could be only less acceptance of Walter's underachievement and social ineptness than we had already experienced in elementary school. If only we could find a program that could address his problems while sheltering him from what we knew would be a disaster during the coming school years.

We found our answer in an unlikely place, *LA Parent Magazine*, a throwaway periodical. In a small corner was an advertisement for Village Glen School, a program for children with social-communication challenges. I arranged three visits to the school. During the last one, the director of special education for our school district accompanied me because she had been previously unaware of the program. Each time I went to Village Glen feeling reluctant about the idea of our gifted child attending a nonpublic school for children with disabilities, and each time I left knowing that this was the right place for Walter for the next few years. The school provides the on-site clinical psychology, communication, and occupational therapy services that Walter needs. We were fortunate to have a caring special education director who facilitated the school district support for Walter's transition to Village Glen School.

Now Walter is in an upper elementary class of 12 students with a highly trained teacher and a teacher's aide. There is constant interaction among his teachers and therapists, and we are informed of problems and successes on a regular basis. This year we are pursuing three areas: (1) to teach Walter social skills such as greeting others and engaging in a conversation, (2) to improve his organizational and study skills, and (3) to instill motivation for academic and interpersonal success.

Probably the most wonderful thing that has happened to Walter at Village Glen has been his teacher. She immigrated from Kenya with her husband and four daughters several years ago. I think it has been a combination of her cultural values, her strong personal attributes, and her devotion to each student in her class that has allowed her to give so much to Walter and his classmates. One of the first things she told Walter was that he should make an effort to know her because it was unlikely that he would ever be so close to someone who grew up in an African village. She has spent hours with Walter, working with him, never giving in when Walter resists completing a project or behaving appropriately. Her husband was the first person to successfully teach Walter to tie his shoes in a conventional manner. He is now Walter's tutor, helping him to focus on completing high-quality homework and using his time efficiently. In the classroom, social and executive skills are emphasized. Walter receives his academic challenges at home through distance learning programs for writing and algebra II, administered by the Johns Hopkins Center for Talented Youth, and learning programming language C with his tutor.

Walter is making progress in his social and study skills this year, but the going is slow. I can't image how he could have flourished in our local public junior high school. To meet the requirements to remain in the Center for Talented Youth Program he took the College Board Exam, the SAT I, last month. He astounded us all by being the 12-year-old kid who scored 710 (out of 800) in both the verbal and math sections, scores that most high school seniors would envy.

In contemplating where we need to go with Walter over the next few years, I think that one of the greatest but most important challenges will be to get him into the real world. Our efforts are aimed at teaching him the social and adaptive skills to navigate, to give him the experience, the practice, to feel comfortable in the real world on a day-to-day basis. At the same time, we hope that he will find a special interest that can benefit others and possibly make a difference. But wherever his path leads, we can't lose sight of the fact that we have a wonderful, unique child, and we must respect . . . and delight in the person he is.

In Walter's words . . .

My intelligence has gotten me out of some situations, allowed me to get good grades, and excel at strategy games. My unsociability has prevented me from joining a mob, or getting into embarrassing situations (if you are unsociable, then you can't get into an embarrassing situation, because you have no social respect to lose). I am not, however, someone to be avoided. I have two good (human) friends and a guinea pig. The guinea pig likes me very much, especially for my magical food-bringing powers. It believes that I am made of food, as it has shown several times.

A View from Inside

LORI S. SHERY

My 12-year-old son, Adam, recently said to me, "Mom, you don't know what it's like to be me."

"You're right," I told him, "I don't. What is it like to be you?"

"It's hard, really hard."

That single statement spoke volumes. I knew firsthand what it was like to be the mother of a child with Asperger syndrome. I knew the feelings of shock and denial upon being told the diagnosis. I knew the anger and sadness that followed closely behind. I knew the constant worry about what the future would hold for this vulnerable child. I knew the guilt that plagued parents, wondering if they did something to cause their child to be born with this disorder, and wondering what the effect that focus on the child with AS had on the other children in the family. I knew the strain that having a child with a disability placed on a marriage. But I didn't know what it was like to *be* the child with Asperger syndrome. I didn't know how much courage it took for him just to get through each day.

As I thought about Adam's first 12 years of life, I realized what it must have been like for this bright, sensitive child who felt lost in the world of "neurotypicals." He was a placid baby, content to just sit quietly. When Adam was a toddler, my husband and I used to joke that we needn't have babyproofed the house because he never "got into" anything. My mother's friends used to remark that they never saw another child sit still for such long periods. We, of course, were convinced it was because he was so well behaved. What we didn't know then was that he was unable to explore the world in the way that other children did. When he became hysterical at the sound of a balloon popping, when he put everything in his mouth until he was 5 years old, when he never stacked blocks but, instead, only knocked down the towers we built for him, we didn't know that he was not experiencing life the way he should have been. He sat for hours pushing the on/off buttons of electronic toys just to hear the sounds they made. At birthday parties, he had no interest in the other children or games, preferring instead to sit on the sidelines, staring at the wheels of a musical cassette tape turning round and round.

His father and I never suspected a problem because Adam was so bright. People constantly told us how gifted he was. He knew his shapes, colors, letters, and numbers by the time he was little more than a year old. He couldn't *say* them because he didn't really start talking until almost 18 months, but he could point to them. At age 2, he could give his grandparents detailed driving directions around town. He taught himself to read at age 2½. He knew all the states and capitals by age 4 and all the countries and U.S. presidents by age 6. How could such a bright child have any problems?

When Adam was not quite 4 years old, we discovered he had a special talent. Within seconds, he could, with 100% accuracy, name the day of the week on which any past or future date would fall. This made him quite popular. People found him fascinating and loved to test his accuracy. Adam never liked the feeling of being different, however, and he soon tired of the "Calendar Game."

He spent most of that school year in the time-out corner. Not surprisingly, his preschool teacher informed us she had serious concerns about his problem behaviors. His father and I felt that the only problem was his teacher. We agreed to have a psychologist observe him in school in order to prove her wrong. I suppose she actually did us a favor. We thought Adam hugged the children in school and on the playground because he came from a loving, affectionate family. We thought he wandered the periphery of the classroom and preferred the company of his teachers over the other children because he was so bright and needed the stimulation. We thought his inability to focus and pay attention was due to his daydreams about future inventions and discoveries. What we didn't realize was that Adam didn't know how to connect with other children. He was content being a spectator rather than a participant. The psychologist told us that Adam did indeed have issues which needed to be addressed, including fine motor problems for which he needed occupational therapy.

We then took him to a pediatric neurologist who expressed concern over his difficulties with socialization. The report we received a week later recommended that Adam be monitored for the possibility of a pervasive developmental disorder. When I looked up the term in my husband's medical books, I became very upset and phoned the doctor. He told me what I needed to hear at that moment. My second child was due to be born in a matter of weeks, and he could read in my voice that I needed reassurance.

And I gladly accepted his reassurances that Adam most likely had some developmental delays and nothing more. That wasn't too bad, I reasoned, they would probably resolve on their own.

Kindergarten was a good year for Adam. He had a teacher who appreciated his uniqueness and enjoyed having him in her class. I was sorry to see her retire at the end of the school year as I had hoped that other children would benefit from her experience.

First grade was the worst. Adam had a teacher who just didn't "get it" but thought she did. The problem was she got it all wrong. Throughout the school year, and even after Adam was diagnosed with attention-deficit/hyperactivity disorder and classified for special education purposes, she used such words as "willful" and "intentional" when describing my son and his actions. He may not have been perfect, but he certainly was not willful, and he never intentionally forgot to turn in any of his assignments. My husband and I should have known it was going to be a bad 10 months when we attended Back to School Night 3 weeks into the school year. Every child had his or her project displayed. Every child, that is, except Adam. When I asked his teacher about it, she said it was a class project which he had plenty of time to complete, and he had apparently decided it just wasn't important enough. I couldn't believe she was saying this about a 6-year-old!

Second grade was a reprieve for all of us. Adam's teacher was a kind, soft-spoken woman who thought he was absolutely wonderful. She gave him countless opportunities to shine in her class, and he adored her.

In third grade, we began to notice new problem behaviors. Adam broke quite a few of our doorknobs from his constant checking to see whether they were locked. He spent hours in the bathroom at home and at school. His teacher, usually a very understanding woman, reported that he was disrupting her class by repeatedly making inappropriate comments. My husband and I decided it was time to take Adam back to the neurologist he had seen 3 years earlier. He referred us to a child psychiatrist who spent a long time with the three of us before making a diagnosis. I can still hear his words, "I believe Adam has something called Asperger. . . . " He and I both said the word, "syndrome" at the same time. I still don't know where I had first seen or heard the name, but we finally had an explanation for our son's difficulties. We were fortunate that this doctor had experience in diagnosing and treating children on the higher-functioning end of the autism spectrum and was able to recognize the signs that had eluded earlier professionals.

The fact that we now had the proper diagnosis didn't ensure our acceptance of it, however. It wasn't made any easier by the fact that the only book I was able to find on the subject painted a very bleak picture. It took 8 months for the news to sink in, at the end of which time we decided to share Adam's diagnosis with the school. Telling Adam's case manager proved to be a wise decision; our school district was appreciative of our honesty and was more than happy to provide Adam with the appropriate accommodations because, as the district put it, they now understood what his needs were.

Ten months after Adam was first diagnosed with Asperger syndrome, we took him to the Yale Child Study Center in New Haven, Connecticut. The center confirmed the diagnosis and told us that the results of the neuropsychological testing also indicated Nonverbal Learning Disabilities, which explained his perceptual and motor difficulties. The Center stressed the importance of social skills training so that Adam could learn cognitively what other children learn intuitively. Team members also recommended a personal aide for Adam to help him navigate through the school day. They asked Adam if he would like to return the following month to participate in their research project. Adam thought about it for a moment and answered, "Yes, perhaps I can help other children by doing this."

That winter, I discovered the Internet. I was a woman on a quest. I wanted to learn everything I possibly could about the two words that were suddenly redefining our lives—Asperger syndrome. It wasn't enough for me to understand my son's needs. I knew that I needed to educate the educators, and I found them to be very receptive.

Fourth and fifth grade saw the emergence of adolescence and, with it, an escalation in Adam's inappropriate behaviors. His teachers were wonderfully patient with him and, I suspect, relied heavily on their sense of humor to get through the school year. Unfortunately, the students were not nearly as tolerant, and his last 2 years of elementary school were filled with a great deal of teasing. This year, Adam entered middle school, and I admit to being as nervous as he was. Everyone with whom I spoke warned that the transition from elementary to middle school was very difficult—for all children. I dreaded the worst. I just wanted us to survive it. I'm happy to say that Adam is doing more than just surviving sixth grade, he is flourishing.

His teachers recognize his disability, but they focus on his possibilities. They won't accept that he *cannot* do something; instead, they design ways for him to succeed.

He is in honors classes and on the All-A Honor Roll. He earned a major part in the school play even though the larger parts usually go to the seventh- and eighth-graders. The drama teacher told us he makes her job easy and is a role model for the other actors.

Just prior to the start of his home economics elective, I expressed concern over Adam's ability to manipulate a sewing needle. His case manager believed he could do far more than we gave him credit for.

I thought about what she said and remembered that he learned to ski when he was 9 years old. I knew how much it meant to him as evidenced by a composition he wrote in fourth grade. The assignment was to write about your greatest personal achievement. He wrote about learning to ski.

I received a phone call from his home economics teacher several weeks later. She was so excited about the beautiful work he did on his pillow that she brought it into the school office to show everyone. I will never forget Adam's beaming face as he proudly handed me his finished masterpiece.

The assistant principal recently announced Adam's name over the public address system. A few months earlier, Adam won the school-level competition of the National Geography Bee. The entire student body was now informed that Adam scored among the top 100 entrants in the state and was chosen to participate in the National Geographic State Finals.

Adam still has difficulty with social situations, but he has made great progress. The boys in the social skills group he has attended for the past 2 years have become his good friends. Last year, on a flight home from Disney World, Adam was seated next to a boy he didn't know. As the plane took off, I could hear Adam making conversation with the youngster.

"Hi, my name is Adam. What's your name?" and then

"Nice to meet you, Tommy. I'm in fifth grade, what grade are you in?" and then

"You're also in fifth grade? What's your favorite subject?"

I smiled to myself. No one but Adam and I knew that this was a well-rehearsed script that he had learned in his group. To anyone listening, it sounded completely natural and spontaneous. They couldn't have known how proud I was of him.

The older Adam gets, the more empathic he becomes. He is learning to read facial cues and body language, although he still misperceives social situations involving children he doesn't know. One such situation occurred when Adam didn't "see" the line of students at the soda machine after school. He inserted his coins only to be angrily told by the next person in line that she had already put her money in the machine, and the soda he had just removed belonged to her.

I credit his shadow aide with making his transition this year a smooth one. She is very attuned to Adam's needs, and we feel fortunate to have her working with him. Because she is with Adam all day, she is able to provide him with continuous social skills training using real-life situations as they arise.

If you ask Adam who his best friend is, he will tell you it's his younger brother, Zachary. Zach loves his older brother unconditionally, while providing (mostly) constructive feedback about his behaviors. I am hopeful that my 8-year-old will grow up to be a kind, understanding, and tolerant adult.

Although it doesn't happen very often, we still occasionally see the return of an old undesirable behavior. It is during those times that I remember the advice of a very dear friend of mine. He taught me to look at them not as setbacks, but instead to see Adam's many accomplishments as the windows to his future. When I do, the view is truly magnificent.

How Did We Get Here?

LINDA RIETSCHEL

A few weeks ago my son and I stood on a beautiful New England college campus. Rather than enjoying the beauty, I found myself observing my son. How did we get here? Could this be possible?

My son received a very late diagnosis of Asperger syndrome (AS). He was 13 years old. He had been called many different things throughout his life. Words such as "eccentric," "gifted," and "shy" come to mind. I was always on the sidelines, though, hoping that they were right and I was wrong. It had always seemed to me to be something more, almost inexplicable or intangible. I would question certain inconsistencies, clumsiness, extreme discomfort around strangers, near hysteria at changes in routine, and, most important, a complete lack of friendships. On the other hand, mastery scores would be quoted to me. Report cards were waved joyfully. There was a sense of what could be the problem with a mind like this. The answer to that is plenty.

When my thoughts return to my child's infancy, I recall an emotionally distant baby. He was our first child, but even as novice parents we realized that this behavior was not what we expected. His attachments were mostly to things, not to people. I was merely a conduit for him to get to whatever toy had his attention at that time. All people seemed to receive the same response from him.

When he was 2 years old I decided that I would have to teach him how to love. My husband is a pilot and can be away from home for several nights. When the baby would awaken in those nights I would take him into my bed without any toys. I lit up the room and talked and talked to him. He had no choice but to look at me and listen. I would hug and kiss him and try to show him that a person could be as valuable as a toy. As his mother I was hoping to teach him to love me. Imagine these first steps that I took as a young mother just on instinct alone.

As my son grew into a toddler, he became comfortable with adults. They were predictable and nonthreatening. Other children did not play a part in his life. His love of learning had already begun and the alphabet and the numbers were learned very rapidly. He was a spontaneous reader whose first book was *Little House on the Prairie*. Golden Books did not play a prominent role in his curriculum! As my only child at this point I was unaware of the unusual nature of this. I did not have a point of comparison.

When he was 3 we moved to a different state. My husband and I already knew that *any* change brought great distress. We dismantled his old room, even pulling up the carpet and recreated the same room for him in the new house. It relieved some of the anxiety, but more anxiety was on its way. New neighbors came to visit, which was very upsetting to my son. He never knew when the doorbell would ring or who would come in. Invariably children would accompany my new neighbors. His behavior was so exaggerated that I did not get off to a good start in the neighborhood. At this point, my child's unknown disability would start to erode not only his life but that of his parents as well. Children's birthday parties, both his own and others, were disasters no matter how much preparation we made. After a while you aren't included anymore. Your heart breaks for your child and yourself.

Kindergarten was a success intellectually for this little boy. However, by October the calls started to roll in. His experienced and wonderful teacher was bewildered. Among other things the child could make a map of the various states out of his sandwich bread. He already knew every state and almost every capital, mountain range, and river. In this class the teacher had to adhere strictly to a schedule. That was his comfort, a predictable schedule. One fateful day, a film strip was shown on crocodiles rather than polar bears. He broke down. The nurse called me to come to the school immediately. Ultimately, it was simple. Her "error" was that she had promised to show a film strip on polar bears but had shown a different one instead. Even at 5, a change so seemingly inconsequential could cause unusual distress. At this point the adults around him began to do almost anything to relieve his anxiety. We were still so far in the dark and we would stay there for 8 more years.

Through the elementary school years, teachers would respond in different ways. At times the child was showered with sympathy. Another year *we* were believed to be somehow causing his behavior. The year after that we were asked why we were "drilling" him on "all these facts." One year we were with a teacher who was so intractable that toward the end of the year we kept him home 1 or 2 days a week. By fifth grade the energy that it took to interpret the world around him was beginning to exhaust him. Many tears were shed after teacher conferences. I had no answers for the questions I was being asked.

How did we evade diagnosis for so long? We coped so well that we did not stand out. In the early years if my son could not work a zipper, snap, or button, we used velcro. We used hooks instead of hangers. If he couldn't tie his shoes, we searched for adult-size velcro sneakers. With the exception of two or three teachers, we were able to adapt his schoolwork to his prodigious academic skills. We ran interference on everything else. For example, during a reading class the assigned book was one he had read many times, many years before. His teacher was unsure of this but my son was able to recite, from memory, part of the first chapter. She gladly handed him a copy of *Of Mice and Men* and told him to have a good time! Also in sixth grade, each month he was asked to fill out a book report on a standard piece of paper. His fine motor skills were always very poor, so I enlarged the teacher's standard form and presented her with almost a scroll and begged her to let him use it. She agreed. I found this type of flexibility more often than not.

At the end of sixth grade I was faced with another endless summer. The librarian and I had become my son's only friends. To give him something to do I called the head of the high school summer school program and asked him to let my son take a high-school level summer course. To this day, I am sure that the head of summer school thinks that this was a part of a master plan to graduate my son early! All I knew was that my son's academic interests were becoming more than I could manage. At 11 years old, my son found himself in a senior-level history class. He loved it and saw nothing unusual in the situation. I can't say the same for the 18-year-olds who were with him! During the school year the cafeteria was an unbearable place for him and so were pep rallies. His teachers and I found alternatives but we were still pinch hitting. We *still* did not know what was wrong. His inflexibility was getting in his way. He became a "selective learner"; if the subject interested him he would work hard, if not he would not work at all. His grades were erratic.

By the time seventh grade began with all the preteen nonverbal methods of communication we were starting to have serious behavioral problems. A child with AS cannot interpret a "certain look." Elementary schools use basic and concrete methods to communicate with students and the students use these with each other as well. There is a big change after the sixth grade. My son became completely confused in making this transition to an environment in which you should know certain things simply by intuition. I still did not have a name for what was wrong and I had exhausted all local doctors. When his anxiety level reached a point that I could not control, I took my son to Yale Children's Hospital. It was there that I heard the words Asperger syndrome for the first time. It was a blessing.

There were no services for him or even an individual education plan

(IEP) without a diagnosis. With diagnosis came the knowledge of the struggle that this child had been fighting every day of his life! All his teachers from preschool to seventh grade were thanked for their compassion even in the absence of an explanation for this mysterious behavior. Most important, we apologized to our son for all the years of confusion on all sides. His reply was that he could not understand why it took us so long to find a doctor who knew the right questions to ask him! We were on our way.

Although I had been living with AS for so many years, it took time to collect all the information I needed to help my son. I knew that he needed to develop more faith in himself. Self-confidence was nonexistent and so were friends or even the ability to form a friendship. His comfort level in the world outside home or school was very poor. I accidentally came across a listing for a camp in *The New York Times*. It stressed social skills, positive self-image, and independence. Could I send a child who had never even had a babysitter to sleepaway camp? I had to try. It was important for him to see that there could be happy times outside his own home. Our family, which included two younger sons, was also in need of a respite. What a special place this camp turned out to be!

Imagine putting him on the bus to the Adirondacks. It ranks right up there with my life's most difficult moments. The director of the camp had come to interview my son and I felt comfortable on the safety aspects, but still as mother I will never know how I got him on that bus. I had signed him up for a month and as we came close to the end, he contacted me to say that he needed to stay with his *friends*! I had never heard this word from him. That was a wonderful day. In addition to all the camp activities, there is another level of training going on. I do not believe that the children are even aware of it. These campers learn to empathize with one another and to share in each other's often hard-won accomplishments. They live together and share lives. To most children it's easy, but to a lonely child with AS it is an experience that we cannot provide at home.

Armed with the camp experience, an IEP and his parents' newly discovered insight into his situation, he began high school. We had to be ever vigilant mainly in situations that had to do with group work or very nonstructured learning assignments. I became very adept at cross-referencing AS symptoms to certain academic occurrences. To be taken seriously, I had to have the published articles that related to whatever assignment had proven impossible for him. At times this became a part-time job for me. The rigidity of AS also becomes problematic when a student is asked to write a paper on something that is a known failure (e.g., he would not "waste his time" writing a paper on the League of Nations). He would not write papers dealing with science fiction or fantasy because these things could not possibly have happened. At this point we were battling AS along with adolescence. It was also important to make teachers aware of the difficulty that my son would have in making intuitive judgments about people's feelings in literature. One of my favorite remarks from my son was, "How do I know how Romeo felt, I'm not Romeo!"

His parents, most teachers, guidance counselors, and vocational counselor had formed an invisible net. To an outsider it would seem that we were making glacier-like progress, but this was not the case. I have always felt that if we set a child with AS on a path alone, he would simply sit down and read a book forever. In my son's case many people were always on that path with him, gently and not so gently prodding him to stand up and move on. He has. He returned to camp for two more summers, growing more confident with each year. He recently told me that he does not need to go back this summer because he has outgrown it! We are moving to a new level.

Last spring I took my dog to a new boarding kennel. My son was with me and he said that it was a place that he would like to work. Once again, words that this mom had never heard. Usually the bustle of a supermarket or discount store would fluster him as a customer let alone as an employee. I spoke with the kennel owner a few weeks later when I felt particularly courageous. She happened to be a psychologist on sabbatical! She knew of AS and was willing to interview my son. My son and I practiced a "job interview unit." He was offered the job and has been working since then. Besides having his own money, it also gives him something in common with the other students. We still have what I call our "Asperger moments." They can send a parent into despair. Ultimately we try to learn from them and build on them rather than be beaten down by them.

As an older teenager he has developed insight into his own disability. After initial anger he might say to me, "That was Asperger's." Progress has recently been made on the social front. Every teenager wanted to see the movie *Titanic* and I agreed with the proviso that he needed to buy his own ticket. He resisted until the film was about to leave the theaters. I wrote on an index card what he should say to the ticket seller and I left to park the car. He is *now* our family's designated ticket buyer. Once taught it is not forgotten. A New England blizzard solved the grocery store problem. I explained that I had only enough time to get a prescription at a drugstore and I would not have time to get milk—a major staple—as the blizzard was coming. Off he went, alone, with $20 for a gallon of milk. Now he is, yes, the designated milk purchaser!

High school will end for my son in June 2000. I have begun a search for colleges with strong support systems for students with social disabilities. There are not too many choices on the college level. I did find one outside Boston that sounded very promising. That is where I was at the beginning of this article. The college has an extraordinary support system for situations such as AS; it even has "quiet dorms" as well as regular ones. The camp experience will enable him to transition to a dorm. His work experience has kept him in the outside world and similar to his peers. Will we be able to do this? Will I feel that his social skills are strong enough? I wish that I could write the real end of this article right now.

This is a trip that is at times heartbreaking and harrowing. We never let him stop on that path for long. Everything that we ever failed at has ultimately helped us later on. We now see how brave our son has been and how our struggle, and the struggle of the many people who know him, might just pay off. I hope that I have presented all my fellow AS parents with hope and ideas. Always remember that we can't change the diagnosis, but we can mold the behavior. Do not ever stop trying. We will find our children in places that we never thought we would see them.

First Advocates

DeANN HYATT-FOLEY
MATTHEW G. FOLEY

When our son, Ryan, was born, Matt and I thought we were parents of a typical child. We expected that Ryan would pass through the developmental milestones as any other child did. Soon we realized we were parents of a child with a disability. When Ryan began school we were thrust into the role of educational advocates. We found ourselves ill equipped for the challenges of this new role. Matt and I discovered that the educators working with Ryan had limited knowledge of autism and how to work with someone with this disorder. We began the long process of becoming informed to persuade the educators to more effectively address Ryan's needs. This process involved becoming knowledgeable about autism, the laws governing special education and appropriate interventions to meet our son's specific needs. As time went on, we began to realize the necessity of developing and maintaining relationships with the people working with Ryan. We discovered that we had to strike a balance between pushing for educational interventions and maintaining healthy, personal relationships.

Obtaining the services and supports that we believed Ryan needed to be successful in school became a time-consuming endeavor. We attended conferences, read information, and talked with other parents. Our knowledge and experience grew to the point to where we felt confident that we understood what Ryan needed. I changed careers and began working for an organization that teaches parents how to advocate for their children. Matt and I decided that we would both go back to school and get master's degrees in education. We felt that having advanced degrees in education would enable us to more effectively advocate for Ryan and also provide us with a livelihood.

I recently attended a conference where a parent/professional stood up and informed the speaker that parents are advocates who look out for the rights of their children. She went on to say, "Parents are the child's first advocates." This statement reminded me that in many ways our experiences with working with professionals in the disability community are not different from those of other parents we know.

During Ryan's first year, the only significant problem was that he had difficulty nursing and as a result his body weight was low. When I switched him to a bottle, he soon reached normal weight. However, when Ryan was about 1 month old, I asked the doctor whether Ryan had a learning disability. Something about Ryan reminded me of my brother who had been diagnosed with a learning disability years earlier. The doctor told me there was absolutely nothing wrong with Ryan. My mom had given us a book on baby's first 12 months. Ryan hit the major milestones either early or right on time, but I continued to feel that something was not right.

It was sometime early in Ryan's second year that Matt and I began to realize he was not developing like other children. Our book on baby's second 12 months indicated that Ryan's progress had slowed; he was no longer hitting the major milestones listed in the book in the normal period of time. By the time Ryan was 18 months old I put the book away because it was too painful to read about all the milestones he should have reached but had not. Ryan exhibited several behaviors that concerned us. He did not display an interest in being with children his age. Ryan would communicate with adults only when he wanted something. He also engaged in a couple of unusual activities. The first was an obsession with opening and closing cabinet doors. He would spend hours at it. My mom joked that Ryan would grow up to be a doorman. The second activity was turning oscillating fans on and off as he watched the fan blades.

Matt and I hoped Ryan would catch up when he was ready. We also hoped he would outgrow his peculiar activities. During this period, Matt and I were completing our undergraduate degrees and we were living in student housing on the university campus. As a result, Ryan's access to children his own age was limited. We thought maybe this lack of access to other children might be contributing to Ryan's slow progress. When Ryan was 3 we decided to enroll him in a highly recommended day care that was run by a psychologist. After Ryan had been in the day care for a couple of weeks, the psychologist asked to meet with us to discuss Ryan. At this meeting we were informed that when Ryan was out on the playground all he would do was stand near the air-conditioning unit and watch the turning fan blade. He would not interact with the other children or staff members. The psychologist suggested getting Ryan's hearing checked because he acted as if he had a hearing problem. When we had his hearing checked we were told his hearing was within normal limits.

After about 6 weeks, Matt and I agreed that this day care was not helping Ryan develop social skills. We decided to enroll him in a smaller day care. Ryan did wonderfully. He learned to ride a tricycle and to swing on a swing set. The day care taught Ryan his alphabet and how to count. We were thrilled to find that he learned some skills before the other children his age. Ryan's vocabulary continued to grow and he began to interact with the other children but in a limited way. Ryan's behavior continued to concern us.

When Ryan was 3½ an incident occurred that demonstrated to us he was not a typical child. One afternoon Ryan shut himself in our bedroom closet. He attempted to open the door but the door was stuck. I immediately opened the door for him. As Ryan exited the closet he stated, "I shut myself in the closet but I didn't realize the door was locked." I wondered how he able to express his thoughts in this way but he could not play with other children or tell us about his day. Because of this incident, I called the local preschool program for children with disabilities and expressed my concerns. After hearing my story, the person on the phone said, "He just has developmental gaps, he'll catch up when he starts school." Just to be sure I checked again with Ryan's doctor and was again told Ryan was fine.

By this time well-meaning friends and family members were becoming concerned. A longtime friend of Matt's family wrote a letter expressing her concern about Ryan. While we were visiting Matt's relatives, a cousin who is a nurse was discreetly asked to observe Ryan's behavior. My mom talked to her physician about Ryan's behaviors and delayed social progress. The physician said it sounded as if Ryan might have autism. Mom purchased a book on autism and gave it to us. We were furious with all of them. Although we did not read the book my mom gave us we did some research on autism. The information we found did not seem to accurately describe Ryan. On the one hand we had professionals saying Ryan would be okay and would catch up to his peers. On the other we had family members saying something was wrong with Ryan. We chose to believe the professionals because the alternative was too difficult to accept.

A month before Ryan started kindergarten we went to the school to talk to his teacher. Matt and I told her something was wrong and we wanted the school to test Ryan. Without realizing it, we began the special education referral process. The testing for Ryan was completed in a couple of months. The teacher's observations reported that Ryan was not interacting with the other students. The school suggested we take him to a psychologist for further testing.

We agreed to have testing administered by a local psychologist who had been referred by the school. After the testing was completed, the psychologist told us she was not sure what Ryan had but she would give him the label that she thought would be most helpful. Several days later the school counselor arranged a meeting in her office. She had the report from the psychologist and told us Ryan had been diagnosed with pervasive developmental disorder not otherwise specified (PDD-NOS). We asked what that was. She told us autism. We were stunned.

We went home and wondered, "Why us?" The next few months are still a haze. In some respects the label was a relief. The label gave us an explanation for some of Ryan's behaviors. It also identified the areas in which he would need interventions and supports. In other respects, we were miserable. We handled our grief in very different ways. Matt withdrew and I tried to act like everything was just fine. We did not want to talk to our families about Ryan so we suffered in silence.

Our first individual education plan (IEP) meeting was held. Everyone read their reports about Ryan. Matt and I just sat and listened. At one point the diagnostician said that Ryan was slightly mentally retarded. We knew she was wrong but we did not say anything. We did not know we could. Ryan was transferred to a different campus from his home school and put in a self-contained classroom. We believed, that because the educators were trained in how to educate children, they would know best how to address Ryan's needs. We did not feel we knew what he needed educationally because we were just his parents. Matt refers to our participation in those first IEP meetings as that of "dashboard dogs." We just sat and nodded our heads, thankful that the school would provide Ryan services to address his special needs. After the meeting we went home and tried as best we could to go on with our lives.

Matt and I felt at last we were on the right track. Ryan was placed in a smaller classroom. There were only eight other boys so the teacher and aide were able to provide a lot of individual attention. Little did we know that in the near future a series of events would not only greatly improve Ryan's education but would also change our lives and the direction of our careers.

Toward the end of kindergarten, Ryan's teacher and a special education administrator suggested that we place Ryan in a class for children with emotional disturbance for first grade. It was a "child management class" (CMC) and it operated on the "level system." The level system involved a child's earning and losing points. The children were allowed certain privileges according to how many points they had earned. We later learned that it was common practice for our school district to place children with pervasive developmental disorders (PDD) in classrooms for children with emotional disorders. We visited the classroom and came away with a bad feeling. Shortly after our visit to the CMC, we went back to the teacher and administrator and said we did not feel the setting was appropriate for our son. The teacher sighed and the administrator said she did not know what else they could recommend for a child like Ryan.

A few days after our meeting about the CMC placement, the administrator suggested we take Ryan to a psychiatrist so Ryan could be placed on Ritalin (methylphenidate). We met with the recommended psychiatrist who spent 20 minutes with the three of us and about 10 minutes alone with Ryan. The psychiatrist also diagnosed Ryan with PDD-NOS and recommended he be placed on Ritalin to help him focus his attention. The doctor recommended counseling, which he could provide on a weekly basis at $90 an hour. The charge to monitor the medication and provide counseling would exceed $490 a month. This amount was well beyond our economic means.

Another IEP meeting was held to discuss the psychiatrist's findings. Prior to this meeting, I had taken the initiative to visit several different classrooms in the school district. Among the classrooms I visited, I found one I felt was appropriate for meeting Ryan's needs. This classroom was for children with learning disabilities. At the IEP meeting, Matt and I insisted that Ryan be placed in this classroom. The IEP committee did not disagree as they had no other suggestions for placement. The committee accepted the psychiatrist's recommendations of Ritalin and counseling. The committee documented in the IEP paperwork that Ryan would be placed on Ritalin to help him focus. Although the IEP committee agreed that counseling was appropriate, this suggestion was not documented in the paperwork. The special education administrator left us with the impression that we were responsible for pursuing the recommended counseling and paying for this service.

After the IEP meeting, I immediately began calling local counselors and psychologists to find someone we could afford. Several of the therapists based their fee on a sliding scale. We were optimistic. The last phone call I made was to a counselor who asked why we were paying for a service the IEP committee recommended. She informed me she had a client with PDD-NOS and the school paid for the counseling sessions. Up to this time, Matt and I believed that we, not the school district, were responsible for paying for assessments, counseling, or any other special interventions.

At this point it became abundantly clear that we needed to become more informed. We had come to realize that the educators on our IEP committee were not sure how to address Ryan's educational needs. We also wondered whether the school district had failed to inform us about other services and supports typically provided to children with PDD-NOS at no expense to the parents. I picked up the phone and started making calls to any organization listed in the phone book that seemed to have a connection with individuals with disabilities. When I called, I asked if there was someone in the office who could tell me what services the school was obligated to provide to Ryan under state law. After several days of making phone calls, I located a Parent Training and Information Center for Texas called the PATH Project. The center gave me the phone number to the PATH office in my area. This office happened to be in our city. I spoke with the Area Development Director and she gave me information about our parental rights and responsibilities in the IEP process.

The Area Development Director had also given me the name and number of a parent of a 16-year-old girl with PDD. It was difficult for me to call a stranger and talk about Ryan's deficits. It did not take long for me to become comfortable talking to this mom. By the end of our first conversation, I was laughing about some of Ryan's peculiar behaviors and situations that seemed tragic before making the phone call.

I spent the summer following kindergarten looking up federal and state regulations. After reading the material, I would place it on Matt's side of the bed. The stack of paper I left for him continued to grow and remained unread. Finally, Matt began to read the information. The next school year began with our being much more informed about educational law.

Over the next 2 years we became very involved with Ryan's education. First grade went smoothly. Ryan received music therapy, one-on-one instruction in the classroom, and in-home training and we received much needed parent training. We felt we were heading in the right direction until the beginning of Ryan's second-grade year. I went to a conference on inclusion where I was persuaded that inclusion in regular education classes was the best placement for Ryan. We spent Ryan's second-grade school year trying to convince the teachers and the IEP committee that the appropriate placement for Ryan was in regular classes. After a great deal of effort we were only able to get him into one regular class. Although we felt that this was a small victory, we were satisfied that we had made some progress. During the next IEP meeting we were told by the committee that Ryan would not be placed in regular classes for the third grade.

As we negotiated with the IEP committee during that time, we continued to learn more about autism and Ryan's educational rights. We also began contacting other parents who had children with autism to find out more about parenting and services their children were receiving in the school and community. Although it had taken me a couple of years, I finally read the book my mother had given me on autism. After talking with other parents about their children and reading about autism we found that Ryan did not fit neatly into this category. Some of the therapists who worked with Ryan said he was not like other children they knew who had autism. In the fall of 1992, Matt found an article on Asperger syndrome (AS) written by Lorna Wing in the university library. This article seemed to accurately describe Ryan. We began asking professionals in our area about this disorder. Some of the professionals recognized the name but were unable to offer specific information about AS.

We met with the special education director and convinced her to pay for an assessment by someone who specialized in autism. We had already found a psychologist in Dallas who worked primarily with children with autism. She assessed Ryan and gave him the diagnosis of high-functioning autism. When she was discussing the results of the assessment, Matt asked her what she knew about AS. She told us she was not familiar with AS.

We continued to educate ourselves about autism by going to several conferences in Dallas. The conferences we attended gave us the opportunity to hear speakers including Temple Grandin and Bernard Rimland. These conferences also provided us an opportunity to network with other parents and discuss intervention strategies and personal experiences.

In early August 1993, we moved to West Texas where I had accepted the position of area development director for the PATH Project. Acquiring this position gave Matt and I greater access to information about educational law and community resources. I also developed skills that made me more effective in working with educators. Matt had contacted the local university and found that they offered a program in counselor education that would provide the necessary course work for licensure as a licensed professional counselor (LPC).

Before we moved to West Texas, I called the special education director and told her we were moving to her district. I asked where we needed to live in her district so Ryan could be in regular classes. The director promised we could move any where in her district and she would provide the necessary services for Ryan to be successful in a regular education classroom. We moved into an apartment within walking distance of an elementary school campus. Ryan and I went to the school and met the principal. Although he expressed reservations about placing Ryan in a regular classroom he said he would work with us.

We made the decision for Ryan to repeat second grade so the IEP focus could be on social skills development without sacrificing academics. Because it had been so difficult to get Ryan into just one regular class in the previous school district we insisted that Ryan not be pulled out for specialized instruction. The first year was the most difficult for all of us, especially Ryan. He would come home with the front of his shirts literally chewed to pieces.

In 1994, Ryan's second grade teacher and the principal expressed their concerns about Ryan's progress. The IEP committee recommended that Ryan receive an educational assessment to establish his academic baseline. The school psychologist administered the testing under the supervision of a local psychologist. After completing the assessment the school psychologist diagnosed Ryan with childhood disintegrative disorder (CDD). We refused to accept the CDD label. Because of our adamant objections the psychologist switched the diagnosis to AS to placate us without administering further testing. Fortunately, we were able to convince the special education director not to put the assessment in Ryan's file. To limit the likelihood of repeating this experience with another professional, Matt and I took graduate-level courses on assessment. We also learned to question how much experience with autism a person has before allowing them to assess Ryan.

During Ryan's elementary school years, the principal and his staff were wonderful. His teachers were carefully chosen by the principal based on their experience and personality. Each year the new teacher would express her concerns about not knowing how to work with a child like Ryan. We provided them with information on autism and told them to treat him like the other children. We had daily conversations with the teachers about how Ryan was doing. We also offered assistance and support when they encountered difficulties. Our daily conversations helped in developing positive relationships. We were fortunate that Ryan was assigned to classrooms of individuals who had a gift for teaching. They found that with prompting and modifications, Ryan could do most of the work.

It was through our experiences with the people on this campus that we learned the value of building relationships. There were many times when we and the educators disagreed on how to work with Ryan, but we always managed to develop a plan everyone could live with. When Ryan's principal retired at the end of fourth grade, he was replaced by one who was not pro-special education. Because we had formed solid relationships with the teachers on the campus, Ryan's supports and services were not adversely affected by the new principal. We expected the transition to junior high to be difficult for both Ryan and his teachers. In the spring of his sixth-grade year we talked with the special education director about bringing in an autism specialist from Houston. We wanted this specialist to assess Ryan and provide information on autism to his teachers. The specialist assessed Ryan, diagnosed him with AS, and provided information on the disorder to his teachers.

We thought it would be a good idea for the new teachers to receive information about Ryan's elementary school years. I developed a portfolio which included a questionnaire in which Ryan's teacher's wrote about their experiences working with him. It also included Ryan's schoolwork samples and information about our family and AS. The principal who retired, all the teachers, and most of the therapists returned the questionnaires. Before school began I gave the notebook to the principal at the junior high school and asked that he pass it along to the teachers.

I also took Ryan up to the school just before the school year began. The principal had Ryan work with other students to help the teachers prepare for their classrooms. This experience gave Ryan the opportunity to meet several of the school staff, kids on the student council, and, most significant to Ryan, several cheerleaders. Preparing the school staff with information on AS and the elementary school teachers' experiences along with acclimating Ryan to the campus helped ease the transition to junior high. We anticipate a successful school year for Ryan and our development of positive relationships with school staff.

When Matt and I were told that Ryan had PDD-NOS we were devastated. We knew this to be a lifetime disability. In the early years Ryan interacted very little with us. We were concerned about him and we did not know what to expect for his future. As he matured and his personality developed we began to experience him as an enjoyable and interesting child. In many ways Ryan is like any other 13-year-old boy. In short, Ryan is a terrific kid, we love him, and we would not change anything about him.

Matt and I began our involvement in the education process like any other parents. We completely relied on the expertise of the educators, believing that they knew what to do. Gradually we came to the conclusion that it was unrealistic to expect them to have all the answers. We were motivated to become involved because the educators did not seem to know what to do with a child like Ryan. It also seemed that the educators were confused about the services Ryan was entitled to receive and who should pay for those services. These experiences demonstrated to Matt and I that we needed to accept the responsibility of ensuring that Ryan receive a free appropriate public education. Now we are informed participating members of Ryan's IEP committee.

Our knowledge and skills were acquired over a long period. When we first became actively involved in the IEP process we focused our attention on the laws and regulations governing special education. Our initial participation in the process was to hold the educators to the law. This approach produced an adversarial relationship between the educators and ourselves. We came to realize that to have a more productive relationship with the school we needed to change our focus away from educational law. After we moved to West Texas we began to focus on developing a positive relationship with the educators. Over time we developed a trusting relationship with the elementary school principal and teachers. Matt, Ryan, and I have developed lifetime friendships with many of the elementary school staff.

The portfolio I put together for the junior high school staff demonstrated the effectiveness of developing relationships with the people who work with Ryan. As I read through the responses I came to realize how much Ryan's teachers and therapists cared for Ryan. Almost every teacher and therapist wrote how much he or she had enjoyed working with Ryan. They also commented on how much they had learned from the experience.

One teacher, who worked with Ryan for several years, wrote that she had heard stories of "parents" which made her leery of working with Ryan. She then states, "Ryan is a joy to work with. He really is a product of good parental support and parents who lobby for what is right for their child. Matt and DeAnn know Ryan better than anyone else and if they hadn't pushed for Ryan's programs and worked hard to build a successful ARD [IEP] team, I don't feel Ryan would be where he is today." We agree.

Useful Internet Addresses

In the past few years, there has been a dramatic increase in the amount of information and number of resources on developmental disabilities available on the World Wide Web. This has been very beneficial to parents, clinicians, and researchers, who can quickly obtain information, search for services, and contact others with similar interests. The following is a limited list of websites providing information on Asperger syndrome. These sites are themselves linked to a very large number of other sites.

Asperger Syndrome Coalition of the United States, Inc. (ASC–U.S.)
(*http://www.asperger.org*)
    A national nonprofit organization committed to providing the most up-to-date and comprehensive information on social and communication disorders, with particular focus on Asperger syndrome and related disorders.

ASPEN® (Asperger Syndrome Education Network, Inc.)
(*http://www.aspennj.org*)
    ASPEN®, Inc. is a nonprofit organization providing families and those individuals affected with Asperger syndrome and related disorders with information, support, and advocacy.

Autism Society of America
(*http://www.autism-society.org*)
    The mission of the Autism Society of America is to promote lifelong access and opportunities for persons within the autism spectrum and their families to be fully included, participating members of their communities through advocacy, public awareness, education, and research related to autism.

Division TEACCH (Treatment and Education of Autism and related Communication handicapped Children, University of North Carolina at Chapel Hill)
(*http://www.unc.edu/depts/teacch*)

The TEACCH website includes information about their program, educational and communication approaches to teaching individuals with autism, their research and training opportunities, as well as information and resources on autism.

Learning Disabilities Association of America
(*http://www.ldanatl.org*)

The LDAA site includes information and resources on many learning disabilities, including learning disabilities involving a significant social component, such as autism and Asperger syndrome.

(United Kingdom's) **National Autistic Society**
(*http://www.oneworld.org/autism_uk*)

NAS is the foremost agency for people with autism, Asperger syndrome and related disorders in the United Kingdom, spearheading initiatives nationally and internationally to advance dissemination of information and provision of services.

OASIS (Online Asperger Syndrome Information and Support)
(*http://www.udel.edu/bkirby/asperger*)

This site provides general information on Asperger syndrome and related disorders, including resources and materials, announcements of major pertinent events and publications, as well as being the major "intersection" for communication among parents, clinicians and educators, and individuals with social disabilities.

Yale Child Study Center
(*http://www.autism.fm*)

This site provides information about clinical and research services at the Developmental Disabilities Section at the Yale Child Study Center, as well as publications on autism, Asperger syndrome, and related disorders; lists of resources organized by state; and links with many clinical and research groups, as well as parent support organizations and advocacy agencies.

Author Index

Subject Index